AIDS in the World II

AIDS
in the
World II

Global Dimensions, Social Roots, and Responses

The Global AIDS Policy Coalition

Edited by

Jonathan M. Mann *and* Daniel J. M. Tarantola

New York   Oxford

OXFORD UNIVERSITY PRESS

1996

Oxford University Press

Oxford   New York
Athens   Auckland   Bangkok
Bogota   Bombay   Buenos Aires   Calcutta
Cape Town   Dar es Salaam   Delhi
Florence   Hong Kong   Istanbul   Karachi
Kuala Lumpur   Madras   Madrid   Melbourne
Mexico City   Nairobi   Paris   Singapore
Taipei   Tokyo   Toronto

and associated companies in
Berlin   Ibadan

Copyright © 1996 by Oxford University Press, Inc.

Published by Oxford University Press, Inc.,
198 Madison Avenue, New York, New York 10016

Oxford is a registered trademark of Oxford University Press

Library of Congress Cataloging-in-Publication Data

AIDS in the world II / the Global AIDS Policy Coalition ; edited by
Jonathan M. Mann and Daniel Tarantola.
p.   cm.
Includes bibliographical references and index.
ISBN 0-19-508994-4 (cloth : alk. paper). — ISBN 0-19-509097-7
(pbk. : alk. paper)
1. AIDS (Disease)—Epidemiology.   2. AIDS (Disease)—Government
policy.   3. AIDS (Disease)—International cooperation.   I. Mann,
Jonathan M.   II. Tarantola, D.   III. Global AIDS Policy Coalition.
[DNLM: 1. Acquired Immunodeficiency Syndrome.   2. World Health.
WD 308 A2883385   1996]
RA644.A25A363582   1996
362.1′969792—dc20
DNLM/DLC
for Library of Congress   96-20008
                                                      CIP

1   3   5   7   9   8   6   4   2

Printed in the United States of America
on acid-free paper

Association François-Xavier Bagnoud

arranged funding for this project

In 1986, François-Xavier Bagnoud lost his life in a tragic helicopter accident at the age of 24, in the desert near Gao, Mali, West Africa. The Association François-Xavier Bagnoud and its Foundation were born out of the desire of his family and friends to continue his joyful spirit of self-giving and loving care for others.

The Foundation develops its activities in François-Xavier's fields of interest, i.e., rescue activities, aerospace, community life in the Swiss Canton of Valais, and through the humanitarian activities of the Association. In the field of aerospace, the Foundation helped finance the François-Xavier Bagnoud Building, home of the Department of Aerospace Engineering at the University of Michigan, from which François graduated in 1982. It also established the biennial $250,000 François-Xavier Bagnoud Aerospace Prize administered by the University for space research that benefits humanity, and it sponsors graduate-level fellowships in aerospace studies.

The Foundation co-financed the François-Xavier Bagnoud Building at the Harvard School of Public Health (to be dedicated in October 1996) to house the François-Xavier Bagnoud Center for Health and Human Rights, established in 1993 as the first academic institute to focus exclusively on health and human rights. A Professorship in Health and Human Rights was endowed by the Foundation to promote, document, research, and analyze the relationships between health and human rights with special attention to children. The Center publishes the Journal, *Health and Human Rights* and organizes international conferences on themes central to its purpose and sponsors fellowships for scholars for study in its mandated fields.

Humanitarian activities of the Association include the promotion of children's rights, the rescue of sexually abused children, and the provision of care and support for children orphaned or infected with the HIV virus and to those with AIDS in the United States, Thailand, India, Colombia, Brazil, Kenya, and Uganda. Innovative activities to rehabilitate former commercial sex workers are sponsored in Myanmar by the Association; and in Uruguay, an effort in poorer neighborhoods educates adolescent street children about their sexuality and promotes healthy sexual practices. The Association is also assisting families in Rwanda whose houses have been destroyed to build new ones and provide a family life for orphaned children.

In its AIDS work, the Association is committed to a global and innovative strategy, integrating information, research, training, prevention, and care. Albina du Boisrouvray, François-Xavier's mother and founding president of the Association, is also a founding member of the Steering Committee of the Global AIDS Policy Coalition (GAPC). In 1991, the Association established the François-Xavier Bagnoud International Pediatric HIV Training Program at the University of Medicine and Dentistry of New Jersey. This program offers training in pediatric HIV/AIDS to physicians, nurses, and social workers from countries throughout the world. It also endowed the François-Xavier Bagnoud Chair in Pediatrics, held by James Oleske, MD, MPH, and the François-Xavier Bagnoud Chair in Pediatric Nursing held by Mary Boland, RN, MSN, FAAN at the same university.

The Association is financed by the foundation and personal contributions of the founding members, who actively seek the projects and programs which it supports. It does not solicit outside requests and proposals but welcomes corporate or private contributions.

The François-Xavier Bagnoud Center for Health and Human Rights Harvard School of Public Health

The Association François-Xavier Bagnoud supported the establishment of the first academic institute to focus exclusively on health and human rights, the François-Xavier Bagnoud Center, at the Harvard School of Public Health, in January 1993. The Center's work combines the academic strengths of research and teaching with a strong commitment to service and advocacy. The Center's mandate includes:

- **research:** to explore and understand the relationships between health and human rights
- **teaching:** to disseminate new knowledge, experience, and ideas
- **service and advocacy:** to stimulate collaboration between the fields of health and human rights, including advocacy and promotion of sound health policies that respect human rights and dignity.

From its position within an academic institution, the Center works at the local, national, and international levels, collaborating with health and human rights practitioners, official and nongovernmental organizations, academic institutions, and international agencies.

Editorial Advisory Board of AIDS in the World

The special contributions of Eka Esu-Williams to the preparation of this volume extended beyond the traditional role of Member of the Editorial Advisory Board. The Editors gratefully acknowledge her work on this project.

Associate Editor: Jeffrey O'Malley

Managing Editor: Carolien Albers

Publication Coordinator: Susan Grady

This book is dedicated to François-Xavier Bagnoud;
to the many whose lives, all too short, live on for us.

Preface

The first edition of *AIDS in the World*, published in November 1992 by the Harvard-based Global AIDS Policy Coalition, tracked the pandemic from the discovery of AIDS in the early 1980s. It described and analyzed the growing gap between the pandemic and the global response and, by uncovering the roots of individual and collective vulnerability to HIV/AIDS, set the stage for a revolutionary personal, community, and global approach to AIDS and health.

This edition, *AIDS in the World II*, continues to track the pandemic and the efforts, successes, and failures encountered as the world attempts to curb its course and mitigate its impact. Yet, this volume is not merely an update; it presents new data, and more importantly, analysis of the pandemic and of what must be done about it. This offers the reader a perspective from which individuals, communities, nations, and international organizations can redefine their response to the pandemic.

Part I provides recent information on the global epidemiology of HIV/ AIDS and analyzes recent trends. The pandemic has become increasingly complex and fragmented, targeting populations characterized by a high degree of social and economic vulnerability.

Part II summarizes the state of scientific progress in HIV/AIDS research. A continuously deepening understanding of the pathogenesis of HIV/AIDS and the development of new drugs and vaccine candidates may contribute additional methods and tools to ongoing prevention and care approaches in a not-so-remote future.

Part III examines how people are responding to the HIV/AIDS pandemic—as individuals or through organized community efforts—and Part IV analyzes the collective efforts of governments, intergovernmental institutions, and nongovernment organizations (NGOs). A series of original surveys provides the most up-to-date account of national and international action against HIV/AIDS.

Then, Part V brings these several threads—epidemiology, research, individual and collective response—together into a new analytic framework to inform a truly modern understanding and response to the pandemic. It shows how risk, risk-taking behaviors, and risk-generating situations are linked to societal environment, and it ties this analytical framework to pragmatic and conceptual dimensions of human rights protections and promotion.

This synthesis is composed of many parts. *AIDS in the World II* includes contributions by 125 authors from a broad array of professional fields. It also required the participation of research assistants, and, through questionnaires, obtained information from over 200 individuals or institutions.

The Editors contributed all chapters or sections that are not specifically attributed to other authors. We also worked closely with many authors to ensure internal consistency and readability. We have sought to fashion a book accessible to a large readership, including people who want to expand their knowledge about the pandemic, health and social workers, people living with HIV/AIDS, and, more generally, those who recognize HIV/AIDS as the pandemic of our time and a defining challenge to our world.

Cambridge, Mass.   J. M. M.
June 1996   D. T.

Contents

CONTRIBUTORS, xxiii
INTRODUCTION, xxxi

PART I   THE STATE OF THE PANDEMIC AND ITS IMPACT, 3

Chapter 1 GLOBAL OVERVIEW: A POWERFUL HIV/AIDS PANDEMIC, 5
  National reporting of AIDS, 5
  National reporting of positive HIV tests, 6
  HIV and AIDS data: AIDS in the World II Survey, 9
  The pandemic has expanded relentlessly: status as of January 1, 1996, 11
  Newly acquired HIV infections in 1995, 18
  New AIDS cases in 1995, 19
  People living with HIV infection and with AIDS as of January 1, 1996, 21
  The future course of the HIV/AIDS pandemic, 24
  What lies behind the first peak of HIV/AIDS epidemics? 37
      Box 1.1 *Living with the Shortcomings of the Pediatric AIDS Case Definition,* 5
          N. Lapointe
      Box 1.2 *Sentinel HIV Surveillance,* 7
          P. A. Sato
      Box 1.3 *Geographic Areas of Affinity,* 9
      Box 1.4 *New Appreciation for Complexities of Perinatally-acquired HIV*
      Infection, 14
          J. M. Oleske
      Box 1.5 *Disease Progression and Mortality following HIV-1 Infection,* 15
          D. Mulder
      Box 1.6 *Status and Trends of the HIV/AIDS Pandemic in Africa,* 28
          AIDSCAP/François-Xavier Bagnoud Center for Health and Human Rights
          at the Harvard School of Public Health

Chapter 2 THE DYNAMIC HIV/AIDS PANDEMIC, 41
          K. A. Stanecki, P. O. Way
  Latin America and the Caribbean, 41

Sub-Saharan Africa, 43
Southeast Asia, 50
    Box 2.1 Urban–Rural Movement and HIV Dynamics, 48
        M. J. Wawer

Chapter 3 THE EVOLVING HIV/AIDS PANDEMIC, 57
        B. G. Weniger, S. Berkley
Traditional risk groups are not monolithic, 57
Increased heterosexual transmission in industrialized countries, 58
Extension into new geographic areas and population groups, 62
Separate epidemics may exist side by side, 62
The effect of political and other events, 63

Chapter 4 THE SPREAD OF HIV AND SEXUAL MIXING PATTERNS, 71
        R. M. Anderson
The incubation period of AIDS, 72
Infectiousness during the incubation period, 75
Shape of the simple epidemic, 77
Mixing patterns and epidemic waves, 77

Chapter 5 THE PANDEMIC OF HIV-ASSOCIATED TUBERCULOSIS, 87
        M. Raviglione, P. P. Nunn, A. Kochi, R. J. O'Brien
    Box 5.1 TB and HIV Coinfection, 91
    Box 5.2 Reversing the Rise in Tuberculosis Morbidity and
    Mortality, 92
        S. J. Heymann, T. F. Brewer

Chapter 6 EPIDEMIOLOGY OF HIV AND SEXUALLY TRANSMITTED INFECTIONS IN
        WOMEN, 97
        B. Vuylsteke, R. Sunkutu, M. Laga
The epidemiology of HIV in women, 97
Biology, behavior, and society, 98
The epidemiology of sexually transmitted infections in women, 101
    Box 6.1 The Interactions between HIV and Other Sexually
    Transmitted Infections, 99
        L. J. Gelmon, P. Piot

Chapter 7 THE ECONOMIC IMPACT IN SELECTED COUNTRIES AND THE SECTORAL
        IMPACT, 110
        A. Whiteside
Literature review, 110
Country case study reviews, 112
Sectoral impact, 114

Chapter 8 SOCIETAL AND POLITICAL IMPACT OF HIV/AIDS, 117
        R. Bayer
    Box 8.1 AIDS and the Arts: Devastation to Democratization, 118
        K. Morrison

   Box 8.2 AIDS: Despair, or a Stimulus to Reform, 122
     D. Shuey, H. Bagarukayo
   Box 8.3 Evolving Impact of HIV/AIDS on India, 124
     P. Mane

PART II   THE FRONTIER OF KNOWLEDGE, 129

Chapter 9 THE CONTRIBUTION OF SOCIAL AND BEHAVIORAL SCIENCE TO HIV/AIDS
     PREVENTION, 131
     P. Gillies
Framing questions and solving problems: the importance of theory, 131
Methodical approaches in research on sexual behavior, 140
Measuring outcomes, 149
   Box 9.1 Sex Research in Response to AIDS, 137
     R. G. Parker
   Box 9.2 Some Lessons from the WHO/GPA Sexual and KABP
   Surveys, 140
     B. Ferry, J. Cleland

Chapter 10 TREATMENT OF HIV DISEASE: PROBLEMS, PROGRESS, AND
     POTENTIAL, 159
     E. C. Cooper

Chapter 11 LONG-TERM SURVIVORS: WHAT CAN WE LEARN FROM THEM? 165
     R. Colebunders

Chapter 12 HIV-2 INFECTION: CURRENT KNOWLEDGE AND UNCERTAINTIES, 171
     K. M. De Cock, F. Brun-Vézinet
Geographic distribution of HIV-2, 171
Disease associations and natural history, 173
Virology of HIV-2 infection and dual reactivity, 173

Chapter 13 HIV HETEROGENEITY IN TRANSMISSION AND PATHOGENESIS, 177
     J. Levy
Biologic features, 177
Serologic features, 179
Molecular features, 180
   Box 13.1 The Global Distribution of HIV-1 Genotypes, 180
     F. E. McCutchan, G. Myers

Chapter 14 HIV VACCINE DEVELOPMENT—PROGRESS AND PROBLEMS, 186
     D. P. Francis
Scientific progress, 186
Scientific concerns, 187
Social concerns, 188
Solutions, 190

Chapter 15 PREPARING FOR HIV VACCINE EFFICACY TRIALS IN DEVELOPING
        COUNTRIES, 193
        W. L. Heyward, S. Osmanov, J. Esparza
    Why conduct HIV vaccine trials in developing countries? 193
    Immediate issues in preparing for field trials, 193
    Additional challenges for the future, 195

Chapter 16 WOMEN-CONTROLLED HIV PREVENTION METHODS, 196
        C. J. Elias, L. L. Heise, E. Gollub

Chapter 17 WHO SETS THE GLOBAL RESEARCH AGENDA FOR BIOMEDICAL
        SCIENCE? 202
        R. Widdus

Chapter 18 AIDS RESEARCH: SOLIDARITY? RIVALRY? FRATERNITY? 205
        A. J. Pinching
    The scientific process, 205
    Early observations on AIDS, 207
    Features of AIDS research, 208

        PART III   RESPONSE: INDIVIDUALS AND POPULATIONS, 213

Chapter 19 HIV/AIDS AMONG WOMEN, 215
        WOMEN AND AIDS: BUILDING A NEW HIV PREVENTION STRATEGY, 215
        G. Rao Gupta, E. Weiss, D. Whelan
    Gender roles and relations, 215
    Assumptions underlying AIDS prevention strategies, 216
    Economic risk factors, 217
    Sociocultural risk factors, 218
    Building a new HIV prevention strategy, 223
        Box 19.1 Relationship between Women's Status and HIV Risk, 222
            D. Whelan

Chapter 20 HIV IN WOMEN: WHAT ARE THE GAPS IN KNOWLEDGE? 229
        Z. A. Stein, L. Kuhn
    HIV transmission, 229
    Prevention programs, 233
        Box 20.1 Gynecologic Disease among Women with HIV/AIDS, 230
            C. Marte

Chapter 21 YOUTH AND HIV/AIDS, 236
        N. D. Hoffman, M. D. Futterman
    A youth-centered approach to HIV/AIDS prevention, 237
    Youth marginalization and disempowerment, 238
    Development of personal behaviors, 240
    Changing roles of young people, 242

Barriers to making choices, 242

Health care and HIV prevention, 242

Partnerships and programs, 243

    Box 21.1 Sex Education: Adolescents' Future versus Adults'
Fears, 238

        M. Baldo

    Box 21.2 Sexual Abuse of Children and HIV/AIDS, 245

        G. A. Gellert

    Box 21.3 Young People, AIDS, and STIs: Peer Approaches in
Developing Countries, 247

        N. Fee, M. Youssef

Chapter 22 MALE HOMOSEXUALITY AND HIV, 252

SECTION 1: BEHAVIOR CHANGES AMONG HOMOSEXUAL MEN, 252

    A. P. M. Coxon

State of knowledge, 252

Changes in sexual behavior, 253

Critical issues, 253

SECTION 2: HIV, HOMOSEXUALITY, AND VULNERABILITY IN THE DEVELOPING WORLD, 254

    D. Altman

Chapter 23 SEXUAL BEHAVIOR AMONG HETEROSEXUALS, 259

    A. A. Ehrhardt

Patterns of sexual behavior and hierarchy of risk, 259

Social context, 260

Barriers to condom use, 260

Prevention, 261

    Box 23.1 Sexuality in Women with HIV Infection, 261

        C. Hankins

Chapter 24 RISK REDUCTION AMONG INJECTING DRUG USERS, 264

    D. C. Des Jarlais, S. R. Friedman

    Box 24.1 Injecting Drug Use: Transition from Heroin to
Semisynthetic Narcotic Analgesic, 265

        S. Sundararaman

Chapter 25 HIV/AIDS IN PRISONS, 268

    T. W. Harding

Clinical AIDS in prison, 268

HIV/AIDS and tuberculosis in prison, 269

Injecting drug use and prison, 269

International guidelines, 270

Chapter 26 PEDIATRIC HIV/AIDS, 273

    BREAST-FEEDING AND HIV/AIDS, 273

    S. Le Coeur, M. Lallemant

Chapter 27 ORPHANS OF THE HIV/AIDS PANDEMIC, 278
        C. Levine, D. Michaels, S. Back
  When parents die of AIDS, where do the children go? 281
  What are the burdens for families related to AIDS orphans? 282
  Organizational support for orphans, 283
Meeting current and future needs, 285
A short- and long-term perspective is needed, 285
        Box 27.1 Projections of Numbers of AIDS Orphans, 278
            D. Michaels, S. Back
        Box 27.2 A Community-Based Program for Orphans and Vulnerable Children,
        Luwero District, Uganda: Strategies for Implementation, 283
            D. Shuey, H. Bagarukayo, S. Senkusu, K. Ryan

Chapter 28 BLOOD AND BLOOD PRODUCT SAFETY, 287
        N. Gilmore
  Screening blood donations, 293
  Excluding infected donors, 294
  Reducing the demand for blood and blood product treatment, 295
  Economic impact of strengthening blood safety, 295
        Box 28.1 The Growing Aftermath of HIV Infection from Blood and Blood
        Component Treatment: Compensation, Litigation, and Public
        Inquiries, 287

Chapter 29 ARE WE LEARNING FROM THE LESSONS OF THE PAST? 302
        J. E. Osborn
  America as a learning ground, 302
  The world as a learning ground, 307

                    PART IV   THE INSTITUTIONAL RESPONSE, 311

Chapter 30 GOVERNMENTAL NATIONAL AIDS PROGRAMS, 315
  Voicing commitment, 317
  Translating commitment into action, 317
  Coalition building, 318
  Planning and coordination, 319
  Managing, 319
  Responding to prevention and care needs, 321
  Securing financial resources and striving towards sustainability, 322
  Evaluating progress and impact, 325
        Box 30.1 Survey of Government National AIDS Programs (GNAP), 315

Chapter 31 HUMAN RIGHTS AND RESPONSES TO HIV/AIDS, 326
        S. Gruskin, K. Tomasevski, A. Hendriks
  Human rights and HIV/AIDS: key principles, 327
  International responses to AIDS and violations of human rights, 328
  Current issues, 334

Human rights aspects of national responses to AIDS: national laws, policies, and practices, 335

Survey of National Laws and Practices, 336

Box 31.1 Updated Chronology of Selected International and Regional Documents on the Human Rights Aspects of HIV/AIDS, 1990–1995, 332

Box 31.2 Assessing the Human Rights Impact, 337
S. Gruskin

Chapter 32 NONGOVERNMENTAL ORGANIZATIONS, 341
J. O'Malley, V. K. Nguyen, S. Lee

The range of NGOs responding to AIDS, 341

NGOs roles and achievements, 344

Needs, capacities, and priorities of service delivery organizations, 346

Identity activism, 347

The greater involvement of people with HIV: principles and problems, 348

The proliferation of NGO activities on AIDS and the dilemmas of funding, 356

Funding trends and their impact on NGOs, 357

Relations between NGOs and governments, 359

Sustaining community action on AIDS, 360

Box 32.1 Society for Women and AIDS in Africa, 342
E. Esu-Williams

Box 32.2 Women Living with HIV/AIDS, 349
W. Chikafumbwa

Box 32.3 Empowerment and Gay Community in Australia, 354
G. Woolcock, D. Altman

Chapter 33 THE PRIVATE SECTOR: HOW ARE CORPORATIONS RESPONDING TO HIV/AIDS? 362
B. Bezmalinovic

Employee assistance programs and services, 364

Corporate policies regarding HIV/AIDS, 364

HIV/AIDS prevention programs, 365

Management information needs, 365

Box 33.1 Workplace Guidelines on HIV/AIDS, 362

Box 33.2 Corporate Response to AIDS in India, 367
A. K. Ganesh, S. Sundararaman

Chapter 34 THE UN RESPONSE, 369
L. Garbus

Box 34.1 Why UNAIDS? 370
P. Piot

Chapter 35 INTERNATIONAL FUNDING OF THE GLOBAL AIDS STRATEGY: OFFICIAL DEVELOPMENT ASSISTANCE, 375
M. Laws

Official development assistance: donor countries, 375

The AIDS in the World II 1994 financing survey: data sources, 376

Survey responses, 378

Development assistance: supply, demand, and fatigue, 387

    Box 35.1 Channels of Official Development Assistance and Sources of Information on AIDS Financing, 379

    Box 35.2 "Donor Fatigue Syndrome," 387

Chapter 36 THE COST OF HIV/AIDS CARE, 390

    A. L. Martin

Country information on the global cost of HIV/AIDS care, 391

  Resource shortfall in developing countries, 394

  Cost of care for HIV/AIDS by stage of illness, 395

  Global cost of care for PWHIV/AIDS, 395

    Box 36.1 Personal Care Strategies of People Living with HIV/AIDS, 398

      R. G. Mota

    Box 36.2 Caring for Persons with AIDS (PWA) in Botswana: Is Home-Based Care the Answer? 405

      C. Cameron, D. S. Shepard, J. Mulwa

    Box 36.3 The San Francisco Care Model, 407

      I. B. Corless, M. Pittman

    Box 36.4 Models of Home-Based Care (HBC): Zambia, 409

      A. L. Martin, E. van Praag, R. Msiska

Chapter 37 GLOBAL SPENDING ON HIV/AIDS PREVENTION, CARE, AND RESEARCH, 414

  Estimated spending on HIV prevention, 425

  Estimated spending on HIV/AIDS care, 425

  Spending on HIV/AIDS research, 425

    Box 37.1 The Cost of HIV Prevention, 414

      J. Broomberg, D. Schopper

PART V   FROM EPIDEMIOLOGY TO VULNERABILITY TO HUMAN RIGHTS, 427

Chapter 38 THE HISTORY OF DISCOVERY AND RESPONSE, 429

  The period of discovery, 429

  The period of early response, 429

  The current period, 430

    Box 38.1 "Risk Groups" or "Risk Behaviors?" 431

      S. Watney

    Box 38.2 The Spread of HIV/AIDS in the World's Indigenous Populations, 434

      R. M. Rowell

Chapter 39 VULNERABILITY: PERSONAL AND PROGRAMMATIC, 441

Chapter 40 SOCIETAL VULNERABILITY: CONTEXTUAL ANALYSIS, 444
    Implementing vulnerability reduction, 453
        Box 40.1 Cultural Influence on Society Vulnerability, 444
            T. Barnett, R. Grellier
        Box 40.2 AIDS as a Challenge to Religion, 447
            D. Defert
        Box 40.3 Country Assessment and Strategic Planning, 453
        Box 40.4 Vulnerability of Young People to HIV/AIDS:
        A Proposed Analytical Framework, 454
        Box 40.5 Societal Context and Response, 457
            J. O'Malley
        Box 40.6 Generating Government Commitment, 458
        Box 40.7 Constraints to Contextual Changes, 461

Chapter 41 FROM VULNERABILITY TO HUMAN RIGHTS, 463
    Background, 463
    Discovery of the human rights basis of vulnerability to HIV, 464
    The human rights analysis of vulnerability to HIV, 469
    Advantages and barriers to the human rights approach, 474
    Conclusion: bringing it all together, 474
        Box 41.1 Tolerance and Discrimination, 466
            J. O'Malley
        Box 41.2 Human Rights Primer, 467
        Box 41.3 Human Rights Underlie Contextual Factors, 469
        Box 41.4 The Human Right to Information: Pathway to Action, 472
        Box 41.5 Example of the Human Rights Analysis, 473

Appendix A AIDS cases reported to the World Health Organization, by GAA and by year,
            1984–1996, 479
Appendix B Method for the estimation and projection of HIV/AIDS, 487
Appendix C Estimated 1994 adult HIV prevalence by country, 491
Appendix D Responses to the survey of Government National AIDS Programs, 496
    Table D-1   AIDS policies and programs: responses of governmental national AIDS programs
    (GNAP), 496
    Table D-2   Countries that responded to AIW II questionnaire on government national AIDS
    program, level of economy, country population, and date of first AIDS case report, 501
    Table D-3   Government national AIDS programs: program structure and partnership, 506
    Table D-4   Government national AIDS programs: estimates and projections of the numbers of
    HIV infections in adults and children (cumulative through the year indicated), 512
    Table D-5   Government national AIDS programs: implementation and impact on other health
    programs, 517
    Table D-6   Government national AIDS programs: financial information, 526
    Table D-7.1   Government national AIDS programs: needs and services: information, medical
    care, and training, 532
    Table D-7.2   Government national AIDS programs: needs and services: reported adequacy of
    condom distribution and outreach and targeted activities, 536

Table D-7.3   Government national AIDS programs: needs and services: projected and reported numbers of condoms distributed and achievement of target, 541

Table D-7.4   Government national AIDS programs: needs and services: condom distribution sites, 1990, 545

Table D-7.5   Government national AIDS programs: needs and services: condom distributions sites, 1992, 550

Table D-7.6   Government national AIDS programs: needs and services: HIV testing and counseling: sites and practices, 555

Table D-8   Government national AIDS programs: behavioral surveys/studies conducted since 1990, 560

Table D-9.1   Government national AIDS programs: evaluation practices, 563

Table D-9.2   Government national AIDS programs: use of evaluation findings, 568

Appendix E Laws and practices in the context of HIV/AIDS: A survey of Government National AIDS Program Managers, 578

Table E-1   Government national AIDS programs: laws and practices regarding HIV/AIDS (as reported by GNAP managers): obligatory testing of specified groups, 578

Table E-2   Government national AIDS programs: laws and practices regarding HIV/AIDS (as reported by GNAP managers): testing of migrants and travelers, 583

Appendix F The Universal Declaration of Human Rights, 588

ACKNOWLEDGMENTS, 593

INDEX, 599

Contributors

DENNIS ALTMAN
La Trobe University and
Asia Pacific Council of AIDS Service
  Organizations
Adelaide, Australia

ROY M. ANDERSON, FRS
Professor
Wellcome Centre for the Epidemiology of
  Infectious Diseases
University of Oxford
Oxford, United Kingdom

SARA D. BACK, MPH
Consultant to the Orphan Project and
Project Director, Women's Interagency HIV
  Study (WIHS)
Bronx Lebanon Hospital Center
New York, New York, United States

HENRY BAGARUKAYO
African Medical and Research Foundation
  (AMREF)
Kampala, Uganda

MARIELLA BALDO, PhD
Global Programme on AIDS
World Health Organization
Geneva, Switzerland

TONY BARNETT
School of Development Studies
University of East Anglia
Norwich, United Kingdom

RONALD BAYER, PhD
HIV Center for Clinical and Behavioral
  Studies
New York Psychiatric Institute and
Professor, School of Public Health
Columbia University
New York, New York, United States

SETH BERKLEY, MD, MPH
Associate Director, Health Sciences
  Division
The Rockefeller Foundation
New York, New York, United States

BEA BEZMALINOVIC, MPP
Consultant to The Global AIDS Policy
  Coalition and
Management Sciences for Health (MSH)
Cambridge, Massachusetts, United States

TIMOTHY F. BREWER, MD, MPH
Channing Laboratory
Brigham and Women's Hospital
Boston, Massachusetts, United States

JONATHAN BROOMBERG, MD, PhD
Health Economics and Financing
  Programme
London School of Hygiene and Tropical
  Medicine
London, United Kingdom

FRANÇOISE BRUN-VÉZINET, Dr. és Sc.
Laboratoire de Virologie
Hôpital Bichat & Claude Bernard
Paris, France

CHARLES CAMERON, MBA, MPH
Management Consultant
Cameron Associates
Barnstead, New Hampshire, United States

WINNIE CHIKAFUMBWA
Coordinator, National Association of
   People with HIV/AIDS in Malawi
   (NAPHAM)
Lilongwe, Malawi

JOHN CLELAND
Demographer, Social and Behavioural
   Studies and Support Unit
Global Programme on AIDS
World Health Organization
Geneva, Switzerland

ROBERT COLEBUNDERS, MD
Institute of Tropical Medicine
Antwerp, Belgium

ELLEN C. COOPER, MD, MPH
American Foundation for AIDS Research
Department of Clinical Research and
   Information
Bethesda, Maryland, United States

INGE B. CORLESS, RN, PhD, FAAN
Institute of Health Professions
Massachusetts General Hospital
Boston, Massachusetts, United States

ANTHONY P. M. COXON, PhD
Project SIGMA
Department of Sociology
University of Essex
Essex, Colchester, United Kingdom

KEVIN M. DE COCK, MD
London School of Hygiene and Tropical
   Medicine
London, United Kingdom

DANIEL DEFERT, MD
Founding Chair
French National Aides Federation
Paris, France

DON C. DES JARLAIS, MD, PhD
Chemical Dependency Institute
Beth Israel Medical Center
New York, New York, United States

ANKE A. EHRHARDT, PhD
Director, HIV Center for Clinical and
   Behavioral Studies
New York State Psychiatric Institute and
Professor of Clinical Psychology
Department of Psychiatry
Columbia University
New York, New York, United States

CHRISTOPHER J. ELIAS, MD, MPH
Senior Associate for Women's
   Reproductive Health
The Population Council
New York, New York, United States

JOSÉ ESPARZA, MD, PhD
Vaccine Development Unit
Global Programme on AIDS
World Health Organization
Geneva, Switzerland

EKA ESU-WILLIAMS, PhD
Society for Women and AIDS in Africa
   (SWAA)
Port-Harcourt, Nigeria

NANCY FEE
Consultant to The Global Programme
   on AIDS,
World Health Organization
Geneva, Switzerland

BENOÎT FERRY
Demographer, Social and Behavioural
   Studies and Support Unit
Global Programme on AIDS
World Health Organization
Geneva, Switzerland
   (Sponsored by ORSTOM, France)

DONALD P. FRANCIS, MD, DSc
Genentech, Inc.
South San Francisco, California,
United States

SAMUEL R. FRIEDMAN, MD
National Development and
Research Institutes, Inc.
New York, New York, United States

DONNA FUTTERMAN, MD
Department of Pediatrics,
    Albert Einstein College of Medicine
Director, Adolescent AIDS Program
Montefiore Medical Center
New York, New York, United States

A. K. GANESH
AIDS Research Foundation of India
Madras, Tamil Nadu, India

LISA GARBUS, MPP
Consultant to The Global AIDS Policy
    Coalition
Cambridge, Massachusetts, United States

GEORGE A. GELLERT, MD, MPH, MPA
Consultant
Philadelphia, Pennsylvania, United States

LAWRENCE J. GELMON, MD, MPH
Departments of Medical Microbiology
University of Manitoba
Manitoba, Winnepeg, Canada, and
University of Nairobi
Nairobi, Kenya

PAMELA GILLIES, PhD
Senior Lecturer in Public Health
    (Hon MFPHM)
Department of Public Health Medicine and
    Epidemiology
University of Nottingham
Nottingham, United Kingdom

NORBERT GILMORE, PhD, MD
McGill Centre for Medicine,
    Ethics, and Law
McGill University
Montréal, Québec, Canada

ERICA L. GOLLUB, DrPH
AIDS Surveillance Unit
AIDS Activities Coordinating Office
    (AACO)
Director of AIDS Epidemiology
Philadelphia Department of Public Health
Philadelphia, Pennsylvania, United States

RACHEL GRELLIER
School of Develoment Studies
University of East Anglia
Norwich, United Kingdom

SOFIA GRUSKIN, JD, MIA
Research Associate and Lecturer in Health
    and Human Rights
François-Xavier Bagnoud Center for
    Health and Human Rights
Harvard School of Public Health
Cambridge, Massachusetts, United States

GEETA RAO GUPTA, PhD
International Center for Research on
    Women
Washington, DC, United States

CATHERINE HANKINS, MD, PhD
Group for Action-Research
McGill AIDS Centre
Montréal, Québec, Canada

TIMOTHY W. HARDING, MD
Professor, University Institute of Legal
    Medicine C.M.U.
University of Geneva
Geneva, Switzerland

LORI L. HEISE
Director, Violence, Sexuality and Health
    Rights Program and Pacific Institute for
    Women's Health
Health and Development
    Policy Project
Washington, DC, United States

AART HENDRIKS, LLA, MA
Faculty of Law
Health Law Section
University of Amsterdam
Amsterdam, the Netherlands

S. JODY HEYMANN, MD, PhD
Department of Health Care Policy
Harvard Medical School
Kennedy School of Government
Cambridge, Massachusetts, United States

WILLIAM L. HEYWARD, MD, MPH
Vaccine Development Unit
Global Programme on AIDS
World Health Organization
Geneva, Switzerland

NEAL D. HOFFMAN, MD
Assistant Professor of Pediatrics
Albert Einstein College of Medicine
Medical Director, Adolescent Health
    Program
Montefiore Medical Center
New York, New York, United States

ARATA KOCHI, MD, PhD
Global Tuberculosis Programme
World Health Organization
Geneva, Switzerland

LOUISE KUHN
HIV Center for Clinical and Behavioral
    Studies
New York State Psychiatric Institute and
Division of Epidemiology
Columbia University
New York, New York, United States

MARIE LAGA, MD
Department of Infection and Immunity and
    Department of Microbiology
Institute of Tropical Medicine
Antwerp, Belgium

MARC LALLEMANT, MD, MPH
Department of Cancer Biology
Harvard School of Public Health
Boston, Massachusetts, United States
    (Sponsored by ORSTOM, France)

NORMAND LAPOINTE, MD, MSc, FRCR(C)
Centre Maternel et Infantile sur le SIDA
Hôpital Sainte-Justine
Montréal, Québec, Canada

MARGARET LAWS, MPP
Consultant to The Global AIDS Policy
    Coalition
Cambridge, Massachusetts, United States

SOPHIE LE COEUR, MD, MPH
Department of Cancer Biology
Harvard School of Public Health
Boston, Massachusetts, United States
    (Sponsored by ORSTOM, France)

SARAH LEE
International HIV/AIDS Alliance
London, United Kingdom

CAROL LEVINE, MD
Executive Director
The Orphan Project
New York, New York, United States

JAY A. LEVY, MD
Professor, Cancer Research Institute and
    Department of Medicine and School
    of Medicine
University of California, San Francisco
San Francisco, California, United States

PURNIMA MANE, PhD
Associate Professor (Reader)
Department of Medical and Psychiatric
    Social Work
Tata Institute of Social Sciences
Deonar, Bombay, India

CAROLA MARTE, MD, PhD
Yale University AIDS Program
New Haven, Connecticut, United States

ANNE L. MARTIN, PhD
President
Health Planning Consultants
Hillsborough, North Carolina, United
    States

FRANCINE E. MCCUTCHAN, PhD
Henry M. Jackson Foundation
Rockville, Maryland, United States

DAVID MICHAELS, MD
Associate Professor of Epidemiology
Medical School
City University of New York
New York, New York, United States

KEN MORRISON
Writer
Communications Consultant
Montréal, Québec, Canada

RUTH GUNN MOTA, MPH
International Health Programs
Santa Cruz, California, United States

ROLAND MSISKA, MD
Joint United Nations Programme on
    HIV/AIDS (UNAIDS)
Country Support, Global Programme
    on AIDS
World Health Organization
Geneva, Switzerland and
Ministry of Health
Lusaka, Zambia

DAAN MULDER, MD, PhD
Medical Research Council (ODA/UVRI)
Programme on AIDS in Uganda
Entebbe, Uganda

JOHN K. M. MULWA, MD
Deputy Permanent Secretary and
Director of Medical Services
Ministry of Health
Gaborone, Botswana

GERALD MYERS, PhD
HIV Sequence Database and
Analysis Project
Los Alamos National Laboratory
Los Alamos, New Mexico, United States

VINH KIM NGUYEN, MD
International HIV/AIDS Alliance
London, United Kingdom

PAUL P. NUNN
Global Tuberculosis Programme
World Health Organization
Geneva, Switzerland

RICHARD J. O'BRIEN, MD
Global Tuberculosis Programme
World Health Organization
Geneva, Switzerland

JAMES M. OLESKE, MD, MPH
François-Xavier Bagnoud Professor of
Pediatrics
Director, Division of Allergy Immunology
and Infectious Diseases UMD—New
Jersey Medical School and
Medical Director, Children's Hospital AIDS
Program (CHAP) United Hospital
Medical Center,
Newark, New Jersey, United States

JEFFREY O'MALLEY, MA
Executive Director
International HIV/AIDS Alliance
London, United Kingdom

JUNE E. OSBORN, MD
Professor of Epidemiology and Pediatrics
The University of Michigan
School of Public Health and Medical
School
Ann Arbor, Michigan, United States

SALADIN OSMANOV, MD, PhD
Vaccine Development Unit
Global Programme on AIDS
World Health Organization
Geneva, Switzerland

RICHARD G. PARKER, PhD
Institute of Social Medicine
State University of Rio de Janeiro
Rio de Janeiro, Brazil

ANTHONY J. PINCHING, MD, FRCP
Louis Freedman Professor of Immunology,
Medical College of Saint Bartholomew's
Hospital
London, West Smithfield,
United Kingdom

PETER PIOT, MD, PhD
Executive Director
Joint United Nations Programme on
HIV/AIDS (UNAIDS)
Geneva, Switzerland

MARY PITTMAN, PhD
President, Hospital Research and
Educational Trust
American Hospital Association
Chicago, Illinois, United States

MARIO RAVIGLIONE, MD, MPH
Global Tuberculosis Programme
World Health Organization
Geneva, Switzerland

RONALD M. ROWELL, MPH
Native American AIDS Prevention Center
Oakland, California, United States

KIM RYAN
African Medical and Research Foundation
(AMREF)
Kampala, Uganda

PAUL A. SATO, MD, MPH
Surveillance, Evaluation, and Forecasting
Unit
Division of Technical Cooperation
Global Programme on AIDS
World Health Organization
Geneva, Switzerland

DORIS SCHOPPER, MD, PhD
Global Programme on AIDS
World Health Organization
Geneva, Switzerland

SAMUEL SENKUSU
African Medical and Research Foundation
    (AMREF)
Kampala, Uganda (born, July 18, 1953;
    died, August 16, 1995)

DONALD S. SHEPARD, PhD
Research Professor, Heller School,
Brandeis University
Waltham, Massachusetts, United States
and
Visiting Professor
Harvard School of Public Health
Cambridge, Massachusetts, United States

DEAN SHUEY, MD, PhD
African Medical and Research Foundation
    (AMREF)
Kampala, Uganda

KAREN A. STANECKI, PhD
Center for International Research
U.S. Bureau of the Census
Washington, DC, United States

ZENA A. STEIN, MD, PhD
HIV Center for Clinical and Behavioral
    Studies
New York State Psychiatric Institute and
Division of Epidemiology
Columbia University
New York, New York, United States

S. SUNDARARAMAN, MD, PhD
Director, AIDS Research Foundation of
    India
Madras, Tamil Nadu, India

ROSE SUNKUTU, MD
Deputy Manager
National AIDS/STD/TB and Leprosy
    Control Programme
Ministry of Health, and
Department of Dermato-Venereology
University Teaching Hospital
Lusaka, Zambia

KATARINA TOMASEVSKI, JD
Danish Centre for Human Rights
Copenhagen, Denmark

ERIC VAN PRAAG, MD
Chief, Health Care and Support Unit
Global Programme on AIDS
World Health Organization
Geneva, Switzerland

BEA VUYLSTEKE, MD
Department of Infection and Immunity
and
Department of Microbiology
Institute of Tropical Medicine
Antwerp, Belgium

SIMON WATNEY
Director
The Red Hot AIDS Charitable Trust
London, United Kingdom

MARIA J. WAWER, MD, MPH
Associate Clinical Professor
Center for Population and Family Health
School of Public Health
Columbia University
New York, New York, United States

PETER O. WAY, PhD
Center for International Research
U.S. Bureau of the Census
Washington, DC, United States

ELLEN WEISS, MPH
International Center for Research on
    Women
Washington, DC, United States

BRUCE G. WENIGER, MD, MPH
Vaccine Safety and Development Activity
National Immunization Program
Centers for Disease Control and
    Prevention
Atlanta, Georgia, United States

DANIEL WHELAN, MA
International Center for Research on
    Women
Washington, DC, United States

ALAN WHITESIDE
Associate Professor
Economic Research Unit
University of Natal
Durban, South Africa

ROY WIDDUS, PhD
Coordinator
Children's Vaccine Initiative
World Health Organization
Geneva, Switzerland

GEOFFREY WOOLCOCK, MD
National Centre for HIV Social Research
Royal Brisbane Hospital
Herston, Brisbane, Australia

MAYADA YOUSSEF, PhD
Health Education Specialist
Global Programme on AIDS
World Health Organization
Geneva, Switzerland

BROUNKER: The city is lacking certain essentials. I will make this known.

LAWRENCE: No one will trade with us. No one will allow us to leave the city. Whole areas of the Isles—all of Scotland forbids any Londoner even to cross the border. We are pariahs in our own country. How are we to live?

BROUNKER: I will make this known. I will make all of this known.

LAWRENCE: It is known. Everyone knows our trouble, that is why we are shunned. Make it felt.

Anthony Clarvoe, from "The Living"
The Kenyon Review, Kenyon College, Gambier Ohio,
Presented by the Harvard and Radcliffe Drama Club at the
Loeb Drama Center,
Cambridge, Massachusetts, May 4, 1995.

It is not thy duty to complete the work, but neither art thou free to desist from it. . . .

Sayings of the Fathers,
II (21)

Introduction

The pathway from the old towards the new is the theme of this book. A coherent new analysis and approach to the pandemic is needed to respond to three interconnected global trends described in this book: the pandemic is intensifying and expanding; the support for anti-AIDS efforts at national and international levels is reaching a plateau; and the impact of current prevention and control efforts, although clearly demonstrated, remains insufficient. It is now clear to people working on, or affected by HIV/AIDS, that the traditional public health approach, even when organized and applied with extraordinary vigor and creativity, lacks sufficient power to combat the pandemic and to mitigate its impact.

To learn from the past and then search for ways to enhance our ongoing response to the pandemic and explore new approaches requires first a clear understanding of the current situation. What is the status of the pandemic? How has it changed as it has matured? What are the nature and extent of the response to the pandemic at the community, national, and international levels, and how have these responses evolved?

Four years ago, *AIDS in the World* (1992) described an expanding and dangerous gap between the pace of the HIV/AIDS pandemic and national and international efforts against it. In the mid-1990s, the pandemic continues to intensify and expand worldwide. Since 1992, the Asian epidemic has rapidly increased, so much so that in 1995, more people living in Asia were newly infected than in any other part of the world, including sub-Saharan Africa. By early 1996, Asia had almost four times more people living with HIV/AIDS than all of the industrialized countries combined. By early 1996, over 30 million people had become HIV infected and 10 million had already developed AIDS. Proving to be more powerful than ever, the pandemic has also become dynamic, volatile, and complex. While some national HIV/AIDS epidemics have slowed, in part as a result of effective prevention, larger analyses using a decades-long frame of analysis suggest that the epidemic is not going away: it is merely shifting its focus onto new vulnerable populations. A temporary decline in HIV/AIDS incidence is only a prelude to a sustained second wave of HIV/AIDS in the world's population.

The impact of the pandemic—in terms of lives, suffering, and financial costs—has deepened substantially. As of January 1, 1996, 20 million people worldwide were living with HIV infection (without AIDS having yet developed) and over one million people were living with clinical AIDS. The number of AIDS orphans exceeds four million and steadily rises; the estimated global cost for medical care has reached $11.6 billion, of which 94 percent is used for treatment in the industrialized world, which contains less than 10 percent of the world's people with HIV infection and AIDS.

The response—in terms of prevention and control efforts—has been largely shaped by a definition of HIV/AIDS as a problem of individual behavior. Proceeding from epidemiological data about individual risk behaviors, a powerful public health strategy was developed in the mid-1980s. This innovative, yet still traditional approach focused on providing individuals with information and education, along with health and social services (such as condoms, testing and counseling, and drug abuse treatment) designed to induce and sustain individual change in behavior. This approach was consolidated into a three-part model for HIV prevention (the third, innovative part was ensuring nondiscrimination towards HIV-infected people and people with AIDS), as developed by the World Health Organization (WHO), and was used as the basis for national AIDS program development worldwide.

Despite major efforts, by the mid-1990s national AIDS programs were having great difficulty fulfilling their role. Major gaps included disregard for the interaction between behavior and social context and the implications of this relationship on effective HIV prevention; the contradiction between the recognition of particularly vulnerable segments of the population by the State and the neglect of their needs; and the insufficient integration of HIV/AIDS work with social, cultural, and economic development. Industrialized and developing countries alike are spending less than one percent of their overall health expenditures on HIV/AIDS prevention, care, and research. Globally, less than one U.S. dollar is spent on HIV/AIDS for every $1,000 of gross development product. There is little doubt that more national resources could be mobilized to face the pandemic more effectively. Initially, developing countries turned to international donors for additional funding. However, the international money supply made available for overall social and economic development and for HIV/AIDS is stagnating: in 1993 overall official development assistance declined from about $60 billion to $54 billion while international financing of the global AIDS strategy leveled off at $250 million, with little prospect for a subsequent increase. In 1993 developing countries financed over 80 percent of the cost of AIDS from their own public and private resources as well as from World Bank loans. Constrained by inadequate policies, insufficient financial support, and weakly coordinated programs, the scope, quality, and impact of existing HIV/AIDS prevention and control efforts have remained inadequate.

Stepping back from the details of the epidemic in any individual community or country, we can see how the pandemic is evolving with time and how it responds to current prevention and control efforts. Certain features of the pandemic have become apparent only recently. A meta-analysis of

maturing epidemics reveals a common societal feature: the increasing concentration of HIV/AIDS among those who before the arrival of AIDS were
already marginalized, stigmatized, and discriminated against within society.
This characteristic of the pandemic is as visible in the United States as it is
in Brazil, France, or Côte d'Ivoire—indeed, it is universal.

Beyond the specifics of particular community or national AIDS programs
is a broad outline of what programs have thus far been unable or unwilling
to do. The fundamental deficiency in HIV/AIDS prevention and control,
which is characteristic of the traditional approach to public health in general, is the lack of meaningful, concrete, coherent action in addressing directly the societal determinants of health, which also influence vulnerability
to HIV. While the tremendous importance of social context for health—and
HIV/AIDS-related behaviors—is readily acknowledged, little is done about
it. Yet because the social context determines to an enormous extent the
lived realities of women, men, and children, social barriers to prevention
must be recognized, understood, and directly addressed.

The lack of linkage between individual life and society is also evident in
the past decade's behavioral research on HIV/AIDS. While useful in describing some features of sexual life, past research efforts have been generally
unhelpful in guiding prevention or in developing more effective prevention
strategies. Consequently, newer conceptual frameworks are increasingly being applied to analysis of sexual behavior; these innovative approaches
share a common concern with extra-individual contexts for sexual behavior
(network, community, and broader society).

How a problem is defined determines what will be done about it. As the
pandemic matures and evolves, as the inherent limits of existing, exces-
sively narrow prevention and control programs become obvious, and as research breaks away from inherited concepts and theories, thus discovering
new territory, so the public health definition of AIDS—and its meaning—
must change. And as the goal of HIV/AIDS prevention and control requires
revised analysis and action on the part of individuals and societies, so must
the tools of analysis and methods of action also change. To ensure that
people can make and effectuate free and informed choices about personal
behavior, public health must simultaneously work *concretely* at personal,
program-related, and social levels. Therefore, to ignore or fail to work at
any of these levels will necessarily lead to a more limited and less successful outcome. Thus a modern understanding of societal vulnerability is required. Beyond the governmental, economic, and sociocultural contexts, the
critical insight from 15 years' experience with HIV/AIDS is that the realization and respect of human rights and dignity is the fundamental, underlying
determinant of societal vulnerability to HIV/AIDS.

We believe that there is something rather unique about the global response to HIV/AIDS. After 15 years of intense efforts, including unprecedented mobilizations of individuals, communities, and institutions, a growing sense of acceptance of an epidemic considered inevitable might have
been expected. Had this occurred, as it has with many public health efforts
in the past, those working against the spread of HIV/AIDS might have

learned to compromise and become satisfied with a partially realized ability to prevent and control the pandemic. At that point, the problem would come to be defined as endemic and then slip inexorably into the background, where it would be relegated to the rank of the many chronic issues of public health. Remarkably, against all odds, those working against the spread of HIV/AIDS remain alert and energetic, eager to find and apply more effective approaches to this difficult task. We all recognize that complacency about HIV/AIDS would be dangerous, that at this early stage in the history of the new phenomenon of global HIV/AIDS, even a decline in HIV incidence cannot be genuinely reassuring, and that the further evolution of the pandemic remains most unclear. Yet the determination to continue and to seek ways to advance further against HIV/AIDS, in the face of enormous challenges, goes beyond a strictly rational calculation of the danger of an epidemic.

Perhaps HIV/AIDS work has drawn together people who refuse to accept the unacceptable and who continue to believe that the world can change. The task we set for ourselves in writing this second edition of *AIDS in the World* was to go beyond describing the status of the pandemic and the response to it, and to go beyond a critique of current approaches (for which we have our share of responsibility). Based on community and national experiences worldwide, available research, and critical analyses of current activities, the central limit in existing prevention and control efforts can be identified: the inability to deal meaningfully with the societal basis of the pandemic. Based on experience in communities and countries around the world, we have developed a framework for analysis of and response to the central, societal reality. This new ability and willingness to identify and respond to the deeper, underlying societal causes of vulnerability to HIV/AIDS as those factors which interfere with people's ability to make and effectuate free and informed choices about their behavior can lead to the potential "uprooting" of the pandemic.

By building upon descriptions of the pandemic and its evolution and current scientific progress while considering responses to the pandemic among specific populations at the national and international levels, *AIDS in the World II* develops an argument for and the basis of a new and expanded approach to HIV/AIDS. Thus, despite the nature and complexity of the challenge ahead, *AIDS in the World II* carries a message of hope and confidence in our collective ability to tame the pandemic and to change our world.

PART I

THE STATE OF THE PANDEMIC AND ITS IMPACT

With time, the HIV/AIDS pandemic is unfolding and revealing its secrets. Paradoxically, the pandemic is becoming simultaneously more difficult and simpler to comprehend. A modern understanding of the pandemic requires two levels of awareness. First, it is essential to appreciate the enormously complex histories of individual HIV/AIDS epidemics at the community or national level. Yet this level of information is insufficient. It is also necessary to recognize the common features among the HIV/AIDS epidemics which, at a deeper level, provide insight into the natural history and the shape of the slowly maturing pandemic.

As emphasized in *AIDS in the World* (1992), the way in which the pandemic is perceived is crucial, for this definition and its associated imagery determine, to a large extent, what will be done about HIV/AIDS and by whom. This section of *AIDS in the World II* uses new and expanded data, including information on numbers of people living with HIV infection and with clinical AIDS, to describe the pandemic's evolution and to outline the larger picture of the phenomenon of global AIDS.

To discover the larger picture, an update of global data and trends is required. The pandemic was previously described as a dynamic, volatile phenomenon that was continuing to spread within all areas already affected and increasingly that was reaching communities and populations previously less affected or even untouched by the pandemic. This general portrait remains valid; the pandemic continues to deepen its hold within already affected populations while it has broadened its geographical and societal reach. In addition, the pandemic was characterized by increasing complexity within each affected community and country. This general feature of the pandemic also remains valid, supplemented by the newly identified role of viral heterogeneity.

The status of the pandemic in the mid-1990s, then, sets the stage for considering its larger picture and global future. The pandemic now has a history from which we can learn. Time was needed for the powerful internal dynamic of the pandemic, its driving force, to become visible. Until now, all HIV/AIDS epidemics were quite recent occurrences; therefore, by definition, only the early history of the epidemic could be known. Unfortunately, in many ways this early history, along with its contingencies and detail, including among whom and when HIV was first introduced into or detected within a population, has continued to dominate public and professional images of the pandemic. Yet, by the mid-1990s, the local and national HIV/AIDS epidemics had evolved, particularly where they had already been underway for a decade or longer.

The first general lesson derived from this analysis is that the world may be poised at the threshold of a larger, second wave of HIV/AIDS. As described in this section of *AIDS in the World II*, the new history of AIDS will likely be dominated by the increasing impact of the epidemic among people with lower levels of risk behavior—levels which previously would not have been characterized as "high risk." Paradoxically, the temporary decline in HIV incidence which is predicted to occur between the first and second waves of the pandemic may seriously mislead the world into a new cycle of mistaken relief and dangerous complacency.

Yet the deeper history of the pandemic is also slowly emerging. The larger commonality among the maturing HIV/AIDS epidemics is societal: the great lesson of the modern pandemic is that certain features of society are fundamental determinants of the epidemic's natural history. This theme, which is vital to our understanding of this pandemic and thus also for future efforts against it, is explored and developed in further chapters of this book.

1

Global Overview:
A Powerful HIV/AIDS Pandemic

National reporting of AIDS

In every country, national health authorities have the responsibility of collecting and reporting health information to the World Health Organization (WHO). Since 1986, WHO has monitored the reporting of AIDS by countries. Official reporting of AIDS provides a broad yet extremely limited indication of the evolution of the pandemic (Appendix A).

The official reporting of AIDS is constrained by several factors. First, national health authorities differ widely in their capability, interest, and willingness to collect or report information about AIDS. Second, even when intentions are ideal, reporting is based on AIDS case definitions that may vary widely among countries or from one reporting period to another. Finally, reporting is often delayed or incomplete and seldom includes pediatric AIDS cases, partly because of the shortcomings of the pediatric AIDS case definition (Box 1-1).

BOX 1-1

Living with the shortcomings of the pediatric AIDS case definition

NORMAND LAPOINTE

The diagnosis of AIDS in children has become increasingly complicated, for several reasons. In the industrialized world, the challenge of reliable diagnosis of symptomatic HIV infection in children is principally technological, as sophisticated laboratory support can generally resolve whether the child is HIV infected and can diagnose AIDS-defining clinical conditions.

However, as this technology is rarely available in the developing world, where the large majority of HIV-infected children live, an alternative approach to diagnosis is required. Accordingly, WHO developed a clinical pediatric AIDS case definition in 1985, which was modified in 1989. However, the major difficulty in creating a useful clinical case definition for pediatric AIDS in the developing world is the high background rate of childhood diseases which are also among the many pediatric manifestations of HIV disease. Thus, a study from Rwanda found the predictive value of the WHO definition to be only 68 percent; in Zaire, the specificity of the clinical definition was 88 percent, with 40 percent sensitivity and a low (30 percent) positive predictive value.[1,2] Suggestions for improving the sensitivity and specificity of the WHO definition have been proposed.[3]

In late 1993, WHO issued *Guidelines for the Clinical Management of HIV Infection in Children,* which uses a diagnostic algorithm, involving signs and symptoms classified as cardinal, characteristic, or associated.[4] The new WHO approach, which also incorporates epidemiological risk factors into the diagnostic algorithms, is being validated in several developing countries.

References

1. P. Lepage, P. Van de Perre, F. Dabis, et al., "Evaluation and simplification of the WHO clinical case definition for pediatric AIDS," *AIDS* 3(1989):221–225.

2. R. Colebunders, A. Greenberg, P. Nguyen-Dinh, et al., "Evaluation of a clinical case definition for AIDS in African children," *AIDS* 1(1987):151–153.

3. L. Belec, F. X. Mbopi Kéou, and A. J. Georges, "Case for the revision of the WHO clinical definition for African AIDS," letter, *AIDS* 6(1992):880–881.

4. World Health Organization, Global Programme on AIDS, *Guidelines for Clinical Management of HIV Infection in Children,* Document WHO/GPA/IDS/HCS/93.3 (1993).

For example, in the United States, about half of AIDS cases are reported to the Centers for Disease Control and Prevention within 3 months after diagnosis, and about 20 percent of cases are not reported until more than 1 year after diagnosis.[1] In the United Kingdom in 1991, an estimated 5 to 20 percent of AIDS cases were never reported.[2] Similarly, in Central America and the Caribbean, an estimated 70 percent of 1992 AIDS cases were unreported.[3] Reporting delays provide flawed data for projections and result in underestimating average survival times.[4]

By the end of 1995, close to 1.3 million AIDS cases had been reported to the World Health Organization since the beginning of the pandemic (Appendix A). One-hundred sixty of the 190 (86 percent) countries and territories had reported at least one case to WHO.[5] However, official AIDS reports can help define general trends but give little information about HIV spread and by definition do not reflect the current status of the epidemic.

National reporting of positive HIV tests

The reporting of HIV infections is mandatory in a number of countries (Chapter 31). However, the quality of such information also varies considerably due to differences in public awareness, commitment to voluntary testing, access to diagnostic services, protection of confidentiality, and actions taken in the event of a positive result. For example, in Sweden almost all pregnant women attend antenatal clinics where they are offered voluntary HIV testing; the acceptance rate has exceeded 97 percent.[6] In addition, an estimated 87 percent of patients attending sexually transmitted infection (STI) clinics in Sweden agreed to be tested. By 1992, one-quarter of men and one-third of women in Sweden had been HIV tested at least once.[7] People more likely to have been tested lived in large urban areas and had higher educational levels.

In the U.S., 25 of the 50 states have laws or regulations requiring confidential, named HIV-reporting, but this reporting is considered to be less complete than the reporting of AIDS cases.[8] In a large number of countries, voluntary testing is at least theoretically offered to adults in the sexually active age-group (Chapter 30). However, access to testing schemes is limited by many factors including the lack of diagnostic facilities and reagents. The persisting gap in both industrialized and developing countries between the capacity to test for HIV and the availability of counseling further limits the coverage of testing schemes and biases the samples of persons who request an HIV test.

Most HIV data originate from blood transfusion centers, diagnostic centers, or screening programs, and are therefore subject to selection and participation bias. This information can provide a general impression about the status and trends of the epidemic, but it is inadequate for defining epidemiological trends in the population. Occasionally, national AIDS programs may overestimate the number of HIV infections as a result of methodological difficulties or, rarely, to stimulate an additional influx of resources to AIDS programs. In most cases, however, national AIDS program estimates should be regarded as conservative.

An increasing number of countries have established *sentinel surveillance systems* along guidelines from the WHO Global Programme on AIDS (WHO/GPA). These systems monitor epidemic trends and are helpful in guiding policy development and management decisions (Box 1-2).

BOX 1-2

Sentinel HIV surveillance

PAUL SATO

A responsive HIV/AIDS prevention and control program requires a surveillance system for monitoring the epidemic's trends over time in different risk populations and in different geographic areas.

Serological surveillance of HIV infections should be designed to provide timely and cost-efficient data of *sufficient* accuracy for planning, implementing, and monitoring national AIDS program (NAP) activities. Large-scale national HIV serosurveys in the community are not recommended for NAPs, given their expense in time, money, and staff resources, and because they do not usually produce data in different risk populations and areas of any greater validity than that obtained through the cost-efficient WHO/GPA method.

The WHO/GPA serosurveillance method involves periodic cross-sectional surveys of HIV seroprevalence in selected "sentinel" populations using the unlinked anonymous (UA) method. Sentinel populations are chosen to provide an indication of HIV trends associated with specific risk behavior or practices in each category.

Typical sentinel sites include: sexually transmitted infection (STI) clinics; injecting drug user (IDU) clinics; and, in high prevalence areas, antenatal clinics.[1] Surveillance of lower-risk groups, such as pregnant women attending antenatal clinics, is generally recommended only when HIV prevalence in higher-risk groups is at least 1–2 percent. The UA method, considered consistent with existing global guidelines on ethics in biomedical research, involves HIV testing of residual blood originally collected for other legitimate purposes, after all identifying information has been removed from the specimen.[2]

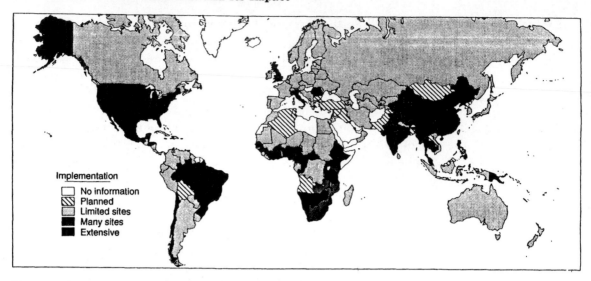

Figure 1-2.1   Sentinel HIV surveillance: status of implementation, early 1995.

Because HIV testing may be associated with discrimination and stigmatization, results may be unreliable where methods other than the UA method (e.g., voluntary testing) are used, since those who agree to HIV testing may differ radically from those who refuse or avoid testing (participation bias). UA testing thereby helps ensure that reliable and valid prevalence estimates are obtained.

WHO/GPA also recommends monitoring results of HIV screening at blood banks for surveillance of blood transfusion safety. Figure 1-2.1 illustrates the status of worldwide implementation of sentinel HIV surveillance, in which Africa, as of late 1995, had the largest experience.

Sentinel HIV surveillance has reminded public health workers of alternatives to the so-called traditional case detection, containment, and control model; the alternative has emphasized that protection of individual rights is required for effective public health work, including for good surveillance. The WHO/GPA approach is flexible: changes in selected sentinel sites can help follow, for example, a transition from HIV spread affecting predominantly highly vulnerable groups to an epidemic transmitted heterosexually in the population at large, or reaching previously less affected geographical areas.

Early in the pandemic, inadequate training or supervision led to poor adherence in some countries to the UA method, causing unintended identification of HIV-infected persons, which in turn led to a loss of credibility by the NAP, and mistrust of the population towards future surveillance efforts. Such experience has confirmed that adequate health worker training and supervision are as crucial to surveillance as good design.[3]

The greatest challenge is the appropriate use of surveillance data for action. Sentinel HIV surveillance was designed to obtain rapid and cost-effective data on HIV distribution and spread. However, since it is based on non-random sampling, sentinel data are not sufficiently accurate for evaluating the effectiveness of prevention programs or for estimating the number of HIV-infected persons in the population as a whole.

Great strides have been made in implementing sentinel HIV surveillance, but additional progress is needed. However, such concerns do not diminish the impressive achievement of many NAPs worldwide in successfully implementing sentinel HIV surveillance and UA testing.

References

1. WHO Global Programme on AIDS, *Training Module: Surveillance of HIV Infection* (June 1993), draft.
2. WHO Global Programme on AIDS, *Unlinked Anonymous Screening for the Public Health Surveillance of HIV Infections*, Proposed international guidelines. Document WHO/GPA/SFI/89.3 (1989).

3. WHO Global Programme on AIDS, *Report of a Meeting on Sentinel HIV Surveillance*, Dakar, December 14–18, 1991. WHO document GPA/CNP/EVA/92.2 (1992).

HIV and AIDS data: *AIDS in the World II Survey*

AIDS in the World II has collected and analyzed information from many sources to estimate incidence and assess trends for HIV infections, AIDS, and AIDS-related deaths throughout the world. The analysis of the status of the HIV/AIDS pandemic which follows provides estimates for 10 geographic areas of affinity (GAAs) and for the world (Box 1-3).

BOX 1-3

Geographic areas of affinity

In the first volume of *AIDS in the World* (1992), the world was divided into ten geographic areas of affinity (GAAs) to facilitate the analysis of both the pandemic and the global response to HIV/AIDS[1] (Figure 1-3.1). The GAA approach grouped together countries with similar HIV/AIDS epidemiology, societal factors, and programs for responding to the pandemic. It attempted to separate areas having historical, ethnic, or cultural similarities, yet distinct patterns of HIV spread and societal responses. For example, the initial behavior of the epidemic was similar in North America, Western Europe, and Oceania, but the approaches to prevention and care and the evolving nature of the pandemic have distinct features in each of these GAAs. In a similar fashion, epidemiological differences between

Figure 1-3.1 Estimated 1995 population, by GAA. Source: estimate based on *The World Bank Atlas, Social Indicators of Development 1991–92.*

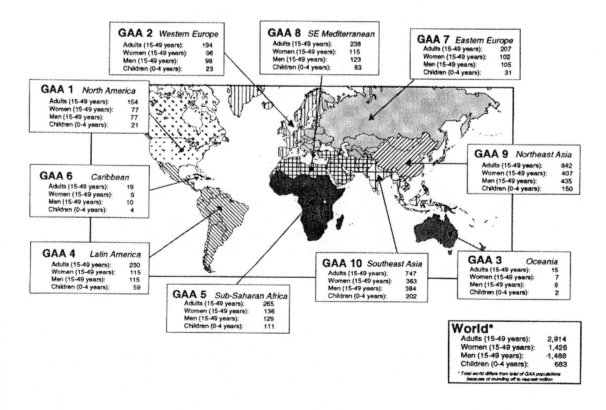

Southeast and Northeast Asia have become increasingly apparent in the last 3 years. Likewise, Latin America and the Caribbean, or Western and Eastern Europe, despite their geographic proximity, continue to experience substantially different patterns of HIV spread, programmatic response, and societal vulnerability to the pandemic.

The GAA concept has distinct advantages and disadvantages. The major disadvantage is that it is insensitive to differences within and between communities and countries. Thus, because they are grouped in single GAAs, important differences between northern and southern Europe, or Australia and the Pacific island nations, are not immediately visible. The main advantage of the GAA approach is in developing broad comparisons, identifying important large-scale trends, and giving shape to the global epidemic. The GAA approach has been retained for this volume of *AIDS in the World*. However, while recognizing the limitations of the GAA system, frequent notes have been made throughout this volume to indicate epidemiological, programmatic, or societal factors that vary in important ways within or between countries from the same GAA.

References

1. J. Mann, D. Tarantola, and T. Netter, eds., "New geography of HIV/AIDS," in *AIDS in the World* (Cambridge, MA: Harvard University Press, 1992):23.

Two HIV viruses are currently involved in the global HIV pandemic: HIV-1 and HIV-2. Found in almost every country around the world since its discovery in 1983, HIV-1 has been extensively researched and its high variability established.[9] Several sub-types of HIV-1, also called *clades*, have now been recognized. They differ in their genetic structure and biological and serological properties (Chapter 13). The geographic mapping of clades isolated from various parts of the world has revealed that certain clades are solely prevalent in certain regions while several other clades may coexist in others (Chapter 3).

In contrast to the widely spread HIV-1, HIV-2 is mostly found in West Africa and in countries that are linked to this region through patterns of population mobility (France, countries in Southern Africa, Latin America, and the Caribbean [Chapter 12]). In addition to structural, serological, and pathogenic differences between HIV-1 and HIV-2, epidemiological studies have shown that the former transmits more efficiently than the latter.[10,11] Thus, in areas where HIV-2 was involved in the majority of infections when it was initially recognized in 1986, the spread of this virus is being overtaken by HIV-1. Since HIV-2 accounts for less than one percent of all HIV infections worldwide, the estimates presented below for HIV-1 may be considered also to include HIV-2. Prevention strategies remain identical for both types of HIV; nevertheless, there are differences in their transmission patterns and pathogenesis.

The methods used to estimate HIV infections, AIDS cases, and AIDS-related deaths were detailed in the first volume of *AIDS in the World*.[12] For the present volume, several variables used in the epidemiological model have been adjusted, based on new knowledge gained from specific features of HIV transmission and of the natural history of HIV disease (Appendix B).

**The pandemic has expanded relentlessly:
status as of January 1, 1996**

From the beginning of the pandemic until January 1, 1996, an estimated 30.6 million people worldwide have been infected with HIV. Of these, 27.4 million were adults (15.8 million men and 11.7 million women) and 3.2 million were children. The largest numbers of HIV-infected people were in sub-Saharan Africa (19.2 million; 63 percent of global total) and Southeast Asia (6.9 million; 23 percent) (Table 1-1). Since the beginning of the pandemic, the large majority of HIV infections (over 28 million; 93 percent) have occurred in the developing world. The number of HIV-infected people in Southeast Asia is now more than three times the total number of infected people in the entire industrialized world (Figure 1-1). The global cumulative number of HIV infections among adults has tripled since the beginning of the decade, from nearly 10 million in 1990 to over 27 million in 1996 (Table 1-2).

An estimated 10.4 million people developed AIDS from the beginning of the pandemic until January 1, 1996. Of these people, 8.4 million (81 percent) were in sub-Saharan Africa, 0.7 million were in Latin America and the Caribbean (7 percent), and 0.7 million were in North America, Western Europe and Oceania combined (7 percent) (Table 1-3). In Southeast Asia, where the pandemic gained intensity more recently, it is estimated that 0.5 million people have already developed AIDS. Of the 2.4 million children with AIDS, the large majority (2 million; 87 percent) were in sub-Saharan Africa.

The life expectancy of people with AIDS—both adults and children—who have access to early and sustained therapy has increased considerably in recent years, largely due to prevention and treatment of opportunistic infections (Box 1-4 and Chapter 11). Detailed information on disease pro-

Table 1-1   Cumulative HIV infections as of January 1, 1996, by geographic area of affinity (GAA)

GAA	Adults	Men	Women	Children*	Total
1 North America	1,269,000	1,087,000	181,000	18,000	1,286,000
2 Western Europe	829,000	691,000	138,000	9,000	838,000
3 Oceania	31,000	28,000	3,000	<1,000	32,000
4 Latin America	1,477,000	1,182,000	295,000	79,000	1,556,000
5 Sub-Saharan Africa	16,550,000	7,881,000	8,670,000	2,672,000	19,222,000
6 Caribbean	467,000	280,000	187,000	36,000	503,000
7 Eastern Europe	37,000	34,000	3,000	<1,000	38,000
8 SE Mediterranean	76,000	63,000	13,000	<1,000	77,000
9 Northeast Asia	179,000	149,000	30,000	2,000	181,000
10 Southeast Asia	6,535,000	4,356,000	2,178,000	380,000	6,915,000
TOTAL WORLD	27,449,000	15,751,000	11,699,000	3,198,000	30,647,000

Source: *AIDS in the World II* survey.
Note: Columns and rows may fail to sum due to rounding to the nearest 1,000.
*HIV infection acquired before or at birth.

Table 1-2 Cumulative adult HIV infections, as of January 1, 1996, by geographic area of affinity (GAA)

Year	North America	Western Europe	Oceania	Latin America	Sub-Saharan Africa	Caribbean	Eastern Europe	SE Mediterranean	Northeast Asia	Southeast Asia	Total world
1978	0	0			0						0
1979	1,000	<1,000		0	<1,000	0					2,000
1980	18,000	1,000	0	1,000	41,000	<1,000					62,000
1981	50,000	6,000	<1,000	18,000	152,000	1,000					227,000
1982	96,000	14,000	<1,000	49,000	373,000	5,000					537,000
1983	156,000	29,000	1,000	96,000	730,000	13,000	0				1,025,000
1984	228,000	50,000	2,000	160,000	1,243,000	25,000	<1,000				1,708,000
1985	310,000	78,000	4,000	238,000	1,921,000	42,000	1,000	0			2,593,000
1986	398,000	115,000	6,000	328,000	2,762,000	64,000	3,000	<1,000	0	0	3,676,000
1987	491,000	160,000	8,000	429,000	3,756,000	91,000	5,000	4,000	<1,000	<1,000	4,944,000
1988	586,000	212,000	10,000	539,000	4,890,000	123,000	7,000	8,000	1,000	7,000	6,384,000
1989	682,000	272,000	13,000	654,000	6,145,000	159,000	10,000	13,000	4,000	41,000	7,993,000
1990	777,000	339,000	16,000	773,000	7,498,000	198,000	13,000	20,000	10,000	138,000	9,782,000
1991	869,000	411,000	19,000	894,000	8,929,000	241,000	16,000	27,000	21,000	357,000	11,784,000
1992	958,000	488,000	21,000	1,015,000	10,414,000	285,000	20,000	36,000	38,000	774,000	14,048,000
1993	1,043,000	570,000	24,000	1,135,000	11,932,000	330,000	24,000	45,000	62,000	1,484,000	16,647,000
1994	1,123,000	654,000	27,000	1,252,000	13,463,000	376,000	28,000	55,000	93,000	2,597,000	19,668,000
1995	1,198,000	741,000	29,000	1,367,000	15,003,000	421,000	33,000	65,000	132,000	4,237,000	23,226,000
1996	1,269,000	829,000	31,000	1,477,000	16,550,000	467,000	37,000	76,000	179,000	6,535,000	27,449,000

Source: *AIDS in the World II* survey.
Note: Columns and rows may fail to sum due to rounding off to the nearest 1,000.

Table 1-3 Cumulative AIDS cases as of January 1, 1996

GAA	Adults	Men	Women	Children[a]	Total
1 North America[b]	443,000	380,000	63,000	7,000	449,000
2 Western Europe	193,000	161,000	32,000	3,000	195,000
3 Oceania	9,000	8,000	1,000	<1,000	9,000
4 Latin America	518,000	414,000	104,000	62,000	579,000
5 Sub-Saharan Africa	6,367,000	3,032,000	3,335,000	2,046,000	8,413,000
6 Caribbean	133,000	80,000	53,000	27,000	160,000
7 Eastern Europe	7,000	7,000	<1,000	<1,000	7,000
8 SE Mediterranean	12,000	10,000	2,000	<1,000	12,000
9 Northeast Asia	12,000	10,000	2,000	<1,000	12,000
10 Southeast Asia	332,000	221,000	111,000	206,000	537,000
TOTAL WORLD	8,024,000	4,321,000	3,703,000	2,351,000	10,375,000

Source: *AIDS in the World II* survey.
Note: Columns and rows may fail to sum due to rounding to the nearest 1,000.
[a]HIV infection acquired before or at birth.
[b]AIDS cases in North America have been estimated on the basis of the 1987 revised CDC AIDS surveillance case definition.

Figure 1-1 Cumulative number of HIV-infected adults, by GAA and by year, 1978–1996 (as of January 1 of each year).

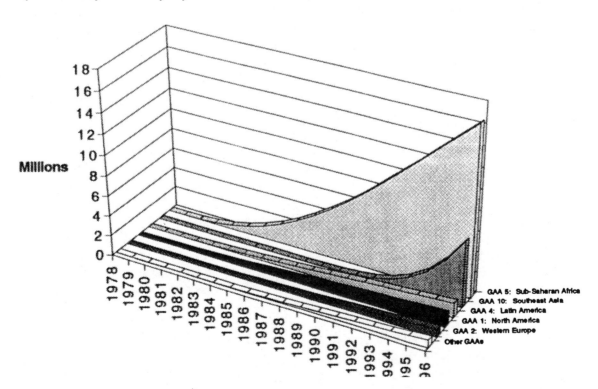

gression rates has been available from the industrialized world through cohort studies of homosexual men and people infected with HIV-1 through blood transfusions. In contrast, relatively little is known about disease progression in developing countries. Studies in Africa, however, suggest that both incubation and symptomatic survival periods are shorter—perhaps far shorter—there than in the industrialized world (Box 1-5). Accordingly, the following estimate of deaths is based on different survival rates applied to each GAA (see Appendix B).

BOX 1-4

New appreciation for the complexities of perinatally-acquired HIV infection

JAMES M. OLESKE

The image of pediatric AIDS has shifted from a focus on the acutely ill infant to a much wider range of age and clinical status than originally perceived. First, the full extent of multiorgan and multisystem impact of HIV infection has become recognized: HIV infection and its associated diseases involve almost every organ system, including the central and peripheral nervous system, the lungs, gastrointestinal tract, liver, pancreas, heart, endocrine system, skin, kidneys, and the hematologic and immunologic systems. In addition to organ impairment directly related to HIV, opportunistic diseases in children include malignancies such as non-Hodgkin's lymphoma and leiomyosarcoma, a tumor almost unique to HIV-infected children.

Second, a bimodal (or even more complex) pattern of clinical response of children to HIV infection has emerged. At the beginning of the epidemic, acute illnesses were recognized in HIV-infected infants and children with early onset of symptoms (prior to 2 years of age). Often severe, these illnesses included progressive encephalopathy, *Pneumocystis carinii* pneumonia, life-threatening bacterial or other opportunistic infections, disseminated cytomegalovirus infection, and severe failure to thrive.[1] These infants frequently died before 6 years of age, although aggressive treatment has improved their chances of surviving for longer periods.

More recently, however, an increasing number of children with onset of HIV symptoms occurring later in life (usually after 4 years of age and as late as 8 years of age), as well as long-term survivors, have been recognized.[2] Delayed clinical disease in these children is progressive, which includes lymphadenopathy, hepatomegaly, non-specific skin lesions, and chronic lymphocyte interstitial pneumonia (LIP). As experience is gained in supportive care, antiretroviral therapy, and in the therapy and prophylaxis of opportunistic diseases, the quality of life and longevity of these perinatally HIV-infected children will increase.[3]

Due both to improved care and to the differential natural history of HIV/AIDS in children, an increasing number of infected children are also living into adolescence and early adulthood. The natural history of HIV/AIDS in infants and children is greatly influenced by availability and access to both supportive (nutrition, immunization, prophylaxis) and specific (antiretroviral, immunological) therapies. Unfortunately, these gains in quality and duration of life have not been extended to most children in the developing world.

In addition, the support and care needs of perinatally infected children have expanded tremendously. Many of the clinical care needs of these children cannot be separated from the overwhelming psychosocial difficulties faced by their families. HIV/AIDS has taken a disproportionate toll among those disadvantaged by poverty, with associated marginalization and difficulties in accessing care and social services. In addition, HIV/AIDS is a multigenerational disease, in which more than one family member is likely to be infected or dying. Thus, unlike other chronic childhood diseases, the HIV-infected child will frequently experience the trauma of losing their primary caretaker.

The challenges of care for perinatally infected children will become ever more complex as longevity increases. It is essential that the gains in life span and quality achieved in the industrialized world be extended to the developing world, where over 90 percent of the perinatally infected children in the world now live.

References

1. G. Scott, C. Mutto, R. Makuch, et al., "Survival in children with perinatally acquired human immunodeficiency virus type 1 infection," *New England Journal of Medicine* 321 (1989):1791–1796.
2. S. Grubman, E. Gross, N. Lerner-Weiss, et al., "Older children and adolescents living with perinatally acquired human immunodeficiency virus infection," *Pediatrics* 95(1995):657–663.
3. S. Grubman and J. Oleske, "The maturation of an epidemic: Update on pediatric HIV infection," *AIDS* 7(1993):S225–S234.

BOX 1-5

Disease progression and mortality following HIV-1 infection

DAAN MULDER

Incubation period and survival in industrialized countries

Early studies on the progression from HIV-1 infection to AIDS suggested rates of 5 to 6 percent per year.[1,2,3] These rates corresponded to a median AIDS-free period of 11 years or longer. More recent studies suggest that in the absence of treatment, half of all infected people will develop AIDS within 9 years after infection.[4] Few individuals develop AIDS during the first 2 years after infection. Thereafter, the annual rate of developing disease increases from about 3 percent in year 3 to 9 percent in year 7. The course of disease beyond 10 years of infection is unknown, but models suggest that the probability of developing AIDS during the eleventh year (after having been AIDS-free for 10 years) may be as high as 15 percent. Some infected individuals have, however, remained apparently healthy for more than 15 years.[5]

Studies of AIDS among adults suggest that survival rates have gradually improved in the industrialized world. In the late 1980s the median survival after diagnosis was approximately 18 months.[6,7] The slowing of disease progression and mortality was concurrent with increased availability and use of prophylactic and therapeutic agents, in particular antiviral drugs and improved prevention and treatment of *Pneumocystis carinii* pneumonia.[8,9] Year of diagnosis and age were independent predictors for survival (earlier year of diagnosis and older age are associated with poorer outcome); race or ethnicity and gender were not.

Incubation period and survival in developing countries

In contrast to the detailed data on progression available from industrialized countries, the data from other geographical areas are scanty and are limited to sub-Saharan Africa. Data are available from six studies, four of which suggest that in Africa, progression rates to AIDS are similar to rates in industrialized countries. Among initially asymptomatic factory employees in Zaire (with unknown dates of seroconversion), the 2-year progression rate to AIDS was 15 percent.[10] A study in Zambia showed a mortality rate of 4 to 6 percent among HIV-seropositive sexually transmitted infection (STI) clinic attendees during an 18-month period.[11] Among HIV-seropositive women in Rwanda who were initially asymptomatic, the 2-year progression rate to death was 7 percent.[12] Finally, of 26 seropositive sex workers in Rwanda who were available for follow-up, 14 had died after 8 years.[13]

Two of the African studies, however, suggest a more rapid progression. In a study of women sex workers in Kenya, the median incubation period from seroconversion to AIDS diagnosis was only 45 months.[14] Computer simulations based on this data suggest that progression to symptomatic disease was considerably more rapid than in industrialized countries.[15] Poor survival among women sex workers in this population may be related to unknown lifestyle factors and frequent reexposure to HIV.[16]

In a prospective cohort study of the population of 15 villages in Uganda, the mortality rate among HIV-seropositive adults was 11.6 percent per year during a 2-year period.[17,18] The 2-year mortality figure of 23.2 percent corresponds to a median progression from seropositivity to death of 5.25 years, which is surprisingly high, particularly in an area where the epidemic has only recently emerged. Moreover, a substantial proportion of those who died progressed from asymptomatic infection or mild disease to death within 6 months, on average.

As data from industrialized countries suggest a median incubation period of about 9 years and a median survival after diagnosis of AIDS of about 18 months, the median survival from infection to death would be about 10.5 years. While the results from some studies in sub-Saharan Africa are consistent with these findings, the combination of studies mentioned above suggests that both the incubation and symptomatic survival periods may be shorter, corresponding to a median survival from infection to death of only 5 to 6 years.

Lack of medical care may affect both the duration of the incubation period (to the extent that nonspecific immune system activation may result from nontreatment of disease), as well as the symptomatic survival period.[19] It is useful to make a distinction between rapid disease progression and premature death when considering the implications of a lack of treatment for, or intense exposure to, high-grade pathogens. If most deaths occur after classical AIDS has developed, rapid disease progression must be occurring. But it seems more likely that what we are seeing is premature death from high-grade infections at a pre-AIDS stage.[20]

In order to document rates of disease progression and changes in markers of progression over time, and to clarify the role of high-grade pathogens in causing premature or rapid death, additional developing country studies are needed—specifically, carefully conducted prospective clinical, virological, and immunological studies of asymptomatic HIV-seropositive individuals.

References

1. H. W. Jaffe, W. W. Darrow, D. F. Eschenberg, et al., "Acquired immunodeficiency syndrome in a cohort of homosexual men. A six year follow-up study," Annals of Internal Medicine 103(1985):210–214.

2. J. J. Goedert, C. M. Kessler, L. Aledort, et al., "Prospective study of human immunodeficiency virus type 1 infection and the development of AIDS in subjects with haemophilia," New England Journal of Medicine 321(1989):1141–1148.

3. C. A. Lee, A. Philips, J. Elford, et al., "Natural history of human immunodeficiency virus infection in a haemophiliac cohort," British Journal of Haematology 73(1989):228–234.

4. J.C. M. Hendriks, G. F. Medley, G. J. P. van Griensven, et al., "Treatment-free incubation period of AIDS in a cohort of homosexual men," AIDS 7(1993):231–239.

5. A. R. Lifson, S. P. Buchbinder, H. W. Sheppard, et al., "Long-term immunodeficiency virus infection in asymptomatic homosexual and bisexual men with normal CD4+ lymphocyte counts: Immunologic and virologic characteristics," Journal of Infectious Diseases 163(1991):959–965.

6. G. F. Lemp, S. F. Payne, D. Neal, et al., "Survival trends for patients with AIDS," Journal of the American Medical Association 263(1990):402–406.

7. S. E. Whitmore-Overton, H. E. Tillett, B. G. Evans, and G. M. Allardice, "Improved survival from diagnosis of AIDS in adult cases in the United Kingdom and bias due to reporting delays," AIDS 7(1993):415–420.

8. Lemp, "Survival trends."

9. L. I. Gardner, J. F. Brundage, J. G. McNeil, et al., "Predictors of HIV-1 disease progression in early- and late-stage patients: The U.S. army natural history cohort," Journal of Acquired Immune Deficiency Syndromes 5(1992):782-793.

10. B. N'galy, R. W. Ryder, B. Kapita, et al., "Human immunodeficiency virus infection among employees in an African hospital," *New England Journal of Medicine* 319(1988):1123–1127.

11. S. K. Hira, N. Ngandu, D. Wadhawan, et al., "Clinical and epidemiological features of HIV infection at a referral clinic in Zambia," *Journal of Acquired Immune Deficiency Syndromes* 3(1990):87–91.

12. C. P. Lindan, S. Allen, A. Serufilira, et al., "Predictors of mortality among HIV-infected women in Kigali, Rwanda," *Annals of Internal Medicine* 116(1992):320–328.

13. M. Bulterys, E. Nzabihimana, A. Chao, et al., "Long-term survival among HIV-1-infected prostitutes," *AIDS* 7(1993):1269.

14. A. Anzala, N. J. D. Nagelkerke, J. J. Bwayo, et al., "Rapid progression to disease in African sex workers with human immunodeficiency virus type I infection," *Journal of Infectious Diseases* 171(1995):686–689.

15. N. J. D. Nagelkerke, F. A. Plummer, D. Holton, et al., "Transition dynamics of HIV disease in a cohort of African prostitutes: A Markov model approach," *AIDS* 4(1990):743–747.

16. J. N. Simonsen, F. A. Plummer, E. N. Ngugi, et al., "HIV infection among lower socioeconomic strata prostitutes in Nairobi," *AIDS* 4(1990):139–144.

17. D. W. Mulder, A. J. Nunn, H. U. Wagner, et al., "HIV-1 incidence and HIV-1 associated mortality in a rural Ugandan population cohort," *AIDS* 8(1994):87–92.

18. D. W. Mulder, A. J. Nunn, A. Kamali, et al., "Two-year HIV-1 associated mortality in a Ugandan rural population," *Lancet* 343(1994):989–990.

19. R. L. Colebunders and A. S. Latif, "Natural history and clinical presentation of HIV-1 infection in adults," *AIDS* 5(suppl. 1)(1991):s103–s112.

20. C. F. Gilks, "Challenge of the HIV epidemic in the developing world," *Lancet* 342(1993):1037–1039.

By January 1, 1996, 9.2 million people were estimated to have died from AIDS worldwide, or 89 percent of all people with AIDS. The total number of people having died from AIDS includes about 7.6 million people in sub-Saharan Africa (83 percent), 0.5 million in Latin America, 0.4 million in Southeast Asia, 358,000 in North America, 144,000 in Western Europe, and 168,000 in the rest of the world (Table 1-4).

Table 1-4   Cumulative AIDS deaths as of January 1, 1996, by geographic area of affinity (GAA)

GAA	Adults	Men	Women	Children[a]	Total
1 North America[b]	352,000	302,000	50,000	6,000	358,000
2 Western Europe	141,000	118,000	24,000	2,000	144,000
3 Oceania	7,000	6,000	<1,000	<1,000	7,000
4 Latin America	458,000	366,000	92,000	60,000	518,000
5 Sub-Saharan Africa	5,611,000	2,672,000	2,939,000	1,999,000	7,610,000
6 Caribbean	115,000	69,000	46,000	27,000	141,000
7 Eastern Europe	5,000	5,000	<1,000	<1,000	5,000
8 SE Mediterranean	7,000	6,000	1,000	<1,000	8,000
9 Northeast Asia	6,000	5,000	1,000	<1,000	6,000
10 Southeast Asia	231,000	154,000	77,000	194,000	425,000
TOTAL WORLD	6,933,000	3,702,000	3,231,000	2,289,000	9,223,000

Source: *AIDS in the World II* survey.
Note: Columns and rows may fail to sum due to rounding off to the nearest 1,000.
[a]HIV infection acquired before or at birth.
[b]AIDS deaths in North America have been estimated on the basis of the 1987 revised CDC AIDS surveillance case definition.

Table 1-5   New HIV infections, January 1, 1995, through December 31, 1995, by geographic area of affinity (GAA)

GAA	Adults	Men	Women	Children*	Total
1 North America	70,000	60,000	10,000	2,000	72,000
2 Western Europe	88,000	73,000	15,000	1,000	89,000
3 Oceania	2,000	2,000	<1,000	<1,000	2,000
4 Latin America	110,000	88,000	22,000	9,000	119,000
5 Sub-Saharan Africa	1,547,000	737,000	810,000	345,000	1,892,000
6 Caribbean	45,000	27,000	18,000	5,000	50,000
7 Eastern Europe	5,000	4,000	<1,000	<1,000	5,000
8 SE Mediterranean	11,000	9,000	2,000	<1,000	11,000
9 Northeast Asia	47,000	39,000	8,000	<1,000	48,000
10 Southeast Asia	2,298,000	1,532,000	766,000	153,000	2,450,000
TOTAL WORLD	4,223,000	2,572,000	1,651,000	516,000	4,739,000

Source: *AIDS in the World II* survey.
Note: Columns and rows may fail to sum due to rounding to the nearest 1,000.
*HIV infection acquired before or at birth.

Newly acquired HIV infections in 1995

New HIV infections, cases of AIDS, and AIDS-related deaths during a calendar year illustrate the current magnitude and global distribution of the epidemic. Worldwide during 1995, 4.7 million new HIV infections occurred (an average of 13,000 new infections each day). Of these, 2.5 million (an average of nearly 7,000 new infections per day) occurred in Southeast Asia and 1.9 million infections (over 5,000 new infections per day) were in sub-Saharan Africa. The industrialized world accounted for about 170,000 new HIV infections (nearly 500 new infections per day; less than 4 percent of the global total). In 1995, 1.7 million women were newly HIV infected (over 4,500 per day; 39 percent of all new adult infections). During 1995 approximately 500,000 children were born with HIV infection (about 1,400 per day); of these children, 67 percent were in sub-Saharan Africa, 30 percent in Southeast Asia, 2 percent in Latin America, and 1 percent in the Caribbean (Table 1-5).

Therefore, in all GAAs, from thousands to millions of people are still becoming infected with HIV each year. The number of adults becoming infected each year seems to have reached a plateau in Western Europe, the Caribbean, and sub-Saharan Africa. The annual number of new infections also appears to have decreased, at least temporarily, in North America, Oceania, and the southeast Mediterranean (Chapter 4). However, in recently affected areas, such as Southeast and Northeast Asia, HIV incidence (new infections per year) is rising steeply (Figure 1-2).

Analysis of HIV incidence in 1995 indicates the comparative rate of increase of the HIV pandemic in various populations. The worldwide incidence of (new) HIV infections in 1995 was estimated at 82.9 per 100,000 population: 145 per 100,000 adults (men and women, 15–49 years old) and

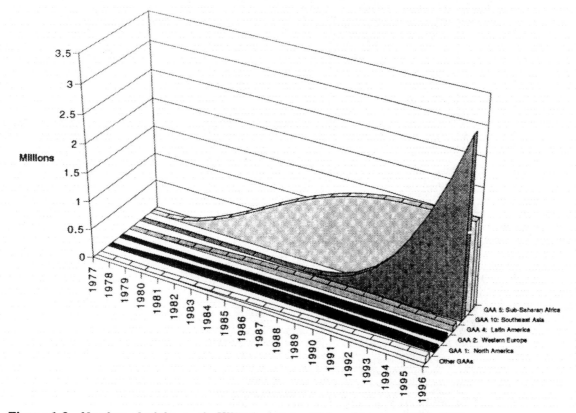

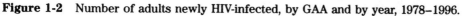

Figure 1-2   Number of adults newly HIV-infected, by GAA and by year, 1978–1996.

75.5 per 100,000 children (under 5 years old). The highest HIV incidence for adults and children combined was in sub-Saharan Africa (318 per 100,000), followed by Southeast Asia (164 per 100,000), and the Caribbean (140 per 100,000). The incidence of HIV in other GAAs was below 50 per 100,000 (Table 1-6).

HIV incidence was higher among women than among men in sub-Saharan Africa (607 vs. 561 per 100,000). However, in all other GAAs, HIV incidence was higher among men. The incidence of HIV infection among children varied among GAAs, from less than one per 100,000 in Eastern Europe, southeastern Mediterranean, and Northeast Asia, to 310 per 100,000 in sub-Saharan Africa. HIV incidence among children in sub-Saharan Africa, Southeast Asia, and the Caribbean was higher than HIV incidence among adults in all other regions of the world.

New AIDS cases in 1995

During 1995, an estimated 1.9 million people developed AIDS, including 1.5 million adults and 400,000 children (Table 1-7). Of people newly developing AIDS, 74 percent were in sub-Saharan Africa, 13 percent were in Southeast Asia and 6 percent in the GAAs which are comprised of industrialized countries. Thus, in 1995, over twice as many people developed AIDS in Southeast Asia than in all the industrialized countries of the world.

Table 1-6 Incidence of HIV infection, January 1, 1995, through December 31, 1995, rates per 100,000, by geographic area of affinity (GAA)

GAA	Adults	Men	Women	Children[a]	Total
1 North America	45.4	77.6	13.0	7.9	24.5
2 Western Europe	45.3	74.7	15.3	5.5	23.2
3 Oceania	15.5	27.1	3.5	1.7	8.3
4 Latin America	47.9	76.7	19.2	15.4	26.7
5 Sub-Saharan Africa	584.1	561.2	606.7	310.1	317.5
6 Caribbean	239.9	289.0	191.1	123.3	140.0
7 Eastern Europe	2.2	4.0	0.4	0.2	1.1
8 SE Mediterranean	4.6	7.4	1.6	0.2	2.2
9 Northeast Asia	5.6	9.0	1.9	0.5	3.2
10 Southeast Asia	307.7	398.9	211.2	75.5	164.3
TOTAL WORLD	144.9	172.9	115.8	75.5	82.9

Source: *AIDS in the World II* survey.
[a]HIV infection acquired before or at birth.

Table 1-7 New AIDS cases, January 1, 1995, through December 31, 1995, by geographic area of affinity (GAA)

GAA	Adults	Men	Women	Children[a]	Total
1 North America[b]	62,000	53,000	9,000	1,000	63,000
2 Western Europe	37,000	31,000	6,000	<1,000	38,000
3 Oceania	2,000	1,000	<1,000	<1,000	2,000
4 Latin America	85,000	68,000	17,000	8,000	93,000
5 Sub-Saharan Africa	1,074,000	511,000	562,000	301,000	1,375,000
6 Caribbean	26,000	16,000	10,000	4,000	30,000
7 Eastern Europe	2,000	1,000	<1,000	<1,000	2,000
8 SE Mediterranean	3,000	3,000	<1,000	<1,000	3,000
9 Northeast Asia	5,000	4,000	<1,000	<1,000	5,000
10 Southeast Asia	160,000	107,000	53,000	87,000	248,000
TOTAL WORLD	1,455,000	795,000	660,000	403,000	1,858,000

Source: *AIDS in the World II* survey.
Note: Columns and rows may fail to sum due to rounding to the nearest 1,000.
[a]HIV infection acquired before or at birth.
[b]AIDS cases in North America have been estimated on the basis of the 1987 revised CDC AIDS surveillance case definition.

Table 1-8 Incidence of AIDS cases, January 1, 1995, through December 31, 1995, rates per 100,000, by geographic area of affinity (GAA)

GAA	Adults	Men	Women	Children[a]	Total
1 North America[b]	39.9	68.3	11.4	5.1	21.5
2 Western Europe	19.2	31.7	6.5	2.2	9.8
3 Oceania	10.2	17.9	2.3	0.8	5.4
4 Latin America	36.9	59.1	14.8	14.0	20.9
5 Sub-Saharan Africa	405.4	389.4	421.1	270.5	230.7
6 Caribbean	138.1	166.4	110.1	105.7	84.6
7 Eastern Europe	0.8	1.4	0.1	<0.1	0.4
8 SE Mediterranean	1.4	2.2	0.5	<0.1	0.6
9 Northeast Asia	0.6	0.9	0.2	0.1	0.3
10 Southeast Asia	21.5	27.8	14.7	43.3	16.6
TOTAL WORLD	49.9	53.5	46.3	59.0	32.5

Source: *AIDS in the World II* survey.
[a]HIV infection acquired before or at birth.
[b]AIDS cases in North America have been estimated on the basis of the 1987 revised CDC AIDS surveillance case definition.

Globally, the estimated incidence of AIDS in 1995 was 32.5 per 100,000 (Table 1-8). The highest incidence occurred among women in sub-Saharan Africa.

People living with HIV infection and with AIDS as of January 1, 1996

On January 1, 1996, an estimated 20.3 million people were living with HIV infection that had not yet evolved into AIDS, including 19.4 million adults (11.4 million men and 8 million women) along with about 850,000 children (Table 1-9). In addition, on January 1, 1996, an estimated 1.2 million people worldwide were living with AIDS, including 1.1 million adults (618,000 men and 472,000 women) and about 62,000 children (Table 1-10).

On January 1, 1996, there were 18 people living with HIV infection for each person living with AIDS (ratio 18:1) (Table 1-11). Depending upon the rate of new HIV infection and the duration of the epidemic, this ratio should gradually decline. The ratio is also influenced by the number of perinatally infected children, since progression from HIV to AIDS and duration of life after the onset of AIDS are shorter in these children than among adults.

Therefore, on January 1, 1996, an estimated 21.4 million people worldwide were living with HIV or AIDS (Table 1-12). Of these, 11.6 million (54 percent) were in sub-Saharan Africa, about 6.5 million (30 percent) were in Southeast Asia, 1 million (5 percent) were in Latin America, 928,000 (5 percent) were in North America, 694,000 (3 percent) were in Western Europe, and 662,000 (3 percent) were in the rest of the world. Forty-one percent of all adults living with HIV and AIDS were women and four percent of all people living with HIV and AIDS were children. The majority of people living with HIV/AIDS were in the developing world (including 92 percent of all adults, 97 percent of all women, and 98 percent of all children).

Table 1-9 Persons living with HIV (not yet progressed to AIDS) on January 1, 1996, by geographic area of affinity (GAA)

GAA	Adults	Men	Women	Children*	Total
1 North America	826,000	708,000	118,000	11,000	837,000
2 Western Europe	636,000	530,000	106,000	6,000	642,000
3 Oceania	23,000	20,000	3,000	<1,000	23,000
4 Latin America	959,000	767,000	192,000	17,000	976,000
5 Sub-Saharan Africa	10,183,000	4,849,000	5,334,000	626,000	10,809,000
6 Caribbean	334,000	200,000	134,000	9,000	343,000
7 Eastern Europe	30,000	27,000	3,000	<1,000	30,000
8 SE Mediterranean	64,000	54,000	11,000	<1,000	65,000
9 Northeast Asia	167,000	139,000	28,000	2,000	169,000
10 Southeast Asia	6,203,000	4,135,000	2,068,000	175,000	6,378,000
TOTAL WORLD	19,425,000	11,430,000	7,995,000	847,000	20,272,000

Source: *AIDS in the World II* survey.
Note: Columns and rows may fail to sum due to rounding to the nearest 1,000.
*HIV infection acquired before or at birth.

Table 1-10 Persons living with AIDS on January 1, 1996, by geographic area of affinity (GAA)

GAA	Adults	Men	Women	Children*	Total
1 North America	91,000	78,000	13,000	<1,000	91,000
2 Western Europe	52,000	43,000	9,000	<1,000	52,000
3 Oceania	2,000	2,000	<1,000	<1,000	2,000
4 Latin America	60,000	48,000	12,000	1,000	61,000
5 Sub-Saharan Africa	756,000	360,000	396,000	47,000	803,000
6 Caribbean	18,000	11,000	7,000	<1,000	19,000
7 Eastern Europe	2,000	2,000	<1,000	<1,000	2,000
8 SE Mediterranean	4,000	4,000	<1,000	<1,000	4,000
9 Northeast Asia	6,000	5,000	1,000	<1,000	6,000
10 Southeast Asia	100,000	67,000	33,000	12,000	112,000
TOTAL WORLD	1,090,000	618,000	472,000	62,000	1,152,000

Source: *AIDS in the World II* survey.
Note: Columns and rows may fail to sum due to rounding to the nearest 1,000.
*HIV infection acquired before or at birth.
*AIDS cases in North America have been estimated on the basis of the 1987 revised CDC AIDS surveillance case definition.

Table 1-11 Ratio of HIV infections to AIDS cases in persons living with HIV/AIDS on January 1, 1996, by geographic area of affinity (GAA)

GAA	HIV prevalence	AIDS prevalence	HIV:AIDS
1 North America*	837,000	91,000	9:1
2 Western Europe	642,000	52,000	12:1
3 Oceania	23,000	2,000	10:1
4 Latin America	976,000	61,000	16:1
5 Sub-Saharan Africa	10,809,000	803,000	13:1
6 Caribbean	343,000	19,000	18:1
7 Eastern Europe	30,000	2,000	13:1
8 SE Mediterranean	65,000	4,000	15:1
9 Northeast Asia	169,000	6,000	30:1
10 Southeast Asia	6,378,000	112,000	57:1
TOTAL WORLD	20,272,000	1,152,000	18:1

Source: *AIDS in the World II* survey.
Note: Columns and rows may fail to sum due to rounding to the nearest 1,000.
*AIDS cases in North America have been estimated on the basis of the 1987 revised CDC AIDS surveillance case definition.

Table 1-12 Persons living with HIV or AIDS on January 1, 1996, by geographic area of affinity (GAA)

GAA	Adults	Men	Women	Children*	Total
1 North America	916,000	785,000	131,000	12,000	928,000
2 Western Europe	688,000	573,000	115,000	6,000	694,000
3 Oceania	25,000	22,000	3,000	<1,000	25,000
4 Latin America	1,019,000	815,000	204,000	19,000	1,038,000
5 Sub-Saharan Africa	10,939,000	5,209,000	5,730,000	673,000	11,612,000
6 Caribbean	352,000	211,000	141,000	10,000	362,000
7 Eastern Europe	32,000	29,000	3,000	<1,000	32,000
8 SE Mediterranean	69,000	57,000	11,000	<1,000	69,000
9 Northeast Asia	173,000	144,000	29,000	2,000	174,000
10 Southeast Asia	6,303,000	4,202,000	2,101,000	186,000	6,490,000
TOTAL WORLD	20,516,000	12,048,000	8,467,000	909,000	21,424,000

Source: *AIDS in the World II* survey.
Note: Columns and rows may fail to sum due to rounding to the nearest 1,000.
*HIV infection acquired before or at birth.

Table 1-13 Prevalence of HIV infection: persons living with HIV who have not yet developed AIDS, January 1, 1996, by geographic area of affinity (GAA) (number of persons infected per 100,000 population)

GAA	Adults	Men	Women	Children[a]	Total
1 North America	534.5	913.9	153.1	52.4	285.9
2 Western Europe	327.4	539.6	110.4	26.2	166.8
3 Oceania	151.9	265.1	34.4	9.4	80.3
4 Latin America	417.2	667.8	166.8	29.3	218.8
5 Sub-Saharan Africa	3845.2	3693.9	3993.9	562.5	1814.0
6 Caribbean	1774.7	2138.2	1414.1	218.5	956.0
7 Eastern Europe	14.5	26.0	2.7	0.7	7.3
8 SE Mediterranean	27.0	43.5	9.3	0.8	12.7
9 Northeast Asia	19.8	32.0	6.8	1.1	11.1
10 Southeast Asia	830.8	1076.9	570.2	86.4	427.7
TOTAL WORLD	666.7	768.3	560.6	124.1	354.6

Source: *AIDS in the World II* survey.
[a]HIV infection acquired before or at birth.

Finally, the point prevalence of HIV infection and AIDS was derived by dividing the number of people living with HIV or AIDS at the beginning of 1996 by the total population. Prevalence provides another perspective on the challenges posed by the pandemic, as it indicates the proportion of the population directly affected by HIV/AIDS. On January 1, 1996, the prevalence of HIV infection in the world—not counting people living with AIDS—was estimated at 355 per 100,000. The highest prevalence was in sub-Saharan Africa (1,814 per 100,000), and the lowest level was in Eastern Europe (7 per 100,000) (Table 1-13).

The global prevalence of AIDS on January 1, 1996 was 20 per 100,000. AIDS prevalence in sub-Saharan Africa was about four times higher than in North America, more than twice the prevalence in the Caribbean and 18 times higher than in Southeast Asia (where a major increase in the prevalence of AIDS is expected by the end of the decade) (Table 1-14). Therefore, the combined global prevalence of HIV infection and AIDS on January 1, 1996 was 375 per 100,000 (Table 1-15). The prevalence of HIV infection and AIDS was 12 times higher in the developing world than in the industrialized world (Table 1-16). Compared with the industrialized world, HIV/AIDS prevalence in the developing world was almost nine times higher among men, 37 times higher among women, and 35 times higher among children.

The future course of the HIV/AIDS pandemic

In 1992, the Global AIDS Policy Coalition projected that by the end of the year 2000, a cumulative total of between 38 million and 110 million adults would have been infected with HIV since the beginning of the pandemic.[13] This broad range took into account major uncertainties prevailing at that time about the future course of the pandemic in Asia, Latin America, and

Table 1-14 Prevalence of AIDS, January 1, 1996, by geographic area of affinity (GAA) (persons living with AIDS per 100,000 population)

GAA	Adults	Men	Women	Children[a]	Total
1 North America[b]	58.6	100.2	16.8	2.8	31.2
2 Western Europe	26.6	43.8	9.0	1.2	13.5
3 Oceania	14.6	25.4	3.3	0.4	7.7
4 Latin America	26.1	41.7	10.4	2.2	13.7
5 Sub-Saharan Africa	285.4	274.2	296.5	42.0	134.7
6 Caribbean	95.9	115.6	76.4	16.3	52.2
7 Eastern Europe	1.1	1.9	0.2	<0.1	0.5
8 SE Mediterranean	1.8	2.8	0.6	0.0	0.8
9 Northeast Asia	0.7	1.1	0.2	<0.1	0.4
10 Southeast Asia	13.4	17.4	9.2	5.8	7.5
TOTAL WORLD	37.4	41.6	33.1	9.0	20.2

Source: *AIDS in the World II* survey.
[a]HIV infection acquired before or at birth.
[b]AIDS cases in North America have been estimated on the basis of the 1987 revised CDC AIDS surveillance case definition.

Table 1-15 Prevalence of HIV infection, including AIDS, January 1, 1996, by geographic area of affinity (GAA) (persons living with HIV or AIDS per 100,000 population)

GAA	Adults	Men	Women	Children[a]	Total
1 North America	593.2	1014.1	169.9	55.3	317.1
2 Western Europe	354.0	583.4	119.4	27.4	180.3
3 Oceania	166.5	290.6	37.7	9.8	88.0
4 Latin America	443.2	709.5	177.2	31.5	232.6
5 Sub-Saharan Africa	4130.6	3968.1	4290.4	604.6	1948.8
6 Caribbean	1870.6	2253.8	1490.5	234.8	1008.2
7 Eastern Europe	15.6	27.9	2.9	0.7	7.8
8 SE Mediterranean	28.8	46.3	9.9	0.8	13.5
9 Northeast Asia	20.5	33.1	7.1	1.2	11.5
10 Southeast Asia	844.2	1094.2	579.4	92.3	435.2
TOTAL WORLD	704.1	809.9	593.7	133.1	374.8

Source: *AIDS in the World II* survey.
[a]HIV infection acquired before or at birth.

Table 1-16 Prevalence of HIV and AIDS in industrialized countries and developing countries, January 1, 1996, by GAA, per 100,000 population

	Adults	Men	Women	Children[a]	Total
Industrialized countries	115.3	190.3	36.2	6.8	61.1
Developing countries	1477.0	1631.9	1317.4	235.8	759.0
TOTAL WORLD	704.8	810.8	594.3	132.2	374.8

Source: *AIDS in the World II* survey.
[a]HIV infection acquired before or at birth.

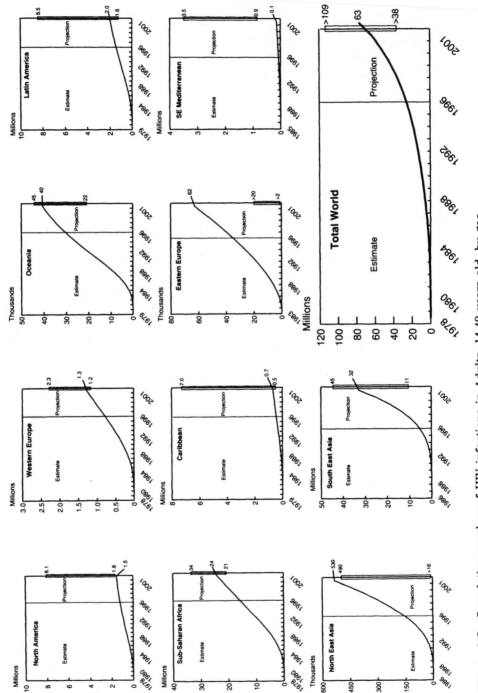

Figure 1-3 Cumulative number of HIV infections in Adults, 14-49 years old, by geographic area of affinity: estimates to 1996 and projections through January 1, 2001.

Eastern Europe, and about the magnitude, quality, and sustainability of the global response.

In December 1995, the WHO Global Programme on AIDS published estimates of HIV prevalence among adults by country (Appendix C).[14] According to these estimates, worldwide, 16.9 million people were living with HIV infection or AIDS by the end of 1994, 11.3 million of whom were in sub-Saharan Africa, 2.9 million in Southeast Asia, 1.1 million in Latin America, 0.2 million in the Caribbean, 1.2 million in North America, Western Europe, and Oceania combined, and 0.2 million in the rest of the world. These estimates, which represent a significant increase of figures published thus far by WHO, are now very consistent with estimates from the Global AIDS Policy Coalition (GAPC) as of January 1, 1995.[15] GAPC estimates for Southeast Asia remain different from those from WHO in that the GAPC figures are higher (4.1 million). The cumulative estimates presented by *AIDS in the World II* in Tables 1-1 and 1-2 are based on the assumption that every HIV infection present in Southeast Asia in January 1995 will generate one new HIV infection within an interval of 2 to 3 years. Thus, according to *AIDS in the World II*'s estimates, the HIV epidemic curve in Southeast Asia is likely to assume a steeper slope, mostly due to the rapid spread of HIV observed in heavily populated India (Figure 1-3).

If current epidemic trends persist through the end of the century, it is most likely that 60–70 million adults will have been infected with HIV by the end of the year 2000. One in every two adults ever infected with HIV will be in Southeast Asia and one in four in sub-Saharan Africa. By the turn of this century, Latin America could also be confronted with a large-scale pandemic, which could emerge from the multiple fragmented epidemics that have been documented in these regions until now.[16] Current trends observed in both Latin America and the Caribbean show that significant shifts are occurring in risk factors associated with reported AIDS cases in these GAAs (Chapter 3).

By the end of the year 2000, more HIV infections are likely to have occurred in adults in Southeast Asia than in any other GAA. The great diversity and complexity of social and cultural networks in Southeast Asia, however, are severe constraints to the accurate forecasting of the course of the pandemic in this heavily and densely populated region.[17] While data suitable for estimating the status and trends of the HIV pandemic are abundant in several countries, particularly in Thailand, they remain fragmentary in other countries in the region, such as India, which accounts for over 70 percent of the adult population in the GAA.[18-21]

In sub-Saharan Africa, where the present estimates assume that HIV incidence peaked in the early 1990s, incidence may decline further if prevention efforts targeting young people and women in particular, are considerably enhanced. In December 1995, a panel of experts meeting in Kampala, Uganda concluded that there were clear signs that the rate of new infection among young adults seemed to have reached a plateau or even to have declined in some areas that had been hard hit by the epidemic in the mid-1980s[22] (Box 1-6). In most parts of sub-Saharan Africa, however, HIV was still spreading with sustained intensity within urban populations as well as in rural populations.

BOX 1-6

Status and trends of the HIV/AIDS pandemic in Africa: report on a workshop held in Kampala, Uganda, December 8–9, 1995*

This workshop preceeded the IXth International Conference on AIDS & STI in Africa. It brought together the following epidemiologists, demographers, economists, and public health and international development experts from Africa, Europe, and North America: Martha Ainsworth, Godwill Asiimwe-Okiror, Edward Brown, John Paul Clark, Kevin M. De Cock, Michel Garenne, Jacob Gayle, Guy-Michel Gershy-Damet, Jaafar Heikel, Hilary Homans, Sam Kalibala, Jean A. Kalilani, Marie Laga, Peter Lamptey, Thierry Mertens, Warren Naamara, Mary O'Grady, Noah Jamie Robinson, Godfrey Sikipa, Cheryl Sönnichsen, Karen Stanecki-Delay, Rand Stoneburner, Don Sutherland, Daniel Tarantola, Maria Wawer, Peter Way, and Vicky Wells.

While remarkable efforts are being made throughout Africa to minimize the spread of HIV and reduce its impacts on individuals, families, communities, and nations, the HIV/AIDS pandemic in Africa continues to thrive relentlessly. It remains powerful and dynamic. It is composed of epidemics that evolve with changing speed in different populations, moving gradually from the silent, emerging stage still observed in North African and Indian Ocean countries to maturity and severity, as seen in several central and eastern African countries.

By the end of 1994, 11 million adults were living with HIV in Africa, representing 65 percent of the world total. As of June 1995, 418,000 AIDS cases had been reported to the World Health Organization by African countries, but these represent only a fraction of the cases that have actually occurred. Thus, this figure projects only a modest image of the heavy toll the epidemics are taking on people's health, on their social and economic well-being, and on their lives. The number of people who have died from AIDS thus far in Africa represents less than one-third of the deaths expected to occur among people who, today, are already infected with HIV.

The major impact of the pandemic on the African population is yet to come. Although the constantly growing HIV/AIDS care needs have already overwhelmed the coping capacity of urban health systems in hard-hit countries, demands for care will fall increasingly on poorly equipped and underfunded rural services, households, and individuals. Already, 80 percent of hospital beds in an infectious disease hospital in Abidjan, Côte d'Ivoire, and 50 percent in a hospital in Kampala, Uganda, are occupied by people with HIV.

The purpose of this document is to summarize the current state of knowledge of the status and trends of HIV/AIDS epidemics in Africa so as to provide national and international policy makers, program managers and the public at large with the information they need to fulfill their responsibilities in the face of one of the most severe human crises of our time.

From silent to mature epidemics

From the emerging, silent stage to that of maturity, HIV epidemics have evolved with a speed that differs among countries and among population groups within geopolitical boundaries.

*On December 8–9, 1995, the AIDS Control and Prevention (AIDSCAP) Project of Family Health International and the François-Xavier Bagnoud Center for Health and Human Rights of the Harvard School of Public Health cosponsored a workshop in Kampala, Uganda, to review the status and trends of HIV/AIDS epidemics in Africa.

HIV/AIDS epidemics are still at their emerging stage in North Africa and in Indian Ocean island countries, accounting for less than 2 percent of all people living with HIV in Africa. There the proportion of women attending urban antenatal clinics and testing positive for HIV remains below one per thousand. The prevalent modes of HIV transmission are similar to those observed in Western Europe, with HIV infection acquired through homosexual contacts and injecting drug use, combined with a slow but steady rise in heterosexual transmission. The large numbers of sexually transmitted infections (STIs) in many of these countries give a measure of the potential for the future growth of the currently silent HIV epidemics

In contrast, HIV epidemics have become severe in Kenya, Malawi, Rwanda, Tanzania, Uganda, Zambia, Zimbabwe and, more recently, Botswana. In these countries, transmission of HIV occurs mainly through heterosexual contact, beginning in the early teen years and peaking before age 25. More than 10 percent of women attending antenatal clinics surveyed in urban areas were found to be HIV infected, with rates that may exceed 30 percent in some surveillance sites. These high rates are associated with growing numbers of HIV-infected newborns. In other countries in Africa, HIV epidemics follow a similar transmission pattern but are currently passing through their intermediate stage: between 1 and 10 percent of women attending urban antenatal clinics are HIV infected.

The rate of HIV infection in sexually active adults continues to rise. Under circumstances that are not yet fully understood, epidemics may suddenly explode with rates of infection increasing severalfold within only a few years, as has been observed recently in Botswana and South Africa. It is clear that population mobility, patterns of sexual behavior, and societal factors influence the potential for such explosions.

Three broadly defined geographic areas, which include countries with severe epidemics and others with epidemics at their intermediate stages, account for almost 90 percent of all current HIV infections in adults and adolescents in Africa. Within these three areas, 19 countries have at least 100,000 people living with HIV. In central and eastern Africa, Cameroon, Ethiopia, Kenya, Rwanda, Sudan, Uganda, and Zaire have 37 percent of all current HIV infections on the continent. A similar proportion is contributed by a second group of countries in southern Africa: Botswana, Malawi, Mozambique, South Africa, Tanzania, Zambia, and Zimbabwe. Finally, West African countries, including Burkina Faso, Côte d'Ivoire, Ghana, Nigeria, and Togo, contribute about 15 percent to the total number of adults and adolescents living with HIV in Africa. These epidemics share a number of characteristics:

- Within each country, HIV epidemics have progressed with different speed in various population groups. Early in the evolution of the epidemics, urban populations and rural communities located along highways have been more rapidly affected. Among them, young adults with multiple sexual partners have high rates of infection. Rates as high as 80 percent have been found among sex workers surveyed in Nairobi and Abidjan.
- As epidemics evolve, they tend to affect younger people with increasing severity, especially young women who acquire infection from older men, and women who assumed they were in a monogamous relationship but have become infected by their spouse or regular partner.
- Over 90 percent of all HIV-infected infants in the world are born in Africa. These children will develop AIDS and die within a few years.
- Demographic surveys in several countries have already noted significant increases in infant and child mortality. Projections for Zambia and Zimbabwe indicate that AIDS may increase child mortality rates nearly threefold by the year 2010. Other estimates point to a more modest impact. In either case, due to high levels of fertility, populations will generally continue to grow but critical deficits will occur in the economically active ages.
- Studies in areas where 8 percent of the adult population is HIV infected have measured a doubling of mortality due to HIV and a decrease of 5 years in life expectancy.

- HIV epidemics will have severe effects on the population age structure indenting the population pyramid in young adults, who are the main contributors to social and economic development.

HIV epidemics of the young

Data obtained from surveillance systems and studies in sub-Saharan Africa demonstrate that HIV/AIDS epidemics are taking an increasing toll on young people, particularly young women.

- The rates of newly acquired HIV infections are highest in the 15–29 age-group among both females and males.
- The peak of new infections occurs 5 to 10 years earlier in young women than in young men.
- Most of the infections in 15- to 19-year-olds are among females. In Masaka, Uganda, for example, HIV prevalence among 13- to 19-year-old females is over 20 times higher than that for males of the same age. Apart from possible biological factors, there are at least two reasons for the disproportionate risk of young women acquiring HIV infection early, including: 1) an earlier age of sexual debut for girls, (in Masaka, the median age at first sexual intercourse is 15 for females and 17 for males); and 2) the patterns of sexual mixing, where young women tend to have sex with older men in the context of marriage or in exchange for money or advantages, whereas young men tend to have sex with young women.
- The high rates of HIV infection in young women and men under 20 years of age (even under 15) call for strong prevention programs in youth and children, prior to—not just after—the onset of sexual activity.
- Even though more HIV infections are found in young women than in young men, women and men are equally likely to acquire HIV infection in their lifetime. When all age-groups are considered, as many women as men are HIV infected, which gives a sex ratio of approximately one woman for one man in the HIV-infected adult population. In Africa, however, the sex ratio can vary considerably with the stage of progression of some of the epidemics. In Abidjan, for example, the sex ratio of reported AIDS cases changed from 4.8 men for every woman in 1988 to a ratio of 1.9:1 in 1993. The sex ratio of the general population in this city which is greatly influenced by migration, combined with sexual mixing patterns, accounts for the initial disparity which, as the epidemic matured, moved gradually toward a more balanced ratio.
- For many women, the major risk factor for HIV is the behavior of their spouse or regular sexual partner. Women in monogamous relationships cannot yet protect themselves against HIV infection if their spouses are not similarly monogamous. This highlights the need for enhancing prevention programs targeted at adult men and for developing effective and safe female-controlled HIV prevention methods such as microbicides.

Continued spread in urban areas and rising infection rates in rural areas

Urban centers generally have substantially higher prevalence of HIV infection than rural areas. This pattern is by no means universal: population displacement, armed conflicts, proximity to highways, or intense migration and population mobility for economic reasons influence strongly the spread of HIV. As a result of a combination of these factors, some rural communities of Kenya, Tanzania, and Uganda have higher infection rates than in neighboring urban populations. In countries where HIV epidemics were initially the attribute of urban areas, rates of HIV infection in rural populations have increased steadily over recent years.

Variations in rates of HIV infection have also been documented within rural areas themselves. In largely rural Rakai District, Uganda, rates of infection are higher in trading centers along the highway than in trading communities on secondary roads, where, in turn, rates are higher than in rural agrarian populations. A similar pattern has been observed in Mwanza, Tanzania.

- The differential between levels of HIV infection in urban populations and in rural populations is narrowing, sometimes rapidly.
- Two out of every three Africans live in rural areas. Thus, although the rate of infection is still lower in most rural populations than in neighboring urban populations, the absolute numbers of HIV-infected persons in rural areas may be expected to equal or surpass the number in urban areas. This projected trend demands renewed attention and resource allocation to rural prevention programs and health care systems, including home-based approaches.
- The soaring growth of the population in major urban centers through internal migration and the sex imbalance within migrant populations have played a key role in increasing the vulnerability of city dwellers and migrants to HIV/AIDS. As the process of urbanization continues through the next century, both the spread of HIV and the unmet demand for care in urban areas will rise further. Unless the response to HIV/AIDS is considerably enhanced and integrated in broader health, social, and economic development policies, the effort to control the epidemics and mitigate their impact will not be successful.

Recent trends in HIV prevalence

Surveillance data show regional variations in patterns of HIV prevalence (proportion of people infected with HIV at a particular time), with respect to the timing and the magnitude of HIV spread.

- Reasons for varying levels of HIV prevalence in different populations are not well understood but are likely to be related to a combination of different sexual mixing patterns, timing of virus introduction, and the presence of other facilitating factors such as STIs.
- A common feature of HIV epidemics is the rapidity of the spread once the virus finds a foothold in a vulnerable population.
- Explosive increases in new infections, as measured in rapidly rising levels of infection over a short period of time, appear to be a predictable pattern of HIV spread for many areas in sub-Saharan Africa. For example, the geographic extension of the epidemics from eastern and central Africa to southern Africa and West Africa during the 1980s and early 1990s resulted in infection levels of 40 to 60 percent in such high-risk behavior populations as STI clinic attendees. This has been followed by increases in HIV infection among antenatal clinic attendees to levels of 15 to 30 percent.
- The epidemics have recently expanded in Botswana, Lesotho, South Africa, and Swaziland, with patterns of spread similar to those observed in nearby Malawi, Zambia, and Zimbabwe.
- A few countries in West and Central Africa still have relatively low levels of HIV prevalence, but these have begun to rise in such countries as Cameroon and Nigeria, which earlier had been relatively spared.
- Although the apparent slow growth of HIV epidemics in areas where low prevalence of HIV infection persists has been credited to social and cultural factors influencing sexual behavior, it may merely reflect a delay in the seeding of the virus.
- The manner in which HIV spreads in a community is now better understood. Explosive growth in new infections occurs over a relatively brief period, with a natural falloff in new infections. This is referred to as *saturation,* which is the stage reached when most of the people at highest risk of acquiring infection have already been infected. This period is then followed by a concentration of

infections in younger age-groups, as young people move into ages of increased sexual activity. Thus, the risk of new infections shifts rapidly to youth.

- While stabilization of infection levels has been observed in an increasing number of mature epidemics, it is important to appreciate that such stabilization can occur as a natural result of a dynamic balance between new infections and deaths. New infections in populations may be balanced, or offset, by deaths occurring in people already infected. An underlying high incidence of HIV infection among younger age-groups may therefore be masked by high numbers of deaths, which removes people who have died of AIDS, or with HIV infection from the sample population. To conclude from stabilizing or even declining prevalence rates either that the epidemic will wane by itself in the absence of prevention or that prevention efforts are no longer necessary, would have tragic consequences for future generations.

- Nevertheless, hope that the number of new infections occurring may have decreased comes from studies of the epidemic in Uganda, a country with one of the older epidemics in Africa. A study of recent trends in HIV infection in women attending several antenatal clinics in Uganda has revealed significant declines in HIV prevalence. Analyses of HIV infection levels by age over time found a consistent decline in levels of infection among the younger age-group (aged 15 to 19), when levels in the early 1990s were compared with levels in late 1994 and in 1995. Since infection levels (or prevalence) in this young age-group reflect more recent patterns in new infections (or incidence), these data suggest a substantial reduction in the incidence of HIV infection in young people over time.

- Modeling of HIV incidence scenarios for studying such findings in 15- to 19-year-olds supports these findings. Similar declines in HIV prevalence among young adults have been reported from another study in the Masaka district in Uganda. These findings could indicate that the growth of the epidemic has been blunted, perhaps temporarily, by behavioral changes that result in decreased spread of HIV in younger age-groups. Behavioral surveys of such populations will assess to what extent behavior change could have led to these apparent declines.

- It has also been suggested that HIV infection might reduce the level of fertility, resulting in fewer HIV-infected women attending antenatal clinics where seroprevalence surveys are conducted.

- If these findings result from behavior modification, it may mean that methods to decrease HIV incidence substantially are within the technical capacity of many countries in sub-Saharan Africa.

- The hope generated by the observed reductions in levels of infection (prevalence) combined with the continuing evidence of new infections (incidence), which are particularly high among young people, should provide additional impetus for enhancing prevention efforts.

Sexually transmitted infections (STIs)

The presence of STIs implies a marked risk of concurrent HIV infection for at least two reasons: (1) the modes of transmission of HIV and other STIs are similar; and (2) the role of STIs in facilitating the transmission of HIV has been clearly established.

- The majority of STIs are treatable. The World Health Organization estimates that 65 million new cases of curable STIs occurred in Africa in 1995.

- STIs are affecting young adults, especially women, with serious consequences. For women these consequences include pelvic inflammatory disease, cervical cancer, infertility, and postpartum endometritis. For infants, maternal STIs may lead to low birth weight, neonatal syphilis, and gonococcal opthalmia.

- STI control programs, through early diagnosis, treatment, and the promotion of safer sexual behavior, have been shown to reduce significantly the rates of STI infections. Successful programs have been documented in Zambia and Zimbabwe and, outside Africa, in Thailand.

- In Mwanza, Tanzania, early treatment of STIs in a rural population has been associated with a 42 percent decline in the rate of newly acquired HIV infections. This important finding supports the revitalization of STI control programs benefiting from new approaches that have already been initiated in several sub-Saharan countries.
- The surveillance of some STIs (syphilis in women and gonorrhea in men) can be used to monitor the risk of HIV infection and to evaluate the effect of HIV/STI prevention programs. As prevention programs for HIV and other STIs move toward integration in most countries, the collection and analysis of STI surveillance data should be conducted concurrently with HIV surveillance.
- STI surveillance data originate mostly from STI and antenatal clinics. However, social and cultural barriers inhibit most women from visiting STI clinics. Antenatal clinics offer STI diagnostic and treatment services to women who are pregnant, existing STI services fail to provide continual and culturally acceptable access to the majority of women. In turn, surveillance of STIs and analysis of their epidemiological patterns remain incomplete. Better understanding of the dynamics of the epidemics of HIV and other STIs and improved prevention and control programs necessitate the creation of integrated services that suit the needs of women.
- Most young women and men do not have access to friendly, effective, and comprehensive STI services. These need to be built within the context of health services targeted toward young people's overall health needs. The information generated from such services will be crucial for understanding and responding to the increased STI/HIV rates now being observed in young people.

HIV/AIDS and mobility

Major political, social and demographic changes have occurred in Africa over the last few decades and have resulted in significant population displacement and migration and rapid urbanization. The improvement in transportation and communication networks, the increased exchange of goods, and the creation of large-scale development programs have stimulated the movement of young men and women within and across national boundaries. Open conflicts, environmental degradation, natural disasters, and low-intensity wars have also led millions of Africans to leave their homes and, in some situations, to turn to survival strategies that increase the practice of unsafe sex. Population mobility facilitates the spread of STIs, including HIV.

- Cross-border migration—of men to South Africa and Côte d'Ivoire from neighboring countries for employment purposes, for example—has been associated with a high risk of HIV infection in the migrant population as well as in their spouses or regular sexual partners upon their return home (e.g., in Burkina Faso, Lesotho, Malawi, Mali, and Swaziland).
- Migration within countries and urbanization (e.g., from rural areas to urban centers or industrial sites) have led to high concentrations of predominantly male communities and increased participation in commercial sex.
- Professional groups characterized by mobility, such as truck drivers, traders, and military personnel, have also been associated with a higher risk of HIV infection.
- Consequences of political and civil unrest and subsequent population displacement have led to an increased spread in HIV transmission; populations displaced from Ethiopia, Liberia, Mozambique, and Rwanda are examples. The movement of troops from West Africa to Angola and Mozambique has been linked to the spread of HIV-2 to these countries.
- Every year, mobility—whether for economic reasons or for survival in conflict situations—affects millions of people throughout Africa, particularly sexually active adolescents and young adults.

Separated from their families and supportive social environments, these young people become more exposed to behaviors that put them at increased risk for HIV and other STIs.

- Intercountry programs targeted at cross-border mobility and national programs aimed at mobile professions and internal migrants should be designed and implemented on the basis of information linking epidemiology and behavioral and social determinants of these populations to HIV and other STIs.
- The design of nationally and internationally funded economic development programs (for example, the construction of highways and creation of new industries or agriculture projects) needs to include an initial appraisal of the potential impact of these projects on the vulnerability of the labor force and the local population to HIV infection and other STIs. Measures to minimize this impact, such as reducing gender imbalance in the labor force, enabling workers to be joined by their families, allowing for regular contacts with distant spouses, and incorporating HIV/STI programs in development schemes need to be built into the project design.
- Even with such initiatives, the sheer dynamic of transition toward increasingly urbanized society brings with it changing behavioral mores that create new needs and present new opportunities for HIV transmission. These changes need to be anticipated and properly addressed through urban-based programs.

Surveillance must improve

Surveillance of HIV prevalence in sentinel populations, whereby sites are selected for the collection of HIV information from carefully selected populations, is fundamental to monitoring the HIV epidemics and guiding policy and programs. HIV prevalence trends in selected populations such as STI and antenatal clinic attendees serve as the standard for measuring the magnitude, growth, and geographic extension of HIV epidemics over time.

The evaluation of trends and their underlying determinants may improve the understanding of changing patterns in HIV incidence (such as the occurrence of new HIV infections) and the impact of interventions while providing better insight into the future course of epidemics in the region.

In sub-Saharan Africa, the quality of HIV surveillance varies widely, from weak attempts to collect data at clinical facilities to overextended sentinel surveillance programs that demand excessive amounts of resources and staff. The establishment of low-cost, well-focused surveillance systems based on anonymous, unlinked HIV testing performed on blood samples collected during service delivery can provide most of the data needed for surveillance purposes.

- During the early stages of HIV epidemics, surveillance at STI clinics has a higher likelihood of detecting HIV infection when prevalence is low in the general population.
- Once HIV prevalence has reached a measurable level among STI clinic attendees, women attending antenatal clinics, whose blood is collected for routine pregnancy monitoring, constitute the most practical and representative population sample to assess the status and trends of HIV infection in the sexually active population.
- The surveillance of AIDS cases has not been used extensively to understand the dynamics of the pandemic, since surveillance is constrained by difficulties inherent to the case definition of AIDS and the general weakness of reporting systems. In mature epidemics, however, the analysis of reported AIDS cases, particularly if reports include information on age and sex, may become increasingly useful. This analysis can provide information relevant to the assessment of trends over time, even if the delay between HIV infection and the onset of AIDS-defining conditions is several years.
- The establishment of these surveillance programs will only succeed if capacity-building through institutional strengthening and skill-building is an integral part of the program. Surveillance will

further improve if regular analysis, feedback, and the use of surveillance information for policy development, program monitoring, and evaluation occur.

- Epidemiological surveillance should be linked to the periodic collection and analysis of behavioral and social data to provide additional clues about the possible association between HIV infection and individual or collective factors influencing the risk of infection.
- National commitments must be made to generate, analyze, and disseminate information on HIV epidemics and international guidance on methods to ensure both the reliability and comparability of the information collected. Such methods should rely on standard procedures, minimum sample sizes, and a limited number of surveillance sites.

Research

Many issues critical to the understanding of HIV epidemics have been incompletely addressed or omitted in ongoing research efforts. Priority research needs include the following:

- Analyzing and interpreting existing epidemiological data in and among countries.
- Validating declines or stabilization of HIV prevalence in some countries. If these declines are real, possible causes should be investigated, including
    - a reduction in incidence due to the natural evolution of the epidemics or the effects of prevention interventions;
    - an increase in AIDS mortality;
    - a reduction in fertility in women infected with HIV who are therefore less likely to be included in antenatal clinic surveillance schemes; and
    - the relative contribution of any of the above factors.
- Determining through behavioral surveys the status and trends of sexual behaviors as they are linked to epidemiological findings.
- Using geographic techniques to study and devise patterns of the current and potential spread of HIV.
- Studying the evolutionary history of HIV/AIDS from the onset of HIV infection to death.
- Exploring the influence of HIV genetic variability on HIV transmission.
- Assessing the effect of viral load and clinical stage of infection on the transmission of HIV.

At a second level of priority, other research needs include the following:

- Evaluating the predictive value of HIV prevalence in antenatal women for estimating HIV prevalence among the general adult population.
- Discovering the type and role of factors responsible for the relatively low prevalence in North African and Indian Ocean countries.
- Assessing the validity of STI incidence as a surrogate for HIV incidence.
- Linking the epidemiology of HIV to the sexual behavior and societal context of young people.
- Comparing and analyzing the biological susceptibility of adult and younger women to HIV infection.

The European Centre for the Epidemiological Monitoring of AIDS, based in Saint-Maurice, France, receives reports of AIDS cases from national reporting centers in 44 countries in Europe.[23] Reported AIDS cases are adjusted by the Centre for delays in reporting, which vary from one mode of transmission to the other. These numbers are not adjusted, however, for the underreporting of those cases which may have been misdiagnosed, nor for those which failed to be reported to national centers.

The Centre estimates that, since the beginning of the pandemic, 165,482 AIDS cases had been diagnosed in Europe by the end of September 1995, including 159,278 among adults and adolescents, and 66,117 among children. According to the Centre's estimates, more than 26,000 new AIDS cases had been diagnosed in Europe in 1994, 16 percent more than in 1993. Of the cases actually reported to the Centre for 1994, 80 percent were among males and 20 percent, females.

Assessing the trends of the HIV/AIDS pandemic on the basis of reported AIDS cases has obvious limitations, particularly because of the time lag between the occurrence of HIV infection and the onset of AIDS-defining conditions. It does, however, provide useful insight into epidemic patterns in a situation such as that prevailing in Europe where the epidemic has matured in most countries, and where the efficiency of reporting, although variable from one country to the next, is generally high in those countries that have been the hardest hit by the pandemic. Based on the Centre's analysis of reported cases, the incidence of AIDS is generally higher in southern Europe than in western and northern Europe where, in turn, it is higher than in central and eastern Europe.

In 1994, France, Italy, Switzerland, Portugal, and Spain were the countries with the highest incidence of AIDS—between 68 per million population (in Portugal) and 191 per million population (in Spain). These five countries accounted for over 75 percent of all AIDS cases diagnosed in Europe in 1994. The incidence of AIDS ranged between 11 and 47 per million in a second group of countries which includes other countries in western and northern Europe, Greece, and Romania. The incidence was below 10 per million in yet a third group of countries which includes countries of central and eastern Europe and the newly independent states.

Since the beginning of the pandemic through September 1995, France, Italy, and Spain, with over 30,000 cases each, accounted for almost 111,000 AIDS cases, or 67 percent of all cases in Europe. Germany, the Netherlands, Switzerland, and the United Kingdom combined reported 36,000 additional cases, or 22 percent of the European total. The remaining 10 percent occurred in other countries in the region. In the early 1990s, the annual trends in AIDS incidence varied considerably from one country to the next, increasing markedly in Italy, Portugal, and Spain; less so in France; leveling-off in Belgium, Denmark, Switzerland, and the United Kingdom; and decreasing in Austria and the Netherlands.

Within Europe, injecting-drug use has become the main mode of transmission involved in newly diagnosed AIDS cases; male homosexual and bisexual transmission now ranks second. Noticeably, the number of AIDS cases attributed to heterosexual transmission in Europe as a whole almost doubled between 1991 and 1994 (from 2,215 to 4,301) while AIDS cases due to injecting drug use increased by 52 percent and those associated with male homosexual/bisexual contact increased by 13 percent during the same period. Injecting drug use was the leading mode of transmission of HIV in newly diagnosed AIDS cases in Italy, Portugal, and Spain, as well as in Poland and Yugoslavia. Male homosexual/bisexual contact was the leading mode of HIV infection in AIDS cases diagnosed in 1994 in Denmark, Germany, Greece, France, Finland, the Netherlands, Norway, and Sweden. Schematically, in that year the majority of AIDS cases in southern as well as central and eastern Europe were attributable to injecting drug use, whereas male homosexual/bisexual contact played this primary role in AIDS cases in northern Europe.

In every country, the incidence of both AIDS cases and newly acquired HIV infections that are attributed to heterosexual contact is on the rise. This rise, however, is not associated with a rise in pediatric AIDS attributable to mother-to-child transmission, the number of which declined from 143 in 1993 to 132 in 1994. The incidence of AIDS in children younger than 13 years of age due to HIV infection acquired through contaminated blood and blood products and through the use of unsterile injection equipment peaked in 1990, then declined gradually. Romania accounts for half of all AIDS cases that occurred in the 0–13-year-old age-group in Europe by the end of 1994.

Based on HIV seroprevalence figures, the European Centre for the Epidemiological Surveillance of AIDS estimates that by the end of 1994, 560,000 adults, adolescents, and children had become infected with HIV since the beginning of the pandemic. Consequently, the needs for care are expected to continue to rise over the next decade. HIV seroprevalence surveys show that the epidemic has not been stopped in any country in the region, underscoring the need for sustained prevention efforts.

In the United States, through June 1995, men who have sex with men continued to account for the largest population of persons with AIDS-defining opportunistic illnesses, but the rate of growth in this risk category has slowed.[24] In contrast, persons infected through injecting drug use and their heterosexual partners accounted for an increasing proportion of persons with AIDS opportunistic infections. Several shifts have been noted through the analysis of AIDS surveillance data: there are emerging trends among women, Black and Hispanic men and women, persons in moderate and small-sized metropolitan areas and in the rural South, persons infected through heterosexual contacts, non-white homosexual and bisexual men, and young men who have sex with men. While overall these data suggest that the AIDS epidemic is reaching a plateau, at least temporarily, its future course will be determined by the strength of prevention programs specifically designed to respond to the needs of marginalized minorities.

What lies behind the first peak of HIV/AIDS epidemics?

When considering the future of the pandemic, a larger and at this stage, somewhat theoretical, approach is required. Consider a hypothetical population has been divided into two subsets: those with higher vulnerability and those with lower vulnerability to HIV infection. People with higher vulnerability are assumed to represent a small fraction of the entire population. In the first phase of the epidemic, people with higher vulnerability become exposed to HIV and the number of new infections rises sharply (Figure 1-4).

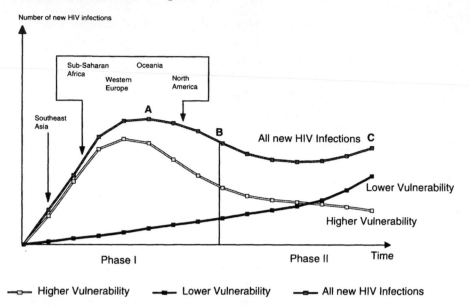

Figure 1-4   New cases of HIV infection over time.

When a substantial portion of the population at higher vulnerability has been infected, the annual increase in the number of new HIV infections gradually declines. However, in this population, the transmission of HIV does not stop abruptly: in addition to a continuing spread of HIV among those more vulnerable to infection, new people may enter this highly vulnerable population. Thus new infections will continue to occur, but at a slower rate. During this phase, a gradually increasing number of people with lower vulnerability will become infected with HIV, depending on the frequency of unprotected sexual encounters between people of higher and lower vulnerability. Accordingly, new HIV infections will begin to occur in the lower vulnerability population. However, because this population is much larger than the population with higher vulnerability, the number of new infections that occur each year in the low-vulnerability population will rise steadily and will likely (eventually) exceed the peak number observed in the higher-vulnerability population subset.

Reflecting the combined effects of the high-vulnerability population and the slow rise in the low-vulnerability population, the number of HIV infections will peak (Figure 1-4, point A). Then, since most highly vulnerable people have already been infected while relatively few lower-vulnerability people become infected, the annual number of new infections will decline (Figure 1-4, point B). At this point, a false impression that the HIV epidemic is under control may develop among policy makers, funders of prevention programs, the media, and the population at large. As a result, prevention programs may be curtailed, funds withdrawn, and public attention and concern diverted, leading to an increase in overall vulnerability to the epidemic. As the epidemic spreads among the low-vulnerability population, a second rise in the number of new HIV infections occurs (Figure 1-4, point C). When and at what level this second epidemic will peak cannot yet be predicted. It will happen over a long period (decades) and it will be determined by the opportunities HIV will find to spread in the population initially considered at lower risk. Within this population, those who are more likely to become infected are members of marginalized groups who have insufficient access to information, education, and health and social services and are stigmatized for reasons of race, ethnicity, gender, or social and cultural factors.

In summary, the global experience of HIV/AIDS is likely only beginning. Available data suggest the possibility that a decrease in annual incidence of new HIV infections may occur; the warning must be sounded that this may only be the "lull before the storm" and that this apparently hopeful outcome may only presage the next phase in a long, sustained struggle with the pandemic.

REFERENCES

1. Centers for Disease Control and Prevention, *HIV/AIDS Surveillance Report*, draft (Atlanta, GA). 1994:6 (No. 1).
2. B. G. Evans, O. N. Gill, and J. A. N. Emslie, "Completeness of reporting of AIDS cases," editorial, *British Medical Journal* 302(1991):1351–1352.
3. Pan American Health Organization, *AIDS/HIV/STD Annual Surveillance Report, 1992* (Washington, DC: PAHO, 1994).
4. S. E. Whitmore-Overton, H. E. Tillett, B. G. Evans, and G. M. Allardice, "Improved survival from diagnosis of AIDS in adult cases in the United Kingdom and bias due to reporting delays," *AIDS* 7(1993):415–420.
5. World Health Organization, "Weekly Epidemiological Record, No. 50, 15, December 1995," 70(1995):353–354.
6. G. Larsson, L. Spangberg, S. Lindgren, and A. B. Bohlin, "Screening for HIV in pregnant women: A study of maternal opinion," *AIDS Care* 2(1990):223–228.
7. A. Blaxhult, C. Anagrius, M. Arneborn, K. Lidman, S. Lindgren, and M. Bottinger, "Evaluation of HIV testing in Sweden, 1985–1991," *AIDS* 7(1993):1625–1631.
8. Centers for Disease Control and Prevention, *HIV/AIDS Surveillance Report* (1994).
9. O. Morton, "Achievements in research," in *AIDS in the World*, J. Mann, D. Tarantola, and T. Netter, eds. (Cambridge, MA: Harvard University Press, 1992):229–258.
10. F. Barré-Sinoussi, "HIV virus variability," in *AIDS in the World*, J. Mann, D. Tarantola, and T. Netter, eds. (Cambridge, MA: Harvard University Press, 1992):267–274.
11. K. de Cock and F. Brun-Vezinet, "The epidemiology of HIV-2 infection," in *AIDS in the World*, J. Mann, D. Tarantola, T. Netter, eds. (Cambridge, MA: Harvard University Press, 1992):275–277.
12. J. Mann, D. Tarantola, and T. Netter, eds., "Methods for the estimation of the number of HIV infections, AIDS cases, and deaths in the world, January 1, 1992, and projections to 1995 and the year 2000," in *AIDS in the World* (Cambridge, MA: Harvard University Press, 1992):871–891.
13. J. Mann, D. Tarantola, T. Netter, eds., *AIDS in the World* (Cambridge, MA: Harvard University Press, 1992) Appendix 2.2, 885–892.
14. World Health Organization, "Provisional working estimates of adult HIV seroprevalences as of end 1994, by country, Weekly Epidemiological Record, No. 50, 15 December 1995," 70(1995):355–357.
15. The Global AIDS Policy Coalition, "Status and trends of the HIV/AIDS pandemic as of January 1995" (Cambridge, MA: Harvard School of Public Health, François-Xavier Bagnoud Center for Health and Human Rights, January 17, 1995).

16. Pan American Health Organization, Regional Program on AIDS/STDs, *Quarterly Report*, March 18, 1995 (Washington, DC: PAHO, 1995).

17. J. Chin, "Scenario for the AIDS epidemic in Asia: Asia-Pacific population," Research Abstracts No. 2 (Honolulu, Hawaii: East-West Center, February 1995).

18. T. Brown and W. Sittitrai, *Estimates of Recent HIV Infection Levels in Thailand*, Research Report No. 9 (Bangkok: Program on AIDS, Thai Red Cross Society, 1993).

19. T. Brown and P. Xenos, *AIDS in Asia: The Gathering Storm*, AsiaPacific Issues series 16 (Honolulu: East-West Center, August 1994).

20. J. Kaldor, P. Effler, R. Sarda, G. Petersen, D. Gertig, and J. Narain: "HIV and AIDS in Asia and the Pacific: An epidemiological overview," *AIDS* 8(1994)(suppl):S165–S172.

21. M. Jain, J. T. Jacob, and G. Keusch, "Epidemiology of HIV and AIDS in India," *AIDS* 8(1994)(suppl):S61–S75.

22. Final Report on the Workshop on the Status and Trends of the HIV/AIDS Epidemic in Africa, co-sponsored by the AIDS Control and Prevention Project of Family Health International and the François-Xavier Bagnoud Center for Health and Human Rights, Harvard School of Public Health, held in Kampala, 8–9 December, 1995.

23. European Centre for the Epidemiological Monitoring of AIDS, Saint Maurice, France, *Quarterly Report* 2(1995):5–10.

24. Centers for Disease Control and Prevention, *HIV/AIDS Surveillance Report* (Atlanta, GA: Centers for Disease Control and Prevention) 1995:7(No. 1).

2

The Dynamic HIV/AIDS Pandemic

KAREN A. STANECKI AND PETER O. WAY

At first glance, the HIV/AIDS situation could appear to have changed little since 1992, with similar countries and population groups most affected and little evidence of impact from intervention programs. Yet a closer look reveals an important broadening and deepening of the AIDS pandemic: in Latin America and the Caribbean, sub-Saharan Africa, and Southeast Asia, the pandemic's impact is intensifying in certain geographic areas and expanding to reach others. Progress in surveillance, particularly through creation of sentinel surveillance systems in sub-Saharan Africa, has also resulted in far better documentation of the pandemic.*

Latin America and the Caribbean

During 1994/1995, HIV epidemics have progressed rapidly in the Caribbean and Latin America. In countries with already existing epidemics, HIV infection rates have typically increased in all population groups previously affected. In countries relatively untouched until recently, substantial increases in levels of infection have generally occurred. While there are still some countries where HIV is rare in the general population, HIV seroprevalence is at or above 2 percent among urban pregnant women in the Bahamas, British Virgin Islands, Haiti, St. Kitts, Guyana, and Honduras (Figure 2-1).

In several countries, the prevalence of HIV among blood donors was the only available evidence of new HIV spread. For example, Chile, El Salvador, Barbados, and St. Vincent have all reported HIV infection levels of 0.3 percent or higher among blood donors, while other population groups either have lower levels or data were not reported. The highest reported infection levels among blood donors were found in Haiti (3.8 percent in 1987; 6.1 percent in 1988; 4.2 percent in 1989; and 3.2 percent in 1990) (Figure 2-2).

In several Central American, South American, and Caribbean countries,

*The data presented in this analysis are drawn from a large number of studies, the reference to which can be found in: HIV/AIDS Surveillance Database; HIV/AIDS Literature Review; International Programs Center, Population Division; U.S. Bureau of the Census; July 1995.

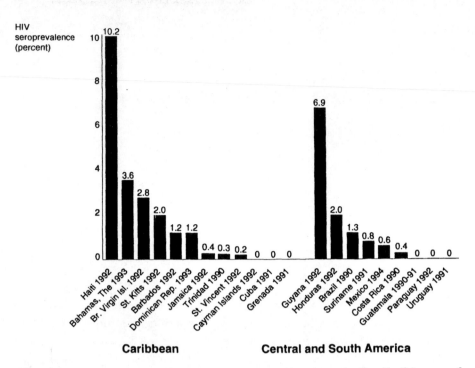

Figure 2-1 HIV seroprevalence among pregnant women in the Caribbean and Latin America, 1990–1994.

Figure 2-2 HIV seroprevalence among blood donors in the Caribbean and Latin America, 1990–1994.

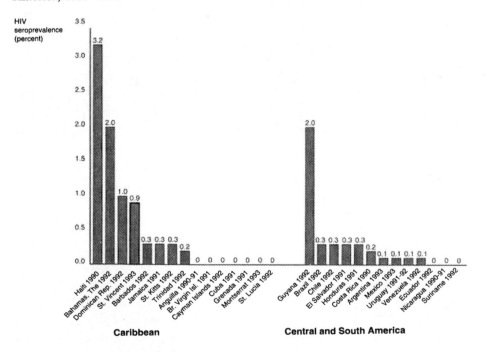

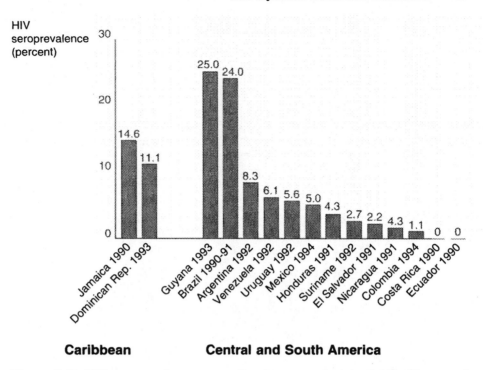

Figure 2-3 HIV seroprevalence among female sex workers in the Caribbean and Latin America, 1990–1994.

HIV infection among sex workers now exceeds 10 percent (Figure 2-3). Only a few countries in this region still report infection levels of less than 1 percent in this population.

HIV infection rates among men attending sexually transmitted infection (STI) clinics indicate the wide geographic spread of HIV: nearly two-thirds of the countries from which data were available report HIV seroprevalence of more than 2 percent in this population. HIV infection levels exceeding 10 percent were documented among STI clinic patients in several countries, including Haiti, the Bahamas, Trinidad, Guyana, and Honduras (Figure 2-4).

Sub-Saharan Africa

Since 1985, repeated HIV seroprevalence studies of pregnant women have been conducted in a number of African countries (Figure 2-5). These generally show a consistent and rapid increase in HIV seroprevalence in this population. For example, in Botswana, HIV seroprevalence increased from less than 10 percent to more than 30 percent in Francistown, and from 6 percent to 19 percent in Gabarone between 1990 and 1993. In the capital cities of Uganda, Zambia, and Malawi, infection levels were 20 percent or greater by 1993. With a reported HIV seroprevalence over 30 percent since 1988, Kigali, Rwanda was another major urban area with already high levels of infection when the civil war broke out in 1994.

However, infection levels among pregnant women vary. In Nigeria, the most populous country in Africa, by the end of 1995 HIV seroprevalence still

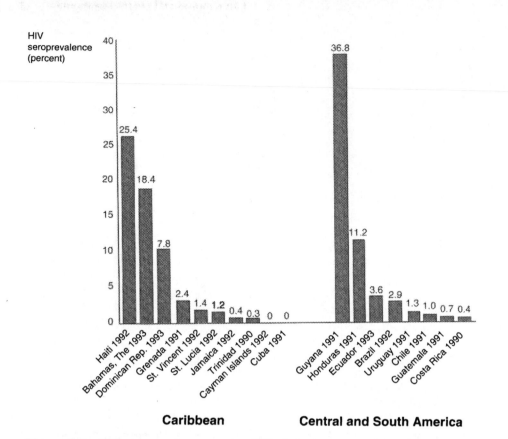

Figure 2-4 HIV seroprevalence among STI clinic patients in the Caribbean and Latin America, 1990–1994.

Figure 2-5 HIV seroprevalence among pregnant women in selected urban areas of Africa, 1985–1994. Infection from HIV-1 and/or HIV-2 is included.

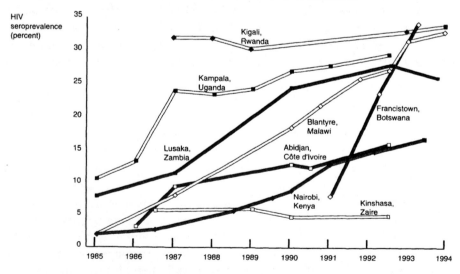

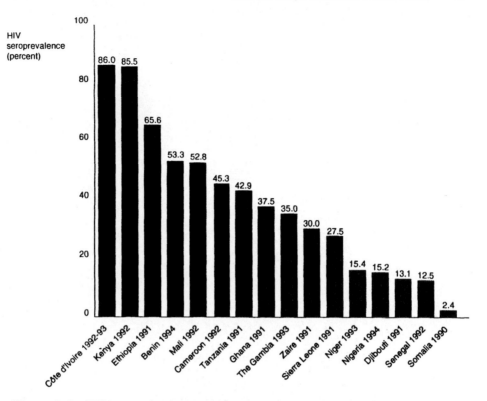

Figure 2-6 HIV seroprevalence among urban women sex workers in sub-Saharan Africa, 1990–1994. Infection from HIV-1 and/or HIV-2 is included.

ranged from 0 to 2 percent. In some areas, such as Bangui (Central African Republic), Brazzaville (Congo), and Kinshasa (Zaire), seroprevalence levels have been relatively stable over the past few years, but concerns have been expressed that stable levels may mask increasing incidence among younger women.

As potential blood donors and health personnel become aware of the risk of HIV infection, more selective standards are increasingly applied in the recruitment of blood donors. Thus, blood donors tend to be less representative of the general population as the epidemic matures. Data from Rwanda demonstrate this phenomenon: between 1985 and 1990, HIV infection among blood donors in Kigali decreased steadily from 13.5 to 2.1 percent, while surveillance data among the general population and pregnant women documented continued increases in HIV prevalence in the population at large.

Data for urban women sex workers show infection levels of greater than 30 percent for many countries (Figure 2-6). In several countries, more than half of urban women sex workers are now infected. Even in heavily affected countries, HIV seroprevalence continues to rise. For example, in Abidjan, Côte d'Ivoire, seroprevalence among women sex workers rose from 69 percent in 1990 to 86 percent in 1992–93.

Patterns of HIV infection among patients attending clinics for sexually transmitted infections are shown in Figure 2-7. Continued increases in HIV

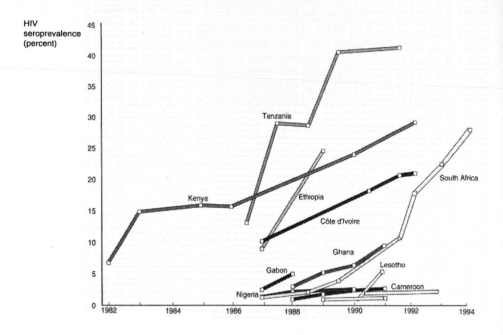

Figure 2-7   HIV seroprevalence among STI patients in urban areas of African countries, 1982–1994.

infection levels have been noted in Tanzania, Kenya, and Côte d'Ivoire, with infection levels of more than 20 percent in the capital cities of these countries. In Botswana, seroprevalence ranges from around 15 percent to as high as 49 percent. Although both Ghana and South Africa (results for black women only) show relatively lower levels of infection, the increases noted in the most recent data are ominous.

In several studies, perhaps due to a combination of selection bias and higher vulnerability of women to STIs, women consulting for STIs had higher HIV infection levels than men (Figure 2-8). In Zambia, for example, seroprevalence ranged from 40 to 70 percent among women, and 35 to 60 percent among men attending STI clinics in 1991.

Patterns of HIV infection by age are influenced by the tendency of men to choose a younger woman as a spouse (as well as a casual sexual partner). This contributes to higher HIV infection levels in younger women than men in the same age-group, while older men tend to have higher infection levels than women of the same age. This pattern is shown in Figure 2-9 for the Rakai District in Uganda.

Urban and rural areas have significantly differing patterns of HIV infection in many sub-Saharan countries. For example, in Bujumbura, the capital of Burundi, 20 percent of pregnant women were HIV infected in 1992, compared with 5 percent in semi-urban areas, and 2 percent in rural areas. Data from the Rakai District in Uganda demonstrate both the urban/rural differentiation in infection levels, as well as the typical age pattern of infection (Figure 2-9). Patterns of mobility and the prevalence of various sexual behaviors determine the spread from urban to rural areas, and from one rural

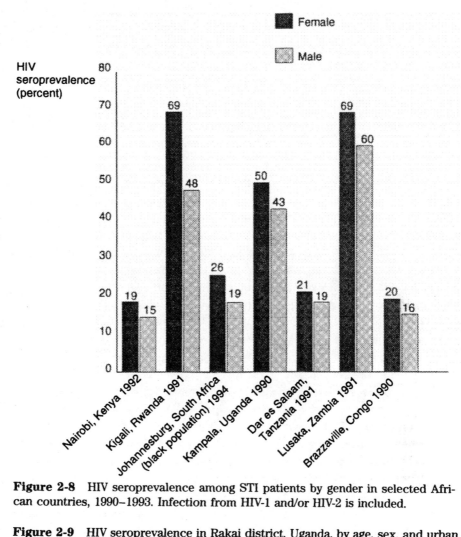

Figure 2-8 HIV seroprevalence among STI patients by gender in selected African countries, 1990–1993. Infection from HIV-1 and/or HIV-2 is included.

Figure 2-9 HIV seroprevalence in Rakai district, Uganda, by age, sex, and urban or rural residence, 1990.

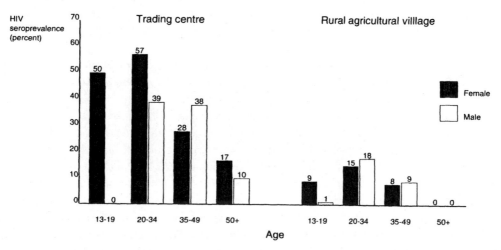

area to another (Box 2-1). The collective violence and consequent population movements that affect rural areas of Sudan, Somalia, Liberia, and Rwanda are likely to increase the vulnerability of these populations to further spread of HIV.

BOX 2-1

Urban–rural movement and HIV dynamics

MARIA J. WAWER

Available urban and rural HIV prevalence data in industrialized and developing countries reveal two major trends: rates of infection are generally higher in larger urban areas, and population movements have contributed to the spread of HIV to rural communities.[1,2,3] HIV is more prevalent among rural persons reporting travel, particularly to urban areas, compared to persons not reporting such travel.[4,5] Accordingly, at the community level, rural villages with populations that have higher rates of travel to urban centers are associated with higher HIV prevalence.[6] Several factors influence the magnitude, policy, and preventive implications of urban-to-rural HIV spread.

Simple definitions of urban and rural residence may be misleading. Although recognized urban settings, such as national capital cities, may have high HIV prevalence, relatively small local or regional towns also may exhibit substantially higher HIV prevalence than the surrounding rural area.[7,8,9] In addition, urban–rural population movement can take several forms, and each can have different impacts upon HIV prevalence, incidence, paths of spread, and economics.

Rapid urbanization is a common phenomenon in many developing countries. This may result in permanent, temporary, or recurring seasonal migration from rural areas to the cities in search of work.[10,11] Although entire families may move to urban areas, it is not uncommon in the early stages of economic/occupational migration for men to constitute the predominant migrant wave.[12] These men often live in low-income neighborhoods or work-provided residences with a preponderance of single men. Although generally less common, women may migrate alone to work in factories or in the entertainment and sex work sector. Thailand offers a paradigm of such migration, which is frequently temporary, with many women returning to their place of origin after earning funds towards a specific financial goal.[13,14] In rapidly urbanizing countries, strong economic, social, and familial ties continue to exist between rural and urban populations, with substantial movement back and forth.[15] Smaller movements within an urban–semirural aggregation, or within a nominally rural area consisting of larger and smaller communities, also can contribute to substantial social and sexual mixing of populations with very different HIV prevalence rates.

The epidemiological implications of such population exchanges for HIV/AIDS are manifold. Migrating and traveling persons are more likely to be young, frequently belong to the economically productive sectors, and are at greatest risk of HIV acquisition.[16] Migration and urbanization dilute pressures on social conformity and erode traditional sexual mores, potentially predisposing these persons to exposure to HIV and other STIs.[17,18] Given their social isolation, the paucity of accompanying permanent female partners, and their cash earnings, young men who migrate in search of work are likely to contact sex workers.[19] The movement of young women into the sex industry presents an important risk for the subsequent transmission of HIV into rural areas.[20,21,22] Marginalization of recent rural migrants is common in the cities, with respect to language, acculturation, and access to health and preventive services. Reaching new migrants with AIDS prevention services may be difficult. In some settings, an international component exacerbates this phenomenon. For example, in one sample, 27 percent of persons living in urban peripheral areas of Abidjan, Côte d'Ivoire, were foreigners, of whom almost one-fifth did not understand French language education campaigns.[23]

Finally, movement of HIV-infected persons to rural areas, in part to seek familial support during periods of deteriorating health, may result in the introduction of the virus and can place economic demands on the receiving families and communities. In the United States, a number of studies have noted migration of HIV-infected individuals to rural states. In addition, "returning to the village to die" is apparently common in many African settings.[24,25,26] Particularly in developing countries, the ill individuals may not know their HIV status nor the etiology of their illness, which increases the difficulty of assessing the magnitude of AIDS-related migration. In the United States, it has been suggested that the cost of medical care for AIDS patients in some rural states may be higher than anticipated on the basis of CDC AIDS surveillance. Because of this, low HIV-incidence regions may need more AIDS-related funding than currently projected.[27]

In order to develop comprehensive HIV/AIDS prevention and care programs, more data are required worldwide regarding urban–rural HIV differentials, urban–rural population mixing, and HIV spread through migration and travel. In many settings, even well-developed survey and surveillance efforts do not adequately cover rural communities, fail to differentiate between rural and urban populations, or do not assess HIV prevalence and informational needs among newly or partially urbanized persons or those planning to migrate to the cities.[28]

An urgent need also exists for HIV prevention programs tailored to migrant and transient communities. Such programs should test novel outreach strategies for individuals who may not normally have contact with existing urban health services because of youth, apparent good health, and cultural and linguistic isolation. Efforts to reach such transitional communities may require coordination by multiple local or national jurisdictions.[29] Background information regarding the social structure and cultural norms of different migrant and transient communities and populations would be invaluable in designing effective programs.

In some settings, it may be desirable to direct HIV prevention messages to rural communities. These messages could stress the need for safe sex and condom use during periods of travel or migration, or during contacts with persons such as travelers and truckers, who have been outside the community. Careful design and implementation of such messages is essential to avoid social stigmatization of all migrants and travelers. Also, it is crucial not to imply that contacts only with migrants are risky. Finally, programs must assist rural families and communities in supporting HIV-infected persons who return to their place of origin.

References

1. J. Bongaarts and P. Way, "Table 1, Estimated HIV seroprevalence among adults 15–49 for cities and rural areas, population aged 15–49, percent of population living in cities, and total number of infected persons, for African countries circa 1987," In *Geographic Variation in the HIV Epidemic and the Mortality Impact of AIDS in Africa*, working paper 1 (New York: Research Division, Population Council, 1989):6–7.

2. J. M. Karon and R. L. Berkelman, "Geographical and ethnic diversity of AIDS incidence trends in homosexual/bisexual men in the United States," *Journal of Acquired Immune Deficiency Syndromes* 4(1991):1179–1189.

3. G.-M. Gershy-Damet, K. Koffi, B. Soro, et al., "Seroepidemiological survey of HIV-1 and HIV-2 infections in the five regions of Ivory Coast," *AIDS* 5(1991):462–463.

4. J. Killewo, K. Nyamurekunge, A. Sandstrom, et al., "Prevalence of HIV-1 infection in the Kagera region of Tanzania: A population-based study," *AIDS* 4(1990):1081–1085.

5. D. Serwadda, M. J. Wawer, S. D. Musgrave, N. K. Sewankambo, J. E. Kaplan, and R. H. Gray, "HIV risk factors in three geographic strata of rural Rakai District, Uganda," *AIDS* 6(1992):983–989.

6. M. J. Wawer, D. Serwadda, S. D. Musgrave, J. K. Konde-Lule, M. Musagara, and N. K. Sewankambo, "Dynamics of HIV-1 infection in a rural district of Uganda," *British Medical Journal* 303(1991):1303–1306.

7. J. Killewo, K. Nyamurekunge, A. Sandstrom, et al., "Prevalence of HIV-1 infection in the Kagera region of Tanzania: A population-based study," *AIDS* 4(1990):1081–1085.

8. Wawer, "Dynamics of HIV-1."

9. C. Obbo, "HIV transmission through social and geographical networks in Uganda," *Social Science and Medicine* 36(1993):949–955.

10. S. H. Preston, "Urbanization: Developing countries," in *International Encyclopedia of Population*, Vol. 2, J. A. Ross, ed. in chief (New York: Free Press, Macmillan Publishing, 1982):650–655.

11. UN, "Table 6, urban and total population by sex 1982–1991," in *Demographic Yearbook 1991* (New York: UN, 1991):134–151.

12. M. T. Basset and M. Mhloyi, "Women and AIDS in Zimbabwe: The making of an epidemic," *International Journal of Health Services* 21(1991):143–156.

13. N. Ford and S. Koetsawang, "Socio-cultural context of the transmission of HIV in Thailand," *Social Science and Medicine* 33(1991):405–414.

14. C. Podhisita, A. Pramualratana, U. Kanungsukkasem, et al., "Sociocultural context of commercial sex workers in Thailand: An analysis of their family, employer and client relations," presented at AIDS Impact and Prevention in the Developing World: The Contribution of Demography and Social Science, the International Union for the Scientific Study of Population (IUSSP) seminar, Annecy, France, December 1993.

15. A. Larson, "Social context of human immunodeficiency virus transmission in Africa: Historical and cultural bases of east and central African sexual relations," *Review of Infectious Diseases* 11(1989):716–731.

16. G.-M. Gershy-Damet, K. Koffi, B. Soro, et al., "Seroepidemiological survey of HIV-1 and HIV-2 infections in the five regions of Ivory Coast," *AIDS* 5(1991):462–463.

17. L. A. Adeokun, "Research on human sexuality in sub-Saharan Africa," Abstract Th.G.O. 11, presented at the V International Conference on AIDS, Montreal, Canada, June 1989.

18. S. H. Ebrahim and D. Hilhorst, "AIDS prevention and its countercurrents in Asia," Abstract Th.H.P.30, presented at the V International Conference on AIDS, Montreal, Canada, June 1989.

19. K. Jochelson, M. Mothibeli, and J.-P. Leger, "Human immunodeficiency virus and migrant labor in South Africa," *International Journal of Health Services* 21(1991):157–173.

20. Podhisita, "Sociocultural context."

21. A. R. Neequaye, L. Osei, J. A. A. Mingle, et al., "Dynamics of human immune deficiency virus (HIV) epidemic—the Ghanaian Experience," in *Global Impact of AIDS*, Proceedings of the First International Conference on the Global Impact of AIDS, A. F. Fleming, M. Carballo, D. W. FitzSimons, M. R. Bailey, and J. Mann, eds. (New York: Alan R. Liss, 1988).

22. F. Denis, F. Barin, G. Gershy-Damet, et al., "Prevalence of human T-lymphotropic retroviruses type III (HIV) and type IV in Ivory Coast," *Lancet* 1(1987):408–411.

23. S. Yelibi, P. Valenti, C. Volpe, et al., "Sociocultural aspects of AIDS in an urban peripheral area of Abidjan (Côte d'Ivoire)," *AIDS Care* 5(1993):187–197.

24. D. Davis and J. Stapleton, "Migration to rural areas by HIV patients: Impact on HIV-related health care use," *Infection Control and Hospital Epidemiology* 12(1991):540–543.

25. A. Vergese, S. L. Berk, and F. Saruvvi, "Urbs in rure: Human immunodeficiency virus infection in rural Tennessee," *Journal of Infectious Diseases* 160(1989):1051–1055.

26. M. Patton, "Virus in our midst," *West Virginia Medical Journal* 85(1989):92–97.

27. K. Davis and J. Stapleton, "Migration to rural areas by HIV patients: Impact on HIV-related health care use," *Infection Control and Hospital Epidemiology* 12(1991):540–543.

28. R. M. Safman, "Projecting the effects of the AIDS epidemic for households and communities in rural Thailand," paper presented at Social and Cultural Context of the AIDS Epidemic in Thailand, the 5th International Conference on Thai Studies, School of Oriental and African Studies (SOAS), University of London, London, 1993.

29. R. Van Duifhuizen and A. Hendriks, "AIDS and mobility: The impact of international mobility on the spread of HIV-AIDS, needs and possibilities for international cooperation," Abstract PoD 5235, presented at the VIII International Conference on AIDS, Amsterdam, The Netherlands, July 1992.

Southeast Asia

Since the early 1990s, HIV epidemics in Asia have expanded substantially. Recent data from countries not previously represented in the *HIV/AIDS Surveillance Database*—Laos and Cambodia—document rapid HIV spread even in countries without the large transnational population movements characteristic of countries such as Thailand and India.

In Thailand, HIV infection levels have increased to over 1 percent among women attending provincial maternity clinics, with levels around 3 percent in some areas (Figures 2-10 and 2-11). Similar rates (or even higher in the

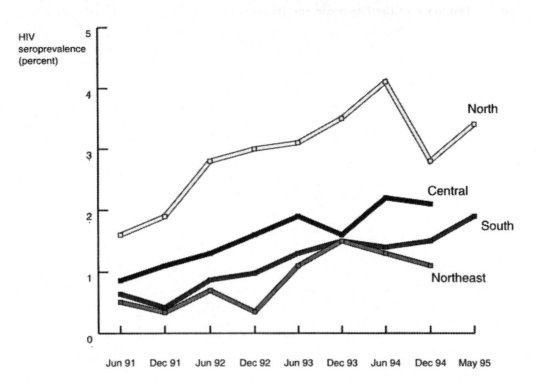

Figure 2-10 HIV seroprevalence among pregnant women in urban areas by region in Thailand, 1991–1995. Source: Division of Epidemiology, Ministry of Public Health, Bangkok, Thailand.

Figure 2-11 HIV seroprevalence among pregnant women in India, Thailand, and Myanmar, 1990–1994.

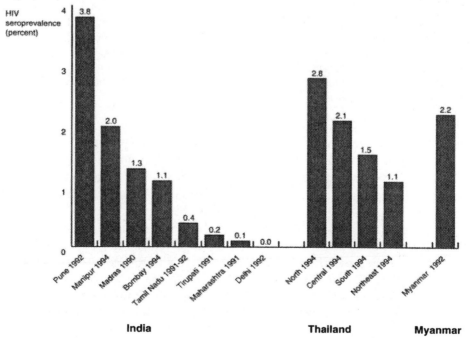

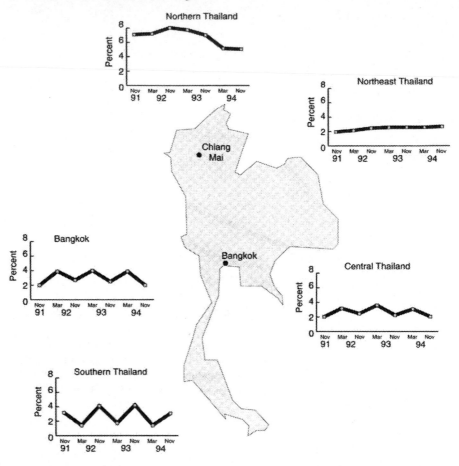

Figure 2-12   HIV seroprevalence among young military service men in Thailand, by year (1990–1994) and by region of assignment. Source: S. Kitsiripornchai, et al., "HIV-1 infection in young men entering the Royal Thai Army: Trends and demographic risk factors," Armed Forces Research Institute of Medical Sciences, Bangkok, Third International Conference on AIDS in Asia and the Pacific, Chiang Mai, Thailand, September, 1995.

northern region of Thailand) have been found among young military service men (Figure 2-12). There is relatively little urban/rural differential in HIV infection rates in this subpopulation. A well-developed transportation infrastructure and high rates of population mobility (including circular migration between rural and urban areas) probably contribute to this finding.

Recent data from urban women in India also show increasing HIV infection levels. Relatively few data are available, however, from the vast rural population of India. The spread of HIV in this country is illustrated by geographic trends (22 of the 32 states in the country have now detected the presence of HIV) (Figure 2-13). Temporal trends emphasize the potential for rapid spread. For example, HIV infection levels among Bombay women sex workers were 20 percent in 1992, but increased to more than 40 percent in this population in 1994. Similar trends are visible in women sex workers in most regions of Thailand, despite successful efforts in promoting condom

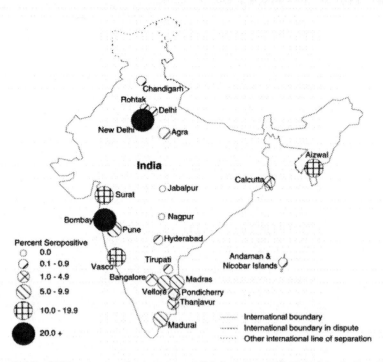

Figure 2-13 HIV seroprevalence among "high-risk populations" in India, 1993–1994.

Figure 2-14 HIV seroprevalence among women sex workers in Thailand, 1990–1994.

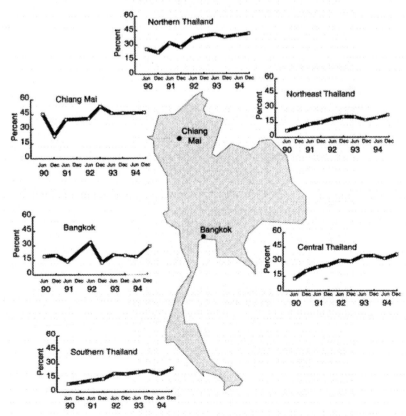

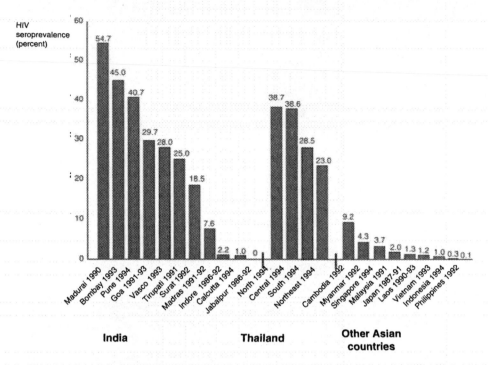

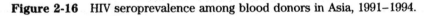

Figure 2-15 HIV seroprevalence among women sex workers in Asia, 1986–1994.

Figure 2-16 HIV seroprevalence among blood donors in Asia, 1991–1994.

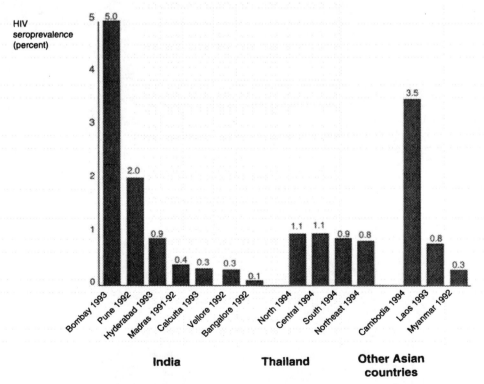

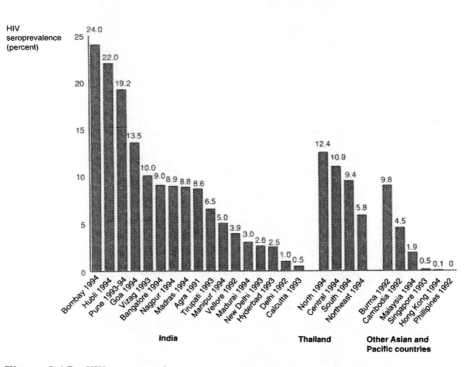

Figure 2-17 HIV seroprevalence among male STI clinic patients in Asia, 1991–1994.

Figure 2-18 HIV seroprevalence among IDU in Malaysia, 1988–1991.

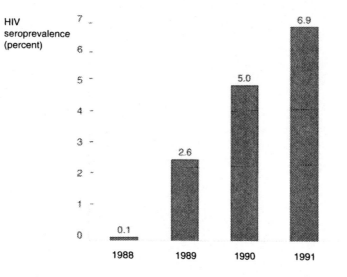

use and widespread media campaigns and declining STI rates in several sex worker populations (Figure 2-14).

HIV infection among sex workers now exceeds 20 percent in all four regions in Thailand and in several areas of India (Figure 2-15). Testing of sex workers in Cambodia and Myanmar shows considerable infection where little had existed before.

Although blood donors may not provide a representative sample of the general population, increasing seroprevalence among blood donors is often an indication of spread of HIV in the population at large. Recent data from Cambodia and Laos confirm the beginnings of epidemics in these countries, and data from India, Thailand, and Myanmar show substantial HIV infection rates in the blood donor population (Figure 2-16).

Male STI clinic patients in selected Asian countries also exhibit high levels of infection: HIV seroprevalence exceeded 16 percent in northern Thailand and 11 percent in Myanmar (Figure 2-17). In India, about one in seven patients was HIV infected at STI clinics in New Delhi and Pune. HIV prevalence rates among STI patients in Thailand are decreasing. In June 1993 rates were over 16 percent. The June 1994 rate fell to 12.4 percent. HIV seroprevalence in injecting drug users in Malaysia increased more than sevenfold between 1988 and 1991 (Figure 2-18).

3

The Evolving HIV/AIDS Pandemic

BRUCE G. WENIGER AND SETH BERKLEY

The HIV pandemic is evolving and becoming increasingly complex. Contrary to what, amazingly, is still popular belief, HIV is not spread predominantly among urban male homosexuals in most countries. By 1992, an estimated 71 percent of all cumulative HIV infections had been acquired heterosexually.[1] The pandemic has also increasingly burdened developing countries, women, and the poor.

The HIV pandemic's increasing complexity has become apparent through the contributions of behavioral sciences (Chapter 9); in reports from populations and regions not previously well studied; through newer techniques of viral analysis; and finally, through reanalysis of its evolution. HIV transmission involves more complex and diverse subpatterns than was originally thought.[2,3] This chapter examines five examples to illustrate the complexity and evolution of the HIV pandemic: (1) traditional "risk-groups" contain multiple subgroups that may differ greatly in their knowledge, perceptions, behaviors, and actual risks for acquiring HIV; (2) HIV transmission persists in populations initially affected (men having sex with men, injecting drug users, and recipients of contaminated blood and blood products) and, globally, is increasingly in the heterosexual population; (3) the pandemic is reaching new populations and geographical areas; (4) separate epidemics may exist alongside with minimal interaction; and (5) economic and political trends may facilitate HIV transmission into new areas and among new population subgroups.

Traditional risk groups are not monolithic

The HIV epidemic was initially recognized among white male homosexuals in large U.S. cities. This relatively affluent and highly educated group championed the initial push for AIDS prevention and care. Later studies of homosexual men in these same cities documented substantial reduction in HIV incidence during the 1980s.[4-6] By the late 1980s, however, it became clear that younger homosexual men—adolescents and men in their early twenties—were engaging in frequent unprotected and multipartner sex. For example, in 1989, 44 percent of homosexual men younger than 30 years old had unprotected anal intercourse during the previous year, compared to only 18 percent of men over 30 years old.[7] It became clear that "risk groups" for HIV infection were neither static nor monolithic populations, but consisted of separate cohorts.

Another recent finding is that high-risk behavior is directly tied to socioeconomic status and is inversely proportional to income, shifting the burden of HIV/AIDS in industrialized countries towards impoverished populations.[8,9] For example, while AIDS prevalence in Philadelphia, Pennsylvania, increased 62 percent from 1988 to 1990, those classified as low income increased by 113 percent, compared with 88 percent and 14 percent increases among middle- and high-income groups.[10] The epidemic's tendency to affect more heavily groups who are discriminated against, have less access to information and services, and lack a supportive social environment has been further substantiated by other reports.[11] In one study, African-American gay and bisexual men in the United States were at higher risk of both STIs and HIV infection than white men with similar behaviors.[12] Another study found HIV seroprevalence among 16–22-year-old African-American gay men in San Francisco and Berkeley, California to be 40 percent, about four times higher than in white gay men of the same age-group.[13]

In Africa, where heterosexual transmission has consistently been the dominant mode of HIV transmission and where seroprevalence among adults in some capital cities exceeds 20 percent, HIV infection is no longer restricted to core high-risk groups.[14] Initially, HIV infection in African men was generally documented among those with higher socioeconomic status. It was postulated that these men could afford multiple sexual partners, pay for sex, and travel away from home. For example, a study among pregnant women in a large urban hospital in Malawi demonstrated an association between a husband's socioeconomic status (as measured by his level of education) and the likelihood of HIV infection in his wife (Figure 3-1).[15] Similar results were found in Tanzania and in other countries in Africa. A possible explanation for this is that their sexual partners belong to the more affluent social class and are more likely (as mentioned above) to have acquired HIV infection early in the pandemic. However, even in the earliest period of the epidemic there was evidence that this pattern did not apply universally and was already changing. Thus, in a well-designed population-based study in Uganda, male heads of poor households were more likely to be HIV infected than heads of wealthier households: infection rates were 13 percent, 11.4 percent, and 7 percent in three strata of increasing household income, respectively.[16] Although comparable studies have not been done in Asia, limited available data and observations suggest that HIV infection is already concentrated in lower socioeconomic groups.[17]

Increased heterosexual transmission in industrialized countries

Over the last 5 years, heterosexual HIV transmission has been rising in industrialized countries—primarily among people in impoverished commu-

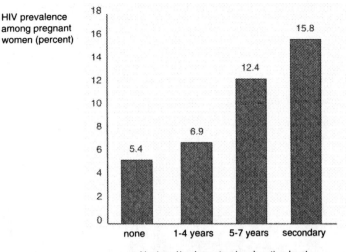

Figure 3-1 Increasing prevalence of HIV infection among pregnant women in Malawi, associated with increased educational level of their husbands or male partners. Source: G.A. Dallabetta, P.G. Miotti, J.D. Chiphangwi, et al., "High socioeconomic status is a risk factor for human immunodeficiency virus type 1 (HIV-1) infection but not for sexually transmitted diseases in women in Malawi: Implication for HIV-1 control," *Journal of Infectious Diseases* 167(1993):36–42.

nities and among people of lower socioeconomic status. In Europe the proportion of AIDS cases attributed to heterosexual transmission of HIV increased from 11.4 percent in 1990 to 16.5 percent in the first 6 months of 1995 (Figure 3-2). In the same period, the proportion of AIDS cases due to transmission through drug use remained stable at around 44 percent, and the proportion of cases involving homosexual and bisexual men declined from 39 percent to 26.5 percent.[18]

In the United States over the last decade, the proportion of AIDS cases who are women has increased steadily: 18 percent of the 79,674 adult and adolescent AIDS cases reported in 1994 were women. Although 41 percent of these women had injected drugs, compared to 38 percent with a risk of heterosexual contact, heterosexual transmission probably constitutes the most frequent route of infection since 19 percent of women had uncertain or unreported risk factors. Upon investigation, two-thirds of these women were found to have been infected sexually.[19] In an STI clinic in the Bronx, New York, HIV seroprevalence was 3.6 percent in men and 4.2 percent in women among clients whose only risk factor was heterosexual activity; having large numbers of sexual partners and the use of crack cocaine elevated risk.[20] A similar pattern has been documented in Detroit and other inner-city communities in the United States.[21]

Studies have shown that African women and men are infected with HIV in relatively equal numbers. In countries with more mature epidemics, like Uganda and Tanzania, HIV infection rates among women exceed rates for men.[22,23] Most of these women, particularly those in traditional marriages or

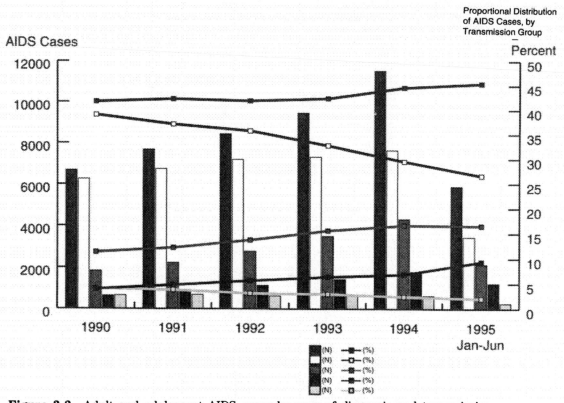

Figure 3-2 Adult and adolescent AIDS cases by year of diagnosis and transmission group, WHO European region, through June, 1995. Source: European Centre for Epidemiological Monitoring of AIDS, *Quarterly Report No. 46* (Saint Maurice, France: European Centre for the Epidemiological Monitoring of AIDS, 1995/2):18–22.

stable partnerships, were probably not infected through their own high-risk sexual activity but rather through the high-risk behaviors of their husbands or partners. One Rwandan study documented infection rates among women with only one lifetime partner at 25 percent.[24] Those women who reported that they knew that their steady partner was not monogamous were more likely to be HIV infected. In a study at an antenatal clinic in Tanzania, more than 50 percent of women reported having only a single sex partner in the last 5 years, yet 9 percent of these women were HIV infected.[25] Many African men became infected through contact with multiple sexual partners, particularly while away from home during trips or seasonal migrations.[26]

In Thailand, husbands are bringing home HIV acquired from extramarital exposures of which wives are often not aware.[27-29] More than one-fifth of Thai males patronize sex workers,[30] and as a result, 1.4 percent of pregnant women surveyed in public hospitals in late 1993 were found to be HIV infected.[31]

In the Americas, women are also at risk of heterosexually acquired infection when their bisexual sexual partners do not inform them of their high-risk behavior. In a Chicago, Illinois (U.S.) study of 333 men who reported sex with both men and women in the previous year, 54 percent reported that none of their female partners knew about their homosexual activities.[32]

The majority of these homosexual encounters were high risk, and the majority of the men did not use condoms with partners of either sex. A study from Costa Rica found that most of the women with AIDS who were surveyed were infected by their male partners who did not generally make known their high-risk sexual behavior.[33]

The shift towards heterosexual transmission throughout Latin America and the Caribbean is well illustrated by AIDS cases that have been reported (Figure 3-3). In Central America, the primary method of transmission in

Figure 3-3 Annual incidence of AIDS cases in the Caribbean and Latin America, by selected risk factors, 1982/1983–1994/1995. 1995 data are incomplete due to delayed reporting. Source: Regional Program on AIDS/STD, Division of Disease Prevention and Control, Pan American Health Organization, *AIDS Surveillance in the Americas*, World Health Organization, PAHO/HCA/Quarterly Report, PAHO/HCA/95-015, September, 1995.

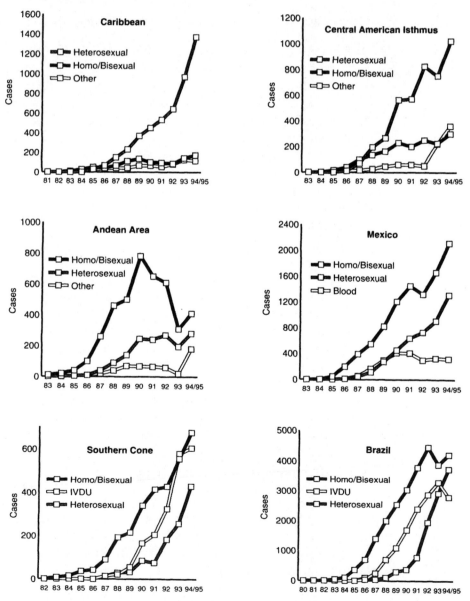

AIDS cases diagnosed over the last 2 years has been through heterosexual intercourse.[34] In the Caribbean, over 80 percent of HIV transmission is already heterosexual. In all these countries, infections are increasingly seen in lower socioeconomic groups. Further south, in 1992 the first anonymous testing unit in Rio de Janeiro, Brazil found an HIV seroprevalence of 22.7 percent among those with the lowest educational levels and 12.2 percent and 8 percent among those with middle and highest levels, respectively.[35] Between 1986 and 1992 the HIV reference center in Belo Horizonte, Brazil documented a tenfold increase in HIV infections. Over this period, the contribution of heterosexual transmission to the total increased from 3.7 percent to 18.6 percent.[36] As elsewhere, this changing pattern was accompanied by a shift in the epidemic's socioeconomic profile: those most recently infected were in a lower income group.

Extension into new geographic areas and population groups

The volatility of the HIV pandemic has also been manifested by its rapid penetration into areas spared during most of the 1980s. As late as 1988, all of Asia was classified as epidemiologic "pattern III," which described areas where few AIDS cases had been reported and relatively little transmission was occurring.[37,38] This classification soon became obsolete, however, and a new epidemiologic pattern appears to have emerged in which IDUs experience rapid HIV transmission, followed by female sex workers and then their clients, their clients' wives, and finally, their offspring.[39-42]

For example, this new epidemiological pattern appeared in 1988 when Thailand experienced an explosive spread of HIV among injecting drug users (IDUs) in Bangkok (from 1 percent HIV infected to over 30 percent in 9 months).[43] By 1989, in its neighbor to the north, Myanmar, 17 percent of IDUs were infected; by 1993 the rate was over 80 percent at several sites.[44] One year later, in 1990, parts of both India and China along the opium routes from Myanmar and the Golden Triangle were affected. In Manipur, in northeast India and just north of Myanmar, HIV infection rates among IDUs increased from zero in early 1989 to over 50 percent in 1990.[45] In the towns of Riuli and Longchuan in China's Yunnan Province on the eastern border of Myanmar, 80 percent of IDUs were found to be infected in 1990.[46,47,48] In 1992 in Malaysia, which borders Thailand to the south, 30 percent of IDUs were HIV infected.[49] Subsequently, in all these countries except China, increasing and alarming HIV rates were also documented among female sex workers and other sentinel heterosexual groups.[50-53]

Separate epidemics may exist side by side

Another feature of the pandemic's complexity is its highly localized impact in which separate epidemics may occur side by side with little interaction. Such a phenomenon may be relatively easy to understand in pre-1994 South Africa, where the structures of apartheid helped sustain separate epidemics among homosexual men in the white community and among heterosexuals in the black population.[54] Furthermore, the intensity of the heterosexual spread of HIV varied according to race: in 1993, the prevalence of HIV infection was 5.6 percent in black women attending antenatal clinics in South Africa, a level more than fivefold higher than among women classified in that country as Asian, Colored, or White.[55]

In New York City, a segregated impact has also occurred; two separate epidemics of HIV have been documented, with little social contact—and thus rare epidemiologic transmission—between them.[56] The first is among men who have sex with men, who are primarily white, but which includes a growing proportion of African-Americans and Hispanics. The second epidemic has occurred among IDUs and their sexual partners and children who live primarily in racially segregated, poverty-stricken, inner-city neighborhoods. As a result, AIDS case rates vary several-fold between different postal districts, reflecting the heterogeneity of risk in New York's diverse economic, ethnic, and social context.[57]

Side-by-side epidemics have also been discovered in Thailand, where the first epidemic wave began among IDUs in 1988, and the second was detected the following year among commercial sex workers.[58] Using technical advances in molecular epidemiology, these two epidemics were found to be unrelated and caused by two distinct genetic variants of HIV-1 circulating in segregated fashion between these two risk groups (Figure 3-4).[59-64] Molecular epidemiology has linked several of the rapidly spreading Asian epidemics (Figure 3-5).[65]

The effect of political and other events

An important source of pandemic dynamism and complexity arises from political and other trends that may enhance transmission in already affected populations or facilitate spread to new geographic areas or to new population subgroups. For example, following the cessation of overt hostilities in the Cambodian civil war in the early 1990s, prostitution increased to service the large number of foreign businessmen, UN troops, and western aid workers who flooded the country to supervise elections, invest in, and help rebuild the country. By the end of 1993, 8 percent of STI clinic patients and 14 percent of women sex workers tested in Cambodia were HIV infected, and at least 2,000 Cambodians were estimated to be HIV infected.[66-68]

In Vietnam and China, decades-long constraints on illicit drugs and prostitution have been partially relaxed as a consequence of economic liberalization, thereby facilitating the arrival and spread of HIV. In Vietnam, 957 HIV infections were reported through November 1993, and mid-1993 serosurveys showed 16 percent (491) of 3,131 IDUs and 1 percent (9) of 1,013 women sex workers infected.[69,70] In China, widespread increases in prostitution have apparently occurred, especially in Guangdong and other southern coastal provinces where free enterprise has most rapidly developed. While IDUs in Yunnan Province constitute 80 percent (899) of the 1,106 HIV infections detected in China through June 24, 1993, there is a paucity of surveys among other high-risk groups elsewhere in China.[71]

Mode of transmission

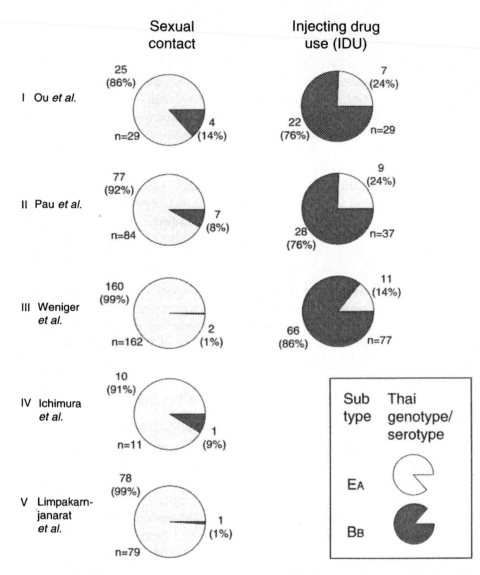

Figure 3-4 Separate epidemics coexist side by side. Source: Molecular Epidemiology of HIV in Asia, B. Weniger, Y. Takebe, Chin-Yih Ou, and S. Yamazaki, *AIDS* 1994, 8(Suppl 2):S19.

International efforts to suppress the narcotics trade may also influence the volatility of the pandemic.[72] More successful law enforcement efforts during the 1980s tended to shift illicit drug refineries closer to the areas of drug cultivation. Police pressure also encouraged smugglers to handle more concentrated forms of drugs, such as heroin and cocaine, which require smaller volumes to conceal than their equivalent in opium or coca paste. With a more valuable product available in areas of cultivation and transshipment, users have an incentive to use more efficient means of drug administra-

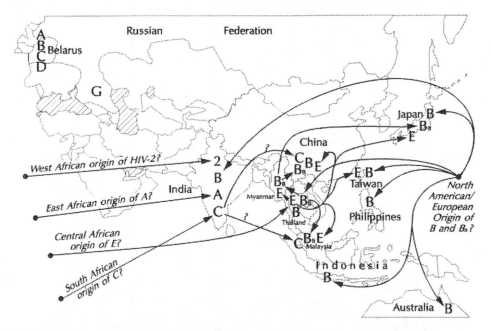

Figure 3-5 Countries where HIV-1 subtypes and HIV-2 have been documented, and probable origins of introductions and hypothesized routes of spread. Adapted from B. G. Weniger et al., "The Molecular Epidemiology of HIV in Asia," *AIDS in Asia and the Pacific, AIDS* 1994; 8(suppl 2):s13–s28. Courtesy of Current Science, Ltd.

tion, such as injection, compared to the use of product by smoking or ingestion. For example, in the Chinese county of Riuli, drug users shifted to the injection of opium and its derivatives between 1983, when none used needles, and 1990, by which time one-third reported injecting drug use (Figure 3-6).[73]

In South America, the cocaine trade routes that ran from the Andean cultivation areas in Peru and Bolivia to Colombia and onwards to North America were increasingly suppressed in the 1980s. As a result, the product was diverted to the east and south, into Argentina and Brazil[74] (Figure 3-7). The southwest Brazilian state of Mato Grosso do Sul, which lies on the cocaine smuggling route between the Andes countries and the great metropolitan areas of São Paulo and Rio de Janeiro, experienced a fivefold increase in AIDS cases between 1987 and 1991.[75] This geographic penetration of the pandemic was accompanied by an extension into the newer risk group of adolescents who were primarily consuming the cocaine. In Mato Grosso do Sul, 58 percent of AIDS cases were attributable to injection of drugs.

In summary, from an epidemic once apparently restricted to certain groups engaging in high-risk behavior in a few world regions, HIV has moved steadily into larger and more diverse populations at risk in many of the world's regions. Adolescents and those living in poverty or suffering discrimination are becoming infected disproportionately in many societies. Young women are at particular risk, even among those who engage in no risky behaviors themselves. Spreading along increasingly complex pathways, the HIV pandemic has penetrated all the major population centers in the world to constitute an enormous and growing challenge.

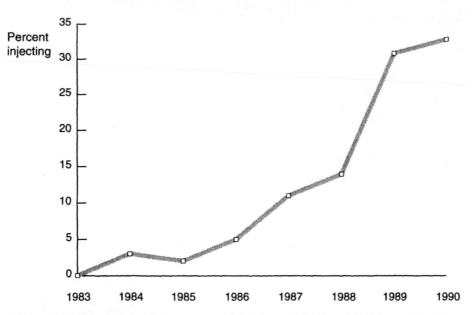

Figure 3-6 Proportion of drug users who inject, Ruili County, Yunnan Province, China. [Source: X. Zheng et al., ref. 46.]

Figure 3-7 Cocaine trafficking routes in the Western hemisphere. [Source: U.S. Department of Justice, ref. 74.]

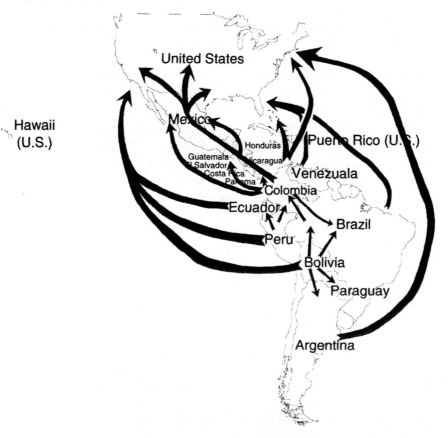

REFERENCES

1. J. Mann, D. Tarantola, and T. Netter, eds., *AIDS in the World* (Cambridge, MA: Harvard University Press, 1992).
2. J. M. Mann, J. Chin, P. Piot, and T. Quinn, "International epidemiology of AIDS," *Scientific American* 259(1988):82–89.
3. P. Piot, F. A. Plummer, F. S. Mhalu, L.-J. Lamborary, J. Chin, and J. M. Mann, "AIDS: An international perspective," *Science* 239(1988):573–579.
4. W. Winkelstein, M. Samuel, N. S. Padian, J. A. Wiley, et al., "San Francisco Men's Health Study III. Reduction in HIV transmission among homosexual/bisexual men, 1982–86," *American Journal of Public Health* 77(1987):685–689.
5. S. C. Hadler, D. P. Francis, J. E. Maynard, et al., "Long-term immunogenicity and efficacy of hepatitis B vaccine in homosexual men," *New England Journal of Medicine* 315(1986):209–214.
6. R. L. Berkelman, W. L. Heyward, J. K. Stehr-Green, and J. W. Curran, "Epidemiology of human immunodeficiency virus infection and acquired immunodeficiency syndrome," *American Journal of Medicine* 86(1989):761–770.
7. R. Stall, D. Barrett, L. Bye, J. Catania, C. Frutchey, J. Henne, G. Lemp, and J. Paul, "Comparison of younger and older gay men's HIV risk-taking behaviors: The Communications Technologies 1989 Cross-Sectional Survey," *Journal of Acquired Immune Deficiency Syndromes* 5(1992):682–687.
8. W. Winkelstein, J. A. Wiley, D. Osmond et al., "San Francisco young men's health study," Abstract WS-C07-3, presented at the IX International Conference on AIDS, Berlin, Germany, June 1993.
9. R. W. Connell, G. W. Dowsett, P. Rodden, et al., "Social class, gay men and AIDS prevention," *Australian Journal of Public Health* 15(1991):178–189.
10. Pan American Health Organization, *AIDS/HIV/STD Annual Surveillance Report, 1992*, draft (Washington, DC: PAHO, 1994).
11. J. Mann, D. Tarantola, and T. Netter, "Assessing vulnerability to HIV infection and AIDS," in *AIDS in the World*, J. Mann, D. Tarantola, and T. Netter, eds. (Cambridge, MA: Harvard University Press, 1992):577–602.
12. S. D. Cochran and V. M. Mays, "STD and HIV incidence in a national sample of U.S. black gay and bisexual men," Abstract PO-CO3-2618, presented at the IX International Conference on AIDS, Berlin, Germany, June 1993.
13. A. M. Hirozawa, D. Givertz, G. Lemp, G. Nieri, L. Anderson, and M. Katz, "Prevalence of HIV-1 among young gay and bisexual men (GBM) in San Francisco (SF) and Berkeley, CA: The second young men's survey," Abstract PO-C12–2875, presented at the IX International Conference on AIDS, Berlin, Germany, June 1993.
14. Final Report on the Workshop on the Status and Trends of the HIV/AIDS Epidemic in Africa, co-sponsored by The AIDS Control and Prevention Project of Family Health International and the François-Xavier Bagnoud Center for Health and Human Rights, Harvard School of Public Health, held in Kampala, 8–9 December, 1995.
15. G. A. Dallabetta, P. G. Miotti, J. D. Chiphangwi, et al., "High socioeconomic status is a risk factor for human immunodeficiency virus type 1 (HIV-1) infection but not for sexually transmitted diseases in women in Malawi: Implications for HIV-1 control," *Journal of Infectious Diseases* 167(1993):36–42.
16. J. A. Seeley, S. S. Malamba, A. K. Nunn, and D. W. Mulder, "Socio-economic status and vulnerability in a rural community in south-west Uganda," Abstract M.D.4030, presented at the VII International Conference on AIDS, Florence, Italy, June 1991.
17. D. E. Bloom and S. Giled, "Who is bearing the cost of the AIDS epidemic in Asia," in

Economic Implications of AIDS in Asia, D. E. Bloom and J. V. Lyons, eds. (New Delhi: UN Development Programme, 1993).

18. European Centre for the Epidemiological Monitoring of AIDS, "HIV/AIDS surveillance in Europe," *Quarterly Report* 46 (Saint Maurice, France: European Centre for the Epidemiological Monitoring of AIDS, 1995):2–18.

19. Centers for Disease Control and Prevention, *HIV/AIDS Surveillance Report*, 6(no.2)(1994):1–39.

20. M. A. Chiasson, R. L. Stoneburner, D. S. Hildebrandt, W. E. Ewing, E. E. Telzak, and H. W. Jaffe, "Heterosexual transmission of HIV-1 associated with the use of smokable freebase cocaine (crack)," *AIDS* 5(1991):1121–1126.

21. L. R. Crane, "Sentinel surveillance for HIV infection in Detroit: Heterosexual transmission in a medium prevalence city. The AIDS Program," Abstract PoC 4013, presented at the VIII International Conference on AIDS, Amsterdam, The Netherlands, July 1992.

22. S. F. Berkley, W. Naamara, S. I. Okware, et al., "AIDS and HIV infection in women in Uganda—are women more infected than males?" *AIDS* 4(1990):1237–1242.

23. L. R. Barongo, M. W. Borgdorff, F. F. Mosha, et al., "Epidemiology of HIV-1 infection in urban areas, roadside settlements and rural villages in Mwanza Region, Tanzania," *AIDS* 6(1992):1521–1528.

24. S. Allen, C. Lindan, A. Serufilira, et al., "Human immunodeficiency virus infection in urban Rwanda," *Journal of the American Medical Association* 266(1991):1657–1663.

25. D. J. Hunter, S. H. Kapiga, G. Lwihula, et al., "Risk factors for HIV-1 infection among family planning clinic clients in Dar-es-Salaam," Abstract PoC 4160, presented at the VIII International Conference on AIDS, Amsterdam, The Netherlands, July 1992.

26. G. Pison, B. Le Guenno, E. Lagarde, C. Enel, and C. Seck, "Seasonal migration: A risk factor for HIV infection in rural Senegal," *Journal of Acquired Immune Deficiency Syndromes* 6(1993):196–200.

27. B. G. Weniger, "Experience from HIV incidence cohorts in Thailand: Implications for HIV vaccine efficacy trials," *AIDS* 8(1994):1007–1010.

28. T. Brown, W. Sittitrai, S. Vanichseni, and U. Thisyakorn, "Recent epidemiology of HIV/AIDS in Thailand," *AIDS* 8(suppl. 2)(1994):s131–s141.

29. W. Sittitrai and T. Brown, "Risk factors for HIV infection in Thailand," *AIDS* 8(suppl. 2)(1994):s143–s153.

30. W. Sittitrai, P. Phanuphak, J. Barry, and T. Brown, *Thai Sexual Behavior and Risk of HIV Infection: A Report of the 1990 Survey of Partner Relations and Risk of HIV Infection in Thailand* (Bangkok: Program on AIDS, Thai Red Cross Society; and Institute of Population Studies, Chulalongkorn University, November 1992).

31. Brown, "Recent epidemiology."

32. J. Stokes, D. McKirnan, B. Burzette, and P. Vanable, "Female sexual partners of bisexual men: What they don't know might hurt them," Abstract WS-D08-5, presented at the IX International Conference on AIDS, Berlin, Germany, June 1993.

33. Pan American Health Organization, *Acquired Immunodeficiency Syndrome in the Americas*, CE111/9 (Washington, DC: PAHO, May 27, 1993).

34. Pan American Health Organization, *AIDS/HIV/STD Annual Surveillance Report*.

35. M. T. A. Fragoso and C. F. Ramos-Filho, "First results from the first anonymous testing unit established in Rio de Janeiro, Brazil," Abstract PO-C30-3277, presented at the IX International Conference on AIDS, Berlin, Germany, June 1993.

36. D. B. Greco, A. C. C. Toledo, H.C.A. Oliveira, and P. R. A. Cordeiro, "Changes in epidemiological characteristics of a population with high risk behavior for HIV infection in Belo Horizonte, Brazil (1986–92)," Abstract WS-CO4-3, presented at the IX International Conference on AIDS, Berlin, Germany, June 1993.

37. J. M. Mann, "International epidemiology of AIDS."

38. P. Pitot, "AIDS: An international perspective."

39. B. G. Weniger, K. Limpakarnjanarat, K. Ungchusak, et al., "Epidemiology of HIV infection and AIDS in Thailand," *AIDS* 5(suppl. 2)(1991):s71–s85 [errata corrected in 7(1993)147].

40. B. G. Weniger, P. Thongcharoen, T. J. John, et al., "HIV epidemic in Thailand, India, and neighboring nations: A fourth epidemiologic pattern emerges in Asia," Abstract PoC 4087, presented at the VIII International Conference on AIDS, Amsterdam, The Netherlands, July 1992.

41. B. G. Weniger, P. Thongcharoen, T. J. John, K. Pavri, M. T. Htoon, and X. Zheng, "Emerging epidemiologic pattern of HIV/AIDS in South and East Asia," Abstract TuP 4-21, presented at the XIII International Congress on Tropical Medicine and Malaria, Pattaya, Thailand, December 1992.

42. T. Brown and P. Xenos, *AIDS in Asia: The Gathering Storm*, AsiaPacific Issues series 16 (Honolulu, Hawaii: East-West Center, August 1994).

43. Weniger, "Epidemiology of HIV infection."

44. M. T. Htoon, H. T. Lwin, K. O. San, E. Zan, and M. Thwe, "HIV/AIDS in Myanmar," *AIDS* 8(suppl. 2)(1994):s105–s109.

45. S. Sarkar, N. Das, S. Panda, et al., "Rapid spread of HIV among injecting drug users in north-eastern states of India," *Bulletin on Narcotics* 45(1993):91–105.

46. X. Zheng, C. Tian, J. Zhang, et al., "Preliminary study of the behavior of 225 drug abusers and the risk factors of HIV infection in Ruili County, Yunnan Province, China," *Chung Hua Liu Hsing Ping Hsueh Tsa Chi (Chinese Journal of Epidemiology)* 12(1991):12–14.

47. X. Zheng, C. Tian, J. Zhang, T. Hall, J. Mandel, and N. Hearst, "Rapid spread of HIV among drug users and their wives in southwest China," Abstract PO-C08-2766, presented at the IX International Conference on AIDS, Berlin, Germany, June 1993.

48. X. Zheng, J. Zhang, C. Tian, et al., "Cohort study of HIV infection among drug users in Riuli City and Longchuan County, Yunnan Province, China" (in Chinese), *Chung Hua Liu Hsing Ping Hsueh Tsa Chi (Chinese Journal of Epidemiology)* 14(1993):3–5.

49. S. Singh and N. Crofts, "HIV infection among injecting drug users in north-east Malaysia," *AIDS Care* 5(1993):273–281.

50. Weniger, "Epidemiology of HIV infection."

51. Htoon, "HIV/AIDS in Myanmar."

52. S. Singh and N. Crofts, "HIV infection."

53. M. K. Jain, T. J. John, and G. T. Keusch. "Epidemiology of HIV and AIDS in India," *AIDS* 8(1994)(suppl. 2):s61–s75.

54. D. J. Martin, B. D. Schoub, G. N. Padayachee, et al., "One year surveillance of HIV-1 infection in Johannesburg, South Africa," *Transactions of the Royal Society of Tropical Medicine and Hygiene* 84(1990):728–730.

55. "Fourth national HIV survey of women attending antenatal clinics, South Africa, October/November 1993," *Epidemiological Comments* 21(4) (Pretoria, April 1994):68–91.

56. J. Gagnon, S. Lindenbaum, A. Jonsen, J. Stryker, and J. Trussel, "HIV/AIDS epidemic in New York City," in *Social Impact of AIDS in the United States*, A. R. Jonsen and J. Stryker, eds. (Washington, DC: National Academy Press, 1993):243–302.

57. *Ibid.*

58. Weniger, "Epidemiology of HIV infection."

59. B. G. Weniger, Y. Takebe, C.-Y. Ou, and S. Yamazaki, "Molecular epidemiology of HIV in Asia," *AIDS* 8(suppl.2)(1994):s13–s28.

60. C.-Y. Ou, Y. Takebe, B. G. Weniger, et al., "Independent introduction of two major

HIV-1 genotypes into distinct high-risk populations in Thailand," *Lancet* 341(1993):1171–1174 [errata corrected in 342(1993):250].

61. C.-P. Pau, S. Lee-Thomas, W. Auwanit, et al., "Highly specific V3-peptide enzyme immunoassay for serotyping HIV-1 specimens from Thailand," *AIDS* 7(1993):337–340.

62. B. G. Weniger, S. Tansuphaswadikul, N. L. Young, C-P. Pau, P. Lohsomboon, W. Yindeeyoungyeon, and K. Limpakarnjanarat, "Differences in immune function among patients infected with distinct Thailand HIV-1 strains," Abstract 012C, presented at the X International Conference on AIDS/International Conference on STD, 7–12 August 1994, Yokohama, Japan.

63. H. Ichimura, S. C. Klicks, S. Visrutratna, C-Y. Ou, M. L. Kalish, and J. A. Levy, "Biologic, serologic, and genetic characterization of HIV-1 subtype E isolates from Northern Thailand," *AIDS Research and Human Retroviruses* 10(1994):261–267.

64. K. Limpakarnjanarat, T. D. Mastro, C-P. Pau, N. L. Young, S. Korattana, and B. G. Weniger, "Prevalence and incidence of Thai HIV-1 genotypes in a cohort of female prostitutes in Northern Thailand," Abstract PO-C02-4435, presented at the IX International Conference on AIDS, Berlin, 6–11 June 1993.

65. B. G. Weniger, "Molecular epidemiology."

66. "Pasteur Institute reports AIDS findings" (in English), *Bangkok Post* (October 31, 1993):20–21, reprinted in *JPRS Report—Epidemiology*, 94WE0083A (Washington, DC: Foreign Broadcast Information Service, March 3, 1994).

67. Agence France Presse, Phnom Penh, "Cambodia: Health ministry estimates 1,000 AIDS virus carriers," broadcast on Hong Kong AFP (in English) (July 25, 1993), printed in *JPRS Report—Epidemiology*, BK2507080493 (Washington, DC: Foreign Broadcast Information Service, August 20, 1993):9.

68. Agence France Presse, Phnom Penh, "Government sets up anti-AIDS commission" (in English) (December 24, 1993), reprinted in *JPRS Report—Epidemiology*, BK24D0504 (Washington, DC: Foreign Broadcast Information Service, February 3, 1994):7.

69. T. H. Nguyen and I. Wolffers, "HIV infection in Vietnam," *Lancet* 343(1994):410.

70. Do Hong Ngoc, personal communication (1993).

71. L. Zheng, "AIDS situation updates" (in Chinese), *Beijing Jian Kang Bao* (June 25, 1993), reprinted in *JPRS Report—Epidemiology* (in English), 93P60311A (Washington, DC: Foreign Broadcast Information Service, August 20, 1993):7.

72. D. C. Des Jarlais, S. R. Friedman, K. Choopanya, S. Vanichseni, and T. P. Ward, "International epidemiology of HIV and AIDS among injecting drug users," *AIDS* 6(1992):1053–1068.

73. Zheng, "Preliminary study."

74. U.S. Department of Justice, *Drugs, Crime, and the Justice System: A National Report from the Bureau of Justice Statistics*, NCJ-133652 (Washington, DC: U.S. Department of Justice, December 1992).

75. L. Guerra de Macedo Rodrigues, "AIDS, e uso de drogas injetíveis no Brasil" ("AIDS, and use of injected drugs in Brazil," in Portuguese), *AIDS Boletim Epidemiológico*, semana epidemiológica 27–30, 6(1993):2–7.

4

The Spread of HIV and Sexual Mixing Patterns

ROY M. ANDERSON

Many have wondered about the likely duration of the HIV/AIDS epidemic, either within a particular risk group or within a country. This short review considers this question with reference to the spread of infection within and between different at-risk groups. Theoretical and empirical studies are employed to assess the degree to which the epidemic will consist of a series of distinct waves of disease as the infection spreads from high-, to medium-, and to low-risk groups.

The historical and epidemiological literature abounds with accounts of infectious diseases invading human communities and of their impact on social organization and historical events.[1,2] We typically think of a new epidemic in a "virgin" population as something that arises suddenly, sweeps through the population in a few months, and then wanes and disappears. Indeed, the classical epidemic curve for many respiratory or intestinal tract viral and bacterial infections is bell-shaped, with an overall duration of a few months to a year or so. Figure 4-1 illustrates a well-documented example, the 1665 plague in London, believed to have killed about one-third of the population in a few months.[3]

The factors determining the shape of these simple epidemic curves have been the focus of much research and controversy, both in the 19th and 20th centuries.[4] Today the consensus is that how rapidly the curve rises is determined by the average number of secondary cases of infection generated by one primary case in a susceptible population. This is called the *basic* or *case reproductive rate* (R_0). After the infection has spread through the population, the prevalence of infection rises, and many of a new case's "contacts" involve people who are either currently infectious or who have recovered from the infection and have acquired a degree of immunity. In a population in which only some are susceptible to infection, the effective reproductive rate (R) may fall below unity (1) in value. That is, each primary case fails to generate at least one secondary case. At this point, the epidemic begins to wane and the curve may decline rapidly.

Even in a densely populated community not everyone will be infected during the course of an epidemic. The fraction infected depends on the

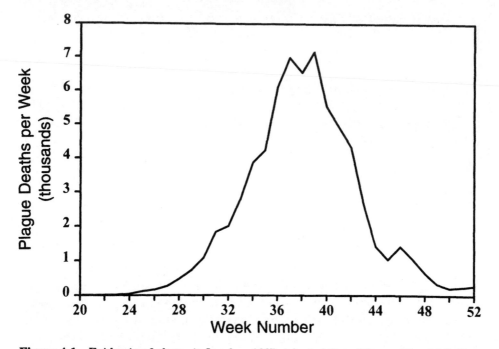

Figure 4-1   Epidemic of plague in London, 1665. Adapted from *Diary of Daniel DeFoe*.

magnitude of the basic reproductive rate, R_0, at the start of the epidemic*
and, in particular, on the value of one of its component parameters, namely,
transmission efficiency. *Transmission efficiency* is expressed as the probability that a contact will occur between infected and susceptible individuals
multiplied by the likelihood that a contact will result in transmission.

The duration of the epidemic is determined by a variety of factors, but the
generation period is of particular importance. That period is defined as the
time from initial infection to the end of the infectious period (whether terminated by recovery or death). For infectious diseases with a 2-week generation period such as measles, an epidemic's duration is typically about 6
months to a year. If the generation period lasts for several years, the epidemic's duration will be from a few to many decades, depending on the
magnitude of the basic reproductive rate R_0. The reproductive number (R)
is essentially defined in units of time of the generation period.

The incubation period of AIDS

As noted above, generation period is a key determinant of the epidemic's
duration. It is important to note that in the case of HIV/AIDS, the generation
time from initial infection to the end of the infectious period is approximately equal to the average incubation period. Current estimates for indus-

---

*For a simple epidemic in a closed population (i.e., no new births, no immigration or emigra-
tion) the fraction infected, (f), is given by the implicit function $1 - f = \exp(-fR_0)$. [J. H.
Gillespie, "Natural selection for resistance to epidemics," *Ecology* 56(1975):493–495, and R. M.
Anderson and R. M. May, "Coevolution of hosts and parasites," *Parasitology* 85(1982):411–426.]

trialized countries suggest a median period of roughly 10 to 12 years in adults aged 20 to 50, irrespective of gender or risk group (Figure 4-2).

The median incubation period is shorter in children and elderly people. In addition, the incubation period may lengthen due to either a change in the definition of AIDS or to improvements in the use of antiviral therapy. The best available data derive from longitudinal studies of people for whom the date of seroconversion is known (at least to within a few months); the longest of these studies have run for approximately 15 years. About 50 to 60 percent of the patients in these cohort studies have developed AIDS by year 12 to 15. Given uncertainties about what fraction of infected people will eventually develop AIDS, the median incubation period may eventually increase or decrease over time, depending on whether the trend in the far right of the lines in Figure 4-2 continues to go up or settles to a stable value less than unity. Data on the incubation period in developing countries is very limited, but recent evidence suggests the median period there may be much shorter in adults[5] (see Appendix B).

These observations are important for assessing the current and future demographic impact of AIDS in the worst afflicted regions of sub-Saharan Africa. Figure 4-3 provides two projections of the impact of AIDS on population growth in a country where a 3 percent annual population growth rate existed prior to the arrival of HIV.[6] The major point of these projections is the relationship between the incubation period, the prevalence of infection in sexually active women over the first 20 years of the epidemic, and the per capita population growth rate. In the early stages of the epidemic (the first 14 years), greater demographic impact and lower HIV prevalence is induced

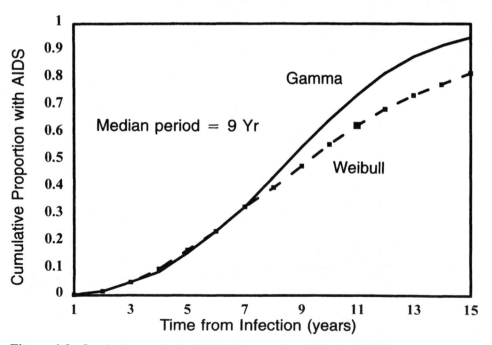

Figure 4-2   Incubation period of AIDS. Source: Hendriks et al. (1993).

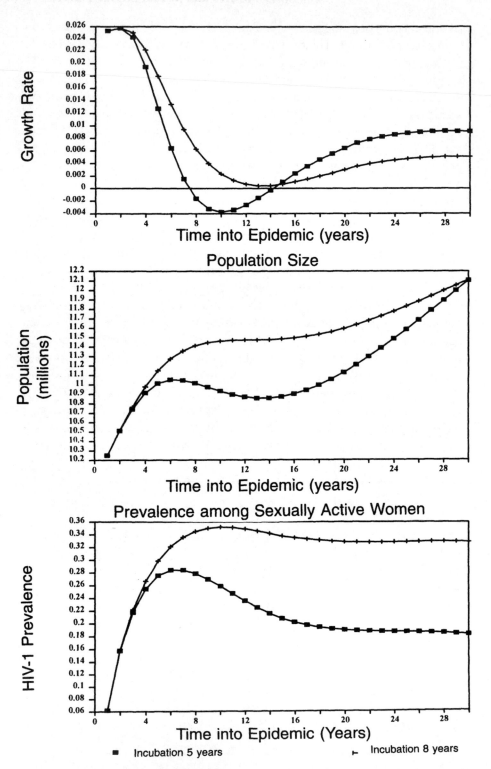

Figure 4-3 Projected impact of AIDS on population growth and population size, and HIV prevalence among sexually active women.

by the shorter incubation period, since the rate of turnover of the infected population is somewhat higher.

Infectiousness during the incubation period

An important determinant of the duration of an AIDS epidemic in a defined community is the manner in which an infected individual's infectiousness varies during the incubation period. For a typical (non-HIV) viral infection, infectiousness is closely correlated with viral abundance in the infected person. Whether this is true for HIV remains unclear, although limited evidence suggests some association between infectiousness and viral burden.

In a typical HIV-infected person, plasma viremia and/or the fraction of infected CD4+ cells varies considerably during the incubation period. Ignoring for a moment the initial phase of primary HIV infection (the few months immediately after infection), a variety of studies have found a steady rise in viremia or the fraction of infected CD4+ cells as a patient progresses to AIDS. More generally, if the burst of viremia associated with primary HIV infection is also taken into account, the pattern of change in viral abundance (or burden) seems to range from high, soon after infection, to low for a period of many years, with a return to high as the patient progresses to AIDS (Figure 4-4).* Irrespective of the mechanisms underlying this pattern, its shape is of great relevance to the duration of the epidemic. Little is understood at present about the relative changes in infectiousness during the two peaks of viremia. Infected individuals may be most infectious during the first peak in viremia, since the virus is more closely related to viral types that were transmitted, in comparison with the virus present in an AIDS patient in whom the virus has evolved for 10 years or more, because selective pressures within the host may be different from those acting in transmission between hosts.

While this remains speculation at present, it can provide a rough idea of how variability of infectiousness may influence the duration of the epidemic. Consider a simple example with two major phases of infectiousness, one early and one late in the incubation period, separated by a long phase of essentially zero infectiousness. Figure 4-5 illustrates three simulated epidemics, with all epidemiological parameters identical except for relative infectiousness in the early and late phases of the incubation period. In one example, the first phase of viremia is a highly infectious period while the late phase is of low infectiousness (A), in the next example, both phases are of equal infectiousness (B), and in the last (C), the early phase is of low and

*The biological processes responsible for this "two-peaked" pattern are the subject of much argument and discussion at present. However, the simplest hypothesis is that it is a direct result of the cytopathic properties of the virus (i.e., killing CD4+ cells), combined with immune selection and antigenic variation. The virus continually generates new "escape" mutants (antigenic variants which are new to the immune system) which are sequentially brought under control by the immune system until CD4+ cell abundance is too low to control the antigenically diverse viral population. [M. A. Nowak, R. M. Anderson, A. R. McLean, T. F. W. Wolfs, J. Goudsmit, and R. M. May, "Antigenic diversity thresholds and the development of AIDS," *Science* 254(1991):963–969.]

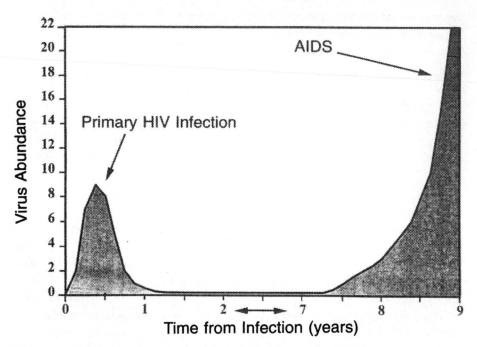

Figure 4-4 Variable viremia over the incubation period of AIDS.

Figure 4-5 Shape of the epidemic based on variable infectiousness.

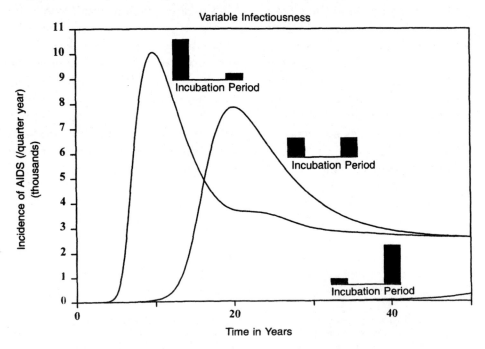

the late phase is of high infectiousness. The epidemic eventually settles to a stable endemic state, *at the same level* in each case. However, the time taken to reach this endemic state varies greatly, being fastest for (A), the case in which the first period is of greatest infectiousness, and slowest in (C), the converse of this case. This simple example contains an important message. While the generation period of the infection is one of the major determinants of the epidemic's duration, the pattern of change in infectiousness (= transmissibility) over this generation period is equally important. Current evidence for HIV is inconclusive concerning which period contributes most to transmission. However, many epidemiologists feel the first period soon after infection is of greatest importance.

Shape of the simple epidemic

Before examining the influence of mixing patterns between and within different risk groups, the predicted shape of the AIDS epidemic in a population which mixes homogeneously is considered. In a homogeneously mixing population, sexual partners are chosen at random, irrespective of their rate of new sexual partner acquisition. Of course, this situation is far removed from reality, but it will provide a useful template for comparison. Theoretical studies of the transmission dynamics of sexually transmitted infections, with the appropriate parameter assignments for HIV infection, suggest that the simple epidemic will be roughly bell-shaped in form but with the prevalence of infection (in the absence of changes in behavior or improvements in treatment) eventually settling at a stable endemic state. As noted earlier, the period of time until the endemic state is reached depends on transmission efficacy (the magnitude of the basic reproductive number). The average number of new cases generated by each primary case of infection can be measured by contact tracing studies or the rate of growth in the epidemic. The intensity of transmission also influences the magnitude of the endemic state. Both these points are illustrated in Figure 4-6, which displays simulated epidemics in a sexually active population under the assumption of high or low transmission intensity. In reality, however, the epidemic is likely to be much more complex in form due to its spread within and between population groups that have different risk factors.

Mixing patterns and epidemic waves

In industrialized countries the three major at-risk groups for HIV infection are homosexual men, injecting drug users (IDUs), and heterosexual men and women. Within each of these broad categories there will be cohorts of individuals at differing degrees of risk. This is illustrated schematically in Figure 4-7. In developing countries, where transmission is predominately among heterosexual men and women, these varying levels of risk will also pertain, depending on sexual behavior and the prevailing patterns of mixing (sexual contact or needle sharing within and between different risk groups).[7]

Consider a simple situation in which three broad categories of risk can be

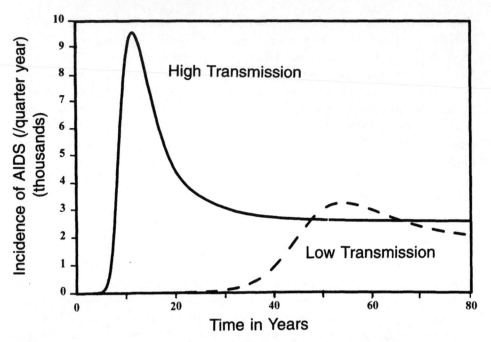

Figure 4-6   Shape of the epidemic, depending on intensity of transmission.

Figure 4-7   Networks of contact between and within vulnerable groups.

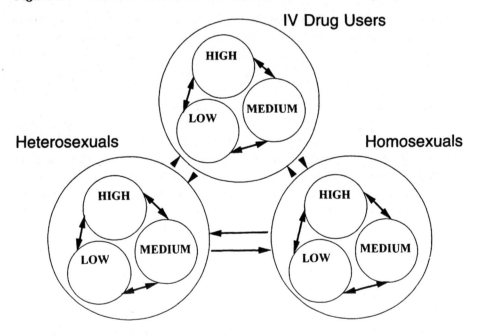

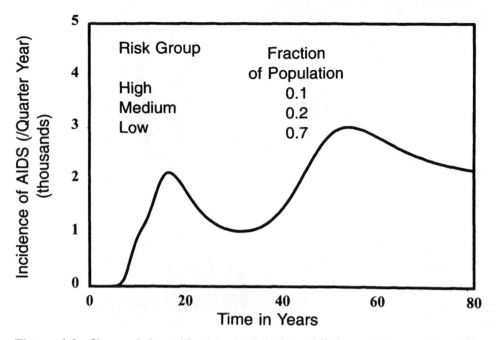

Figure 4-8   Shape of the epidemic—combination of high-, medium-, and low-risk groups.

identified (high, medium, and low), and where little or no mixing occurs between these three risk segments within any of the broader risk categories (i.e., heterosexuals, male homosexuals, or IDUs). If the high-risk category constitutes 10 percent of this total population, the medium group 20 percent, and the low-risk group 70 percent, then the combination of the three separate epidemics in each segment will result in a multiple peaked epidemic curve as illustrated in Figure 4-8. The epidemic wave in the high-risk group is visible in the far left part of the first epidemic peak. Note the complex nature of the composite epidemic, in which a period of declining incidence of AIDS after the first peak is followed by a much larger epidemic of longer duration in the low-risk group. There are many lessons to be learned from this simple illustration. The most important is that a phase of decline in AIDS incidence may not herald the end of the epidemic. Therefore, great caution must be exercised in interpreting current patterns in industrialized countries, where, for example, the epidemic in male homosexuals appears to be approaching its peak (e.g., in the United States and the United Kingdom).

Worldwide, the majority of HIV infections are occurring among heterosexuals in developing countries, particularly in sub-Saharan Africa, Southeast Asia, Latin America, and the Caribbean. Thus, the remainder of this section focuses on heterosexual transmission in these areas. Before examining patterns of HIV infection in these regions, it is worth comparing the longitudinal trends in HIV seroprevalence in highly vulnerable groups such as female sex workers, as an illustration of how waves of the epidemic appear in a community. As shown in Figure 4-9, HIV seroprevalence has begun to

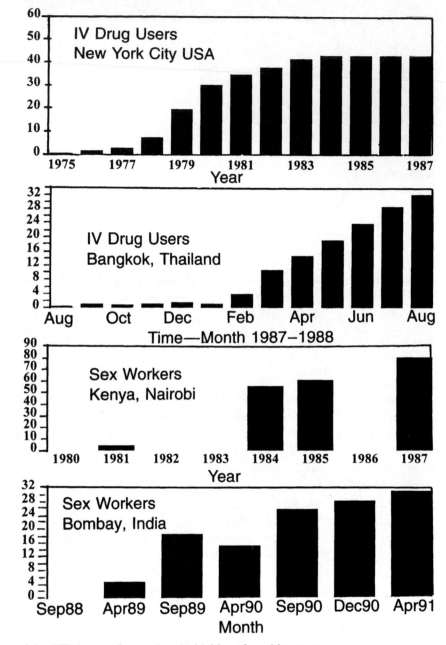

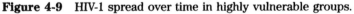

Figure 4-9   HIV-1 spread over time in highly vulnerable groups.

plateau in a number of communities. This implies that the incidence of AIDS in these groups will in turn reach a plateau in 5 to 10 years' time. (A plateau in seroprevalence does not mean zero incidence of new infections, rather it implies that new infections balance losses due to mortality or emigration from a particular community.) In these examples, the period from the introduction of HIV to the beginning phase of the plateau is short, involving only a few years. This is exactly what is to be expected on theoretical grounds for the first wave of the epidemic in the highest-risk groups. In the severely afflicted regions of the developing world, women sex workers typically represent one of the highest at-risk groups.[8] For example, in Nairobi, Kenya, HIV seroprevalence in this group appeared to plateau at very high levels (60–90 percent) in the early 1980s. Now the next major wave of the Kenyan epidemic is taking place, involving pregnant women (regarded as "low-risk" individuals). As illustrated in Figure 4-10, there is about a 5- to 6-year gap between the attainment of a plateau of HIV prevalence among the women sex workers and the suggestion of the appearance in 1989 of a plateau in the low-risk group (pregnant women). Patterns similar to those recorded in sub-Saharan Africa are now emerging in India and Thailand (Figure 4-11).

Men seeking treatment at sexually transmitted infection clinics form an intermediary group between these high- and low-risk groups. They provide or represent a bridge in the sexual contact network that permits spread between the different at-risk categories. The degree to which the different waves of the epidemic in each risk group are distinct will depend on the pattern of mixing between the groups.

In broad terms, the pattern of mixing ranges along a continuum from fully assortative (like-with-like) to fully disassortative (like-with-unlike).[9,10] Random mixing falls between these extremes. If mixing is fully assortative (i.e., those in high sexual activity groups only choose their sexual partners from within that group), then the epidemic waves are likely to be distinct (provided the population can actually be stratified into segments having very different rates of sexual partner acquisition).

The quantitative data available from industrialized and developing countries support this idea, and reported patterns of sexual partner acquisition

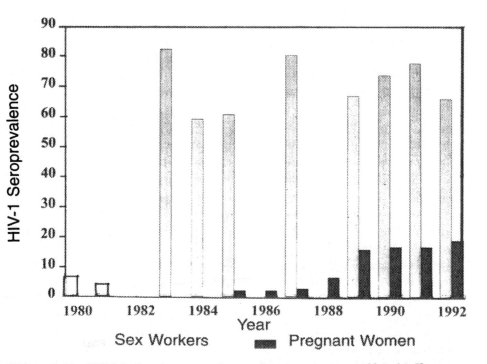

Figure 4-10   HIV-1 in female sex workers and pregnant women, Nairobi, Kenya.

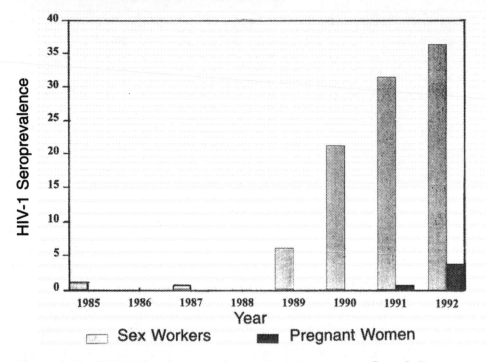

Figure 4.11   HIV-1 in female sex workers and pregnant women, Pune, India.

suggest that most people have few partners and a few have very many.[11,12,13] However, if mixing is weakly assortative, then the waves of infection may be less distinct in the overall epidemic curve. This point is illustrated in Figure 4-12, which presents an example of a simulated HIV epidemic in a heterosexual community in a developing country. In this figure, mixing is moderately assortative; HIV saturation in the high-activity group (sex workers) occurs about 40 years before saturation is reached in the general population (low-activity women). If mixing had been weakly assortative to random mixing, HIV saturation in the low-risk group would have occurred much earlier, shortly after saturation in the high-risk group. The observed patterns recorded in Figures 4-10 and 4-11 suggest that moderate levels of assortative mixing may be what is actually occurring.

Over the past decade, much progress has been made in the quantitative study of patterns of sexual behavior in human societies. However, our understanding of sexual contact networks and the associated patterns of mixing between high- and low-risk groups remains quite limited. Improved knowledge in this area will be vital both to assess observed epidemiological patterns (i.e., will the epidemic consist of a series of distinct waves?) and to analyze the potential demographic impact of AIDS. To illustrate this last point, Figure 4-13 shows the simulated trajectories of an HIV epidemic in a community in a developing country. Three variables are plotted over the time course of the epidemic: the prevalence of infection in sexually active women, the net population growth rate per annum in the community (3 percent prior to the arrival of HIV), and the fraction of orphans in the population. Three epidemics are illustrated for which parameter assignments were identical, except for the degree to which mixing was assortative (high, moderate, and weak) between high and low sexual activity classes (stratified on the basis of rates of sexual partner acquisition). The more assortative the pattern of mixing, the less the degree of spread and the less the impact of the HIV epidemic. Given an overall mean rate of sexual partner acquisition in the population, the greater the degree to which those with high rates of sexual partner acquisition choose their partners from within their own activity class, the less the infection will spread in the majority of the community (who belong to the lower sexual activity classes).[14]

Once it became apparent that the average incubation period of AIDS ranged from a few to many years, the question of the overall duration of the epidemic was resolved. In general, the major growth phase will last for a few to many decades, depending on the mix of risk groups in different countries and the prevailing patterns of sexual activity and mixing between risk groups. In those at highest risk, with highly assortative mixing within the group, the epidemic can move from very low prevalence to saturation at very high levels within 1 to a few years (Figure 4-13). In low-risk groups with limited contact with higher-risk groups, it will take a few decades before HIV seroprevalence plateaus or begins to decline. The reduction of the epidemic to an endemic state arises as the effective reproductive rate (R) settles to unity (1), i.e., where each new case of infection generates, on average, only one secondary case.

It is not possible in any given community to ascertain with precision

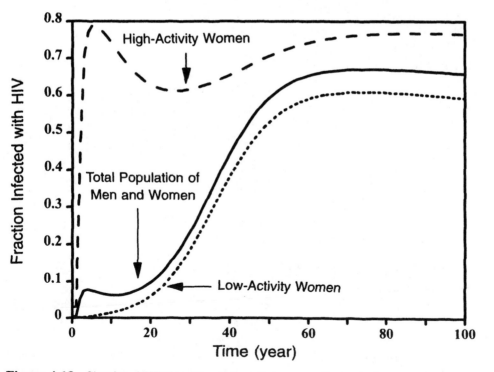

Figure 4-12   Simulated HIV-1 epidemic in a heterosexual population in a developing country.

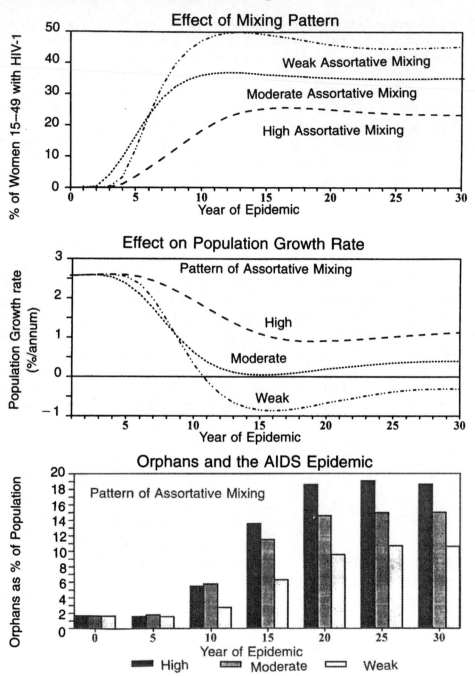

Figure 4-13   Influence of sexual mixing patterns.

whether the passage of infection through the different at-risk groups or activity classes within a group will result in distinct waves of infection marked
by discernible peaks in the overall epidemic. Although this is likely, as yet it
is too early to document specific examples. The epidemic of the longest
duration is probably in sub-Saharan Africa, but the absence of detailed longitudinal cohort surveys from any but a few locations makes the detection
of waves of infection difficult at present. The emerging patterns in indus-

trialized countries have been better documented via sophisticated disease surveillance systems and will, in time, reveal the complex nature of the composite epidemic curve.

In practical terms, three major messages arise from an understanding of the likely complexity of longitudinal patterns in HIV and AIDS incidence in behaviorally heterogeneous populations or communities. First, a declining phase in AIDS or HIV incidence should not be interpreted as the "beginning of the end" of the epidemic. It may well be the trough between epidemic peaks within risk groups with differing degrees of exposure to infection. Second, the study of patterns of mixing and sexual contact within and between different at-risk groups is an important component of analysis and interpretation of epidemiological patterns. Understanding in this area can provide important insights into how best to target education or condom distribution in order to reduce the overall magnitude of the epidemic. Third, irrespective of the composition of risk groups and the pattern of mixing, the overall duration of the epidemic phase will be many decades. Following this period, the infection is likely to become endemic with persistence in the small fraction (the "core") of highly sexually active individuals.

Over this long scale of many decades, viral evolution will play a significant role in many aspects of transmission and pathogenicity. Conventional wisdom suggests that highly pathogenic organisms will evolve over time to become less harmful to their hosts, as this benefits both species in the host–parasite interaction, but this wisdom is false. Evolution will favor enhancing the pathogen's success in transmission.[15] This efficacy of transmission may or may not be linked to reduced virulence. In the case of HIV, the pattern of occurrence of HIV-1 and HIV-2 in parts of West Africa suggests that the greatest transmission success is achieved by the more virulent strain (HIV-1). HIV-1 has invaded communities in which HIV-2 was already established, and appears to be replacing the older inhabitant. Current epidemiological data suggest that HIV-1 is both more pathogenic (shorter average incubation period) and more transmissible.[16] The coming decade will provide many insights into questions concerning the shape of the epidemic curve and the direction of viral evolution. Hopefully, however, it will also see signs that education effort and the promotion of safer sex practices have had a beneficial impact on the epidemic's magnitude and its likely level of endemic persistence.

REFERENCES

1. C. Creighton, *History of Epidemics in Britain*, Vols. I and II (Cambridge, U.K.: Cambridge University Press, 1894).
2. W. H. McNeill, *Plagues and Peoples* (Oxford: Basil Blackwell, 1977).
3. D. Defoe, *Journal of the Plague Year, or, Memorials of the Great Pestilence in London in 1665*, E. W. Brayley, ed. (London: Thomas Tegg, 1722).
4. R. M. Anderson and R. M. May, *Infectious Diseases of Humans: Dynamics and Control* (Oxford: Oxford University Press, 1991).
5. D. Mulder, A. Nunn, H. Wagner, A. Kamali, and J. Kengeya-Kayondo, "HIV-1 incidence and HIV-1 associated mortality in a rural Ugandan population cohort," *AIDS* 8(1994):87–92.

6. S. Gregson, G. P. Garnett, and R. M. Anderson, "Is HIV-1 likely to become a leading cause of adult mortality in sub-Saharan Africa?" *Journal of Acquired Immune Deficiency Syndromes* 7(1994):839–852.

7. G. Garnett and R. M. Anderson, "Factors controlling the spread of HIV in heterosexual communities in developing countries: Patterns of mixing between different age and sexual activity classes," *Philosophical Transactions: Biological Sciences. The Royal Society of London, Series B* 342(1993):137–159.

8. M. Laga, N. Nzila, and J. Goeman, "Interrelationship of sexually transmitted diseases and HIV infection: Implications for the control of both epidemics in Africa," *AIDS* 5(suppl. 5)(1991):s55–s63.

9. J. Jacquez, C. Simon, J. Koopman, L. Sattenspiel, and T. Perry, "Modelling and analysing HIV transmission: The effect of contact patterns," *Mathematical Biosciences* 92(1988):119–199.

10. S. Gupta, R. M. Anderson, and R. M. May, "Networks of sexual contacts: Implications for the pattern of spread of HIV," *AIDS* 3(1989):807–817.

11. Analyse des Comportements Sexuels en France, Investigators, "AIDS and sexual behaviour in France," *Nature* 360(1992):407–409.

12. A. M. Johnson, J. Wadsworth, K. Wellings, S. Bradshaw, and J. Field, "Sexual lifestyles and HIV risk," *Nature* 360(1992):410–412.

13. R. M. Anderson, "Epidemiology of HIV infection: Variable incubation plus infectious periods and heterogeneity in sexual activity," *Journal of the Royal Statistics Society, Series A, Statistics in Society* 151(1988):66–93.

14. G. Garnett and R. M. Anderson, "Factors controlling the spread of HIV."

15. R. M. Anderson and R. M. May, "Coevolution of hosts and parasites," *Parasitology* 85(1982):411–426.

16. K. M. De Cock, F. Zadi, G. Adjorlolo, M. O. Diallo, M. Sassan-Morokro, E. Ekpini, T. Sibailly, R. Doorly, V. Batter, K. Brattegaard, and H. Gayle, "Retrospective study of maternal HIV-1 and HIV-1 infections and child survival in Abidjan, Côte d'Ivoire," *British Medical Journal* 308(1994):441–443.

5

The Pandemic of HIV-Associated Tuberculosis

MARIO RAVIGLIONE, PAUL P. NUNN,
ARATA KOCHI, AND RICHARD J. O'BRIEN

As people live with HIV, they become vulnerable to a variety of opportunistic infections and other diseases, one of the most important of which is tuberculosis (TB). The historical rebound of tuberculosis, starting in the 1980s, following decades of arduous and often successful prevention and control efforts, poses new challenges to public health. The association of the two pandemics—HIV and tuberculosis—has occurred in a context of general complacency about tuberculosis.

In most developing countries, tuberculosis is the most important opportunistic infection observed among HIV-infected patients because it occurs frequently, is transmissible to both HIV-infected and uninfected persons, is relatively easily treated, and can be prevented.[1]

The World Health Organization (WHO) estimates that 8.8 million new cases of TB and 3 million deaths due to TB occurred worldwide in 1995.[2] These numbers are predicted to increase further, such that more than 10 million TB cases and 3.5 million TB-related deaths could occur in the year 2000. It is anticipated that the HIV epidemic will be responsible for 20 percent of the projected increase in global TB.[3]

Four main lines of evidence support the strong association of tuberculosis and HIV infection. First, in countries where both infections are common, HIV seroprevalence is much higher among tuberculosis patients than in the general population.[4] For instance, in Uganda during 1990–1992, the incidence of HIV infection among tuberculosis patients was 5.9 times greater than among women attending antenatal clinics at the same hospitals.[5] In Lusaka, Zambia, as many as 37 percent of hospitalized children with tuberculosis were HIV infected, compared to 11 percent among non-tuberculosis controls.[6] The HIV seroprevalence in tuberculosis patients in several countries is provided in Table 5-1.

Second, active TB occurs frequently among patients with AIDS in populations where concurrent TB and HIV infections are common (Table 5-2).

Third, cohort studies have shown that the risk of developing active TB among persons infected with *Mycobacterium tuberculosis* is much higher in HIV-infected persons than in HIV-seronegative persons. For a person coin-

Table 5-1 HIV seroprevalence among patients with tuberculosis in selected countries*

Selected country	Year	Total no. of TB cases in sample	HIV(+) (%)
Kampala, Uganda[1]	1988/89	59	66
Four sites, Uganda[2]	1990/92	1,770	44
Lusaka, Zambia[3]	1988/89	345	60
Abidjan, Côte d'Ivoire[4]	1989/90	2,043	40
Tanzania[5]	1991/93	6,154	32
Cité Soleil, Haiti[6]	1989/90	143	39
Rio de Janeiro, Brazil[7]	1989	136	5.2
U.S.[8]	1992	n.s.	12.5(0–66)
France[9]	1991	4,181	6
Thailand[10]	1994	n.s.	10(1.4–4.0)
Manipur State, India[11]	1992/93	148	11.5
Bombay, India[12]	1992/93	684	8.9

*n.s., non-specified.

[1]P. P. Eriki, A. Okwera, T. Aisu, et al., "Influence of human immunodeficiency virus infection on tuberculosis in Kampala, Uganda," *American Review of Respiratory Diseases* 143(1991):185–187.

[2]T. Aisu, M. C. Raviglione, J. P. Narain, et al., "Monitoring HIV-associated tuberculosis in Uganda," presented at the World Congress on Tuberculosis, Bethesda, Maryland, November 16–19, 1992.

[3]A. M. Elliott, N. Luo, G. Tembo, et al., "Impact of HIV on tuberculosis in Zambia: A cross sectional study," *British Medical Journal* 301(1990):412–415.

[4]K. M. De Cock, E. Gnaore, G. Adjorlolo, et al., "Risk of tuberculosis in patients with HIV-I and HIV-II infections in Abidjan, Ivory Coast," *British Medical Journal* 302(1991):496–499.

[5]H. L. Chum, R. J. O'Brien, T. M. Chonde, P. Graf, and H. L. Rieder, An Epidemological Study of HIV infection and tuberculosis in Tanzania, 1991–1993. AIDS 1996 (in press).

[6]H. C. Clermont, R. E. Chaisson, H. A. Davis, et al., "HIV-1 infection in adult tuberculosis patients in Cité Soleil, Haiti," Abstract TH.B.490, presented at the VI International Conference on AIDS, San Francisco, California, June 1990.

[7]A. L. Kritski, E. Werneck-Barroso, M. Armandas Vieira, et al., "HIV infection in 567 active pulmonary tuberculosis patients in Brazil," *Journal of Acquired Immune Deficiency Syndromes* 6(1993):1008–1012.

[8]I. Onorato, S. McCombs, M. Morgan, and E. McCray, "HIV infection in patients attending tuberculosis clinics, United States, 1988–1992," presented at the 33rd Interscience Conference on Antimicrobial Agents and Chemotherapy, New Orleans, Louisiana, October 17–20, 1993.

[9]B. Marshall, C. Moyse, and A. Lepoutre, "Cas de tuberculose déclarés en France en 1991," *Bulletin Epidémiologique Hebdomadaire* 53(1992):247–249.

[10]V. Payanandana, B. Kladphuang, N. Talkitul, and S. Tornee, Information in preparation for an external review of the National Tuberculosis Programme, Thailand. (Bangkok: Tuberculosis Division, Department of Communicable Disease Control, Ministry of Public Health, 1995.) (ISBN: 974-7960-73-7)

[11]I. Ibopishak Singh, "HIV infection amongst tuberculosis patients at tuberculosis hospital, Chingeirong, Manipur," presented at the 17th Eastern Regional Conference on Tuberculosis and Respiratory Diseases of the IUATLD, Eastern Region, Bangkok, Thailand, November 1–4, 1993.

[12]K. C. Mohanty, R. M. Sundarani, and R. B. Pasi, "Changing trend of HIV infection in tuberculosis and pulmonary diseases patients, since 1988, at Bombay," presented at the 17th Eastern Regional Conference on Tuberculosis and Respiratory Diseases of the IUATLD, Eastern Region, Bangkok, Thailand, November 1–4, 1993.

fected with HIV and tuberculosis, the annual risk of developing active TB ranges from 5 to 15 percent, whereas the *lifetime* risk for people with tuberculosis infection in the absence of HIV infection is only 5 to 10 percent.[7–12]

Fourth, TB case notifications in many countries have increased with the HIV epidemic. For example, TB notification rates in Malawi have increased fourfold over the past 4 or 6 years, largely due to the rapid increase in HIV-associated tuberculosis.[13] In the U.S., after 30 years of decline, the number of tuberculosis cases reported yearly increased regularly between 1985 and 1992.[14]

WHO has estimated the number of persons latently infected with *tubercle bacilli*, but without disease, to be 1.7 billion, or one-third of the global population in 1990.[15] Most of these TB-infected people (approximately 1.3 billion) live in Asia, sub-Saharan Africa, and Latin America, where about half of the adult population is TB infected.[16] In these areas, the impact of HIV will likely have devastating consequences for already overburdened national tuberculosis programs. For example, in Chiang Mai and Chiang Rai (northern Thailand), where HIV has progressed rapidly, a 5 to 7 percent increase in tuberculosis registrations occurred during 1990–1992.[17] In Chiang Mai and the northern provinces, HIV seroprevalence among tuberculosis cases increased from 5 percent in 1989 to 40 percent in 1992.[18]

The extent of overlap between the populations infected with HIV and tuberculosis determines the number of coinfected persons in each area. In

Table 5-2 Frequency of TB among AIDS patients

Country/region	Source	Percent of persons with AIDS having TB
Africa[1,2,3]	Clinical/autopsy	20–54
Latin America: Brazil,[4] Mexico[5]	Autopsy	24–28
Caribbean: Haiti[6]	Clinical	23
Southeast Asia: India,[7] Thailand[8]	Clinical	52–68
Europe: Italy,[9] England and Wales[10]	Surveillance	5–11
U.S.[11]	Surveillance	4

[1]J. M. Mbaga, K. J. Pallangyo, M. Bakari, and E. A. Aris, "Survival time of patients with acquired immunodeficiency syndrome: Experience with 274 patients in Dar-es-Salaam," *East African Medical Journal* 67(1990):95–99.

[2]S. B. Lucas, A. Nounnou, C. Peacock, et al., "Mortality and pathology of HIV infection in a West African city," *AIDS* 7(1993):1569–1579.

[3]D. T. McLeod, P. Neill, W. Robertson, et al., "Pulmonary diseases in patients infected with the human immunodeficiency virus in Zimbabwe, Central Africa," *Transactions of the Royal Society of Tropical Medicine and Hygiene* 83(1989):691–697.

[4]K. Sanches, E. Almeida, M. Pinto, and A. Sole-Cava, "AIDS and tuberculosis in the state of Rio de Janeiro, Brazil," Abstract TH.C.731, presented at the VI International Conference on AIDS, San Francisco, California, June 1990.

[5]J. Jessurum, A. Angeles-Angeles, and N. Gasman, "Comparative demographic and autopsy findings in acquired immunodeficiency syndrome in two Mexican populations," *Journal of Acquired Immune Deficiency Syndromes* 3(1990):579–583.

[6]J. W. Pape, B. Liautaud, F. Thomas, et al., "Acquired immunodeficiency syndrome in Haiti," *Annals of Internal Medicine* 103(1985):674–678.

[7]A. Kaur, P. G. Babu, M. Jacob, et al., "Clinical and laboratory profile of AIDS in India," *Journal of Acquired Immune Deficiency Syndromes* 5(1992):883–889.

[8]S. Tansuphaswasdikul, "Thai experiences on the diagnostic approaches and management of pulmonary complications in HIV infection," presented at the 17th Eastern Regional Conference on Tuberculosis and Respiratory Diseases of the IUATLD, Eastern Region, Bangkok, Thailand, November 1–4, 1993.

[9]E. Girardi, G. Antonucci, O. Armignacco, et al., "Tuberculosis and AIDS: A retrospective, longitudinal, multicenter study on Italian AIDS patients," *Journal of Infection* 28(1994):261–269.

[10]J. M. Watson, S. K. Meredith, E. Whitmore-Overton, et al., "Tuberculosis and HIV: Estimates of the overlap in England and Wales," *Thorax* 48(1993):199–203.

[11]G. M. Cauthen, A. B. Bloch, and D. E. Snider, "Reported AIDS patients with tuberculosis in the United States," Abstract TH.C.725, presented at the VI International Conference on AIDS, San Francisco, California, June 1990.

Table 5-3 Estimated number of 15–49-year-old persons coinfected with HIV and *M. tuberculosis* in 1995 and 2000

Region	Mid-1995			2000		
	HIV-infected (thousands)	TB-infected (%)	HIV/TB co-infected (thousands)	HIV-infected (thousands)	TB-infected (%)	HIV/TB coinfected (thousands)
Sub-Saharan Africa	8,500	47	4,000	>9,000	47	>4,230
Latin America and Caribbean	>1,500	28.5	>430	>2,000	24	>480
Asia and Pacific	>3,000	45	>1,380	8,000	36	2,880
North America, Europe, Australasia	>1,250	12	>120	1,000	9	90
TOTAL	14–15,000	—	>5,900	>20,000	—	>7,680

developing countries, where young adults have high rates of infection with both HIV and *M. tuberculosis*, risk of coinfection is correspondingly high. In industrialized countries, the large majority of TB-infected people are elderly and at lower risk of HIV infection. However, among certain population groups, such as injecting drug users, the proportion of tuberculosis-infected young adults may be similar to that in developing countries.[19]

The size of the HIV-associated tuberculosis epidemic can be estimated using two methodologies. First, given WHO's global estimates of HIV infection and tuberculosis infection in the age-group at highest risk of HIV infection (15–49 years), and assuming that the risks of being infected with *M. tuberculosis* and HIV are independent, it is estimated that 6 million persons were coinfected by mid-1995.[20] Assuming an annual risk of developing tuberculosis of 5 to 15 percent, 300,000 to 900,000 new cases of HIV-attributable tuberculosis could have occurred in this age-group in 1995 (Box 5-1). By the year 2000, with nearly 8 million coinfected people worldwide, the annual number of HIV-attributable tuberculosis cases in this age-group may be as high as 400,000 to 1,200,000 (Table 5-3).[21]

A second method for determining the HIV-associated tuberculosis epidemic combines WHO's estimates of the global tuberculosis burden with reported HIV seroprevalence data among patients with tuberculosis.[22,23] Using this method, an estimated 4.2 percent of all new tuberculosis cases were attributable to HIV infection in 1990. Because of anticipated changes in HIV seroprevalence among tuberculosis patients through the year 2000, and assuming that 95 percent of HIV-associated tuberculosis cases are attributable to HIV infection, this proportion is expected to increase to 8.4 percent in 1995 and 13.8 percent by the year 2000, when more than 1.4 million cases of tuberculosis may be attributable to HIV infection.[24] Thus, over the 10-year period 1990–1999, it is estimated that more than 88 million people will develop tuberculosis, and that 8 million of these cases will be attributable to HIV infection.[25] This method of estimation yields a higher number, but it includes TB cases expected in the pediatric and older adult populations, and assumes more realistically that the risks of being infected with *M. tuberculosis* and HIV are related.

BOX 5-1

TB and HIV coinfection

When the estimates of adult HIV infections presented in *AIDS in the World II* (Chapter 1) are combined with the rates of tuberculosis infection estimated by the WHO Tuberculosis Program, a picture of a severe, dual pandemic emerges. As of January 1, 1996, approximately 20.5 million adults were living with HIV infection or diagnosed AIDS. Approximately 8.7 million had both HIV/AIDS and TB infection: 59 percent of dual HIV/TB infections were in sub-Saharan Africa, 32.5 percent in Southeast Asia, 3.5 percent in Latin America, and 5 percent in the rest of the world (Table 5-1.1).

Table 5-1.1 HIV/AIDS and coinfection TB based on *AIDS in the World II* estimates, adult cases, January 1, 1996

GAA	Adult HIV/AIDS prevalence January 1, 1996	% TB infected	HIV/TB coinfected
1 North America	916,000	15	137,000
2 Western Europe	688,000	15	103,000
3 Oceania	25,000	15	4,000
4 Latin America	1,019,000	30	306,000
5 Sub-Saharan Africa	10,939,000	47	5,141,000
6 Caribbean	352,000	30	106,000
7 Eastern Europe	32,000	15	5,000
8 SE Mediterranean	69,000	15	10,000
9 Northeast Asia	173,000	45	78,000
10 Southeast Asia	6,303,000	45	2,836,000
TOTAL WORLD	20,516,000		8,726,000

Source: Adult HIV/AIDS prevalence figures, *AIDS in the World II* survey; TB infection rate, Dr. M. Raviglione.

In 1995, deaths from HIV-associated TB were estimated at 266,000 (8.9 percent of the 3 million TB deaths worldwide). By the year 2000, half a million deaths (almost 15 percent of the 3.5 million deaths due to tuberculosis) may be attributed to HIV-associated tuberculosis.[26] Therefore, in the decade 1990–99, an estimated three million of 30 million total tuberculosis deaths worldwide may be attributable to HIV.[27]

This bleak outlook could worsen with the emergence and spread of multidrug resistant (MDR) strains of tuberculosis, which result from inadequate TB treatment. HIV has not caused the MDR-TB problem but has heightened its recognition. Also, unlike most people, persons immunosuppressed with HIV infection who then become infected with *M. tuberculosis* have an extraordinarily high risk of developing active tuberculosis within a short time.[28] Thus, HIV infection can "telescope" a tuberculosis epidemic of both MDR and susceptible strains, permitting its clinical manifestations to be seen in months rather than years.

MDR-TB has been noted in the United States and other industrialized countries, where the infrastructure for treating tuberculosis was essentially dismantled in the years prior to the AIDS epidemic.[29] Fortunately, proper application of tuberculosis control principles, including the use of directly observed therapy, can diminish and eventually eliminate the problem.[30]

Clearly, the scale of the current tuberculosis pandemic exceeds the present HIV/AIDS problem. In low-income countries, tuberculosis is generally not under control, nor has it ever been. Before attending to the additional problems created by HIV, the essentials of tuberculosis control must be in place and functioning (Box 5-2). Without these elements it will be impossible to successfully address the additional problems created by HIV.

BOX 5-2

Reversing the rise in tuberculosis morbidity and mortality

S. JODY HEYMANN AND TIMOTHY F. BREWER

Past approach

For the past 20 years, countries have tended to use one of two strategies to control tuberculosis. Both strategies emphasized the importance of treating active cases, but differed in their approach to prevention. The first strategy relied on vaccination of infants with Bacillus Calmette-Guerin (BCG).[1] The second relied on tuberculin screening of case contacts with chemoprophylaxis for tuberculin-positive individuals. General population tuberculin screening has also been done.[2] Though BCG has been used in many industrialized countries, some have curtailed or considered curtailing their BCG programs.[3,4] Most developing countries have never had national chemoprophylaxis programs.

A growing epidemic

Over the past decade, tuberculosis cases have risen in both developing and industrialized countries.[5,6] HIV-infected persons are more likely to develop active tuberculosis, and rising tuberculosis case rates have been found particularly in populations most affected by the HIV/AIDS pandemic.[7,8,9] At the same time, tuberculosis resistant to chemotherapy has become more prevalent.

Rethinking approaches to preventing the spread of tuberculosis

The rise in tuberculosis infections and cases requires countries to rethink their tuberculosis control strategies. Without new prevention strategies, tuberculosis control programs in developing countries may be unable to meet the needs of HIV and *M. tuberculosis*-infected persons.[10] Continued emphasis on treatment of smear positive cases and BCG vaccination as the only means of control overlooks the realities of high rates of developing active tuberculosis coupled with the much more common treatment complications, relapses, and deaths, despite treatment in dually infected patients.[11,12,13] Chemoprophylaxis decreases the risk of active disease and death in this population and when the benefits to the patient's contacts are taken into account, it has been shown to be effective and feasible in developing as well as industrialized countries.[14,15,16] The use of chemoprophylaxis for dually HIV-tuberculosis infected individuals should be expanded in both developing and industrialized countries. Tuberculosis chemoprophylaxis can contribute critically both to the health of dually infected individuals and to decreasing the spread of tuberculosis.

Some medical and public health professionals have raised concerns about apparent variability in BCG efficacy. However, a recent meta-analysis of BCG efficacy showed that the effectiveness of BCG is maintained across time, strains, and populations.[17] Because chemoprophylaxis regimens of proven efficacy for the prevention of multiple drug resistant tuberculosis (MDR-TB) do not exist, the use of BCG in populations at high risk for MDR-TB is particularly important.

In countries where BCG is not yet routinely given, for non–HIV-infected persons BCG vaccination should be expanded to include all at high risk for infection with MDR-TB, strongly considered for those at high risk for infection with drug sensitive TB, and reviewed for the general population. Because of the risk of disseminated BCG, expanding the use of BCG in HIV-infected individuals in countries with low overall rates of tuberculosis requires further study.[18] However, increasing rates of BCG vaccination in non–HIV-infected persons will, by leading to decreased spread, lower the risk of new TB infection for HIV-infected individuals.

Rethinking approaches to preventing multiple drug-resistant tuberculosis

In non–HIV-infected patients, MDR-TB has a mortality rate despite aggressive treatment almost equal to that of untreated tuberculosis; HIV-infected patients have mortality rates as high as 72–89 percent.[19,20] Fear over the spread of MDR-TB has led to the implementation of policies that dramatically restrict the rights of persons infected with tuberculosis, such as the forced confinement of patients who do not complete their treatment in some cities in the U.S.

To date, there is no evidence that confinement is effective in preventing the spread of MDR-TB. While confinement removes a small number of infected individuals from having contact with others, it may also discourage other contagious individuals from seeking treatment. The net result may not be a decrease in the number of contagious untreated patients. To justify confinement of tuberculous patients, this practice needs to be more effective than less restrictive alternatives of increasing patient adherence to treatment. This has not been shown. In fact, a comprehensive medical program designed to meet the needs of patients has been highly effective in successfully treating tuberculosis patients who previously failed to complete therapy.[21] In both developing and industrialized settings, tuberculosis treatment programs using enablers and incentives were cost-effective and highly successful, even among patients chronically non-adherent to previous treatments.[22,23]

Finally, the rationale made for confinement is based on the assumption that patient non-adherence to therapy is the reason for MDR-TB. Insufficient attention has been paid to physician error, including failure to identify MDR-TB and prescribing or changing to inadequate therapies, which is a known important cause of MDR-TB.[24] Educating physicians in the treatment of tuberculosis with the availability of specialists to treat patients with MDR-TB might reduce the rate of MDR-TB more effectively without restricting human rights.

Need for a global approach

Developing countries with the greatest burden of tuberculosis often have insufficient resources to cover prevention and care for all affected. Over a quarter of preventable adult deaths in developing countries are due to tuberculosis.[25] The rise of tuberculosis is a global problem which requires a global commitment of resources to its reversal.

References

1. H. G. ten Dam, "Research on BCG vaccination," *Advances in Tuberculosis Research* 21(1984):79–106.
2. American Thoracic Society, "Control of tuberculosis in the United States," *American Review of Respiratory Diseases* 146(1992):1623–1633.
3. K. M. Citron, "BCG vaccination against tuberculosis: International perspectives," *British Medical Journal* 306 (1993):222–223.
4. V. Romanus, "Tuberculosis in Bacillus Calmette-Guerin immunized and unimmunized children in Sweden: A ten-year evaluation following the cessation of general Bacillus Calmette-Guerin immunization of the newborn in 1975," *Pediatric Infectious Disease Journal* 6(1987):272–280.

5. American Thoracic Society, "Control of tuberculosis in the United States," *American Review of Respiratory Diseases* 146(1992):1623–1633.

6. J. F. Murray, "Emerging global programme against tuberculosis: Agenda for research, including the impact of HIV infection," *Bulletin of the International Union of Tuberculosis and Lung Disease* 66(1991):207–209.

7. C. L. Daley, P. M. Small, G. F. Schecter, et al., "Outbreak of tuberculosis with accelerated progression among persons infected with the human immunodeficiency virus," *New England Journal of Medicine* 326(1992):231–235.

8. P. A. Selwyn, D. Hartel, V. A. Lewis, et al., "Prospective study of the risk of tuberculosis among intravenous drug users with human immunodeficiency virus infection," *New England Journal of Medicine* 320(1989):545–550.

9. A. M. Elliot, N. Luo, G. Tembo, et al., "Impact of HIV on tuberculosis in Zambia: A cross sectional study," *British Medical Journal* 301(1990):412–415.

10. S. Grzybowski, "Preventive treatment for tuberculosis control in developing countries. The case for preventive chemotherapy," *Bulletin of the International Union Against Tuberculosis and Lung Disease* 66(suppl)(1990):25.

11. P. Nunn, D. Kibuga, S. Gathua, et al., "Cutaneous hypersensitivity reactions due to thiacetazone in HIV-1 seropositive patients treated for tuberculosis," *Lancet* 377(1991):627–630.

12. M. Hawken, P. Nunn, S. Gathua, et al., "Increased recurrence of tuberculosis in HIV-1-infected patients in Kenya," *Lancet* 342(1993):332–337.

13. J. H. Perriens, R. L. Colebunders, C. Karlhunga, et al., "Increased mortality and tuberculosis treatment failure rate among human immunodeficiency virus (HIV) seropositive compared with HIV seronegative patients with pulmonary tuberculosis treated with 'standard' chemotherapy in Kinshasa, Zaire," *American Review of Respiratory Diseases* 144(1991):750–755.

14. S. J. Heymann, "Modelling the efficacy of prophylactic and curative therapies for preventing the spread of tuberculosis in Africa," *Transactions of the Royal Society of Tropical Medicine and Hygiene* 87(1993):406–411.

15. J. W. Pape, S. S. Jean, J. L. Ho, et al., "Effect of isoniazid prophylaxis of the incidence of active tuberculosis and progression of HIV infection," *Lancet* 342(1993):268–272.

16. T. Aisu, M. C. Raviglione, E. Van Praag, et al., "Preventive chemotherapy for HIV-associated tuberculosis in Uganda: A feasibility study," Abstract WS-B09-3, presented at the IX International Conference on AIDS, Berlin, Germany, June 1993.

17. G. A. Colditz, T. F. Brewer, C .S. Berkey, et al., "Efficacy of Bacillus Calmette-Guerin vaccination in the prevention of tuberculosis: Meta-analyses of the published literature," *Journal of the American Medical Association* 271(1994):698–702.

18. M. Besnard, S. Sauvion, C. Offredo, et al., "Bacillus Calmette-Guerin infection after vaccination of human immunodeficiency virus infected children," *Pediatric Infectious Disease Journal* 12(1993):993–997.

19. M. Goble, M. D. Iseman, L. A. Madsen, et al., "Treatment of 171 patients with pulmonary tuberculosis resistant to isoniazid and rifampin," *New England Journal of Medicine* 328(1993):527–532.

20. P. C. Hopewell, "Impact of human immunodeficiency virus infection on the epidemiology, clinical features, management, and control of tuberculosis," *Clinical Infectious Diseases* 15(1992):540–547.

21. R. J. McDonald, A. M. Memon, and L. B. Reichman, "Successful supervised ambulatory management of tuberculosis treatment failures," *Annals of Internal Medicine* 96(1982):297–302.

22. P. Farmer, S. Robin, S. L. Ramilus, and J. Y. Kim, "Tuberculosis, poverty, and 'compliance': Lessons from rural Haiti," *Seminars in Respiratory Infections* 6(1991):254–260.

23. C. Pozsik, J. Kinney, D. Breeden, et al., "Approaches to improving adherence to antituberculosis therapy—South Carolina and New York, 1986–1991," *Morbidity and Mortality Weekly Report* 42(1993):74–81.

24. A. Mahmoudi and M. D. Iseman, "Pitfalls in the care of patients with tuberculosis: Common errors and their association with the acquisition of drug resistance," *Journal of the American Medical Association* 270(1993):65–68.

25. K. Klaudt, ed., *World Health Organization Report on the Tuberculosis Epidemic* (Geneva: WHO, 1993).

The HIV-associated TB epidemic has led to a huge increase in the number of patients in TB treatment centers in high HIV prevalence countries. These numbers threaten the ability to provide adequate supervision of TB chemotherapy, which is essential for adherence to the full regimen and an acceptable cure rate. Inadequate supervision will result predictably in unnecessarily high mortality rates during treatment, fatal adverse effects of therapy, high rates of recurrence, and potential increases in drug resistance. This largely reflects chronic neglect of tuberculosis control. Cost-effective approaches for treatment of TB exist and have been shown to be feasible and effective in the poorest countries. The message—to governments of low-income countries especially, and to donor agencies—is that in the era of AIDS, continued neglect of tuberculosis control is unacceptable.

REFERENCES

1. J. P. Narain, M. C. Raviglione, and A. Kochi, "HIV-associated tuberculosis in developing countries: Epidemiology and strategies for prevention," *Tubercle and Lung Disease* 73(1992):311–321.

2. P. J. Dolin, M. C. Raviglione, and A. Kochi, "Global tuberculosis incidence and mortality during 1990–2000," *Bulletin of the World Health Organization* 72(1994):213–220.

3. *Ibid.*

4. Narain, "HIV-associated tuberculosis."

5. T. Asiu, M. C. Raviglione, J. P. Narain, et al., "Monitoring HIV-associated tuberculosis in Uganda," presented at the World Congress on Tuberculosis, Bethesda, Maryland, November 16–19, 1992.

6. C. Chintu, G. Bhat, C. Luo, et al., "Seroprevalence of human immunodeficiency virus type 1 infection in Zambian children with tuberculosis," *Pediatric Infectious Disease Journal* 12(1993):499–504.

7. P. A. Selwyn, D. Hartel, V. A. Lewis, et al., "Prospective study of the risk of tuberculosis among intravenous drug users with human immunodeficiency virus infection," *New England Journal of Medicine* 320(1989):545–550.

8. P. A. Selwyn, B. M. Sckell, P. Alcabes, et al., "High risk of active tuberculosis in HIV-infected drug users with cutaneous anergy," *Journal of the American Medical Association* 268(1992):504–509.

9. S. Allen, J. Batungwanayo, K. Kerlikowske, et al., "Two-year incidence of tuberculosis in cohorts of HIV-infected and uninfected urban Rwandan women," *American Review of Respiratory Diseases* 146(1992):1439–1444.

10. A. Guelar, J. M. Gatell, J. Verdejo, et al., "Prospective study of the risk of tuberculosis among HIV-infected patients," *AIDS* 7(1993):1345–1349.

11. G. Antonucci, E. Giradi, M. C. Raviglione, et al., "Risk factors for tuberculosis in HIV-infected subjects: A prospective cohort study," *Journal of the American Medical Association* 274(1995):147–169.

12. I. Sutherland, "Recent studies in the epidemiology of tuberculosis, based on the risk of being infected with tubercle bacilli," *Advances in Tuberculosis Research* 19(1976):1–63.

13. Narain, "HIV-associated tuberculosis."

14. Centers for Disease Control, "Tuberculosis morbidity—United States, 1994," *Morbidity and Mortality Weekly Report* 44(1994):387–395.

15. P. Sudre, H. G. ten Dam, and A. Kochi, "Tuberculosis: A global overview of the situation today," *Bulletin of the World Health Organization* 70(1992):149–159.

16. *Ibid.*

17. T. Bamrungtrakul, P. Akarasewi, and D. Viriyakittja, "Trends of HIV-1 coinfection among tuberculosis patients, Thailand, 1989–1992," presented at the 17th Eastern Regional Conference on Tuberculosis and Respiratory Diseases of the International Union Against Tuberculosis and Lung Disease (IUATLD), Eastern Region, Bangkok, November 1–4, 1993.

18. V. Payanandana, B. Kladphuang, N. Talkitkul, and S. Tornee, "Information in preparation for an external review by the National Tuberculosis Programme, Thailand" (Bangkok:

Tuberculosis Division, Department of Communicable Disease Control, Ministry of Public Health, 1995) (ISBN: 974–7960–73–7).

19. D. Altarac, B. Raucher, S. Back, and S. E. Nichols, "Reevaluation of PPD testing in a high risk cohort," presented at the 33rd Interscience Conference on Antimicrobial Agents and Chemotherapy, New Orleans, Louisiana, October 17–20, 1993.

20. WHO, Global Programme on AIDS, "The current global situation of the HIV/AIDS pandemic," *Weekly Epidemiological Record* 70(1995):193–196.

21. WHO, Global Programme on AIDS, *HIV/AIDS Pandemic: 1993 Overview*, WHO/GPA/CNP/EVA/93.1 (Geneva, 1993).

22. Dolin, "Global tuberculosis."

23. Narain, "HIV-associated tuberculosis."

24. Dolin, "Global tuberculosis."

25. *Ibid.*

26. *Ibid.*

27. *Ibid.*

28. C. L. Daley, P. M. Small, G. F. Schecter, et al, "Outbreak of tuberculosis with accelerated progression among persons infected with the human immunodeficiency virus. An analysis using restriction-fragment-length polymorphisms," *New England Journal of Medicine* 326(1992):231–235.

29. K. Brudney and J. Dobkin, "Resurgent tuberculosis in New York City. Human immunodeficiency virus, homelessness, and the decline of tuberculosis control programs," *American Review of Respiratory Disease* 144(1991):745–749.

30. T. R. Frieden, P. I. Fujiwara, R. M. Washko, and M. A. Hamburg, "Tuberculosis in New York City—turning the tide," *New England Journal of Medicine* 333(1995):229–233.

6

Epidemiology of HIV and Sexually Transmitted Infections in Women

BEA VUYLSTEKE, ROSE SUNKUTU, AND MARIE LAGA

Throughout the industrialized and developing world, the proportion of women infected with HIV is increasing. This section focuses on the epidemiology of HIV and sexually transmitted infections (STIs) in women, with an emphasis on studies conducted from 1990 to the present. Data from six geographic areas of affinity (GAAs) are included: North America, Western Europe, Latin America, sub-Saharan Africa, the Caribbean, and Southeast Asia. In the other GAAs, levels of HIV infection among women are fortunately still very low.

The epidemiology of HIV in women

The expanding pandemic of HIV infections in women

Recent data on the female-to-male ratio of HIV infection and AIDS cases worldwide indicate that an increasing proportion of infections and AIDS cases are occurring among women. In the industrialized world, AIDS was primarily a disease of men during the first decade of the pandemic. But in sub-Saharan Africa, where HIV has always been spread predominantly by heterosexual contact, the female/male ratio was nearly equal during the first decade of the pandemic. Today, the female/male ratio in industrialized countries is growing steadily. In Colombia in 1987, the female/male HIV-infection ratio was 1:75; by 1992, the ratio had narrowed to 1:5.[1] Among young people entering the U.S. Job Corps in 1988, the female/male HIV-infection ratio was 1:1.6; by 1992 it had reversed and risen to 1.8:1.[2] In sub-Saharan Africa, population-based studies in Uganda and Tanzania show that infection rates for women now substantially exceed those for men, with female/male ratios ranging from 1.3:1 to 1.7:1.[3,4,5]

Women are not only being infected with HIV more frequently than men, they are becoming infected at a younger age. Numbers of new infections peak among women between the ages of 15 and 25 years, while for men this peak occurs a decade later, between 25 and 35 years old.[6,7] Moreover, data on HIV prevalence among different groups of women are, not surprisingly, quite complex.

Female sex workers

Among female sex workers, one of the most severely affected groups in the world, HIV prevalence rates vary widely (Chapter 2). In North America and Europe, HIV infection in female sex workers is related almost entirely to injecting drug use. Thus, a multicenter European study involving nine countries found that 31.8 percent of female sex workers who also injected drugs were HIV infected compared to only 1.5 percent of non-injectors.[8] In contrast, HIV prevalence rates among female sex workers in sub-Saharan Africa and, more recently, Asia, are uniformly high—ranging between 40 and 90 percent. Incidence rates as high as 38 per 100 person-years and 10 percent per month have been found among female sex workers in Nairobi, Kenya and Chiang Mai, Thailand, respectively.[9,10]

Pregnant women

Among pregnant women, HIV prevalence remains below 1 percent in Western Europe, most of North America, and many Latin American countries.[11-14] In the Caribbean, seroprevalence among pregnant women ranges from 0 percent in Martinique to 8 percent in a slum of Port-au-Prince, Haiti.[15,16] In sub-Saharan Africa, however, very high levels of infection have been found among pregnant women in urban areas of Rwanda (33 percent), Uganda (29 percent), Malawi (23 percent), and Zambia (33.6 percent); seroprevalence is lower in neighboring countries such as Mozambique (0.8 percent) and appears stable in Zaire (5 percent).[17-22]

In Southeast Asia, by 1994, HIV seroprevalence among pregnant women was 2 percent or above in several studies conducted in India, Myanmar, and Thailand. However, given the rapid progression of HIV infection in these countries, these percentages can be expected to increase substantially.

Biology, behavior, and society

Biological, behavioral, and societal factors are all responsible for the gender differences in HIV epidemiology. Innate and acquired biological factors may help explain women's vulnerability to HIV infection. First, even in the absence of any other enhancing factors, HIV transmission from men to women seems to be more effective than from women to men.[23] Second, enhancing factors such as other sexually transmitted infections (STIs) are more likely to be present in women. This is because women are more susceptible than men to STIs and because these infections are more likely to go undetected and untreated in women. A few studies have suggested an association between the use of certain contraceptives (oral contraceptives, the intrauterine device [IUD], a diaphragm) and increased risk for HIV infection.[24,25,26] However, these associations have not been confirmed in other studies.[27,28,29]

A combination of behavioral and biological factors could also account for the gender difference in the age at which HIV infection rates peak. Girls become sexually active at a younger age than boys, and their youth may make them more susceptible than adult women to STIs and HIV. This is possibly due to a larger area of cervical ectopy, trauma, a less resistant vaginal epithelium, or some other biological features related to the lack of maturation of the genital tract.

Finally, over the past decade it has become increasingly clear that HIV and other STIs interact with and amplify each other. The presence of an ulcerative or non-ulcerative STI enhances the transmission of HIV, while HIV itself alters the clinical presentation and natural history of other STIs (Box 6-1).[30]

BOX 6-1

The interactions between HIV and other sexually transmitted infections

LAWRENCE J. GELMON AND PETER PIOT

The first volume of *AIDS in the World* noted that "persons who have histories of STI are at increased risk of acquiring HIV, while HIV-infected persons are likely to have a greater susceptibility to infection with other STIs and, if co-infected, may experience them in an unusually severe and protracted course." Little has changed in the past 3 years to warrant a revision of this statement.

In the past few years, additional reports on the prevalence of certain STIs have been published. However, they provide STI prevalence data in populations of STI clinic patients, who by definition are likely to have an STI or to be among a known high-risk group for STIs, such as sex workers. These data estimate the proportion of various STIs in the population sampled but cannot indicate the STI burden in the general population. These reports are also sometimes taken out of context and erroneously reported in the media as applying to the whole population. In addition, most studies are cross-sectional, one-time events; few populations are being followed to determine STI trends. Trends would help establish associations between changes in STI prevalence and increasing HIV infection rates or to measure the effectiveness of interventions.

The associations between HIV infection and STIs have been studied in a variety of settings over the past decade. In 1992, a figure in *AIDS in the World* showed that the relationship between HIV and STIs was "synergistic," in that both ulcerative and non-ulcerative STIs increased the risk of HIV transmission, while HIV infection could prolong or augment the infectiousness of people with STIs.[1]

At that time, only genital ulcer disease (GUD), especially chancroid and syphilis, had been consistently shown to facilitate the acquisition of HIV infection; recent studies have confirmed this relationship in both HIV-1- and HIV-2-infected people.[2-11] In addition, there is more recent evidence of an association between HIV infection and urethritis or urethral discharge, such as in gonorrhea.[12-15] However, the evidence for this association is not as solid, although a recent prospective study from Zaire found that non-ulcerative STIs (gonorrhea, chlamydia, and trichomoniasis) were risk factors for sexual acquisition of HIV-1 in women.[16-18] The increased risk of HIV acquisition associated with GUD, chlamydia, gonorrhea, or trichomonas has been confirmed.[19,20]

The presence of GUD or non-ulcerative inflammations of the cervix also increases the amount of HIV in the infected woman's genital tract, but whether this is directly associated with an increased risk of HIV transmission to the male partner is unclear.[21,22]

Earlier research found that HIV-1 infection was associated with an increased frequency of gonorrhea, chancroid, genital herpes, papilloma virus, and even early signs of cervical cancer, all of which may be related to immunodeficiency. Recent studies have also shown that the presence of HIV-1 infection may reduce the effectiveness of standard treatments for STIs such as chancroid and syphilis.[23,24]

From a public health perspective, what might be the effect of improved STI control on the HIV epidemic? Few studies have examined this question directly, although there have been attempts to predict its effects using mathematical models.[25,26] These calculations quantify the *attributable risk,* which is a measure of the proportion of disease that could be prevented by eliminating a certain exposure. For example, one study concluded that the attributable risk of HIV-1 transmission for women with gonorrhea was 44 percent, with chlamydia 22 percent, with trichomonas 18 percent, and with genital ulcer only 4 percent.[27] Does this mean that 44 percent of cases of HIV-1 could be prevented by control of gonorrhea? Unfortunately, the answer is, not necessarily. Calculations of attributable risk are influenced not only by the size of the study population but also by the underlying prevalence of the disease in question. In the case of STIs and HIV, such calculations are extremely complex and subject to conflicting interpretation.[28]

The first conclusive randomized trial demonstrating the impact of STI treatment on the incidence of HIV was conducted in a rural population of Tanzania between 1991 and 1995. It showed that improved STI treatment reduced the incidence of HIV infection by about 40 percent, although no change in sexual behavior had been observed over time in the study or the control population.[29] Such information is invaluable in emphasizing the critical impact that STI treatment can have on the HIV pandemic.

References

1. J. N. Wasserheit, "Epidemiological synergy: Inter-relationship between HIV infection and other STDs," in *AIDS and Women's Reproductive Health,* L. Chen J. S. Amar, and S. J. Segal eds. (New York: Plenum, 1992), reprinted in *Sexually Transmitted Diseases* 19(1992):61–77.

2. L. R. Barongo, M. W. Borgdorff, and F. F. Musha. "Epidemiology of HIV-1 in urban areas, roadside settlements and rural villages in Mwanza Region, Tanzania," *AIDS* 6(1992):1521–1528.

3. M. W. Borgdorff, L. R. Barongo, and E. van Jaarsveld, "Sentinel surveillance for HIV-1 infection: How representative are blood donors, outpatients with fever, anaemia, or sexually transmitted diseases, and antenatal clinic attenders in Mwanza Region, Tanzania?" *AIDS* 7(1993):567–572.

4. L. Zekeng, D. Yanga, and A. Treburg, "HIV prevalence in patients with sexually transmitted diseases in Yaounde, Cameroon in 1989 and 1990: Necessity of an STD control programme," *Genitourinary Medicine* 68(1992):117–119.

5. P. M. V. Martin, G. Gresenguet, and M. Massanga, "Association between HIV-1 infection and sexually transmitted disease among men in Central Africa," *Research in Virology* 143(1992):205–209.

6. S. Suwangool, S. Seripinan, and A. Sonjai, "HIV infection in male patients attending a sexually transmitted disease clinic," *Journal of the Medical Association of Thailand* 75(1992):293–298.

7. M. O. Diallo, A. Amouzou, K. T. Zunon, et al., "Trends in HIV-1 and HIV-2 infections in men attending an Abidjan sexually transmitted diseases clinic, 1990–1992," presented at VII International Conference on AIDS in Africa, Yaounde, Cameroon, 1992.

8. M. Temmerman, F. M. Ali, E. N. Chomba, and J. Ndinya-Achola, "Rapid increase of both HIV-1 infection and syphilis among pregnant women in Nairobi, Kenya," *AIDS* 6(1992):1181–1185.

9. T. Nopkesorn, T. D. Mastro, and S. Sangkharomya, "HIV-1 infection in young men in northern Thailand," Abstract PO-C11-2832, presented at the IX International Conference on AIDS, Berlin, Germany, June 1993, reprinted in *AIDS* 7(1993):1233–1239.

10. A. L. S. Patullo, J. Nasio, and M. Malisa, "Increased HIV-1 prevalence in women with genital ulcer disease presenting to an STD clinic in Nairobi, Kenya," Abstract PO-C20-3091, presented at the IX International Conference on AIDS, Berlin, Germany, June 1993.

11. J. Pepin, D. Dunn, and I. Gaye, "HIV-2 infection among prostitutes working in the Gambia: Association with serological evidence of genital ulcer diseases and with generalized lymphadenopathy," *AIDS* 5(1991):69–75.

12. Barongo, "Epidemiology of HIV-1."

13. P. M. V. Martin, G. Gresenguet, and M. Massanga, "Association between HIV-1 infection and sexually transmitted disease among men in Central Africa," *Research in Virology* 143(1992):205–209.

14. Diallo, "Sexually transmitted diseases."

15. Nopkesorn, "HIV-1 infection in young men."

16. Suwangool, "HIV infection in male patients."

17. Temmerman, "Rapid increase."

18. M. Laga, A. Manoka, and M. Kivuvu, "Non-ulcerative sexually transmitted diseases as risk factors for HIV-1 transmission in women: Results from a cohort study," *AIDS* 7(1993):95–102.

19. F. A. Plummer, J. N. Simonsen, and D. W. Cameron, "Cofactors in male-female sexual transmission of HIV-1," *Journal of Infectious Diseases* 163(1991):233–239.

20. Laga, "Non-ulcerative sexually transmitted diseases."

21. J. K. Kreiss, R. Coombs, and F. A. Plummer, "Isolation of HIV-1 from genital ulcers in Nairobi prostitutes," *Journal of Infectious Diseases* 160(1989):380–384.

22. D. R. Clemetson, G. B. Moss, and D. M. Willerford, "Detection of HIV DNA in cervical and vaginal secretions. Prevalence and correlates among women in Nairobi, Kenya," *Journal of the American Medical Association* 269(1993):2860–2864.

23. M. Tyndall, M. Malisa, and F. A. Plummer, "Ceftriaxone no longer predictably cures chancroid in Kenya," *Journal of Infectious Diseases* 167(1993):469–471.

24. D. M. Musher, "Syphilis, neurosyphilis, penicillin, and AIDS," *Journal of Infectious Diseases* 163(1991):1201–1206.

25. N. J. Robinson, R. Hayes, et al., "STD cofactor effects, and associations between HIV and other STDs: Stochastic simulation exercise in SW Uganda," presented at the VIII International Conference on AIDS in Africa, Marrakech, Morocco, December 1993.

26. K. F. Schulz, R. Hayes, and F. Plummer, personal communication.

27. Laga, "Non-ulcerative sexually transmitted disease."

28. T. E. Mertens, R. Hayes, and P. G. Smith, "Epidemiological methods to study the interaction between HIV infection and other STDs," *AIDS* 4(1990):57–65.

29. H. Grosskurth, F. Mosha, J. Todd, E. Mwijarubi, A. Klokke, K. Senkoro, P. Mayaud, J. Changalucha, A. Nicoll, G. ka-Gina, J. Newell, K. Mugeye, D. Mabey, and R. Hayes, "Impact of improved treatment of sexually transmitted diseases on HIV infection in rural Tanzania: Randomized controlled trial," *Lancet* 346 (1995): 530–535.

For both men and women, the most important behavorial risk factors for acquiring HIV are the number of sex partners and the number of unprotected sexual contacts.[31,32] For women, however, an additional risk is created by their relative lack of control over the conditions of their lives in general, and specifically, the conditions under which they have sex. This problem applies to sexually active females across the spectrum from sex workers to monogamous, married women.

Women who must trade sex for necessities are a less well-studied risk group than sex workers, but they too are at high risk of HIV infection. For example, economic necessity has led women in Zambia to become fish traders—traditionally a male-dominated activity. Recognizing that the women are disadvantaged within this professional group, the fishermen have used their position of power to demand sex in exchange for fish.[33]

Other behavioral factors that may increase women's risk of HIV infection, especially in Africa, include traditional sexual practices such as dry sex and ritual sexual cleansing.[34] Dry sex is the practice of inserting certain herbs or topical mixtures into the vagina to dry up vaginal secretions before intercourse. This is said to enhance the male's pleasure during intercourse. However, the practice irritates the vaginal epithelium and cervical mucosa, increasing vulnerability to HIV and other STIs.[35] The tradition of ritual sexual cleansing requires a widow to have sexual intercourse with a male relative of her deceased husband shortly after the funeral. This transfers responsibility for the woman and her children from the deceased to his relative. In some countries the advent of HIV/AIDS has led to questioning the wisdom and advisability of this tradition.[36]

The epidemiology of sexually transmitted infections in women

Syphilis

The high rate of syphilis in some populations and its re-emergence in others is particularly disconcerting given that it is easily detected by a simple labo-

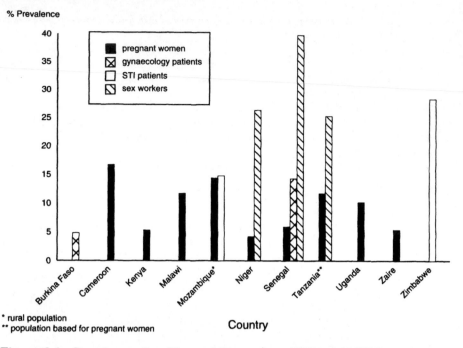

% Prevalence

* rural population
** population based for pregnant women

Country

Figure 6-1   Prevalence of positive syphilis serology (RPR+ and TPHA+) in different female urban populations in sub-Saharan Africa, 1990–1993.

ratory test and can be treated cheaply and reliably. Figure 6-1 summarizes syphilis prevalence data (based on rapid plasma reagent/*Treponema pallidium* hemagglutinin [RPR/TPHA] seroreactivity) for different female urban populations in sub-Saharan Africa. High syphilis infection rates are not confined to Africa. In Porto Alegre, Brazil, 2.3 percent of newborns were found to have clinical and/or laboratory evidence of syphilis.[37]

Among sex workers, the syphilis seroprevalence rate was 40 percent in Senegal, 45 percent in Brazil, 33 percent in Puerto Rico, and in Thailand it was 11 percent in a northern town and 15 percent in a southern town.[38–41]

Currently, syphilis is rare in most European countries, including Sweden, France, and Belgium.[42,43,44] There was, however, an injecting drug–associated increase in the incidence of syphilis among female sex workers in the Netherlands which peaked in 1989.[45] A re-emergence of syphilis is even more apparent in the U.S., where cases among African-American women more than tripled between 1985 and 1990 from 35 per 100,000 to 116 per 100,000.[46]

Other genital ulcer disease

The incidence of genital ulcers is far higher in developing countries than in industrialized countries. *Haemophilus ducreyi*, the causative agent of chancroid, remains an important cause of genital ulcers in sub-Saharan Africa and Asia. Twenty percent of pregnant women in a rural area in Mozambique had antibodies against *H. ducreyi*, and 15 percent of South African women seeking medical care for genital ulcers were suffering from chancroid.[47,48] In Latin America, however, syphilis is far more prevalent than chancroid and accounts for the largest percentage of genital ulcers. In Brazil, for example, only 7 percent of genital ulcers registered between 1989 and 1992 were due to chancroid, whereas 49 percent were caused by primary syphilis.[49]

Finally, wherever HIV is widespread, genital herpes is becoming an increasingly important etiologic agent of genital ulcers. For example, in Kigali, Rwanda, in 1984, the most common cause of genital ulcer syndrome in women was syphilis; by 1991 it was genital herpes.[50]

Gonococcal and chlamydial infections

Severe complications of gonorrhea and chlamydial infection are more likely to occur in women than in men. Unlike syphilis, these two STIs are often asymptomatic in women, and infected women may not seek medical care. The consequence of an untreated, ascending infection of the cervix is pelvic inflammatory disease (PID), a common cause of gynecologic admission to hospitals. The long-term effects of PID include chronic abdominal pain, extrauterine pregnancy, and infertility.[51] Gonorrhea rates vary sharply worldwide, but the rate of chlamydial infections is remarkably homogeneous.

As with HIV infection, there is a considerable variation in gonorrhea rates from country to country, but most striking is the large difference in prevalence rates among developing countries. Among low-risk women, high rates of gonorrhea were found in Kenya (10 percent) and Mozambique (7 percent).[52,53] Among high-risk women, gonorrhea prevalence exceeded 20 percent in Bolivia, Côte d'Ivoire, Niger, and northern Thailand.[54-57] In Western Europe (Belgium, France, the Netherlands, and Sweden), reported cases of gonorrhea in both males and females decreased continuously between 1980 and 1990, and the prevalence rarely exceeded 0.3 percent in low-risk women and 5 percent in high-risk women.[58-65]

The epidemiology of chlamydial infection differs from that of gonorrhea and this difference remains to some extent unexplained. In contrast to other STIs, the prevalence rates of chlamydia in developing countries have often been comparable to the rates in industrialized countries. The reported number of chlamydial infections in North America and Western Europe increased in the 1980s, but this was in part because new diagnostic tests were developed and screening programs were established.[66,67,68] Evidence of chlamydial infection was found in about 8 percent of low-risk women in some parts of North America, Western Europe, and sub-Saharan Africa.[69-74] Comparable prevalence has been found among low-risk women in Latin America and the Caribbean: 4 percent among pregnant women in Nicaragua, 10 percent among women at an antenatal clinic in Haiti, and 16 percent among women at a family planning clinic in Martinique.[75,76,77] Moreover, although a high prevalence of chlamydial infection was noted among high-risk women, the difference between low-risk and high-risk groups was less striking than for gonorrhea. The fact that there is a short-lived immunity after infection could explain both this and the strong association between chlamydial infection and young age.[78] Chlamydial infection has also repeatedly been associated with new or multiple sex partners and with hormonal contraception.[79,80,81]

Trichomoniasis and bacterial vaginosis

Trichomoniasis and bacterial vaginosis account for most cases of sexually transmitted vaginitis. Its symptoms (abnormal vaginal discharge, vaginal itching) are among the most frequent complaints presented by women at STI clinics.

A striking feature of trichomoniasis is its consistently high prevalence among low-risk pregnant women in many developing countries (e.g., over 30 percent in Haiti, Malawi, and Uganda).[82,83,84] In sub-Saharan Africa, very small differences in trichomoniasis prevalence were noted between low-risk and high-risk women. In Mozambique, trichomoniasis was present in 23 percent of pregnant women and 24 percent of female STI patients.[85] For pregnant women and sex workers, respectively, its prevalence rate was 12 percent and 13 percent in Niger, and 16 percent and 18 percent in Senegal.[86,87] In industrialized countries, trichomoniasis is much less prevalent.[88] There are several reasons for the high trichomoniasis prevalence among pregnant women in many developing countries. The infection can be asymptomatic and so may only be detected where screening is done. In some cultures, women may not seek treatment because symptoms of vaginal discharge are not perceived as a health problem. And finally, even when a woman is symptomatic and perceives her symptoms as a problem, health services may be inaccessible and/or stigmatizing—especially for STIs.

REFERENCES

1. M. Marino, L. D. Castano, J. Suarez, et al., "Spread of HIV/AIDS to the female population in Colombia," Abstract PO-C06-2721, presented at the IX International Conference on AIDS, Berlin, Germany, June 1993.

2. G. A. Conway, M. R. Epstein, C. R. Hayman, et al., "Trends in HIV prevalence among disadvantaged youth," *Journal of the American Medical Association* 269(1993):2887–2889.

3. S. Berkley, W. Naamara, S. Okware, et al., "AIDS and HIV infection in Uganda—are more women infected than men?" *AIDS* 4(1990):1237–1242.

4. J. Killewo, K. Nyamuryekunge, A. Sandström, et al., "Prevalence of HIV-1 infection in the Kagara region of Tanzania: A population-based study," *AIDS* 4(1990):1081–1085.

5. L. R. Barongo, M. W. Borgdorff, F. F. Mosha, et al., "Epidemiology of HIV-1 infection in urban areas, roadside settlements and rural villages in Mwanza Region, Tanzania," *AIDS* 6(1992):1521–1528.

6. *Ibid.*

7. Berkley, "AIDS and HIV."

8. European Working Group on HIV Infection in Female Prostitutes, "HIV infection in European female sex workers: Epidemiological link with use of petroleum-based lubricants," *AIDS* 7(1993):401–408.

9. D. M. Willerford, J. J. Bwayo, M. Hensel, et al., "Human immunodeficiency virus infection among high-risk seronegative prostitutes in Nairobi," *Journal of Infectious Diseases* 167(1993):1414–1417.

10. T. Siraprapasiri, S. Thanprasertsuk, A. Rodklay, et al., "Risk factors for HIV among prostitutes in Chiangmai, Thailand," *AIDS* 5(1991):579–582.

11. S. C. Wasser, M. Gwinn, and P. Fleming, "Urban-nonurban distribution of HIV infection

in childbearing women in the United States," *Journal of Acquired Immune Deficiency Syndromes* 6(1993):1035–1042.

12. Y. Brossard, M. Larsen, L. Meyer, et al., "HIV epidemiological trends (1987–1991) among pregnant women in the Paris area," Abstract WS-C04-1, presented at the IX International Conference on AIDS, Berlin, Germany, June 1993.

13. P. J. E. Bindels, "Resultaten van de screening op HIV-antistoffen bij zwangere vrouwen, bezoeksters van infertiliteitspoliklinieken en abortusklinieken in de regio Amsterdam in 1990," *Nederlands Tijdschrift der Geneeskunde* 135(1991):2123–2128.

14. I. L. Chrystie, S. J. Palmer, A. Kenney, et al., "HIV seroprevalence among women attending antenatal clinics in London," Abstract PoC 4360, presented at the VIII International Conference on AIDS, Amsterdam, The Netherlands, July 1992.

15. R. Chout, D. Quist, S. Vaton, et al., "*Chlamydia trachomatis* in asymptomatic female adolescents and young adults in Martinique," Abstract 331, presented at the X International Meeting of the International Society for STD Research, Helsinki, Finland, August–September 1993.

16. R. Boulos, E. Holt, P. Kissinger, et al., "Stable HIV-1 seroprevalence rates in pregnant women residing in a Haitian urban slum," Abstract M.C.3015, presented at the VII International Conference on AIDS, Florence, Italy, June 1991.

17. A. De Clercq, V. Leroy, C. Zilimwagabo, et al., "Prévalence des maladies sexuellement transmissibles (MST) et statut immunitaire chez les femmes enceintes infectées par le VIH, Kigali (Rwanda), 1992–1993," Abstract Th.R.T 033, presented at the VIII International Conference on AIDS in Africa, Marrakech, Morocco, December 1993.

18. J. E. Zelaya, G. Tembo, W. Naamara, et al., *AIDS Surveillance Report: June 1992*, unpublished report (Entebbe, Uganda: Ministry of Health, AIDS Control Programme Surveillance Unit).

19. G. A. Dallabetta, P. G. Miotti, J. D. Chiphangwi, et al., "High socioeconomic status is a risk factor for human immunodeficiency virus type 1 (HIV-1) infection but not for sexually transmitted diseases in women in Malawi: Implications for HIV-1 control," *Journal of Infectious Diseases* 167(1993):36–42.

20. K. Flykness, M. Roland, and B. Belge, "Current HIV/AIDS situation and future demographic impact," background paper 1, Socio-economic impact of AIDS in Zambia (1994).

21. J. Barreto, J. Liljestrand, C. Palha de Sousa, et al., "HIV-1 and HIV-2 antibodies in pregnant women in the city of Maputo, Mozambique," *Scandinavian Journal of Infectious Diseases* 25(1993):685–688.

22. B. Vuylsteke, M. Laga, M. Alary, et al., "Clinical algorithms for the screening of women for gonococcal and chlamydial infection: Evaluation of pregnant women and prostitutes in Zaire," *Clinical Infectious Diseases* 17(1993):82–88.

23. European Study Group on Heterosexual Transmission of HIV, "Comparison of female to male and male to female transmission of HIV in 563 stable couples," *British Medical Journal* 304(1992):809–813.

24. F. A. Plummer, J. N. Simonsen, D. W. Cameron, et al., "Cofactors in male-female sexual transmission of human immunodeficiency virus type 1," *Journal of Infectious Diseases* 163(1991):233–239.

25. S. H. Kapiga, J. F. Shao, G. K. Lwihula, et al., "Risk factors for HIV infection among women in Dar-es-Salaam, Tanzania," *Journal of Acquired Immune Deficiency Syndromes* 7(1994):301–309.

26. G. S. Bernstein, R .M. Nakamura, R. Frezieres, et al., "Vaginal trauma related to use of contraceptive diaphragms. Relevance to transmission of HIV," Abstract PO-C02-2593, presented at the IX International Conference on AIDS, Berlin, Germany, June 1993.

27. Kapiga, "Risk factors."

28. Bernstein, "Vaginal trauma."

29. S. Allen, P. Van de Perre, A. Serufilira, et al., "Human immunodeficiency virus and malaria in a representative sample of childbearing women in Kigali, Rwanda," *Journal of Infectious Diseases* 164(1991):67–71.

30. M. Laga, N. Nzila, and J. Goeman, "Interrelationship of sexually transmitted diseases and HIV infection: Implications for the control of both epidemics in Africa," *AIDS* 5(suppl. 1)(1991):s55–s63.

31. Barongo, "Epidemiology of HIV-1."

32. T. Siraprapasiri, S. Thanprasertsuk, A. Rodklay, et al., "Risk factors for HIV among prostitutes in Chiangmai, Thailand," *AIDS* 5(1991):579–582.

33. C. Mushinge, W. Chama, and Muliekelela, *Investigation of High Risk Situations and Environments and Their Potential Role in the Transmission of HIV in Zambia, The Case of the Copperbelt and Luapula Provinces* (Lusaka: Population Council of Zambia, 1992).

34. R. McNamara, *Female Genital Health and the Risk of HIV Transmission*, issue paper 3 (Geneva: UN Development Programme, 1993).

35. A. O. Runganga, "Vaginal use of herbs/substances, an HIV transmission facilitatory factor?" Abstract M.P.C 085, presented at the VIII International Conference on AIDS in Africa, Marrakech, Morocco, December 1993.

36. M. Bulterys, F. Musanganire, A. Chao, et al., "Traditional mourning customs and the spread of HIV-1 in rural Rwanda," correspondence, *AIDS* 8(1994):858–859.

37. P. Naud, L. Bergmann, M. Genehr, et al., "Prevalence of congenital syphilis in a Brazilian center in 1992," Abstract PO-C10-2815, presented at the IX International Conference on AIDS, Berlin, Germany, June 1993.

38. N. D. Samb, F. Van Der Veen, M. Sene, et al., "Sentinel surveillance of STDs, and its implications for AIDS control in Senegal," Abstract PoC 4328, presented at the VIII International Conference on AIDS, Amsterdam, The Netherlands, July 1992.

39. M. E. Fernandes, A. Reingold, N. Hearst, et al., "HIV in commercial sex workers in São Paulo, Brazil," Abstract PoC 4190, presented at the VIII International Conference on AIDS, Amsterdam, The Netherlands, July 1992.

40. M. Alegria, M. Vera, R. Robles, et al., "What have we learned from adolescent prostitutes in the Caribbean that adult prostitutes did not tell us?" Abstract WS-C08-2, presented at the IX International Conference on AIDS, Berlin, Germany, June 1993.

41. N. Chaistri, V. Danutra, and B. Limanonda, "Prevalence of syphilis and anti-HIV-1 seropositive among prostitutes in two urban areas of Thailand," Abstract PO-C14-2896, presented at the IX International Conference on AIDS, Berlin, Germany, June 1993.

42. D. Danielsson, "Gonorrhoea and syphilis in Sweden—past and present," *Scandinavian Journal of Infectious Diseases* 69(1990):69–76.

43. L. Meyer, V. Goulet, V. Massari, et al., "Surveillance of sexually transmitted diseases in France: Recent trends and incidence," *Genitourinary Medicine* 70(1994):15–21.

44. D. Walckiers, P. Piot, A. Stroobant, et al., "Declining trends in some sexually transmitted diseases in Belgium between 1983 and 1989," *Genitourinary Medicine* 67(1991):374–377.

45. H. F. Treurniet and W. Davidse, "Sexually transmitted diseases reported by STD services in the Netherlands, 1984–1990," *Genitourinary Medicine* 69(1993):434–438.

46. Centers for Disease Control, "Primary and secondary syphilis—United States, 1981–1990," *Morbidity and Mortality Weekly Report* 40(1991):314–323.

47. B. Vuylsteke, R. Bastos, J. Barreto, et al., "High prevalence of sexually transmitted diseases in a rural area in Mozambique," *Genitourinary Medicine* 69(1993):427–430.

48. N. O'Farrell, A. A. Hoosen, K. D. Coetzee, et al., "Genital ulcer disease: Accuracy of clinical diagnosis and strategies to improve control in Durban, South Africa," *Genitourinary Medicine* 70(1994):7–11.

49. National HIV/STD program, *DST, Boletim Epidemiológico* 1(Brazil: Ministry of Health, 1993).

50. Jos Bogaerts, personal communication.

51. J. N. Wasserheit, "Significance and scope of reproductive tract infections among third world women," *International Journal of Gynaecology and Obstetrics* (suppl. 3)(1989):145–168.

52. J. N. Mungai, G. M. Maitha, M. Z. Kitabu, et al., "Prevalence of HIV and other STDs in three populations in Nairobi for year 1991," Abstract PoC 4714, presented at the VIII International Conference on AIDS, Amsterdam, The Netherlands, July 1992.

53. Vuylsteke, "High prevalence."

54. J. Vega, W. Levine, M. Estenssoro, et al., "High STD prevalence among commercial sex workers in La Paz, Bolivia," Abstract PO-C10-2818, presented at the IX International Conference on AIDS, Berlin, Germany, June 1993.

55. P. D. Ghys, M. O. Diallo, V. Traoré-Ettiegne, et al., "Evaluation of simple screening criteria for the diagnosis of cervicitis in commercial sex workers (CSWS) in Abidjan, Côte d'Ivoire," presented at the X International Meeting of the International Society for STD Research, Helsinki, Finland, August–September 1993.

56. A. Hassane, R. Paradis, A. Mounkaila, et al., "Estimation rapide de prévalence des MST/VIH à Niamey, Niger," Abstract Th.P.C 087, presented at the VIII International Conference on AIDS in Africa, Marrakech, Morocco, December 1993.

57. K. Limpakarnjanarat, T. D. Mastro, W. Yindeeyoungyeon, et al., "STDs in female prostitutes in northern Thailand," Abstract PO-C10-2820, presented at the IX International Conference on AIDS, Berlin, Germany, June 1993.

58. D. Walckiers, P. Piot, A. Stroobant, et al., "Declining trends in some sexually transmitted diseases in Belgium between 1983 and 1989," *Genitourinary Medicine* 67(1991):374–377.

59. Meyer, "Surveillance."

60. H. F. Treurniet, W. Davidse, "Sexually transmitted diseases reported by STD services in the Netherlands, 1984–1990," *Genitourinary Medicine* 69(1993):434–438.

61. Danielsson, "Gonorrhoea."

62. D. Guerreiro, F. Bivar, M. Palma, et al., "Study on sexually transmitted diseases in prenatal and family planning clinics in an area of Lisbon," Abstract PoC 4669, presented at the VIII International Conference on AIDS, Amsterdam, The Netherlands, July 1992.

63. I. Kallings, C. Brihmer, B. Sikström, et al., "History and prevalence of sexually transmitted diseases among Swedish women attending family planning clinics," Abstract 24, presented at the X International Meeting of the International Society for STD Research, Helsinki, Finland, August–September 1993.

64. A. Stary, W. Kopp, and J. Söltz-Szöts, "Medical health for Viennese prostitutes," *Sexually Transmitted Diseases* 18(1991):159–165.

65. H. Ward, S. Day, J. Mezzone, et al., "Prostitution and risk of HIV: Female prostitutes in London," *British Medical Journal* 307(1993):356–358.

66. J. Schachter, "Future problems for Chlamydia control programmes," Abstract 11, presented at the X International Meeting of the International Society for STD Research, Helsinki, Finland, August–September 1993.

67. H. F. Treurniet and W. Davidse, "Sexually transmitted diseases reported by STD services in the Netherlands, 1984–1990," *Genitourinary Medicine* 69(1993):434–438.

68. Meyer, "Surveillance."

69. J. Sellors, L. Pickard, A. Gafni, et al., "Effectiveness and efficiency of selective vs. universal screening in women attending family planning clinics," Abstract C22106, presented at the International Society for STD Research, IX International Meeting, Banff, Canada, October 1991.

70. T. V. Ellerbrock, S. Lieb, P. E. Harrington, et al., "Heterosexually transmitted human immunodeficiency virus infection among pregnant women in a rural Florida community," *New England Journal of Medicine* 327(1992):1704–1709.

71. Kallings, "History and prevalence."

72. Vuylsteke, "High prevalence."

73. P. S. J. Nsubuga, W. Roseberry, F. Judson, et al., "Rapid assessment of STD prevalence: The validity of STD rapid indicators in Uganda," Abstract 141, presented at the X International Meeting of the International Society for STD Research, Helsinki, Finland, August–September 1993.

74. N. D. Samb, F. Van Der Veen, M. Sene, et al., "Sentinel surveillance of STDs, and its implications for AIDS control in Senegal," Abstract PoC 4328, presented at the VIII International Conference on AIDS, Amsterdam, The Netherlands, July 1992.

75. F. Espinoza, M. Egger, B. Herrmann, et al., "STD in Nicaragua: Population rate estimates and health seeking behaviour," Abstract PO-C06-2702, presented at the IX International Conference on AIDS, Berlin, Germany, June 1993.

76. J. Desormeaux, F. Behets, H. Hamilton, et al., "Sexually transmitted diseases (STD) among pregnant women living in Haitian shantytowns: A first baseline study," Abstract WS-C06-5, presented at the IX International Conference on AIDS, Berlin, Germany, June 1993.

77. R. Chout, D. Quist, S. Vaton, et al., "*Chlamydia trachomatis* in asymptomatic female adolescents and young adults in Martinique," Abstract 331, presented at the X International Meeting of the International Society for STD Research, Helsinki, Finland, August–September 1993.

78. J. N. Arno, B. P. Catz, R. McBride, et al., "Age and clinical immunity to infections with *Chlamydia trachomatis*," *Sexually Transmitted Diseases* 21(1994):47–52.

79. B. Vuylsteke, M. Laga, M. Alary, et al., "Clinical algorithms for the screening of women for gonococcal and chlamydial infection: Evaluation of pregnant women and prostitutes in Zaire," *Clinical Infectious Diseases* 17(1993):82–88.

80. M. Alary, J. R. Joly, J.-M. Moutquin, et al., "Strategy for screening pregnant women for Chlamydial infection in a low-prevalence area," *Obstetrics and Gynecology* 82(1993):399–404.

81. M. J. W. van de Laar, Y. T. H. P. van Duynhoven, J. A. R. van den Hoek, et al., "Prevalence and risk factors of *Chlamydia trachomatis* infection among visitors of a STD outpatient clinic in Amsterdam," Abstract 360, presented at the X International Meeting of the International Society for STD Research, Helsinki, Finland, August–September 1993.

82. J. Desormeaux, F. Behets, H. Hamilton, et al., "Sexually transmitted diseases (STD) among pregnant women living in Haitian shantytowns: A first baseline study," Abstract WS-C06–5, presented at the IX International Conference on AIDS, Berlin, Germany, June 1993.

83. G. A. Dallabetta, P. G. Miotti, J. D. Chiphangwi, et al., "High socioeconomic status is a risk factor for human immunodeficiency virus type 1 (HIV-1) infection but not for sexually transmitted diseases in women in Malawi: Implications for HIV-1 control," *Journal of Infectious Diseases* 167(1993):36–42.

84. P. S. J. Nsubuga, W. Roseberry, F. Judson, et al., "Rapid assessment of STD prevalence:

The validity of STD rapid indicators in Uganda," Abstract 141, presented at the X International Meeting of the International Society for STD Research, Helsinki, Finland, August–September 1993.

85. Vuylsteke, "High prevalence."
86. A. Hassane, R. Paradis, A. Mounkaila, et al., "Estimation rapide de prévalence des MST/VIH à Niamey, Niger," Abstract Th.P.C 087, presented at the VIII International Conference on AIDS in Africa, Marrakech, Morocco, December 1993.
87. Samb, "Sentinel surveillance."
88. Guerreiro, "Study on sexually transmitted diseases."

7

Economic Impact in Selected Countries and the Sectoral Impact

ALAN WHITESIDE

As the speed and extent of HIV spread differs greatly among countries and geographical areas, so too will its economic impact. Assessing and predicting the economic impact of HIV/AIDS is difficult, for in no country has the epidemic run its course, national and sectoral economic impacts are not felt until AIDS cases appear in significant numbers, and the full economic impact will take time to appear. This chapter reviews the relevant literature and work in progress and illustrates the economic impact of HIV/AIDS through a review of six country case studies.

Literature review

Literature on the economic impact of AIDS is broadly divided into macroeconomic and microeconomic studies. Macroeconomics relates to whole economic systems and normally refers to a country's economy. Microeconomics examines individual consumers, groups of consumers, and firms. Between the two lie regional economies (state, province, and county) and analyses of individual sectors such as agriculture or transport.

Economic analysis during the first years of the HIV/AIDS epidemic was speculative, and assumed that AIDS would adversely affect economies at all levels, from national to household. In 1988, the First International Conference on the Global Impact of AIDS included presentations on HIV-related direct and indirect costs; its impact on food production in East and Central Africa and on the mining industry; and the impact on families and development.[1] Yet few data were available.

Economists and policy makers knew the epidemic would have a complex impact: "Because the infection is concentrated in the 20–40 age group, AIDS is attacking the most sexually active and the most economically productive populations. The 20–40 age group carries an enormous economic burden in societies in which nearly 50 percent of the population is under 15 years of age. . . ."[2]

However, methods were not then available to assess the economic impact of HIV/AIDS, nor was there much information on the effect of any specific disease on economies. Research had been done on the costs of disease, premature death, and morbidity; however, literature on the effect of these health factors on economic growth and development was lacking. Accordingly, AIDS, with its far-reaching impact and magnitude, has stimulated new interest and research in health economics. In the early 1990s, studies began to demonstrate how AIDS might affect economies.

The World Bank approach

In the 1993 *World Development Report*, in order to establish a sense of the scale of health problems, the concept of a global burden of disease was developed. This combines a measure of mortality (premature death) and morbidity (the loss of healthy life due to disability) into units of disability-adjusted life years (DALYs).[3] By calculating the cost of ill-health and premature death, the DALY concept facilitates comparisons among diseases and helps identify costs associated with patterns of disease.

Using this methodology, the 1993 *World Development Report* documents enormous regional and global inequalities in health status. In sub-Saharan Africa in 1990, ill-health and accidents led to the loss of 575 DALYs per 1,000 population, of which HIV and sexually transmitted infections (STIs) accounted for 8.8 percent. In industrialized countries there were only 117 DALYs lost per 1,000 population; HIV accounted for 3.4 percent of these, the highest level being in the communicable disease category. Finally, in extending the concept of DALYs to prevention and control, the report suggests that HIV "can be substantially controlled with cost-effective intervention; less than $100 per DALY [can be] saved" in developing economies.[4]

The macroeconomic literature

Two seminal papers provide methodologies for assessing the macroeconomic impact of AIDS. The first attempts to identify and analyze the main channels through which HIV will affect economic and social systems, establishes an economic case for effective policies of HIV prevention, and reviews a selection of methodologies and empirical evidence on the impact of HIV on households, productive sectors, and the government.[5]

The second paper provides an overview of the macroeconomic impact of HIV/AIDS, concentrating on sub-Saharan Africa. This study postulates that the effect of AIDS will be felt in two ways. First, it will have an impact on human capital, the skills base of an economy. Economic growth is closely correlated with increases in urban, skilled populations. If these populations are adversely affected, this will have a disproportionate and negative impact on economic growth. Second, HIV/AIDS will affect savings, which are essential for economic growth, as they allow new and replacement investment. If AIDS patients finance their treatment costs from savings, and if this is not offset by an inflow from foreign sources, then investment and future growth will suffer. The overall message is bleak—AIDS has the potential to slow economic growth significantly, a real concern in much of Africa where growth has, at best, been minimal.[6]

An inherent problem with studies of the macroeconomic impact is the complexity both of economies and HIV/AIDS. In Zambia, for example, one of the main banks recorded a rise in staff mortality, largely due to AIDS, from 0.4 percent in 1987 to 2.2 percent in 1992. The greatest number of deaths (29.5 percent) occurred among 36–40-year-olds, while this group accounted for only 19 percent of employees.[7] The loss of relatively senior staff causes major problems for the bank, and the effects extend into the national economy: branches of the bank may have to close; the bank may operate less efficiently, adversely affecting the business climate; and employees may cash insurance policies and pension funds, reducing investment funds. Where skilled and experienced staff is in short supply, increases in morbidity and mortality may have severe ripple effects throughout the entire economy.

The microeconomic literature

To date, microeconomic research has concentrated on rural agriculture in Africa, and in Asia to a limited extent.[8,9,10]

As of mid-1995, two ambitious and important studies were underway. The World Bank and University of Dar-es-Salaam are conducting a longitudinal survey of 800 households in Kagera, Tanzania. The households are interviewed at 18-month intervals to measure the impact of morbidity and mortality on household composition and migration of members; individual and household labor supply; health care utilization and expenditure; school enrollments and expenditure; economic activities and income of household members; individual and household consumption expenditure; transfers into and out of the household; savings; and assets, including housing, durable goods, land and animals. Analysis of the data is in progress.[11]

In addition, the International Children's Centre in Paris has initiated a study of the socioeconomic evolution of children and families affected by AIDS, involving 200 households with AIDS patients in each of three countries: Burundi, Côte d'Ivoire, and Haiti. Information is collected on the socioeconomic characteristics of household members, sources of modern and traditional medical treatment, direct and indirect treatment costs, and community infrastructure. Subsequently, 120 households in each country will be followed longitudinally for a year, with a more detailed questionnaire administered every 2 months. Unfortunately, all three study countries have been affected by political problems.[12]

Country case study reviews

Tanzania

The World Bank developed a framework for analyzing the effects of AIDS on the growth of gross domestic product (GDP), using a simple model that incorporates the increase in morbidity and mortality due to AIDS. The model examines labor productivity lost per AIDS case and AIDS costs met from reduced savings.

According to this study, AIDS in Tanzania will reduce the average real GDP growth rate in the period 1985–2010 from 3.9 percent without AIDS to between 2.8 and 3.3 percent with AIDS. The result is that by 2010, the economy will be between 15 and 25 percent smaller because of the epidemic. Although the projected effects are large, the study warns that estimates may actually be too conservative because of interactions not predicted.[13]

Cameroon

In another study, a computable general equilibrium model was developed for Cameroon. On the production and supply side, the model included three agricultural, five manufacturing, and three service sectors. The labor market was divided into three skills categories: rural unskilled, urban unskilled, and urban skilled. The model also considered foreign trade, income generation and production demand, investment and savings, and supply–demand equilibrium. The model suggested that, in the worst case, the average annual GDP growth rate for the period 1987–1991 could fall dramatically from 4.3 percent to 2.4 percent.[14]

Swaziland

In 1993, the Swaziland Government commissioned a report on the socioeconomic impact of HIV/AIDS on human resources, education, employee benefits, health care, and social welfare. The report suggests that the government should begin planning for increased morbidity and mortality among its personnel. For example, currently civil servants are able to take up to 1 year of sick leave (6 months with full pay and 6 months with half pay). This policy will have adverse effects on the payroll and efficiency of government, as posts will remain unfilled or are occupied by people in an acting capacity only, or additional staff will have to be recruited.[15]

Thailand

A study was undertaken here to project HIV infection and AIDS cases and deaths, and then to consider the associated direct and indirect costs. Direct costs include personal health care expenditure and the cost of prevention. Indirect costs were calculated by assuming an average loss per AIDS death of 25 years, the cost of which was then discounted. The least total cost (direct plus indirect) was estimated to rise from U.S. $97 million in 1991 to $1.8 billion in the year 2000, a higher total cost from $100 million in 1991 to $2.2 billion in 2000.[16]

The study notes that "unless significant behavior changes occur the AIDS epidemic is likely to alter the performance of the Thai economy." A labor shortage—in terms of both quality and quantity—may occur with an increase in AIDS.[17] Other areas of concern are foreign investment and the migration of labor. The nation's saving rate may be reduced, and tourism, a major economic activity, may decline.

South Africa

The research conducted here also projected future AIDS cases and estimated the associated direct and indirect costs. The indirect costs were developed using the human capital approach, using lost earnings as a proxy measure for lost production. The study found that low estimates of the direct cost of AIDS would be $21.5 million in 1991, rising to $1.2 billion in the year 2000. In higher estimates, direct costs would increase from $32 million in 1991 to $2.9 billion in the year 2000.

Indirect costs were adjusted to show the difference between skilled and unskilled workers. The conclusion is that the total costs of the epidemic have the potential to grow to enormous proportions with an impact on consumption, but the overall economic impact will be sustainable to the end of the decade. However, the study warned that the macroeconomic view hides devastating economic consequences at the microeconomic level.[18]

Republic of Korea

The study conducted here calculated the number of HIV infections and AIDS cases, and then concentrated on a typical 30-year-old man or woman. The cost of premature death was US $227,572 for a man and $114,200 for a woman, including direct medical expenditure and indirect costs (at a discount rate of 3 percent). The limited scope of this study suggests that the countries of East Asia are lagging behind in their economic assessment of AIDS.[19]

Sectoral impact

The effect of AIDS will be felt first at the microeconomic, or household level. The next stage will occur when sectors of an economy feel its impact. Sectors can be defined as similar types of economic activity; for example, transport would include airlines, railways, freight on roads and shipping, and mining would include extraction of minerals and quarrying. Later, impacts on the national economy would be detected. The effects are cumulative: AIDS will continue to have an impact on individual households while affecting the macroeconomy.

At present, the sectoral impact is the least-researched area. To date, the only sector-specific study involves transport in Thailand. This study first estimated how many workers will be infected. AIDS-related costs were then evaluated and the proportion to be borne by the industry was established.[20] The study estimated that in 1992, there were 10,000 HIV-infected truck drivers in the country, few of whom had developed AIDS or had died. By the year 2000, the study projected that 67,000 truck drivers will have been HIV infected, 2,680 of whom will have died. The annual cost, including absenteeism and replacement cost, was estimated at $28,000 in 1991 and projected to reach $11.3 million by the year 2000. These figures are helpful in motivating the transportation sector to enhance HIV prevention efforts.

Conclusion

Studying the impact of AIDS on national economies and sectors in these economies should lead to action. This type of work can be valuable for two reasons: it provides tools for advocacy and it permits planning. One of the major problems in dealing with the epidemic is that many people do not believe it will affect them. The challenge is to take economic information to policy makers, politicians, and the leadership in countries to help persuade them to take action.

Second, it is a harsh and unfortunate reality that many people have been infected and will become ill and die from AIDs in the years ahead. Responding to this can occur in one of two ways: either reactively, or proactively, by anticipating future care needs and costs.

Economic impact analysis should enhance appreciation for the value of people. People make economies work and people will have to bear the burden of this disease. Perhaps economic development will once again focus on people.

REFERENCES

1. A. F. Fleming, M. Carballo, D. W. FitzSimons, M. R. Bailey, and J. Mann, eds., *Global Impact of AIDS* (New York: Alan R. Liss, 1988).
2. N. Miller and R. C. Rockwell, eds., *AIDS in Africa: The Social and Policy Impact* (New York: Edwin Mellen Press, 1988):xxvi.
3. World Bank, *World Development Report 1993: Investing in Health* (New York: Oxford University Press, 1993).
4. *Ibid.*
5. D. Cohen, *Economic Impact of the HIV Epidemic* (New York: HIV and Development Programme, UN Development Programme, 1992).
6. M. Over, *Macroeconomic Impact of AIDS in Sub-Saharan Africa*, Technical Working Paper 3 (Washington, DC: Population, Health and Nutrition Division, Africa Technical Department, World Bank, June 1992).
7. Data provided to the author by a major bank in Zambia.
8. T. Barnett and P. Blaikie, *AIDS in Africa: Its Present and Future Impact* (London: Belhaven Press, 1992).
9. S. Gillespie, "Potential impact of AIDS on farming systems: A case-study from Rwanda," *Land Use Policy* 6(1989):301–312.
10. A. M. Zola, "Implication of AIDS for the agricultural sector in Laos P.D.R.," in *Economic Implications of AIDS in Asia*, D. E. Bloom and J. V. Lyons, eds. (New Delhi: UN Development Programme, 1993).
11. M. Ainsworth and A. M. Over, "Economic impact of AIDS in Africa," in *AIDS in Africa*, M. Essex, S. Mboup, P. J. Kanki, and M. R. Kalengayi, eds. (New York: Raven Press, 1994):565.
12. *Ibid.*
13. World Bank, Tanzania, *AIDS Assessment and Planning Study, A World Bank Country Study* (Washington, DC: World Bank, 1992).
14. G. Kambou, S. Devarajan, and M. Over, "Economic impact of the AIDS crisis in sub-Saharan Africa: Simulation with a computable general equilibrium model," *Journal of African Economies* 1(1992):109–130.
15. A. Whiteside and G. Wood, *Socio-Economic Impact of HIV/AIDS in Swaziland*, AIDS Issues Paper, (Mbabane, Swaziland: Government of Swaziland, 1994).
16. M. S. Viravaidya, A Obremskey, and C. Myers, "Economic impact of AIDS on Thailand," in *Economic Implications of AIDS in Asia*, D. E. Bloom and J. V. Lyons, eds. (New Delhi: UN Development Programme, 1993).
17. *Ibid.*

18. J. Broomberg, M. Steinberg, P. Masobe, and G. Behr, "Economic impact of the AIDS epidemic in South Africa," in *Facing Up to AIDS, The Socio-Economic Impact in Southern Africa*, S. Cross and A. Whiteside, eds. (Basingstoke, U.K.: Macmillan Press, 1993).

19. B.-M. Yang, "Economic impact of AIDS on the Republic of Korea," in *Economic Implications of AIDS in Asia*, D. E. Bloom and J. V. Lyons, eds. (New Delhi: UN Development Programme, 1993).

20. P. Giraud, "Economic impact of AIDS at the sectoral level: Developing an assessment methodology and applying it to Thailand's transport sector," in *Economic Implications of AIDS in Asia*, D. E. Bloom and J. V. Lyons, eds. (New Delhi: UN Development Programme, 1993).

8

Societal and Political Impact of HIV/AIDS

RONALD BAYER

"In the beginning there was America." This striking formulation, used to describe the impact of the American response to AIDS in Germany, could well have been extended to other advanced industrial nations.[1] It was in the United States that AIDS was first identified; more importantly, the epidemic of HIV infection took hold there in the late 1970s and early 1980s, before anyone could anticipate how many people would be affected by the new infectious disease threat. How America responded and did not respond provided an object lesson to the industrial nations where the epidemic came later and where the numbers of infected people were smaller.

In the formative years, the period from 1981 to 1986—when the precise dimensions of the AIDS epidemic in the United States remained uncertain and the extent to which populations not initially infected might be exposed was unclear—analysts often predicted that no geographical region and no aspect of social life would remain untouched. Thus, when in 1985 the prospect of widespread heterosexual transmission of HIV became the subject of anxiety, a popular U.S. magazine carried the headline "Now No-one is Safe from AIDS."[2] Yet, by 1993, after more than a decade of living with AIDS, a very different, more nuanced picture had emerged.

In 1986, the U.S. Public Health Service estimated that between one and 1.5 million Americans were already infected with HIV.[3] Seven years later estimates of cumulative HIV infection suggest that those earlier figures were overstated.[4] Indeed, estimates of HIV infections now hover at one million or less. While heterosexual transmission has occurred, and while the incidence of new infection among heterosexual women continues to rise at disturbing rates, HIV in the United States has remained largely an epidemic among gay and bisexual men, injecting drug users, and their sexual partners. As the incidence of infection declined dramatically among gay men, the relative significance of drug use in the U.S. epidemic has increased. As a consequence, the U.S. epidemic has become increasingly focused in populations of color—African-Americans and Latinos—and its impact is evidenced by the grim statistics on the role of AIDS as a leading cause of death among young African-American men and women.[5]

The configuration of American politics in the 1980s, in the grip of a profoundly conservative national administration, and the fact that this was an epidemic of the socially marginalized, concentrated in certain geographical locations, shaped the impact of AIDS on the United States. The response to AIDS has been greatest where both epidemiology and politics permitted gay men and their allies to press for changes, to elicit sympathetic responses, and to wrest sometimes grudging concessions.[6] In contrast, the efforts of drug users and those who speak on their behalf to evoke such concern have been far less effective.

It is not surprising that AIDS, which has taken the lives of so many young artists and performers, and which has had so dramatic an impact on life in New York, San Francisco, and Los Angeles, would have generated some response from those culturally dominant cities (Box 8-1). In the theater, the trajectory from Larry Kramer's angry, early play, *The Normal Heart*, to Tony Kuschner's *Angels in America*, the two-part, award-winning drama, tells much about the willingness of theater audiences and critics to confront the impact of AIDS. Perhaps more crucial is the box office success of *Philadelphia*, a film that depicts the struggle of a white gay lawyer dying of AIDS against his former employers, who dismissed him because of his disease. Whatever its limitations, and the relative safety of its subject in 1993, the reception given to both the film and its Academy Award–winning star, Tom Hanks, again tells a great deal about the impact of AIDS in America over the decade. Even the ever-cautious medium of television first commissioned and then broadcast the film version of Randy Shilts' book *And the Band Played On*.

BOX 8-1

AIDS and the arts: devastation to democratization

KEN MORRISON

> "asked for three hundred words, I found three thousands names"*

AIDS has been characterized by devastation and discord. In the midst of death and dismay, art has depicted the devastation, heralded dawn, and embraced democratization.

The cultural world is being decimated. AIDS has taken the well-known and the rising: Manuel Puig, Argentinean author; Philly Bongoley Lutaaya, Ugandan musician; Amanda Blake, American television star; Reinaldo Arenas, Cuban novelist; Tina Chow, fashion model/designer; Denholm Elliot, British actor; Michel Foucault, French philosopher; Freddie Mercury, rock singer; Robert Mapplethorpe, photographer; Rudolf Nureyev, ballet dancer; Keith Harring, graffiti artist; Michael Lynch, poet; Leonard Bernstein, conductor; Cyril Collard, French writer-cineaste; Rene Highway, Canadian dancer; and the list goes on.

The relationship between AIDS and the arts and its reciprocal impact might be summarized in these terms: bearing witness, affirmation, and galvanization.

- Bearing witness entails the testimonies of mourning, remembrance, and reverence, and includes elements ranging from red ribbons to elegy, from the Names project quilt to the photos of hope and sadness.

*Excerpt from the author's reply to the editors inviting his contribution.

- Affirmation is part of a general process of moving the traditional boundaries from prevention to promotion. From the southern African *Puppets against AIDS* to the cartoons of the German Ralph Koenig, from melodrama like *Philadelphia* to musical comedy like *Patient Zero,* from the songs of Michael Callen to cabarets of Malaysia's Pink Triangle, from T-shirts to children's drawings; in all of these, art has been instrumental in prevention and sensitization, as we redefine learning and loving.

- Galvanization is the essence of activism. The arts have been part of the process of democratization of health and education, and part of the process of empowerment through community mobilization, training, and fundraising. Whether used to confront authorities, to articulate desires, or to challenge beliefs, art and AIDS embody partnerships and community action.

But despite the willingness of Hollywood to embrace an actor who portrayed a gay man with AIDS, and of his willingness to speak out on behalf of gay men to a worldwide audience on the night of his award, America's attitude toward homosexuality remains profoundly ambivalent, moving toward greater tolerance yet also exhibiting deeply homophobic actions. In 1986, the U.S. Supreme Court upheld the constitutionality of criminal sanctions against men who engaged in consensual sexual activities with each other.[7] In 1993, the effort on the part of President Bill Clinton to overcome the military's bar to service on the part of openly homosexual men and women met with ignominious defeat.

However, it is striking that AIDS did not produce a widespread anti-homosexual reaction. Certainly there were acts of discrimination, and reports of violence directed at gay men increased. In addition, the torpid response of the Reagan administration to AIDS can be traced, at least in part, to its anti-homosexual attitude. Yet, as Altman has so acutely observed, the AIDS epidemic quite paradoxically has served as the occasion for the incorporation of gay organizations into the pluralistic fabric of American political life.[8] This was not a gift but rather a hard-won achievement. Further, even during the Reagan years (1980–88), public health officials at the national level were compelled to engage representatives of gay organizations in wide-ranging discussions about AIDS policy. Thus it was possible for gay groups to thwart widespread HIV testing without consent and to win the support of Centers for Disease Control (CDC) officials to the banner of anti-discrimination and confidentiality.[9] More strikingly, activist organizations like ACT-UP, made up primarily of gay men, were remarkably effective in forcing the consideration of radical changes in the policies for approval of new therapeutic agents.[10] Here the agenda of the gay community and the anti-regulatory ideology of the Reagan-Bush administrations were quite compatible. However, there was less success in overcoming resistance to explicit AIDS education efforts, for in this instance, the social conservatism of the nation's political leadership and the anti-welfare state ideology of the national government provided the grounds for resistance.

Both the achievements and failures of the efforts by the gay community must be set against the profound impact of the AIDS epidemic: more than

200,000 people have died in the U.S. Entire friendship networks have vanished and residential communities have been devastated; AIDS has required living in the face of death. In this context, gay men have established a remarkable network of organizations—political, social, and service—to meet their needs and protect their interests.

The capacity of drug users for self-organization stands in stark contrast, as does the capacity of those who speak on their behalf to affect public policy.[11] Since the mid-1980s it has been clear that a failure to provide effective treatment to injecting drug users would represent a virtual death sentence to tens of thousands who would be exposed to HIV through the sharing of injection equipment.[12] Yet on neither federal nor state levels have the necessary resources been forthcoming. This politics of neglect is a direct consequence of profound fear and suspicion evoked by drug users as well as identification of drug use with the African-American and Latino underclass.

Yet even here, AIDS has had a striking and paradoxical impact. Despite the commitment of federal and state officials to a law enforcement approach to drug use in the 1980s, some progress occurred in the implementation of programs based on radically different principles. Drawing from the experience of Europe—the Netherlands and Britain—a number of public health officials and researchers began to assert in the mid-1980s that injecting drug users had to be assured access to sterile equipment.[13] Ultimately, the demand for needle exchange won the support of gay AIDS activists, although not of the African-American community.[14] Ultimately, the struggle for "harm reduction" pitted conservative law enforcement constituencies and representatives of the African-American community against white AIDS activists, a number of public health officials, and researchers. Despite such opposition, needle exchange programs were established, legally in some smaller communities in the American West and as underground efforts in other, more heavily impacted cities.

With evidence about the potential efficacy of needle exchange mounting, the pitched ideological battles subsided. The election of Bill Clinton brought to Washington a national administration that was assumed would be more sympathetic to needle exchange. But political timidity and the grip of conservative forces on the Congress, even before the election of 1994, made a major departure in policy unlikely. Needle exchange, on a national scale that could make an impact, would remain a forlorn hope.

In the years since the epidemic first emerged, the U.S. federal government's expenditures have risen dramatically. Although far short of what many believe would be necessary to undertake adequate prevention efforts and to fund fully the programs designed to meet the social and medical needs of those who are sick, the resources being devoted to AIDS are substantial. Reflecting both the number of persons with AIDS and HIV infection in need of care, federal expenditures for treatment alone in 1993 were $2.5 billion. When expenditures for research, prevention, and income support (for those incapable of work) are added, the federal government spent $5.1 billion in 1993. It is an indication of both the size of the U.S. federal budget and of the U.S. economy that such expenditures do not represent a major burden. Thus early fears that the AIDS epidemic would have a profound impact on the U.S. economy have not been realized.

Here there is a striking paradox: despite the relatively large number of AIDS cases, compared to other industrial nations, and the suffering it has imposed on those communities that have borne the burden of disease, the epidemic has not had a major impact on the institutions of American society. In 1993, the National Research Council (NRC) explained this situation by stating that the "limited response [to the AIDS epidemic] can in part be explained because the absolute numbers of the epidemic, relative to the U.S. population, are not overbearing, and because U.S. social institutions are strong, complex and resilient."[15] More important, however, was the "concentration of the epidemic in socially marginalized groups." Although AIDS had spared no region of the country, "many geographical areas and strata of the population are virtually untouched by the epidemic and probably never will be; certain confined areas and populations have been devastated and are likely to continue to be."[16] The report concluded with a dire prediction: "HIV/AIDS will disappear not because, like smallpox, it has been eliminated, but because those who continue to be affected are socially invisible, beyond the sight and attention of the majority population."[17]

The response provoked by the NRC report reflected the complexity of efforts to shape an adequate response to an epidemic that has primarily affected marginalized populations. In San Francisco one commentator summed up his understanding of the report with the headline, "National Academy of Sciences to Gays, Blacks and Junkies: Drop Dead."[18] Both the Chair and Co-Chair of the National AIDS Commission voiced their disapproval as well: "The report subtly encouraged the vast majority of people outside those specific neighborhoods [most affected by the epidemic] to deny the epidemic's threat, and thus accelerate the virus' spread through all segments of society. . . . It is difficult to describe what a devastating impact that cruel influence had on those living with HIV and their families and loved ones."[19]

Why would the NRC's characterization of the epidemiological trends and its predictions have provoked such a response? In part, the disagreement was over how to understand the epidemiological trends. More important, there was great fear that if the U.S. believed that AIDS no longer threatened every town and every citizen, the fragile political basis for the support of AIDS prevention and research would be shattered. From this perspective, it was felt that only by universalizing the threat of AIDS could the needs of those who were truly vulnerable be met.

On March 7, 1993, *The New York Times* published a front-page story headlined "Targeting Urged in Attack on AIDS: A Neighborhood Focus Could Halt Spread, Some Urge."[20] This suggestion also provoked a bitter encounter. In brief, the controversy centered on whether an undifferentiated strategy for dealing with the AIDS epidemic—one that in some ways suggested universal vulnerability—entailed a misallocation of resources and effort. Instead of such an approach, some proposed an intensive effort focused on those communities where the HIV epidemic had taken root. The significance of this controversy was highlighted by an NRC panel member, Allan Brandt, who stated, "Targeting would require a reconceptualization of the problem, a fundamental rethinking of the epidemic."[21]

Crucial ethical and policy issues are raised by the targeting debate; they will become central in the U.S. and other countries with similar epidemiological configurations. Does current AIDS prevention policy in the U.S. suffer because of a "scatter shot" approach, which is not epidemiologically grounded? Are those most at risk for HIV infection poorly served by current approaches? Would a shift towards a more targeted approach place those outside current centers of HIV at risk? Would a more targeted approach to prevention foster stigmatization? Would it weaken the political alliance that currently supports HIV prevention, research, and care?

In the end, the policy challenge is to articulate an ethic of social solidarity in the face of an epidemic that does not affect all equally. This issue must also be joined on a global level. How will the wealthy industrial nations with relatively small or stable HIV epidemics respond to the nations of the world that are poor and medically impoverished and that face the burden of an ever-increasing prevalence of HIV infection? It is in the answer to these questions that the future of the global epidemic of HIV/AIDS will lie.

BOX 8-2

AIDS: despair, or a stimulus to reform?

DEAN SHUEY AND HENRY BAGARUKAYO

The first cases of AIDS were recognized in south central Uganda in the mid-1980s. After a brief initial period of denial and attempts to minimize the problem, Uganda has been remarkably open in recognizing and confronting the epidemic.

As of 1995, it is estimated that 1–1.5 million Ugandans are HIV infected in a total population of 17 million. AIDS has penetrated all socioeconomic classes and all geographic locations in Uganda.[1] Yet, statistics do not reflect the daily impact or the ever-present influence of AIDS in Uganda. Part of the impact is actually due to massive efforts to educate the populace about AIDS. Multiple studies have shown almost universal awareness (over 98 percent) that there is a disease called AIDS, a high degree of awareness (over 92 percent) that it is spread by sexual intercourse, and a high level of knowledge (over 90 percent) that having one partner or being sexually abstinent may stop the spread of AIDS.[2]

As the epidemic progresses, almost every family in Uganda will be affected. For example, in 1989, none of 311 primary level 7 students in one southwestern district had seen anyone with AIDS. Three years later, 75 percent of a similar sample knew someone with AIDS, and 27 percent had a family member with AIDS.[3] Data from another district in the north, considered less affected by AIDS, found that 59 percent of mothers of children under the age of two knew someone with AIDS, and that 6 percent had family members with AIDS.[4]

Many anecdotal reports document the effect of AIDS on the lives of Ugandans. Daily life is disrupted, traditional habits and beliefs are challenged, and a new level of uncertainty is injected into an already uncertain existence. The most common social events in Uganda today are said to be funerals, the costs of which place a tremendous burden on the meager resources of families. As funerals become more frequent, even their nature changes. Traditional funeral practice in rural areas was for all work in the community to stop for 3 days. This practice has been discontinued in many places, as funerals are occurring at a pace that would endanger production.

Agricultural practice is also altered as labor availability changes with the death of family members. Crops raised have been switched from labor-intensive, high-value crops, such as maize or millet, to less labor-intensive, lower-value crops, such as cassava and plantains.[5]

The 15–45-year-old population is most affected by AIDS. In Uganda, due to the combination of AIDS and a high birth rate, the dependency ratio (the number of dependents, mainly children and the elderly, to the number of producers) is 1.07:1, one of the most unfavorable ratios in the world.[6] The increased dependency ratio has complicated preparation of the next generation for life as adults. Children are caring for children. The elderly are caring for children. School attendance and vocational education are jeopardized.

Employers are affected by the loss of personnel, particularly those who are trained. Quietly, people are suggesting that it is advisable to invest in shorter training courses for more people rather than longer courses for fewer people, as it is unwise to depend on any single individual with so many likely to be lost to AIDS. People feel a sense of impermanence and vulnerability, and there is already a perception expressed at both community and policy-making levels that family planning is less of a priority, due to the AIDS epidemic.

AIDS is omnipresent and necessarily affects the political system. Concerns about loss of personnel, including politicians, are frequently expressed. The perception that AIDS disproportionately affects the educated and the elite, although not borne out by the census, probably reflects the personal experience of senior politicians and civil servants. Some political leaders have proposed repressive measures, such as mandatory testing for HIV as a requirement for civil service promotion, but fortunately these have not been adopted. National policy supports the rights to privacy and self-determination, and the principle of nondiscrimination regarding AIDS.[7]

Uganda has recognized that AIDS is a multisectoral problem.[8] Ministries other than health are being encouraged to develop specific AIDS control programs, and individual districts are doing the same. Further work is needed to make this multisectoral approach more effective, but a foundation has been established.

Many of the effects of AIDS are not quantifiable. Who can enumerate the impact of almost constant grieving and of widespread uncertainty? The statement that "AIDS will finish us all" evidences a fatalism which can paralyze a society. There is often a sense of desperation, as those affected seek any and all cures, expending scarce family resources on both modern and traditional medicines, often compromising the economic well-being of the family unit.

Yet, perhaps not all of the social effects of AIDS are negative. AIDS is triggering a re-examination of the role of women and children in society. AIDS has provoked much discussion and the beginning of action on women's reproductive and sexual rights. Women are beginning to demand the right to have sex be safe. A process of recognizing the advantages of marital fidelity to family and economic life has started. The government of Uganda had already established structures to increase women's participation in political and social processes, such as mandatory women's representatives at all levels of the political system. AIDS has made it obvious that the concerns expressed by these women must be taken seriously in national policy-making.[9]

The abuse of children and adolescents as sexual partners has also been highlighted as a problem. One study found that half of sexually active female primary level 7 students stated they had been forced at least once to participate in sex, and 22 percent stated they had been given a gift or reward in exchange for sex.[10]

In addition, the failure of society to protect the property rights of orphans and widows has been recognized. A review of Ugandan law pertaining to children was conducted during 1990–1993. Changes have been recommended in laws regarding marriage to minors, the protection of the property rights of children, and the protection of children from sexual defilement, all of which are becoming much higher priorities of the government of Uganda.[11] Past acceptability that those in positions of power, such as teachers or employers, would extort sexual favors from those in subordinate positions is waning. AIDS has been a stimulus for Ugandans to confront the issue of adolescent sexuality in a more mature and open fashion than in many industrialized nations. In Uganda, religious leaders, although many are still opposed to condoms, debate the issue openly, and condom use in general and the instruction of adolescents about how to use condoms is an accepted national strategy.[12]

Another positive effect is that AIDS has been the impetus for cooperative efforts, involving multiple organizations and sectors in society, based on humanitarian impulses, to deal with the problems of those afflicted by AIDS, to care for the dependents of those lost to AIDS, and to prevent infection in those not infected.

Political structures have changed due to the impact of AIDS. A multisectoral AIDS Commission formed in 1991 has been a key to drawing many non–health sector ministries, such as information, defense, and education, into the effort against AIDS.[13]

Thus, Uganda has been affected widely and profoundly by AIDS. In even the most optimistic scenarios, the effects will continue for decades to come. But Uganda will survive, and in many respects, AIDS has catalyzed a process of societal self-examination and cooperation which will stand Uganda in good stead for the future. As important as international aid and cooperation may be in combating the epidemic of AIDS, the future will depend on Ugandans.

References

1. Ministry of Health, *AIDS Control Programme Surveillance Report* (Entebbe, Uganda: Ministry of Health, June 1993).
2. African Medical and Research Foundation, *Kabale KAP Study* (Kampala, Uganda: AMREF, March 1992).
3. *Ibid.*
4. AMREF, *Soroti Baseline PHC Survey* (Kampala, Uganda: AMREF, August 1992).
5. T. Barnett and P. Blaikie, *AIDS in Africa: Its Present and Future Impact* (London: Belhaven Press, 1992).
6. World Bank, *Uganda Social Sector Strategy*, draft report 10765-UG (Washington, DC: Population and Human Resources Division, Eastern Africa Department, World Bank, July 24, 1992).
7. Statistics Department, *Results of the 1991 Population and Housing Census* (Entebbe, Uganda: Statistics Department, Ministry of Finance and Economic Planning, October 1992).
8. Uganda AIDS Commission, *AIDS Control in Uganda: The Multisectoral Strategy* (Kampala, Uganda: Uganda AIDS Commission Secretariat, April 1992).
9. Uganda AIDS Commission, *Uganda National Operational Plan for AIDS Prevention, Care, and Support* (Kampala, Uganda: Uganda AIDS Commission Secretariat, August 1993).
10. H. Bagarukayo, B. Babishangire, K. Johnson, and D. Shuey, "Sexuality and AIDS prevention among primary school students in Kabale district of Uganda," poster presented at the VIII International Conference on AIDS in Africa, Marrakech, Morocco, December 1993.
11. Uganda National Programme of Action for Children, *Priorities for Social Services Sector Development in the 1990's and Implementation Plan 1992/93–1994/5* (Kampala, Uganda: Ministry of Finance and Economic Planning, September 1992).
12. Uganda AIDS Commission, *The Multisectoral Strategy.*
13. *Ibid.*

BOX 6-3

Evolving impact of HIV/AIDS on India

PURNIMA MANE

It is not easy to trace the development of HIV/AIDS in India, for the epidemic continues to be relatively neglected and the response is hidden. Yet, by the year 2000, India will probably have the largest number of HIV-infected persons in any single country. It is evident that with its enormous population and the multifarious problems of development, the impact of HIV/AIDS in India will be severe and will necessitate monumental efforts on the part of all sectors.

In the World Bank's *World Development Report 1993,* the HIV/AIDS scenario for India has been described as potentially one of the worst.[1] Current rates of infant mortality, maternal mortality, average life expectancy, and morbidity already paint a dismal picture of the Indian health situation.[2] The established health facilities are inadequate for the population they are expected to serve, and they are not sought eagerly by the Indian population.[3] The private health sector, which employs two-thirds of the medical human resources and is responsible for two-thirds of the total expenditure on health in India, is poorly regulated.[4] For example, many private hospitals in Bombay have recently made HIV testing mandatory for all surgical patients, and several force HIV-infected individuals to leave the hospital, refusing to treat them despite national policy which categorically opposes such practices.[5] Unethical medical practices abound and jeopardize plans for infection control.[6] Folk medicine is popular but little is known about practices that occur in alternative systems of medicine, leaving them outside the realm of current activities related to HIV/AIDS education.

The growing epidemic of HIV/AIDS will place severe pressure on the health infrastructure. Anecdotes describe attempts by lower-level health care workers, to blackmail HIV-infected persons, and instances of discrimination and exploitation are likely to increase.

It is also useful to examine the Indian situation regarding sexually transmitted infections (STIs) and tuberculosis. In a report of baseline surveys conducted in different parts of India (Calcutta, Jaipur, Madras, and a rural area in Tamil Nadu), STIs were more common than previously assumed.[7] For example, in Calcutta, 70 percent of 450 sex workers surveyed reported having an STI during the previous year. On physical examination, 81 percent were found to be infected with at least one STI; of 151 asymptomatic women sex workers, 82 percent were infected with an STI. Fairly high STI prevalence was also reported in Madras among a large (n = 1,500) and diverse group that included prisoners, industrial workers, transport workers, antenatal clinic attendees, and primary health center attendees. Similar findings were reported in Jaipur in a survey of workers from the industrial and transport sector and women attending antenatal clinics.[8] Though the HIV prevalence was low in these studies, the high prevalence of STIs clearly indicates the potential for future HIV transmission.

A serious situation is also observed with regard to tuberculosis. Sixty percent of people with AIDS in India are also reported to be infected with tuberculosis.[9] The combined impact of these diseases on a country like India will be serious. The stigma and fear around tuberculosis have abated only marginally in India so that the nexus between tuberculosis and HIV is likely to create even stronger barriers to the integration of HIV-infected persons in society.

Looking beyond health, other factors contribute to raising the level of HIV risk among different sections of the Indian population. The literacy rate of the population is as low as 48 percent with a distinct urban–rural and gender difference, skewed unfavorably against the rural population and women.[10] Illiteracy implies relatively low access to information, support, and care, seriously undermining the chances of the illiterate to protect themselves and their loved ones from HIV. The illiterate are also underprivileged in other ways: they constitute an exploited and marginalized population, which is deprived of the relative protection of formal institutions. Already there is a tendency to view people who are multiply disadvantaged, such as sex workers, devadasis (women who are dedicated to the gods and are unable to have one partner), and hijras (castrated men who live in closed communities, have a female identity and are often involved in prostitution for a living), as vectors of transmission. While HIV/AIDS has compelled public acknowledgment of these sections of society, their social and cultural marginalization has persisted and has even been enhanced.

For those who are literate, other cultural differences create serious problems in communicating about HIV. The Indian subcontinent is known for its diversity, and remote pockets of the country and rural areas, not currently seen as high prevalence areas, are particularly neglected in terms of HIV education.

Other than the formal media, much has been expected from the educational sector in terms of raising awareness on HIV/AIDS. The educational sector, however, is crippled by large-scale budgetary cuts and deficits, overwhelmed by the vast numbers it is expected to serve, and often unable to cope with the cultural differences and socioeconomic disadvantages. Education on HIV/AIDS has further added to its responsibilities and not surprisingly, receives scant attention. In the wake of AIDS, sex education through the educational sector has been called for, yet many religious groups are sensitive about and resist open discussions on sex. The debate over sex education and HIV education rages on, and political uncertainties further delay action.

Several other aspects of the sociocultural life of India are likely to be significant in understanding the impact of HIV/AIDS. Of particular concern are the implications for women. It is now generally acknowledged that women are vulnerable to HIV/AIDS and yet are often powerless to ensure needed behavior change for protection against HIV/AIDS.[11] Women's health needs are generally neglected in India and few women access health care services. Therefore, there is a strong likelihood that HIV prevalence and AIDS among women in India is underrecognized and underreported. This is a country where studies found that over 90 percent of some groups of tribal women have gynecological or sexually transmitted infections and a majority have never received treatment for these conditions.[12]

The Indian woman is likely to be at a special disadvantage if she becomes HIV infected; she will be viewed as the vector of transmission and as the "guilty" one, transgressing cultural norms of fidelity and womanliness, and thus deserving a "just" punishment. Special efforts will need to be made to avert tragedies, such as desertion of women with AIDS. Ironically, the spotlight on sex workers among women in the HIV/AIDS epidemic has not only stigmatized them further but has led to a neglect of programs for women who are not identified as such. This increases the vulnerability of all women, not just sex workers.

This perspective on the sociocultural impact of HIV/AIDS has focused on the negative aspects for specific sections of the population and the sociocultural lives of the Indian people. However, the recognition of the HIV/AIDS epidemic in India has also led to increasing openness on the issues of sex and sexuality, which is essential to create an environment conducive to discussing safer behavior. It has also brought about an acknowledgment—even if reluctant and half-hearted—of the existence of sexual practices and identities that have hitherto been dismissed as nonexistent and irrelevant to the "culture." It has highlighted the vulnerability of marginalized sections of Indian society even though this has often led to victimization. Services for counseling and initiation of community-based care are beginning to be developed by the National AIDS Control Organization (NACO) and the State AIDS Cell to reduce the impact of HIV.[13] More significantly, AIDS has caused an emergence of a range of non-governmental organizations and social activists who grapple with the complexities of the issues surrounding HIV/AIDS, particularly those related to human rights, the impact of HIV/AIDS, and needed efforts. Undoubtedly, the impact of HIV/AIDS is mainly experienced by the informed minority who perceives AIDS as a genuine problem for India. For the majority, however, AIDS remains an alien phenomenon that is not recognized as having an impact on their world. Undoubtedly, acknowledgment of the "Indianness" of HIV/AIDS will come when the numbers of those affected rise sharply and the epidemic visibly affects all strata of Indian society and diverse aspects of Indian life, beyond health.

References

1. World Bank, *World Development Report 1993: Investing in Health, World Development Indicators* (New York: Oxford University Press, 1993).

2. P. Mane and S. A. Maitre, *AIDS Prevention, The Socio-Cultural Context in India* (Bombay: Tata Institute of Social Sciences, 1992).

3. Directorate General of Health Services, Central Bureau of Health Intelligence, *Health Information India 1990* (New Delhi: Ministry of Health and Family Welfare, Government of India, 1991).

4. R. Duggal, "Private health sector, regulation and control," *Foundation for Research in Community Health (FRCH) Newsletter, Special Issue on Medical Malpractice* V(1991):6–8.

5. Staff Correspondent, "AIDS tests," *Times of India* (March 7, 1994).

6. N. H. Antia, "Misuse of medicine," *FRCH Newsletter* V(1991):1–2.

7. National AIDS Control Organization, "Some highlights of STD prevalence studies in India," *AIDS in India, Newsletter of the National AIDS Control Organization* (June 1993):15–16.

8. *Ibid.*

9. Staff Correspondent, "State warned of HIV epidemic," *Times of India* (January 10, 1994).

10. Government of India, *Census of India Provisional Population Tables 1991* (New Delhi: Government of India, 1992).

11. C. Elias and L. Heise, *Development of Microbicides: A New Method of HIV Prevention for Women,* working paper (New York: Population Council, 1993).

12. R. Bang and A. Bang, "Why women hide them: Rural women's viewpoints on reproductive tract infections," *Manushi* 69(1992):27–30.

13. National AIDS Control Organization, *National AIDS Control Programme India: Country Scenario An Update April 1993* (New Delhi: Ministry of Health and Family Welfare, Government of India, 1993).

REFERENCES

1. G. Frankenberg, "Germany: The uneasy triumph of pragmatism," in *AIDS in the Industrialized Democracies: Passions, Politics, and Policies,* D. Kirp and R. Bayer, eds. (New Brunswick, NJ: Rutgers University Press, 1992): 99–133.

2. "Now No-one is Safe from AIDS," cover headline, *Life* (August 1985).

3. U.S. Public Health Service, "Public health service plan for the prevention and control of AIDS and the AIDS virus," *Public Health Reports* (July–August 1986):341–348.

4. Centers for Disease Control and Prevention, "Estimates of HIV prevalence and projected AIDS cases: Summary of a workshop, October 31–November 1, 1989," *Morbidity and Mortality Weekly Report* 39(1990):110–119.

5. Centers for Disease Control and Prevention, "Update: Mortality attributable to HIV infection among persons aged 25–44 years—United States, 1991 and 1992," *Morbidity and Mortality Weekly Report* 42(1993):869–872.

6. R. Bayer, *Private Acts, Social Consequences: AIDS and the Politics of Public Health* (New Brunswick, NJ: Rutgers University Press, 1991).

7. U.S. Supreme Court decision, S.Ct.2841(1986), following *Bowers v. Hardwick.*

8. D. Altman, "Legitimacy through disaster," in *AIDS: The Burdens of History,* D. Fox and E. Fee, eds. (Berkeley, CA: University of California Press, 1988).

9. R. Bayer, "Public health policy and the AIDS epidemic: An end to HIV exceptionalism?" *New England Journal of Medicine* 324(1991):1500–1504.

10. C. Levine, "Has AIDS changed the ethics of human subjects research?" *Law, Medicine and Health Care* 16(1988):167–173.

11. S. Friedman, J. L. Sotheran, A. Abdul-Quader et al., "AIDS epidemic among blacks and Hispanics," *Milbank Quarterly* 65(suppl. 2)(1987):490.

12. Presidential Commission on the Human Immunodeficiency Virus Epidemic, *Final Report* (Washington, DC: Presidential Commission on the Human Immunodeficiency Virus, 1988).

13. Institute of Medicine, National Academy of Sciences, *Confronting AIDS* (Washington, DC: National Academy Press, 1986).

14. H. Dalton, "AIDS in black face," *Daedalus* (Summer 1986):205–227.

15. National Research Council, *Monitoring the Social Impact of AIDS in the United States* (Washington, DC: National Academy Press, 1993).

16. *Ibid.*

17. *Ibid.*

18. R. Morse, "Read the news today, oy veh," *San Francisco Examiner* (February 7, 1993):A3.

19. J. Osborn and D. Rogers, "AIDS policy: Two divisive issues," *Journal of the American Medical Association* 270(1993):494–495.

20. G. Kolata, "Targeting urged in attack on AIDS: A neighborhood focus could halt spread, some urge," *New York Times* (March 7, 1993):1.

21. *Ibid.*

PART II

THE FRONTIER OF KNOWLEDGE

Progress in the sciences of AIDS has continued at a remarkable pace. This part of *AIDS in the World II*, describes current progress in important research areas such as human sexuality, treatment of HIV infection, virological study, and vaccine development.

Yet these chapters share commonalities beyond their contributions to knowledge about HIV/AIDS, for the role and influence of society weighs heavily on these scientific endeavors. AIDS has highlighted the social context within which scientific methods, priorities, and goals are established and realized.

Societal support for research clearly illustrates this issue. Thus, Francis identifies slow progress towards an AIDS vaccine with a lack of political and social commitment for such a vaccine (Chapter 14), while Widdus illustrates how the political processes outside and within major governmental research agencies influence research funding (Chapter 17).

Ongoing research and HIV

Significant progress has been noted by Cooper in the development of new therapies for HIV disease (Chapter 10). The hope generated by preliminary results of ongoing research in the industrialized world should not overshadow the fact that as more effective and safer drugs are developed, their availability and affordability to the majority of the world's people living with HIV and AIDS will necessitate major improvements in the ways health care systems are designed, operated, and funded.

In Chapter 11 of this volume, Colebunders comments on the slow progression of HIV infection reported in industrialized countries as well as in Rwanda in the mid-1980s. De Cock and Brun-Vézinet go on to summarize the current knowledge and uncertainties regarding HIV-2 infection from studies conducted primarily in West Africa, several of which were in collaboration with overseas research teams (Chapter 12). Elias, Heise, and Gollub review the progress achieved in devising women-controlled HIV prevention methods that are being developed and tried concurrently in industrialized and developing countries (Chapter 16). These studies all underscore the need for HIV/AIDS research to transcend institutional and national boundaries, each effort helping to piece together the mosaic of knowledge and understanding that will ultimately enable us to bring the pandemic under control.

Several chapters return to the fundamental problem of global inequity, expressed both as developing countries' virtual lack of access to the products of scientific research (i.e., drugs for antiretroviral therapy or prophylaxis/treatment of opportunistic infections) as well as their unequal participation in research itself. Widdus examines how the HIV/AIDS research agenda, largely driven by and for industrialized countries, is drawn up (Chapter 17). Yet as over 90 percent of the HIV/AIDS pandemic is occurring in the developing world, Heyward and colleagues describe the efforts undertaken to ensure that vaccine research in developing countries conforms to international technical and ethical standards (Chapter 15).

To Anton Chekov's famous dictum that national science doesn't exist, for if it is only national, it is not science, the HIV/AIDS pandemic adds the dimension of global interdependence. Levy, McCutchan, and Meyers establish the virological case for the necessity of a global perspective on the epidemic and its future course (Chapter 13). The discovery of HIV-1 subtypes (*clades*) means, bluntly, that HIV prevention and control—whether involving vaccine, treatment, or behavior-based prevention—must take virological evolution around the world into account. For a vaccine tailored to only one clade would likely be substantially less effective in areas of the world where other clades predominate. In addition, the viral strains less prevented by vaccine could well migrate to, and then flourish in, an area where transmission had been reduced by an effective, although clade-specific vaccine.

In social and behavioral research, Gillies and Parker identify yet another important societal dimension relevant to HIV/AIDS prevention (Chapter 9). For their devestating critique of concepts and methods initially (and sometimes, still) used to study sexual behavior in the context of HIV/AIDS underscores the absolute need to account for societal influences on human behavior. They issue a clarion call for new research frameworks and methods that are able to link the personal and the collective, always anchored in the lived, highly diverse realities of people.

While clearly identifying the societal problems and obstacles to progress in their fields, each of the following chapters also expresses hope for progress and improvement. Despite clear awareness of the scientific and social challenges ahead, none are overcome by despair. In this regard, it is also fitting that this part concludes with Pinching's eloquent essay about the process and progress of science in the era of AIDS (Chapter 18). Pinching is not impressed by superficial vanities, disputes, or appearances; his is a larger and more humane vision of people working hard in genuinely complex territory. He is convinced that sharing, communicating, and struggling together is already building the better, future path.

The Contribution of Social and Behavioral Science to HIV/AIDS Prevention

PAMELA GILLIES

The contribution of social scientific research to HIV/AIDS prevention and care has been questioned repeatedly. Reasons for frustration and dissatisfaction have included reliance on quantitative survey research, lack of exploration into the social context of behavior, limited discussion of national and local policies, limited evaluation, inadequate consideration of diverse processes for preventing HIV infection, and poor elaboration of concepts of sexuality.[1]

It is therefore important to assess the content, quality, and direction of this research and to consider the critique of social science's contribution to HIV/AIDS prevention and control. To do so, this section reviews, in a systematic yet selective manner, HIV-related social and behavioral research published from 1991 to 1993. The first part identifies and discusses the conceptual frameworks that have been used in social science research on HIV/AIDS. The second part examines methodological approaches thus far applied to the study of sexual behavior in the context of HIV/AIDS. The final part considers the role of social science in evaluating outcomes of HIV prevention efforts.

Framing questions and solving problems: the importance of theory

Conceptual models for organizing and integrating information can comprise many theories from a range of disciplines (see, for example, Table 9-1). In HIV/AIDS–related research, conceptual models have frequently been applied to explain specific types of behaviors, for example, condom use in specific contexts. Since models may derive from many theories, they can be cross-disciplinary. Theories, on the other hand, tend to be discipline specific, originating in such fields as psychology, sociology, or mathematics. These conceptual models and theories help to explain the world and actions, and if they are close to the "truth," they should help to predict the future. Since a future that can be predicted may be influenced, theory is a powerful tool for constructive action. It guides the focus of scientific attention in framing the questions which research must ask. Theory establishes

Table 9-1 Examples of conceptual models and theories proposed or applied in sexual behavior studies in the social sciences, 1991–1993

Country	Author and year of publication	Model name	Typology	Key variables	Authors reported explanatory power
A. Psychology					
United Kingdom	Abraham et al.[1] 1991	Health belief model	Social psychology	Attitudes, beliefs, perceived severity, expectations, intentions	Intentions were not found to predict safer sexual practice over time.
United States	Boyer and Kegeles[2] 1991	AIDS risk reduction model (ARRM)	Social psychology	Problem perception, susceptibility, intentions, motivation, individual and other social determinants	Not tested.
United States	Brown et al.[3] 1991	Health belief model	Social psychology	Attitudes, beliefs, perceived severity, expectations, intentions	Of limited use in predicting HIV preventive behavior.
United Kingdom	Davies and Weatherburn[4] 1991		Psychology	Dyadic interaction, negotiation, interpersonal skills	Not tested.
Germany	Eich et al.[5] 1991	Social support	Social psychology	Psychological well-being	Supportive social network correlates with psychological well-being.
Uganda	McGrath et al.[6] 1991	Social support	Social psychology	Well-being and social activities	Lack of social support and stigma outside the household results in withdrawal of individuals from activities outside the home.
United States	Nabila et al.[7] 1991	Social support	Social psychology	Communication	Good support is associated with feeling comfortable discussing safe sex.
United States	Ostrow et al.[8] 1991	Social support	Social psychology	Perceived material and emotional support, self-affirmation, objective and subjective social integration and conflict	Positive relation in white men between social support and low risk-taking, and between social support and mental health; some evidence of negative influence of social support and mental health in black men.
United States	O'Reilly and Higgins[9] 1991	Stages of change	Social psychology	Perception of risk susceptibility; expectations, roles, norms, skills, intentions, attitudes, values, beliefs	Limited influence on psychological states.

United States	Petosa and Jackson[10] 1991	Health belief model	Social psychology	Perception of risk susceptibility; expectations, roles, norms, skills, intentions, attitudes, values, beliefs	Accounted for 43% of variance in safer sex intentions.
United States	Basen-Engquist and Parcel[11] 1992	Attitudes, norms, and self-efficacy model	Social psychology	Attitudes, intentions, self-efficacy, norms	Weak associations between intentions and behaviors.
Netherlands	Schaalma, Kok, and Peters[12] 1993	Theory of reasoned action and self-efficacy theory	Social psychology	Norms, attitudes, intentions, self-efficacy, expectations	Attitudes, norms, and knowledge are all associated with intentions.

B. Psychology/Sociology

United States	Kelly et al.[13] 1992	Diffusion theory	Sociology/social psychology	Skill, acquisition behavior, roles, norms	Reductions in unprotected anal intercourse between 15% and 25% of men; increases in social norm perception rating.
Thailand	Maticka-Tyndale et al.[14] 1994	Health belief model, theory of reasoned action, and Rothman and Topman's community participation model	Sociology/social psychology	Attitudes, beliefs, norms; perceptions of severity; self-efficacy intentions; village resources, especially sexual health services	In progress.

C. Sociology and Other Categories

South Africa	Jochelson, Mothibeli, and Leger[15] 1991	Systems theory	Sociology/social psychology	Heterosexual relationships network; description of familial/marital sexual experiences, perceptions, behaviors, beliefs, and attitudes; conditions in hostels; separation anxiety	Migrant labor system facilitates HIV transmission.
United States	Wallace[16,17] 1991, 1993	Sociogeographic network model	Social geography	Relationships, population mix and distribution, social network structure	To be tested.

(continued)

Table 9-1 Examples of conceptual models and theories proposed or applied in sexual behavior studies in the social sciences, 1991–1993—continued

Country	Author and year of publication	Model name	Typology	Key variables	Authors reported explanatory power
Brazil	Parker[18] 1992	Social construction drawing on scripting theory	Anthropology	Meanings of sexual behavior and sexuality; emotional power, desire, eroticism, language; symbolic constraints and cultural representations	Improved understanding of erotic meetings outlined appropriate ways to eroticize risk reduction strategies.
Uganda	Ankrah[19] 1993	"Clanship"	Anthropology	Family ties and activities in a cultural context, kinship systems	Understanding of family coping mechanisms in AIDS treatment and care in Africa.
United Kingdom, Brazil, and Dominican Republic	Gillies and Parker[20] 1993	Social construction	Sociology/ anthropology	Language, identity, behaviors, emotional relationships, economics	Demonstrates importance of cultural meanings and emotional power of relationships and fluidity of category.
United Kingdom	Coxon[21] 1993	Social construction and network theory	Sociology	Sexual roles in couples relationships	In progress.
Netherlands	Duyves[22] 1994	Social construction, spatial theory of desire	Cultural geography	Spatial relations in desire, imagination, emotion, public space, sexual preferences	In progress.
United States	Laumann, Gagnon, and Michael[23] 1994	Social construction, scripting theory, network theory	Sociology	Interpsychic variables; interpersonal and cultural scenarios in respect to social and sexual relationships	Increasing understanding of symbolic meanings in relation to sexuality.

[1]C. Abraham, P. Sheeran, D. Abrams, et al., "Young people learning about AIDS: A study of beliefs and information sources," *Health Education Research* 6(1991):19–29.

[2]C. B. Boyer and S. M. Kegeles, "AIDS risk and prevention among adolescents," *Social Science and Medicine* 33(1991):11–23.

[3]L. K. Brown, R. J. DiClemente, and L. A. Reynolds, "HIV prevention for adolescents: Utility of the health belief model," *AIDS Education and Prevention* 3(1991):50–59.

[4]P. Davies and P. Weatherburn, "Towards a general model of sexual negotiation," in *AIDS: Responses, Interventions and Care,* P. Aggleton, G. Hart, and P. Davies, eds. (Bristol, U.K.: Falmer Press, 1991).

[5]D. Eich, A. Dobler-Mikola, and R. Luthy, "Psychosocial well-being in asymptomatic HIV positive individuals is associated with age and social networks," Abstract W.B.2395, presented at the VII International Conference on AIDS, Florence, Italy, June 1991.

[6]J. W. McGrath, E. M. Ankrah, D. A. Schumann, M. Lubega, and S. Nkumbi, "Psychosocial impact of AIDS in urban Uganda families," Abstract M.D.4261, presented at the VII International Conference on AIDS, Florence, Italy, June 1991.

[7]E. B. Nabila, H. Gilbert, and R. F. Schilling, "Social support networks and sexual risk taking in female IV drug users," Abstract W.D.4026, presented at the VII International Conference on AIDS, Florence, Italy, June 1991.

[8]D. G. Ostrow, R. E. D. Whitaker, K. Frasier, C. Cohen, J. Wan, C. Frank, and E. Fischer, "Racial differences in social support and mental health in men with HIV infection: A pilot study," *AIDS Care* 3(1991):55–63.

[9]K. R. O'Reilly and D. L. Higgins, "AIDS community demonstration projects for HIV prevention among hard-to-reach groups," *Public Health Reports* 106(1991):714–720.

[10]R. Petosa and K. Jackson, "Using the health belief model to predict safer sex intentions among adolescents," *Health Education Quarterly* 18(1991):463–476.

[11]K. Basen-Engquist and G. S. Parcel, "Attitudes, norms and self-efficacy: A model of adolescents' HIV-related sexual risk behavior," *Health Education Quarterly* 19(1992):263–277.

[12]H. P. Schaalma, G. Kok, and L. Peters, "Determinants of consistent condom use by adolescents: The impact of experience of sexual intercourse," *Health Education Research* 8(1993):253–269.

[13]J. A. Kelly, J. S. St. Lawrence, Y. Stevenson, A. C. Hauth, S. C. Kalichman, Y. E. Diaz, T. L. Brasfield, J. J. Koob, and M. G. Morgan, "Community AIDS/HIV risk reduction: The effects of endorsements by popular people in three cities," *American Journal of Public Health* 82(1992):1483–1489.

[14]E. Maticka-Tyndale, M. Haswell-Elkins, R. Kuyyakanond, M. Kiewying, and D. Elkins, "Research based HIV health promotion intervention for the mobilization of rural communities in Northeast Thailand," *Health Transition Review* 4 (suppl)(1994): 349–367.

[15]K. Jochelson, M. Mothibeli, and J. P. Leger, "HIV and Migrant Labor in South Africa," *International Journal of Health Services* 21(1991):157–173.

[16]R. Wallace, "Traveling waves of HIV infection on a low dimensional 'sociogeographic' network," *Social Science and Medicine* 32(1991):847–852.

[17]R. Wallace, "Social disintegration and the spread of AIDS-II. Meltdown of sociogeographic structure in urban minority neighborhoods," *Social Science and Medicine* 37(1993):887–896.

[18]R. G. Parker, "Sexual diversity cultural analysis and AIDS education in Brazil," in *Time of AIDS: Social Analysis, Theory and Method*, G. H. Herdt and S. Lindenbaum, eds. (Newbury Park, CA: Sage Publications, 1992).

[19]E. M. Ankrah, "Impact of HIV/AIDS on the family and other significant relationships: The African clan revisited," *AIDS Care* 5(1993):5–22.

[20]P. A. Gillies and R. G. Parker, "Cross cultural perspectives on sexual behavior and prostitution," *Health Transition Review*, 4 (suppl)(1994):257–271.

[21]A. J. Coxon, "Network and nemesis: The use of social networks as method and substance in researching gay men's response to HIV/AIDS," presented at the ARHN Working Group on Sexual Behavior Research Conference, International Perspectives in Sex Research, Rio de Janeiro, Brazil, April 22–25, 1993.

[22]M. Duyves, "Framing preferences, framing differences: Investing Amsterdam as a gay capital," in *Conceiving Sexuality: Sex Research in a Postmodern World*, R. G. Parker and J. H. Gagnon, eds. (New York and London: Routledge, 1994).

[23]E. O. Laumann, J. H. Gagnon, and R. T. Michael, "Sociological perspective on sexual action," in *Conceiving Sexuality: Sex Research in a Postmodern World*, R. G. Parker and J. H. Gagnon, eds. (New York and London: Routledge, 1994).

the key factors for investigation and provides the intellectual structure for analysis and interpretation of findings. However, if models or theories are slavishly adhered to they may prove restrictive, limiting the imagination and denying competing, credible conceptual bases for research.

The following review of social science models and theories describes the approaches used for an understanding of sexual behavior in the context of HIV/AIDS.

Conceptual models and theories, 1991–1993

In Table 9-1, selected examples of conceptual models and theories proposed or applied in sexual behavior studies related to HIV/AIDS and presented in the scientific literature from 1991 to 1993 are classified under the headings: A Psychology; B Psychology/Sociology; and C Sociology and Other Categories. In any review of this type, a cautionary note on publication bias should be made. It is also important to remember that scientists in developing countries may experience great difficulty in preparing articles for submission, thus data from these areas are insufficient. Of the 22 studies in which models and theories were explicitly addressed, 12 were derived principally from psychology (or social psychology), 2 involved both psychology and sociology, and 8 came from sociology and other categories.

Psychology emerged as the dominant conceptual approach used in these studies of HIV prevention, emphasizing individual determinants of sexual behavior and assuming that behavior is rational. Important factors in these analyses included beliefs, attitudes, perceptions, motivations, and intentions. The notion of the "social" is expressed in a relatively unsophisticated manner that is limited to providing reinforcing "cues" for individual behavior.

Of the 22 studies in Table 9-1, 16 were from industrialized countries; 1 involved both Western and Latin-American researchers; 3 were from Africa (with one of these led by a Western researcher); 1 was from Asia (led by a Western researcher); and 1 was from Latin America (from a Western researcher who had lived in Brazil for over 10 years). Only 2 studies involved principal researchers from developing countries.

A social approach to sexuality "examines the range of behavior, ideology and subjective meaning within and between human groups," mediated by culture.[2] To understand individual behaviors, the social approach to sexuality requires a better understanding of social and cultural systems and symbols (Box 9-1). Yet, while social factors should play a central role in framing questions about the spread of HIV, Table 9-1 demonstrates that social science thinking remains governed by conceptual approaches that emphasize the individual.

BOX 9-1

Sex research in response to AIDS

RICHARD G. PARKER

Few areas of behavioral research have been as neglected as the study of human sexuality. For nearly 50 years prior to the emergence of the HIV/AIDS pandemic, sex research had been marginalized and received low priority for research funding. Only a few centers focused on research on sexual behavior; this lack of an established research community seriously limited the potential for a rapid and powerful response to an epidemic closely linked with sexual behavior.[1,2,3]

The HIV/AIDS pandemic promptly raised awareness of the need for an understanding of sexual behavior. Unprecedented research funding became available for studies of sexual behavior in relation to HIV transmission—particularly in the United States, Australia, and a number of Western European countries, but also in many developing countries affected by the HIV/AIDS epidemic. By the late 1980s, new centers for HIV/AIDS–related behavioral research had been founded at several major universities and studies of sexual behavior were initiated by the World Health Organization's Global Program on AIDS and other organizations.[4,5]

Given the serious limits of pre-existing data, early research sought to quantify sexual attitudes and behaviors in different communities.[6] Baseline behavioral data were collected, such as numbers of sexual partners, criteria for partner selection, the prevalence of condom use, and attitudes toward HIV infection and AIDS.[7] Through quantifiable data, these studies sought to document the statistical frequency of behavioral factors linked to HIV infection and to improve understanding of the dynamics of HIV transmission in different societies.[8,9]

However, these surveys provided little insight into many of the issues associated with effective intervention.[10,11] One of the most consistent findings in many knowledge, attitudes, beliefs, and practices (KABP) surveys has been the limited impact knowledge of HIV infection seems to have on risk behavior.[12,13] These surveys documented the low level of behavioral change that had occurred in response to early HIV prevention efforts.[14,15] Furthermore, even in those settings where widespread behavioral change was reported, such as among gay communities in some developed countries, it appeared that a range of factors (like the development of community support structures and the restriction of AIDS-related discrimination) were as important as AIDS information in stimulating personal behavioral change.[16]

As the epidemic has continued to expand, dissatisfaction with current sexual behavior research has increased. Sexual behavior research must now go beyond the rate of particular attitudes and reported sexual practices to examine the contexts in which sexual activity is shaped; the social, cultural, political, and economic systems in which behavior occurs and becomes meaningful must also be considered.[17,18] It is increasingly clear that a range of contextual factors, such as the structure of gender power relations and the formation of sexual identities, play a fundamental role in shaping both sexual behavior and behavioral responses to HIV/AIDS.[19,20] Thus, social and behavioral research in response to AIDS has evolved dramatically, leading to a new emphasis on research methods and theoretical frameworks that might be applied to better understand the relations between HIV/AIDS and sexual behavior.[21,22]

In light of these developments, large-scale KABP surveys have increasingly been replaced by more focused, small-scale, qualitative studies of sexual culture, examining the social representations, symbols, and meanings that shape and structure sexual experience in different settings.[23,24] Research attention has shifted to the structures of power in gender relations and the experience of sexual violence and discrimination.[25] Models of sexual behavior change have gradually shifted from a focus on the individual to approaches aimed at understanding the collective responses of different communities.[26,27] Epidemiological questions have been supplemented by an effort to identify the social, cultural, economic, and political dimensions of sexual behavior in relation to the HIV/AIDS epidemic. Methodologies from the different disciplines have evolved due to increasing linkage with other social sciences, such as anthropology.

The next phase of sexual research will be critical. To offer useful guidance for HIV prevention, it must combine traditional approaches and new methods to provide a new understanding of sexual behavior. And, as sex research develops further, it will draw renewed, and hopefully productive, attention to the fundamentally social dimensions not only of sexual conduct, but of the entire range of human behavior.

References

1. C. F. Turner, H. G. Miller, and L. E. Moses, eds., *AIDS: Sexual Behavior and Intravenous Drug Use* (Washington, DC: National Academy Press, 1989).

2. A. Chouinard and J. Albert, eds., *Human Sexuality: Research Perspectives in a World Facing AIDS* (Ottawa, Canada: International Development Research Centre, 1989).

3. J. H. Gagnon, "Sex research and sexual conduct in the era of AIDS," *Journal of Acquired Immune Deficiency Syndromes* 1(1988):593–601.

4. P. Abramson and G. Herdt, "Assessment of sexual practices relevant to the transmission of AIDS: A global perspective," *Journal of Sex Research* 27(1990):215–232.

5. M. Carballo, J. Cleland, M. Caraël, et al., "Cross-national study of patterns of sexual behavior," *Journal of Sex Research* 26(1989):287–299.

6. P. Abramson and G. Herdt, "Assessment of sexual practices relevant to the transmission of AIDS: A global perspective," *Journal of Sex Research* 27(1990):215–232.

7. Carballo, "Cross-national study,"

8. Turner, *AIDS: Sexual Behavior.*

9. Carballo, "Cross-national study."

10. R. G. Parker, G. Herdt, and M. Carballo, "Sexual culture, HIV transmission, and AIDS research," *Journal of Sex Research* 28(1991):77–98.

11. R. G. Parker, "Sexual cultures, HIV transmission, and AIDS prevention," *AIDS* 8(suppl.1)(1994):s309–s314.

12. Turner, *AIDS: Sexual Behavior.*

13. G. Herdt and S. Lindenbaum, eds., *Time of AIDS: Social Analysis, Theory and Method* (Newbury Park, CA: Sage Publications, 1992).

14. Turner, *AIDS: Sexual Behavior.*

15. Herdt, *Time of AIDS.*

16. S. Kippax, R. W. Connell, G. W. Dowsett, and J. Crawford, *Sustaining Safe Sex* (London: Falmer Press, 1993).

17. Parker, "Sexual cultures, HIV, and AIDS prevention."

18. Herdt, *Time of AIDS.*

19. WHO, Global Programme on AIDS, Social and Behavioural Studies and Support Unit, *Social and Contextual Factors Affecting Risk-Related Sexual Activity Amongst Young People in Developing Countries, General Protocol,* WHO/GPA/SSB (Geneva, 1993).

20. WHO, Global Programme on AIDS, Social and Behavioural Studies and Support Unit, *Sexual Negotiation, the Empowerment of Women, and the Female Condom, General Protocol,* WHO/GPA/SSB (Geneva, 1993).

21. J. H. Gagnon and R. G. Parker, "Conceiving sexuality," in *Conceiving Sexuality: Approaches to Sex Research in a Postmodern World,* R. G. Parker and J. H. Gagnon, eds. (New York and London: Routledge, 1994).

22. M. Boulton, "Methodological issues in HIV/AIDS social research: Recent debates, recent developments," *AIDS* 7(suppl.1)(1993):s249–s255.

23. Parker, "Sexual culture, HIV, and AIDS research."

24. Parker, "Sexual culture, HIV, and AIDS prevention."

25. Gagnon, "Conceiving sexuality."

26. Kippax, *Sustaining Safe Sex.*

27. P. M. Davies, F. C. I. Hickson, P. Weatherburn, and A. J. Hunt, *Sex, Gay Men and AIDS* (London: Falmer Press, 1993).

Alternative conceptual approaches

Fortunately, the challenges of HIV prevention have stimulated an increasing number of researchers to approach human behavior from a variety of creative and innovative perspectives. For example, social construction theory has been applied to studies of sexual culture in Brazil.[3,4] This approach posits that the data obtained through traditional sexual behavior surveys has been of greater use in epidemiological modeling of the spread of HIV than for designing educational and other forms of intervention.

As an alternative, the emotional significance of certain sexual acts and the wider systems of meanings that made these behaviors important have been described. Using qualitative techniques, the erotic significance of sexual practices in different social and cultural contexts was examined. This research indicated that transgressing normative rules and regulations is a potent erotic force in Brazilian sexual life. The concept of transgression suggests consideration of an extremely wide range of sexual behaviors that are perceived as exciting, satisfying, and meaningful. For example, anal intercourse, although socially proscribed, is commonly practiced by both sexes from adolescence through adulthood. It is therefore not surprising that "the *bunda* (literally, the "behind" or "ass") of both men and women is treated as almost a national fetish, reproduced in a whole range of images and media."[5] These findings demonstrate the need for understanding of local sexual culture in developing HIV prevention programs. For as in Brazil, strategies advocating risk reduction and safer sex may clash with culturally influenced activities linked with sexual satisfaction. To be effective, health education will need to modify behavior in ways that remain culturally attractive.

Other research considers that traditional values maintain strong influence in contemporary cultures. Accordingly, the importance of the African kinship, or "clanship," system in local community responses to HIV/AIDS has been emphasized.[6] The clanship grouping is a traditional social unit in sub-Saharan Africa. Clan structures have been ignored in AIDS prevention efforts in Africa, in part because of the way in which the industrialized country funders of HIV prevention programs have conceptualized the problem. Imaginative new approaches will be required to work with existing social systems and to emphasize strengths within communities, thereby engaging clan members in HIV prevention and AIDS care.

Researchers in South Africa have used systems theory to investigate the effect of the migrant labor system on heterosexual relationships around mines.[7] They found that the migrant labor system created geographic networks of sexual relationships between urban and rural communities and a market for prostitution in mining towns. Migrant laborers are separated from wives, earn low wages, and live in poor conditions. Men reported that contact with sex workers and brief casual encounters offered not only sexual satisfaction but the pleasure of female company and comfort from the harsh reality of the mining world. These researchers provide a picture of how the economic system shapes behaviors, which suggests that preventive efforts must include addressing the economic system itself.

In summary, sociological theories are opening new avenues in research on sexuality and HIV/AIDS prevention. Conceptual approaches drawing from sociological theory could be strengthened by theories from political science, and by theories of justice and political democracy. Frameworks that successfully integrate these varied components will help communities develop more informed responses to the HIV/AIDS epidemic and can help policy makers respond more effectively to the rich diversity and meaning of behaviors across cultures.

Methodical approaches in research on sexual behavior

The study of sexual behavior is essential for HIV/AIDS prevention and control. Many sexual behavior surveys have been carried out; for example, of the 827 published abstracts on social impact and response from the 1992 International AIDS Conference, 31 percent (N = 269) contained information from sexual behavior, attitude, and knowledge surveys.[8]

Quantitative sexual behavior surveys

General population surveys. During the 1980s, demographic and health surveys (DHS) were widely used for fertility and family planning purposes. These surveys, directed at women, inquired about marriage, fertility, contraception, and child health, but produced very limited information on sexual behavior.[9] Recently, the DHS Program recognized that its surveys could contribute to greater understanding of sexual behavior and incorporated detailed questions on male and female sexual behaviors.[10]

Despite the need for information on sexual practices to guide public health responses to HIV/AIDS, sexual behavior surveys of general populations were uncommon in both industrialized and developing countries until the later 1980s. From 1987 to 1990, the WHO Global Programme on AIDS (WHO/GPA) supported national and city-wide surveys of sexual behavior in adults (ages 15 to 49) in developing countries. Of 40 such surveys undertaken, the findings from 15 have been published, including 12 country-wide surveys (Box 9-2).[11]

BOX 9-2

Some lessons from the World Health Organization Global Programme on AIDS (WHO/GPA) sexual behavior surveys and knowledge, attitudes, beliefs, and practices (KABP) surveys

BENOÎT FERRY AND JOHN CLELAND

Between 1980 and 1994, sexual behavior surveys were conducted among the general population or specific population groups in 67 countries (Table 9-2.1). Fifteen of these sexual behavior and KABP

Table 9-2.1 Countries indicating that they conducted at least one sexual behavior survey, 1980–1994

GAA	Country	A	B	C	D	E	F	G	H	I	J	K
1	Canada			•								
1	USA											•
2	Belgium	•	•	•			•					•
2	France	•	•	•	•	•	•		•		•	•
2	Germany	•		•	•		•		•	•	•	
2	Liechtenstein									•		
2	The Netherlands	•	•	•	•	•	•		•		•	•
2	Norway			•	•	•	•				•	
2	Sweden			•			•	•	•			
2	Switzerland	•		•	•		•	•			•	
2	United Kingdom										•	
3	Australia	•	•	•	•		•	•	•		•	•
3	Vanuatu											•
4	Brazil	•	•	•	•						•	
4	Colombia										•	
4	Costa Rica	•	•	•			•	•	•		•	
4	Ecuador	•		•			•	•			•	
4	Guatemala	•					•			•		
4	Mexico	•	•	•		•		•			•	•
4	Peru	•					•	•				•
4	Surinam	•		•			•	•	•			
5	Benin	•					•			•	•	•
5	Botswana						•	•				•
5	Burkino Faso	•					•		•	•	•	
5	Cameroon	•					•			•	•	
5	Comoros	•										
5	Congo						•					
5	Côte d'Ivoire	•							•		•	•
5	Djibouti	•										
5	Gabon						•				•	
5	Ghana	•					•			•	•	•
5	Guinea						•					
5	Madagascar	•					•				•	
5	Mali	•					•			•	•	
5	Mauritania										•	
5	Mauritius										•	
5	Senegal	•	•	•	•	•	•		•	•	•	•
5	South Africa	•	•	•	•	•	•	•	•		•	
5	Togo	•										•
5	Uganda						•	•		•		•
5	Zaire	•					•				•	
5	Zambia	•					•	•	•	•		•

(continued)

Table 9-2.1 Countries indicating that they conducted at least one sexual behavior survey, 1980–1994—continued

GAA	Country	A	B	C	D	E	F	G	H	I	J	K
5	Zimbabwe	•					•	•		•	•	•
6	Antigua and Barbuda						•					
6	Barbados										•	
6	Grenada						•		•		•	
6	Jamaica	•		•			•				•	•
6	St. Lucia						•	•				•
6	Trinidad and Tobago						•					•
7	Czech Republic	•			•		•	•				
7	Estonia			•								
7	Hungary	•									•	
7	Kyrgyz Republic						•	•		•		•
7	Lithuania						•	•				
7	Turkmenistan										•	
7	Ukraine			•			•	•	•	•	•	•
7	Yugoslavia, Fed. Rep.				•		•			•		•
8	Jordan						•	•				•
8	Morocco	•					•					•
8	Tunisia	•	•				•			•	•	•
9	China	•			•						•	
9	Hong Kong	•		•	•	•	•	•			•	•
9	Viet Nam	•			•		•				•	
10	India	•	•	•	•	•	•	•	•	•	•	•
10	Malaysia	•	•	•	•	•		•	•	•		
10	Singapore	•	•									
10	Thailand	•			•		•	•	•	•		•
	TOTAL	40	12	21	17	9	46	26	18	17	39	28

Code for column headings: A: female sex workers; B: male sex workers; C: homosexual/bisexual males; D: injecting drug users; E: drug users who do not inject; F: young people; G: students; H: people with HIV; I: military personnel; J: general population through large-scale surveys; K: general population through small-scale surveys.

surveys have been reviewed and summarized by the Global Programme on AIDS (GPA) of the World Health Organization.[1] These surveys were all conducted during 1989–1990 in developing countries. While not all are of publishable quality, they provide insight into knowledge, attitudes, beliefs, and practices concerning HIV/AIDS.

For example, awareness of HIV/AIDS was high in the late 1980s, yet incorrect beliefs regarding modes of transmission were alarmingly prevalent (Table 9-2.2). The large majority of women and approximately two-thirds of men professed faithfulness to their regular sexual partner (Table 9-2.3). However, there was considerable variability among sites, ranging from 5 percent to more than 50 percent of men reporting at least one such contact. The percentage of men reporting five or more such sexual partners was consistently low, ranging from 0 to 11 percent. Unfortunately, however, among men who reported five or more nonmarital partners in the last 12 months, a substantial proportion (20 to 50 percent) perceived no risk of HIV infection to themselves. Also, these surveys did not support the common assumption that towns and cities are more conducive than rural areas to nonregular sexual relationships.

Large variations in condom awareness were also apparent. In some locations, almost everyone had

Table 9-2.2 Selected indicators of knowledge, beliefs, and attitudes from 15 WHO Global Programme on AIDS sexual behavior and KABP surveys, 1989–1990*

Survey location	Percentage of all respondents aware of AIDS	Among respondents aware of AIDS, percentage believing that touching someone with AIDS can transmit infection	Percentage of all men aware of condoms and source of supply	Among respondents aware of AIDS, percentage reporting themselves to be at moderate or high risk of HIV infection
Central African Republic	83	60	43	60
Côte d'Ivoire	90	51	46	37
Guinea Bissau	75	69	31	30
Togo	64	40	48	27
Burundi	96	77	48	6
Kenya	89	75	54	13
Lesotho	98	67	67	8
Tanzania	96	66	N/A	5
Lusaka[a]	98	88	60	10
Mauritius	92	49	79	3
Manila[a]	98	76	64	5
Singapore	95	79	93	0
Sri Lanka	77	39	N/A	2
Thailand	99	63	89	19
Rio de Janeiro[a]	100	93	85	9

*Note: National surveys of knowledge, attitudes, beliefs, and practices (KABP) unless otherwise indicated. N/A, not applicable.
[a]City sample.

Table 9-2.3 Selected behavior indicators from 15 WHO/Global Programme on AIDS sexual behavior and KABP surveys, 1989–1990[a]

Survey location	Percentage of all respondents reporting sex outside their regular partnership in last 12 months		Percentage of all men reporting 5 or more partners outside their regular partnership in last 12 months	Among men who reported having obtained commercial sex in last 12 months, percentage who always used condoms on these occasions
	Men	Women	Men	Men
Central African Republic	14	5	2	18
Côte d'Ivoire	51	13	10	11
Guinea Bissau	44	21	1	N/A
Togo	20	1	2	8
Burundi	7	2	2	26
Kenya	31	12	4	N/A
Lesotho	24	19	8	15
Tanzania	32	14	5	8
Lusaka[a]	36	10	8	25
Mauritius	10	0	N/A	N/A
Manila[a]	15	1	1	21
Singapore	10	1	3	28
Sri Lanka	4	3	0	N/A
Thailand	28	2	11	33
Rio de Janeiro[a]	44	10	10	5

[a]Note: National surveys unless otherwise indicated. N/A not applicable.
[a]City sample.

heard of condoms while in others more than half of the respondents were completely ignorant about them. Clearly, awareness of condoms must be complemented by knowledge of a source of supply. In these surveys, fewer than half of persons in most of the African sites had sufficient knowledge and access for condom use. Finally, the percentage of men who reported consistent use of condoms for commercial sexual contacts ranged from 5 percent to over 30 percent.

References

1. J. Cleland and B. Ferry, eds., *Sexual Behaviour and Knowledge about AIDS in the Developing World—Findings from a Multisite Study,* scientific report, WHO/GPA/SSB (Geneva, 1994).

From 1991 to 1993, surveys have been published and reported from 21 countries, mainly from industrialized nations, but also from developing countries.[12-20] The significance of national surveys that receive publicity cannot be overestimated. They place sexual behavior on the national policy and research agendas and help create a political climate in which policy development and in-depth research can proceed.

However, the sexual survey approach has been criticized for several reasons. First, there is concern about the quality of the data produced; two-thirds of the surveys funded by WHO/GPA were not of sufficient scientific quality to be published. However, improvements in methodological rigor clearly can yield reliable and valid data.[21,22,23] Second, the utility of survey data for understanding HIV/AIDS epidemiology and modeling has been questioned.[24,25] Finally, the usefulness of survey data for designing of prevention programs has been unclear. This problem is amplified by the use of core protocols to investigate sexual practices. For while population-based sexual behavior surveys can offer simple descriptions of sexual practices, they are not designed to explore cultural diversity or the social context of behavior. Based on individualistic models of behavior and using questionnaires or structured interviews, these surveys can only provide superficial answers to such questions as who does what, with whom, how many times, and with how many recent partners. They cannot, however, address why people engage in behaviors.

Surveys of the sexual behavior of target populations. In contrast to the relatively small number of surveys of general populations, numerous sexual behavior surveys have been conducted for specific groups, such as female sex workers, gay men, and injecting drug users. Surveys of "target" populations are popular because they cost less and are usually less politically controversial, as they often involve socially marginalized groups. For example, Table 9-2 shows that in 1991–93, sexual behavior surveys of female sex workers from 30 countries were presented at international AIDS conferences. There is only limited evidence, however, that findings from these surveys have been translated into effective public health interventions.

Table 9-2   Countries presenting sexual behavior surveys of female sex workers at the International AIDS Conferences, 1991–1993

GAA		Countries
1	North America	Canada, United States
2	Western Europe	Austria, Belgium, Denmark, France, Greece, Italy, Spain, United Kingdom
3	Oceania	Australia
4	Latin America	Argentina, Barbados, Brazil, Dominican Republic, Mexico, Peru
5	Sub-Saharan Africa	Ghana, Kenya, Nigeria, Tanzania, Zaire, Zambia, Zimbabwe
9	Northeast Asia	Hong Kong
10	Southeast Asia	Indonesia, Philippines, Singapore, Thailand, Sri Lanka

Source: Abstracts of the VII, VIII, and IX International AIDS Conferences.

Qualitative studies of sexual behavior

Little qualitative research on sexuality in the context of HIV/AIDS existed until the early 1990s.[26] Using several examples of recent qualitative studies, Table 9-3 summarizes the questions formulated, the conceptual basis of the study, research methods, and key findings. Two general characteristics of these studies were that psychology did not provide the dominant conceptual framework and that questions related not only to individuals, but also to social, cultural, political, and economic factors. In the questions asked, there is a new emphasis on the complexity of sexual life, associated with the challenge of developing innovative responses for effective HIV prevention.

Experiencing sexuality. Asking questions about how men and women experience their sexuality leads research beyond stereotypes. For example, one study of young women in a Western culture showed that sexual behaviors were not necessarily due to acceptance of male dominance, but involved social considerations and fear of expressing sexual feelings. Even though young women were concerned about pregnancy, they tended not to resist male pressure for penetrative sex—partly because of love, but mostly because of fear of losing the boyfriend.[27] They "did" sex to keep the boyfriend and to keep him happy, and they trusted the boyfriend to protect their reputation as part of the bargain. Penetrative sex had considerable emotional and social significance for women, but it was governed by unspoken cultural rules.

Another Western study described how the "male technique" of sex stimulated young men's fantasy and erotic desire, yet produced anxiety when it failed to arouse the female.[28] Thus, attempts to alter the cultural notion of technique to include safer sex practices might be more appropriate for HIV prevention than exhorting people to specific actions, such as putting on condoms, that conflict with men's sense of what is erotic or masculine. However, while harnessing the existing concept of technique may facilitate changes in some behaviors, challenges such as anal sex and transgression of sexual norms still remain.[29,30]

Constructing sexual identities and roles. Studies of gay men in the Philippines, the U.K., and Canada have shown that sexual identity and sexual role are not immutable characteristics of persons or self.[31,32] They may shift over time and may be shaped by such factors as age, place, relationships, and social class.[33] Static categories that use sexual practices to define identity or role should therefore be avoided. Questions about social, cultural, and historical influences and their influence on a person's sexual identity and role challenge notions that sexuality has a purely biological basis and that a "sex drive" is an exclusively physiological imperative.

Table 9-3 Selected qualitative studies of sexuality published 1991–1994

Country/author and year	Questions asked	Theoretical framework; methods used	Main findings
United Kingdom/ Holland et al.,[1] 1991	How do young women experience their sexuality?	Social construction; structured questionnaires with 496 14–16-year-olds, in-depth interviews with 150 of same group	Social context of sex, gender role, and young girls' reluctance to accept their sexuality are important factors.
Nigeria/Orubuloye et al.,[2] 1993	How do adult women experience their sexuality?	Sociology/anthropology; in-depth interviews with a probability sample of 600 women	Women have control over their sexuality in a variety of circumstances, especially when a partner has an STI or AIDS.
United States/ Kline et al.,[3] 1992	How do adult women experience their sexuality?	Sociology/anthropology/social psychology; 16 focus groups with 134 women	Culture and economic conditions affect sexual life. Women can negotiate safe sex under certain circumstances.
Australia/Waldby et al.,[4] 1990	How do adult men experience their sexuality?	Social construction; volunteer, in-depth interviews with 8 men aged 23–37	Male desire, fantasy, sex roles, and sexual techniques could be harnessed for HIV preventive programs.
United Kingdom/ Coxon et al.,[5] 1993	How is male sex role related to behavior?	Social construction; sexual diaries from 385 active gay men	Sexual practices vary widely as do sexual roles in active/passive domain.
Philippines/Tan,[6] 1994	How is sexual identity constructed?	Social construction; focus groups, interviews, and questionnaires	Sexual identity is not an essential characteristic. Meanings of behaviors and identity vary by class.
Papua New Guinea/Leavitt,[7] 1991	What is the effect of sexual ideology on sexual life?	Unclear; not adequately described	Cultural analysis on its own is insufficient to explain sexual life.
Brazil/Raffaelli et al.,[8] 1993	How does sexual culture influence sexual behavior?	Social construction; focus-group discussions with 53 youths. Open-ended discussion with 15 youths. Life-history discussions with 6 young people, field observations, structured interviews with 413 young people	Cultural and social processes shape sexual behavior.
Australia/Dowsett et al.,[9] 1992	How does class influence sexual behavior?	Sociology; 28 life-history interviews, 4 group discussions	Homosexuality needs to be problematized; the category should not be taken for granted. Information and sexual preventive practices vary by social class.

(continued)

Table 9-3   Selected qualitative studies of sexuality published 1991–1994—continued

Country/author and year	Questions asked	Theoretical framework; methods used	Main findings
Thailand/Manderson,[10] 1992	What role has the erotic in commercial performances?	Anthropology/social construction; ethnography	The body is a means of production rather than a mirror to the self.
Nigeria/Orubuloye et al.,[11] 1993	How are transport and commercial systems related to sexual behavior?	Unclear; interviewed 258 truck drivers and 467 itinerant female hawkers	Occupational demands result in a multiple network of sexual relationships.
South Africa/Jochelson et al.,[12] 1991	How do migrant and labor systems affect sexual life?	Anthropology/sociology; 44 men and women were interviewed	The labor system influences sexual life.

[1]J. Holland, C. Ramazanoglu, S. Scott, S. Sharpe, and R. Thomson, "Risk, power and the possibility of pleasure: Young women and safer sex," *AIDS Care* 4(1991):273–283.

[2]I. O. Orubuloye, J. C. Caldwell, and P. Caldwell, "African women's control over their sexuality in an era of AIDS," *Social Science and Medicine* 37(1993):859–872.

[3]A. Kline, E. Kline, and E. Oken, "Minority women and sexual choice in the age of AIDS," *Social Science and Medicine* 34(1992):447–457.

[4]C. Waldby, J. Kippax, and S. Crawford, "Heterosexual men negotiating safe sex: A case study," Abstract 4119, presented at the VI International Conference on AIDS, San Francisco, California, June 1990.

[5]A. P. M. Coxon, N. H. Coxon, P. Weatherburn, et al., "Sex role separation in sexual diaries of homosexual men," *AIDS* 7(1993):877–882.

[6]M. Tan, "From Bakla to Gay: Shifting gender identities and sexual behaviours among Philipino men who have sex with men," in *Conceiving Sexuality: Sex Research in a Postmodern World*, R. G. Parker and J. H. Gagnon, eds. (New York and London: Routledge, 1994): 85–97.

[7]S. C. Leavitt, "Sexual ideology and experience in a Papua New Guinea Society," *Social Science and Medicine* 33(1991):897–907.

[8]M. Raffaelli, R. Campos, A. P. Merritt, et al., "Sexual practices and attitudes of street youth in Belo Homzonte, Brazil," *Social Science and Medicine* 37(1993):661–670.

[9]G. W. Dowsett, M. D. Davis, and R. W. Connell, "Working class homosexuality and HIV/AIDS prevention: Some recent research from Sydney, Australia," *Psychology and Health* 6(1992):313–324.

[10]L. Manderson, "Public sex performances in Patpong and exploration of the edges of imagination," *Journal of Sex Research* 4(1992):451–475.

[11]I. O. Orubuloye, P. Caldwell, and J. C. Caldwell, "Role of high risk occupations in the spread of AIDS: Truck drivers and itinerant market women in Nigeria," *International Family Planning Perspectives* 2(1993):43–48.

[12]K. Jochelson, M. Mothibeli, and J. P. Leger, "HIV and migrant labor in South Africa," *International Journal of Health Services* 21(1991):157–173.

Systems and sexual life. Studies of the way in which social, occupational, and economic systems shape sexual life have emphasized that preventing HIV spread must address these issues to be effective. In Nigeria, the working and social life of long-distance highway truckers, coupled with the economic vicissitudes of female traders on route who provide sexual and domestic services, influences sexual networks and activity.[34]

These examples demonstrate that qualitative and multidisciplinary approaches have started to enrich the understanding of sexuality through the elaboration of its social, cultural, and historical meanings. Social science is beginning to find answers in studies that situate human behaviors within the diverse and sophisticated contexts in which they operate. This new approach is moving towards a greater coherence with inevitable changes in emphasis for the public health approach to the AIDS epidemic.

Measuring outcomes

How has social science contributed to the evaluation of prevention programs?

Evaluating interventions with schools and youth groups

While HIV/AIDS education programs for schools and youth groups have proliferated, the scientific foundation for such programs is quite limited and an evaluation of their impact has been rare, in both industrialized and developing countries.[35]

Table 9-4 shows that among seven trials published from 1991 to 1993 which examined the impact of school health education, only three (from the U.K., U.S., and Tanzania) randomly allocated subjects to experimental and control groups with pre- and post-testing.[36,37,38] Three of the remaining trials were controlled; however the study by Kirby et al. only involved post-testing, which limits the extent to which conclusions can be drawn.[39–42] The studies all attempted to make interventions relevant to young people, and several reinforced learning through discussion sessions and role playing.

The outcomes of these seven intervention trials (Table 9-5) include

- evidence that such programs increase knowledge of HIV/AIDS and about preventive practices;
- some evidence that intervention has a small effect on attitudes, beliefs, and perception of risk;
- limited evidence that intervention changes intentions to engage in risky sexual practices;
- very limited and equivocal data on the impact on young people's behavior in terms of condom use and number of sexual partners.

Evaluating interventions with female sex workers

As shown in Table 9-6, most of the research among female sex workers has occurred in developing countries.[43] Many of these studies were methodologically flawed (principally due to the lack of control groups).

Evaluating interventions among injecting drug users

Recent studies of injection drug users demonstrate that while most interventions have some impact on needle-injecting practices, sexual behaviors are more difficult to change. As Table 9-7 shows, needle exchange programs, counseling, and outreach community-based peer efforts can reduce needle-sharing practices in many drug users. However, even in well-conceived and executed programs, approximately two in three drug users did not change their behavior.

Evaluating interventions among gay men

Studies have consistently shown that gay men have responded to the threat of HIV by changing their behavior. Table 9-8 lists recent evaluation studies,

Table 9-4 School health education program evaluation, 1991–1993

Location/author and year	Age	Intervention	Sample size	Study method
Nottingham, United Kingdom/Bellingham, Gillies,[1] 1993	16–19	Streetwise package for out-of-school youth: streetwise comic, role-playing, tutor-led active learning activities	337	Randomized controlled trial (RCT), YTS center trainees randomly allocated by center; pre-posttest with 2-week follow-up; focus-group discussions
Philadelphia, United States/Jemmott et al.,[2] 1992	15	5-hour program including videotapes, games, exercises to encourage correct use of condoms, role-plays for safer sex	157	RCT; individuals randomized to groups; pre-post questionnaires with 3-month follow-up
Northern Tanzania/Klepp et al.,[3] 1993	11–12	Lecture or film (45 minutes duration)	Not given	RCT schools randomly assigned; pre-post questionnaire
Spain/Ordonana et al.,[4] 1992	High school	Information package	115	4 matched groups, 3 experimental, and 1 control; pre-post questionnaire with 2-week and 3-month follow-up
United States/Boyer et al.,[5] 1991	13–15	Skills-building lesson	513	Controlled trial; schools allocated to experimental and control conditions; pre-post questionnaire
Berlin, Germany/Schutte et al.,[6] 1991	12–18	Teacher-led education program	1105	Controlled trial; schools allocated to experimental or control groups; pre-post questionnaire
United States/Kirby et al.,[7] 1991 (Muskegon, Michigan; Gary, Indiana; Jackson, Mississippi; Quincy, Massachusetts; Dallas, Texas; and San Francisco, California)	—	Counseling on sexual issues, pregnancy prevention, school-based clinic, vouchers for free contraceptives at a nearby family planning clinic	—	Matched schools compared; post-test after intervention only (poorest design reported here)

[1]K. Bellingham and P. A. Gillies, "Evaluation of an AIDS education programme for young adults," *Journal of Epidemiology and Community Health* 47(1993):134–138.

[2]J. B. Jemmott, L. S. Jemmott, and G. T. Fong, "Reductions in HIV risk associated with sexual behaviours among black male adolescents: Effects on AIDS prevention intervention," *American Journal of Public Health* 82(1992):372–377 [errata corrected in 82(1992):684].

[3]K. I. Klepp, S. Ndeki, A. Irena, et al., "Evaluation of AIDS education for primary school children in Northern Tanzania," Abstract WS-D02-3, presented at the IX International Conference on AIDS, Berlin, Germany, June 1993.

[4]J. Ordonana, J. Guiterex, P. Martinez, et al., "Health education in high schools: Effectiveness of short-term interventions," Abstract PoD 5875, presented at the VIII International Conference on AIDS, Amsterdam, The Netherlands, July 1992.

[5]C. Boyer, M. Shafer, and J. Tschamm, "Evaluation of an STD/HIV education and skills building intervention for high school students," Abstract W.D.4135, presented at the VII International Conference on AIDS, Florence, Italy, June 1991.

[6]E. Schutte and H. Oswald, "Evaluation of an AIDS-prevention programme in West Berlin schools," Abstract W.D.4218, presented at the VII International Conference on AIDS, Florence, Italy, June 1991.

[7]D. Kirby, C. Waszak, and J. Zeiglar, "Six school based clinics: Their reproductive health services and impact on sexual behaviour," *Family Planning Perspectives* 23(1991):6–16.

Table 9-5 Impact of school programs of HIV/AIDS education, 1991–1993

Author and year	HIV/AIDS knowledge	HIV/AIDS attitudes and beliefs	Ability to talk about sex with partner	Perception of risk	Behavioral intentions	Sexual behavior
Bellingham, Gillies,[1] 1993	Significant increase	No effects	Increase (not statistically significant)	Significant changes	No effect	No effect.
Jemmott et al.,[2] 1992	Significant increase	Less favorable attitudes towards risky sex	Not recorded	Not recorded	Weaker intentions to engage in risky sex	Fewer sexual partners; increase in condom use; less anal sex
Klepp et al.,[3] 1992	Significant increase	Small increase in positive attitudes to prevention	Not recorded	Not recorded	Significantly less likely to have sex	Not recorded
Ordonana et al.,[4] 1992	Significant increase	No effects	Not recorded	Not recorded	—	No effect
Boyer et al.,[5] 1992	Significant increase	No data	Not recorded	Not recorded	Not recorded	Increase in skills related to preventive behavior; no effect on actual behaviors
Schutte et al.,[6] 1991	Significant increase	More positive attitudes towards people with AIDS	Not recorded	Decrease in unreasonable fears	Not recorded	No effect
Kirby et al.,[7] 1991	No data	No data	Not recorded	No data	No data	Increase in condom use; increase in oral contraceptive pill use

[1]K. Bellingham and P. A. Gillies, "Evaluation of an AIDS education programme for young adults," *Journal of Epidemiology and Community Health* 47(1993):134–138.

[2]J. B. Jemmott, L. S. Jemmott, and G. T. Fong, "Reductions in HIV risk associated with sexual behaviours among black male adolescents: *Effects on AIDS prevention intervention," American Journal of Public Health* 82(1992):372–377 [errata corrected in 82(1992):684].

[3]K. I. Klepp, S. Ndeki, A. Irena, et al., "Evaluation of AIDS education for primary school children in Northern Tanzania," Abstract WS-D02-3, presented at the IX International Conference on AIDS, Berlin, Germany, June 1993.

[4]J. Ordonana, J. Guiterex, P. Martinez, et al., "Health education in high schools: Effectiveness of short-term interventions," Abstract PoD 5875, presented at the VIII International Conference on AIDS, Amsterdam, The Netherlands, July 1992.

[5]C. Boyer, M. Shafer, and J. Tschamm, "Evaluation of an STD/HIV education and skills building intervention for high school students," Abstract W.D.4135, presented at the VII International Conference on AIDS, Florence, Italy, June 1991.

[6]E. Schutte and H. Oswald, "Evaluation of an AIDS-prevention programme in West Berlin schools," Abstract W.D.4218, presented at the VII International Conference on AIDS, Florence, Italy, June 1991.

[7]D. Kirby, C. Waszak, and J. Zeiglar, "Six school based clinics: Their reproductive health services and impact on sexual behaviour," *Family Planning Perspectives* 23(1991):6–16.

Table 9-6 Results from selected studies of interventions among female sex workers, 1991–1993

Country/author and year	Intervention	Evaluation	Results
Kenya/Moses et al.,[1] 1991	Condom distribution program at an STI clinic with health education	Comparison of control versus experimental group (controlled trial)	Reduction in HIV transmission through increased condom use
Nigeria/Williams et al.,[2] 1992	Peer-led health education and condom promotion in an STI clinic	Pre-posttest design	Increase in knowledge, condom use, and clinic attendance
Mexico/De la Vega et al.,[3] 1992	Community-based peer education program with 99 peer educators working in a "red light" district	Pre-post intervention interviewing	Increase in condom use; in 7/10 sexual acts undertaken, condom use increased by 20%
Tanzania/Matasha et al.,[4] 1992	Community nurse providing medical services and health education to sex workers in their workplace	Reported condom use	Increase in those reporting regular condom use
Thailand/Rojanapitahyakorn,[5] 1992	All-condom policy in the sex industry; non-compliance increased financial penalties for brothel keepers, such as fines and closure	Not clear; pre-post design	Proportion of sex workers reporting using condoms increased by 50% in one year (from 30% to 80%)
Cameroon/Tchupo et al.,[6] 1993	Peer distribution of condoms, i.e., sex workers to sex workers	Number of condoms sold/distributed	Ongoing study, but increase in distribution of condoms by 180% from first to second year
Ivory Coast/Kale et al.,[7] 1993	Neighborhood peer-led health education and condom promotion	Count of number of condoms distributed	Ongoing, but 16-fold increase in condom distribution in the first 6 months of the project
Bali, Indonesia/Tuti Merati et al.,[8] 1993	Flyers, posters, and brochures in brothels displaying information about AIDS and promoting condom use	Pre-post test design	30% increase in proportion of sex workers who said they used condoms with clients (from 65% to 95%); those willing to ask clients to use condoms increased by 15% (5% to 20%)

Singapore/Chan et al.,[9] 1993	Videos in negotiation skills and correct condom use at an STI clinic, plus distribution of posters, stickers, and pamphlets describing correct use of condoms	Condom sales and interviews	84%–95% increase in monthly condom sales at the clinic; high levels of understanding of the video
Singapore/Archibald et al.,[10] 1993	Lectures and role-play workshops	Comparison of control versus experimental groups (controlled trial)	Increase in STI knowledge in comparison group, but no change in reported condom use

[1]S. Moses, F. A. Plummer, E. N. Ngugi, "Controlling HIV in Africa: Effectiveness and cost of an intervention in a high frequency STD transmission group," *AIDS* 5(1991):407–411.

[2]A. Williams, N. Lamson, and S. Efem, "Implementation of an AIDS prevention programme among prostitutes in the Cross River State of Nigeria," *AIDS* 6(1992):229–242.

[3]G. De la Vega, E. Suarez y Toriello, and G. de la Rosa, "Community based AIDS prevention in Cuidad, Juarez, Mexico," in *Effective Approaches to AIDS Prevention* (Geneva: WHO/Global Progamme on AIDS, 1992):23.

[4]E. Matasha et al., "Commercial sex workers intervention programme: A pilot project in Northern Tanzania," Abstract PoD 5639, presented at the VIII International Conference on AIDS, Amsterdam, The Netherlands, July 1992.

[5]W. Rojanapitahyakorn, "Promoting a hundred percent condom use in sex entertainment establishments in Thailand," in *Effective Approaches to AIDS Prevention* (Geneva: WHO/Global Programme on AIDS, 1992):16–22.

[6]J. P. Tchupo et al., "Importance of peer distribution of condoms to prostitutes," Abstract WS-D10-4, presented at the IX International Conference on AIDS, Berlin, Germany, June 1993.

[7]K. Kale, G. Mah-bi, K. N'da et al., "Prevention of STD/AIDS among prostitutes and clients in Abidjan: Initial phase of implementation," Abstract PO-C14-2901, presented at the IX International Conference on AIDS, Berlin, Germany, June 1993.

[8]K. Tuti Merati, "AIDS education among female commercial sex workers in Bali, Indonesia: A pilot intervention study," Abstract PO-D09-3661, presented at the IX International Conference on AIDS, Berlin, Germany, June 1993.

[9]R. K. W. Chan, A. Goh, G. L. Goh et al., "'Project Protect'—An STD/AIDS intervention programme for sex workers and establishments in Singapore," Abstract PO-C14-2904, presented at the IX International Conference on AIDS, Berlin, Germany, June 1993.

[10]C. P. Archibald, R. K. W. Chan, Mi. L. Wong et al., "Improved knowledge but unchanged behaviour following a safe sex intervention among prostitutes in Singapore," Abstract PO-D09-3645, presented at the IX International Conference on AIDS, Berlin, Germany, June 1993.

Table 9-7   Results from selected studies of interventions among injecting drug users, 1991–1993

Country/authors and year	Intervention	Proportion who changed drug-related behavior or sexual behavior
United States/Poane et al.,[1] 1993	Syringe exchange	12% decrease in sharing works
United States/Caslyn et al.,[2] 1992	Safer sex messages for those enrolled in a methadone program	Unspecified increased condom use from low level; 22% decrease in those reporting multiple sex partners
United States/Friedman et al.,[3] 1991	Peer pressure group meeting and counseling	9% mean increase in acts with condoms
United States/Tross et al.,[4] 1991	Outreach intervention comprising self-efficacy and peer support programs	37% decrease in sharing works
United States/Stephens et al.,[5] 1991	Education program with risk reduction counseling	43% decrease in sharing works; 21% decrease in injecting; 29% increase in bleach use
Italy/Nicolosi et al.,[6] 1991	Counseling and testing	25% decrease in sharing works

[1]D. Poane, D. C. Des Jarlais, C. Caloir, et al., "AIDS risk reduction behaviours among participants of syringe exchange programs in New York City," Abstract PO-C24-3188, presented at the IX International Conference on AIDS, Berlin, Germany, June 1993.

[2]D. A. Caslyn, A. J. Saxon, E. A. Wells, and D. M. Greenberg, "Longitudinal sexual behavioural changes in injecting drug users," *AIDS* 6(1992):1207–1211.

[3]S. R. Friedman, B. Jose, and A. Neaigis, "Peer mobilization and widespread condom use by drug injectors," Abstract W.D.54, presented at the VII International Conference on AIDS, Florence, Italy, June 1991.

[4]S. Tross, A. Abdul-Quader, and H. M. Schvert, "Determinants of needle-sharing change in street recruited New York City IV drug users," Abstract S.D.4115, presented at the VII International Conference on AIDS, Florence, Italy, June 1991.

[5]R. S. Stephens, T. E. Feucht, and S. W. Roman, "Effects of an intervention program on AIDS-related drug and needle behaviour among intravenous drug users," *American Journal of Public Health* 81(1991):568–571.

[6]A. Nicolosi, S. Molinari, and M. Musicco, "Positive modifications of injecting behaviour among intravenous heroin users from Milan and Northern Italy 1987–1989," *British Journal of Addiction* 86(1991):91–102.

including an extremely well-designed investigation conducted by Kelly and colleagues.[44]

Towards different models of intervention?

The targeting of groups as described has made some contribution towards the prevention and control of HIV infection worldwide. There is, however, little room for optimism that further refinements of current interventions will make a substantive additional impact. Best estimates suggest that from *one in four* to *one in three* individuals may change their sexual or drug-injecting practices in response to community participation programs. It would appear that targeted interventions derived primarily from psychological theories of behavior can be usefully supported by changes of service provision or policy.[45] The example of the "all condom" policy in Thailand apparently required draconian enforcement measures and this model may not be readily applied in other contexts or cultures.[46] These difficulties notwithstanding, changes to the "system" may potentiate targeted efforts for behavioral change.

There are substantial drawbacks, however, to the targeting approach. Such targeting inevitably excludes other subgroups; those most obviously excluded are the poor. Indeed, exploring AIDS as a disease of absolute or relative poverty would require a shift in the current discourse from the individual and groups to society. It would require greater effort in understand-

Table 9-8 Selected studies evaluating HIV preventive interventions among gay men, 1991–1993

Country/author and year	Intervention	Evaluation	Key findings
United States/Kelly et al.,[1] 1991	Popular opinion leaders in the gay community trained to engage with peers in safer sex conversations; follow-up by telephone	Randomization of 2 city sites in a controlled evaluation (total N = 659), pre-post testing	30% fewer men engaged in unprotected anal intercourse compared with controls
United States/Kelly et al.,[2] 1992, 1993	Distribution of AIDS education posters and materials in gay bars; social norm/peer opinion leaders influence program, opinion leaders nominated by bars	Randomized trial involving 16 city sites; pre-post testing	Up to year 1, 20–25% reported decrease in unsafe sex compared with controls; up to year 2, frequency of unprotected intercourse was reduced by 50%
United States/Kegeles et al.,[4] 1992	Community peer outreach in gay bars and venues	Pre-post test	26% were able to avoid unsafe sex when aroused; 8% had increased sexual communication skills and 8% encouraged each other to have safe sex
Netherlands/de Kooning et al.,[5] 1993	Videos	Pre-post test	Increase in knowledge and self-efficacy and in intentions to have safer sex; better attitudes towards condoms and decrease in oral unsafe sex with steady partners

[1] J. A. Kelly, J. S. St. Lawrence, Y. E. Diaz, et al., "HIV risk behaviour reduction following intervention with key opinion leaders of population: An experimental analysis," *American Journal of Public Health* 81(1991):168–171.

[2] J. A. Kelly, K. J. Sikkema, R. A. Winnett, et al., "Outcomes of a 16 city randomized field trial of a community level HIV risk reduction intervention," Abstract TuD 0543, presented at the VIII International Conference on AIDS, Amsterdam, The Netherlands, July 1992.

[3] J. A. Kelly, R. A. Winnett, R. A. Roffman, et al., "Social diffusion models can produce population-level HIV risk behaviour reduction: Field trial results and mechanisms underlying change," Abstract PO-C23-3167, presented at the IX International Conference on AIDS, Berlin, Germany, June 1993.

[4] S. M. Kegeles, R. Hays, and T. Coates, "Community level risk reduction intervention for young gay and bisexual men," Abstract PoD 5749, presented at the VIII International Conference on AIDS, Amsterdam, The Netherlands, July 1992.

[5] D. de Kooning, W. Debets, C. Blom, and T. G. M. Sandfort, "Evaluation of a small scale AIDS prevention activity for men with homosexual contacts," Abstract PO-C23-3175, presented at the IX International Conference on AIDS, Berlin, Germany, June 1993.

ing contextual factors and the meanings of systems, symbols, and processes for people around the world. It would then lead to a need for public health models of prevention to include community development. Such approaches, informed by theories of political democracy, economy, and justice, would require a comprehensive view of the problem and a vision for resolution grounded in cohesiveness rather than fragmentation, at an intellectual and practical level. Evaluating the outcomes of individually oriented projects may seem easy in contrast to the difficulties of establishing "development" outcomes from projects that cross the sectoral boundaries of health, education, social welfare, law, trade, and industry. Technical expertise in this important field of measurement is needed to contribute to cohesive analysis. It should be obvious that counting small behavior changes in individuals in the short-term cannot be a means for measuring the value of long-term programs that build on the strengths of communities to promote civic engagement, networks of communication, partnerships in small business ventures in disadvantaged communities, retraining initiatives, and collective actions on health and welfare issues.

Conclusion

This brief review of social science's response to HIV/AIDS suggests that an initial period of overreliance on certain conceptual frameworks and research methodologies is giving way to innovative and creative efforts to understand the diversity of human behavior. HIV/AIDS has clearly catalyzed and is an important part of a dynamic new phase of research, particularly in the field of human sexual behavior.

REFERENCES

1. S. E. Lucas and M. W. Ross, guest eds., "Berlin conference review," *AIDS Care* 5(1993):471–525.
2. C. S. Vance, "Anthropology rediscovers sexuality: A theoretical comment," *Social Science and Medicine*, 8(1991):875–884.
3. R. G. Parker, *Bodies, Pleasures, and Passions: Sexual Culture in Contemporary Brazil* (Boston, MA: Beacon Press, 1991).
4. R. G. Parker, "Sexual diversity, cultural analysis, and AIDS education in Brazil," in *Time of AIDS: Social Analysis, Theory and Method*, G. H. Herdt and S. Lindenbaum, eds. (Newbury Park, CA: Sage Publications, 1992).
5. *Ibid.*
6. E. M. Ankrah, "Impact of HIV/AIDS on the family and other significant relationships: The African clan revisited," *AIDS Care* 5(1993):5–22.
7. K. Jochelson, M. Mothibeli, and J. P. Leger, "HIV and migrant labor in South Africa," *International Journal of Health Services* 21(1991):157–173.
8. VIII International Conference on AIDS/III STD World Congress, Amsterdam, The Netherlands, 19–24 July 1992, *Published Abstracts & Indices*, 3(1992):197–230.
9. D. Schopper, S. Doussantousse, and J. Orav, "Sexual behaviors relevant to HIV transmission in a rural African population. How much can a KAP survey tell us?," *Social Science and Medicine* 37(1993):401–412.

10. N. Rutenberg, A. K. Blanc, and S. Kapiga, "Sexual behaviour, social change and family planning among men and women in Tanzania," *Health Transition Review* 4(suppl.)(1994):173–196.

11. M. Caraël and J. Cleland, "Extra-marital sex, implications of survey results for STD/HIV transmission," *Health Transition Review* 4(suppl.)(1994):153–172.

12. A. M. Johnson, J. Wadsworth, K. Wellings, and J. Field, *Sexual Attitudes and Lifestyles* (Oxford, U.K.: Blackwell Scientific Publications, 1994).

13. J. Chetwynd, "Changes to sexual practices amongst the general population of New Zealand," in VIII International Conference on AIDS/III STD World Congress, Amsterdam, The Netherlands, July 19–24, 1992). D439. Vol. 2, *Poster Abstracts.* Abstract number POD5314.

14. B. C. Leigh, M. T. Temple, and K. F. Trocki, "Sexual behaviour of U.S. adults: Results from a national survey," *American Journal of Public Health* 83(1993):1400–1408.

15. M. Melbye and R. J. Biggar, "Interactions between persons at risk for AIDS and the general population in Denmark," *American Journal of Epidemiology* 135(1992):593–602.

16. Analyse des Comportements Sexuels en France, Investigators, "AIDS and sexual behaviour in France," *Nature* 360(1992):407–409.

17. P. K. Lui, J. F. Lau, P. C. Li, et al., "KABP Study on AIDS in Hong Kong," Abstract PO-D01-3426, presented at the IX Conference on AIDS, Berlin, Germany, June 1993.

18. R. Munakata and T. Kazuo, "Cross national study—implications for STD/HIV transmission," in *Proceedings of the IUSSP Working Group on AIDS Conference: AIDS Impact and Prevention in the Developing World: The Contribution of Demography and Social Science* (Annecy, France: December 5–9, 1993).

19. G. Thimothe, A. Adrien, and M. Cayenites, "High risk sexual behavior related to HIV transmission in Haiti," in VIII International Conference on AIDS/III STD World Congress, Amsterdam, The Netherlands, 19–24 July 1992: D531. Volume 2, Abstract number POD-5857,

20. P. Sawanpanyalert and W. Wongkraisritong, "Sexual and AIDS attitudes and behaviour among Thai population: Findings and implications from the first telephone survey," Abstract PO-D01-3391, presented at the IX International Conference on AIDS, Berlin, Germany, June 1993.

21. Schopper, "Sexual behaviours."

22. Johnson, *Sexual Attitudes.*

23. O. Dare and J. G. Cleland, "Reliability and validity of survey data of sexual behaviour," *Health Transition Review* 4(suppl.)(1994):93–110.

24. Johnson, *Sexual Attitudes.*

25. H. L. Smith, "On the limited utility of KAP styled survey data in the practical utility epidemiology of AIDS with reference to the AIDS epidemic in Chile," *Health Transition Review* 3(1993):1–16.

26. C. S. Vance, "Anthropology rediscovers sexuality: A theoretical comment," *Social Science and Medicine* 33(1991):875–884.

27. J. Holland, C. Ramazanoglu, S. Scott, S. Sharpe, and R. Thomson, "Risk, power and the possibility of pleasure: Young women and safer sex," *AIDS Care* 4(1991):273–283.

28. C. Waldby, S. Kippax, and J. Crawford, "Heterosexual men negotiating safe sex: A case study," Abstract 4119, presented at the VI International Conference on AIDS, San Francisco, California, June 1990.

29. M. Raffaelli, R. Campos, A. P. Merritt, et al., "Sexual practices and attitudes of street youth in Belo Homzonte, Brazil," *Social Science and Medicine* 37(1993):661–670.

30. Parker, "Sexual diversity."

31. M. Tan, "From Bakla to gay: Shifting gender identities and sexual behaviours in the Philippines," in *Conceiving Sexuality: Approaches to Sex Research in a Postmodern World*, R. G. Parker and J. H. Gagnon, eds. (New York and London: Routledge, 1995):85–97.

32. A. P. M. Coxon, N. H. Coxon, P. Weatherburn, et al., "Sex role separation in sexual diaries of homosexual men," *AIDS* 7(1993):877–882.

33. T. Myers, G. Godin, L. Calzavara, J. Lambert, D. Locker, and the Canadian AIDS Society, *The Canadian Survey of Gay and Bisexual Men and HIV Infection: Men's Survey* (Ottawa: Canadian AIDS Society, 1993).

34. I. O. Orubuloye, P. Caldwell, and J. C. Caldwell, "The role of high risk occupations in the spread of AIDS: Truck drivers and itinerant market women in Nigeria," *International Family Planning Perspectives* 2 (1993):43–48.

35. M Baldo, P. Aggleton, and G. Slutkin, "Does sex education lead to earlier or increased sexual activity in youth?," Abstract PO-D02-3444, presented at the IX International Conference on AIDS, Berlin, Germany, June 1993.

36. K. Bellingham and P. A. Gillies, "Evaluation of an AIDS education programme for young adults," *Journal of Epidemiology and Community Health* 47(1993):134–138.

37. J. B. Jemmott, L. S. Jemmott, and G. T. Fong, "Reductions in HIV risk associated with sexual behaviours among black male adolescents: Effects on AIDS prevention intervention," *American Journal of Public Health* 82(1992):372–377 [errata corrected in 82(1992):684].

38. K. I. Klepp, S. Ndeki, A. Irena, et al., "Evaluation of AIDS education for primary school children in Northern Tanzania," Abstract WS-D02-3, presented at the IX International Conference on AIDS, Berlin, Germany, June 1993.

39. J. Ordonana, J. Guiterex, P. Martinez, et al., "Health education in high schools: Effectiveness of short-term interventions," Abstract PoD 5875, presented at the VIII International Conference on AIDS, Amsterdam, The Netherlands, July 1992.

40. C. Boyer, M. Shafer, and J. Tschamm, "Evaluation of an STD/HIV education and skills building intervention for high school students," Abstract W.D.4135, presented at the VII International Conference on AIDS, Florence, Italy, June 1991.

41. E. Schutte and H. Oswald, "Evaluation of an AIDS-prevention programme in West Berlin schools," Abstract W.D.4218, presented at the VII International Conference on AIDS, Florence, Italy, June 1991.

42. D. Kirby, C. Waszak, and J. Zeiglar, "Six school based clinics: Their reproductive health services and impact on sexual behaviour," *Family Planning Perspectives* 23(1991):6–16.

43. D. E. Woodhouse, J. J. Potterat, J. B. Muth, et al., "Street outreach for STD/HIV prevention—Colorado Springs, Colorado, 1987–91," with editorial note, in *Behavioral and Prevention Research Branch Summary of MMWR Articles, 1992–1993* (Atlanta, GA: Centers for Disease Control, Feb. 14, 1992, Vol. 41, No. 6, pp. 94–97).

44. J. A. Kelly, K. J. Sikkema, R. A. Winnett, et al., "Outcomes of a 16 city randomised field trial of a community level HIV risk reduction intervention," Abstract TuD 0543, presented at the VIII International Conference on AIDS, Amsterdam, The Netherlands, July 1992.

45. World Bank, "Investing in Health," in *World Bank World Development Report* (New York: Oxford University Press, 1993):99–107.

46. W. Rojanapitahyakorn, "Promoting a hundred per cent condom use in sex entertainment establishments in Thailand," in *Effective Approaches to AIDS Prevention* (Geneva: GPA/WHO, 1992): 16–22.

10

Treatment of HIV Disease: Problems, Progress, and Potential

ELLEN C. COOPER

In 1984, when HIV (then called HTLV-III or LAV) was discovered and subsequently established as the cause of AIDS, the search began to find drugs that could inhibit the replication and growth of this retrovirus and to test the safety and efficacy of these drugs in people with HIV infection. Amazingly, a drug first tested in patients with AIDS in July 1985 proved so effective in delaying disease progression that in March 1987, less than 2 years later, the U.S. Food and Drug Administration (FDA) approved it for marketing.

The drug was a nucleoside analog called *azidothymidine*, or AZT. (A nucleoside analog is a chemical that is very similar to one of the building blocks of DNA, a nucleic acid essential to most forms of life, including retroviruses such as HIV.) In a placebo-controlled trial involving fewer than 300 patients, AZT's effectiveness in delaying the onset of opportunistic infections and the death of patients with HIV disease was so definitive that the trial was terminated after less than 6 months.[1] A New Drug Application was submitted to the FDA in December 1986 and approval for marketing was granted in less than 4 months.

The expedited but scientifically rigorous testing and approval of this first drug raised expectations for rapid progress in developing a cure for HIV disease. However, in the decade since the discovery of HIV, only four antiretroviral drugs (zidovudine, didanosine, zalcitabine, and stavudine)—all nucleoside analogs with limited efficacy and significant toxicity—have been licensed by regulatory authorities in the United States and Europe for the management of patients with HIV. Several more drugs, including at least two protease inhibitors, are expected to be approved relatively soon. Nevertheless, all these drugs are at best partially effective, so at the present time, cure is still a distant dream.[2]

Immune-based therapeutic strategies to delay or reverse HIV disease progression are even less advanced. The finely tuned human immune system has proven very difficult to manipulate pharmacologically for the benefit of patients with HIV disease, and no immunomodulatory drug for treatment of persons with HIV is licensed in the U.S. Even a highly active immunomodulator such as interleukin-2, which causes a significant increase in the peripheral blood CD4 count in patients with early-to-moderate stage HIV disease (i.e., CD4 count over 200), must still be tested in long-term, controlled clinical trials before its clinical benefit can be assessed.[3]

More encouragingly, substantial progress has been made in developing and testing drugs to treat or prevent the many otherwise fatal opportunistic infections caused by bacteria, fungi, protozoa, or other viruses in people with HIV-weakened immune systems. As a result of these advances, many people with HIV are living longer and more productive lives than 10 years ago; tragically, the vast majority still succumb eventually to the disease.[4,5] Rather than dying quickly from *Pneumocystis carinii* pneumonia (PCP) or cryptococcal meningitis, for example, patients are suffering from "the wasting syndrome" (severe weight loss, chronic diarrhea, and fever) or from the more difficult to treat opportunistic infections, such as *Mycobacterium avium* complex (MAC) or cytomegalovirus (CMV).[6]

The lack of certain important information, such as how best to use specific therapeutically active drugs, has led to some troubling events. For example, the results of the European "Concorde" trial of AZT therapy in asymptomatic HIV-infected patients, reported for the first time in 1993, caused increased uncertainty about when to begin antiretroviral therapy.[7] When asymptomatic patients who started AZT immediately upon entry into the study were compared with those who deferred therapy until the initial symptoms of HIV disease developed, no difference in the progression to AIDS or death after 3 years was detected. Unfortunately, many people misinterpreted these data as meaning that AZT is of little or no benefit in asymptomatic individuals. However, the correct conclusion is that the beneficial effects of AZT—when it is used alone early in the disease—are of limited duration, i.e., 1 to 2 years, a result which has also been seen in other trials.[8,9] In addition, the benefits of initiating AZT treatment in patients with advanced disease have been clearly established; the Concorde results are not directly relevant to these patients.

The next logical research question was whether AZT in combination with another active antiretroviral drug, such as ddI (didanosine) or ddC (zalcitabine) would be superior to AZT alone. Clinical results from two large controlled trials designed to answer this question, one conducted in the United States (referred to as ACTG 175) and the other in Europe and Australia (the Delta trial), were reported in late 1995. ACTG 175 was a 3-year study in which two combinations of nucleoside antiretroviral drugs (AZT + ddI and AZT + ddC) were compared with two monotherapies (AZT and ddI) in almost 2,500 people with CD4 counts between 200 and 500 at entry. Results indicate that the treatment of moderately immunocompromised persons with antiretroviral drugs delays progression to AIDS and death, although zidovudine (AZT) monotherapy did not provide as much benefit as either combination therapy or monotherapy with didanosine (ddI).[10]

The Delta trial of over 3,000 patients with entry CD4 counts between 50 and 350 was stopped prematurely, after an average follow-up of 26 months, because of a highly significant difference in the proportion of AZT-naive patients (who had taken no prior AZT) who died on AZT monotherapy compared to either of the combination therapies. Progression to AIDS was also slower in the patients receiving one of the combination therapies.[11] (Didanosine monotherapy was not included in this trial.) In contrast to ACTG 175, however, patients in the Delta trial who were AZT experienced (over half had taken AZT for longer than 1 year prior to enrollment) had a rate of progression to AIDS and death that was similar across all three drug regimens. In ACTG 175, AZT-experienced patients on either ddI alone or on AZT + ddI (but not AZT + ddC) did better than those who continued on AZT alone.

Thus, together the Delta trial and ACTG 175 demonstrate the superiority of both AZT + ddI and AZT + ddC compared to AZT alone in patients who have not previously taken antiretroviral drugs. The value of ddI alone is less clear, since it was studied in only one of the trials. Likewise, recommendations for the management of AZT-experienced patients are not clear at this time, since one trial (ACTG 175) showed a benefit of changing regimens whereas the other trial (Delta) did not. The results of a third large study in the U.S., conducted by the NIH-supported Terry Beirn Community Programs for Clinical Research on AIDS, will be available in 1996. This trial of 1,200 people compares the same three regimens as the Delta trial, but studies an even more advanced patient population (CD4 under 200 at entry). Since most of these patients were AZT experienced at enrollment, this study should provide important information to help explain the different outcomes in ACTG 175 and the Delta trial in this important group of patients.

Although the results of these trials are encouraging for the future of combination treatment, there are several important caveats. First, it would be inappropriate to conclude from either study that *any* combination therapy is better than *any* monotherapy. One can only conclude that these two particular combinations, AZT + ddI and AZT + ddC, are better than AZT monotherapy, particularly in AZT-naive patients. Also, these results should not be interpreted as recommending that any of these regimens can be taken indefinitely or that they are appropriate for everyone. Many questions remain, which will only increase in number and complexity as more antiretroviral drugs become available.

One obvious unanswered question is whether any of the promising new drugs, which were not available at the time when ACTG 175 and the Delta trial were designed, will be of even greater benefit to patients. For example, the combination of AZT and lamivudine (3TC, another nucleoside analog expected to be licensed in late 1995) has been evaluated in four clinical trials in 1993–1994, two in the United States and two in Europe. All were relatively short (6 months of comparing AZT alone with the combination, after which all patients were offered the combination) and small (fewer than 100 patients in each treatment group). All studies showed desirable effects on laboratory markers (increase in CD4 and decreased viral load) that were more pronounced and sustained than as yet seen with any other nucleoside analog alone or in combination with AZT.[12] However, these trials were not designed to determine whether changes in laboratory markers would translate into clinical benefit. An overall assessment of risks and benefits of new drugs and combinations intended for the long-term treatment of HIV disease require large long-term studies in which clinical outcome, i.e., the effect of the treatment on progression of disease, is carefully monitored.

Protease (or proteinase) inhibitors are a promising, potent new class of antiretroviral drugs.[13] These drugs inhibit the activity of protease, an enzyme of HIV that is essential for viral replication. At least four protease inhibitors are currently being evaluated in controlled clinical trials (i.e., saquinavir, indinovir, ritonavir, and Virasept). Non-nucleoside reverse transcriptase inhibitors (NNRTIs) are another class of drugs in development. Resistance to all of these drugs develops over time, especially when given as monotherapy.[14] Nevertheless, the existence of additional classes of drugs opens many more opportunities for new drug combinations, as well as new treatment options.

Significant progress has been made in our understanding of HIV pathogenesis and in development of effective therapies. However, many questions remain—questions that can only be answered through large, well-designed and well-conducted clinical trials. Therefore, in addition to identifying new active drugs and drug combinations, the research goals for clinical trials of antiretroviral drugs should include:

- the development of better management strategies to optimize the use of available drugs;
- the identification of "surrogate" markers that accurately reflect treatment success or failure in the individual patient;
- a better understanding of the clinical significance of drug resistance; and
- the development of better methods for defining drug interactions.

HIV disease manifests itself differently and proceeds at a different pace in different individuals. Such diversity results from the complex interaction of at least three variables: the route of acquisition of HIV by the individual; the particular mix of strains—including drug resistant strains—of HIV that infect the individual at a given time; and the specific characteristics of the individual's metabolism, immune system, and general state of health. Specific but as yet unidentified co-factors may also play a role. The rapidity with which HIV replicates and mutates in infected individuals is unprecedented; thus, the need for primary care physicians to find useful surrogate markers of impending disease progression is urgent. Ideally, in individual patients, these markers would indicate—*before* the occurrence of irreversible clinical or immunological deterioration—when the therapy being used is beginning to lose its effectiveness. If reliable indicators of the need to change to another potentially effective antiretroviral regimen can be identified before the patient becomes sicker, the progression of disease might be further delayed.

Even though currently available drugs are limited in number and potency, a significant prolongation of the asymptomatic state in HIV-infected people is a realistic outcome. In addition to the goals identified above, more collaborative, community-based research is needed, ideally on an international scale; in the community setting different medical management approaches to the treatment of a large number of patients can be compared for periods long enough to yield clinically meaningful results.

This research, however, should not overshadow the acute health care needs faced by developing countries where even the access to simple preventive and curative drugs remains a problem. In the industrialized world, new treatment approaches can find their place with relative ease in the existing health care systems, reaching most, although not all, potential beneficiaries. To make these therapies available to people living with HIV/AIDS in the developing world would require a major improvement in the health care systems and critical financial and political decisions. The clear need for improvement of HIV/AIDS care in developing nations, however, may create the opportunity and provide the impetus needed to reconsider resource allocation and use in the economic and social development sectors as well as to redress the insufficiencies of existing health systems.

The challenge of developing a cure for AIDS remains squarely before us. We are morally and medically committed not only to developing new therapeutics, but also to devising more effective treatment strategies using the drugs already available, to prolong and improve the lives of people currently infected with HIV. Through collaborative, community-based research, the goal of changing HIV from a relentlessly progressive disease in most people living with HIV/AIDS to one in which they can be maintained in good health for long periods of time will become practical and will perhaps lead to a cure.

REFERENCES

1. M. A. Fischl, D. D. Richman, M. H. Grieco, et al., "The efficacy of azidothymidine (AZT) in the treatment of patients with AIDS and AIDS-related complex: A double-blind, placebo-controlled trial," *New England Journal of Medicine* 317(1987):185–191.

2. J. E. Osborn, "The rocky road to an AIDS vaccine: An editorial," *Journal of Acquired Immune Deficiency Syndromes and Human Retrovirology,* 9(1995):26–29.

3. J. A. Kovacs, M. Baseler, R. J. Dewar, et al, "Increases in CD4 T lymphocytes with intermittent courses of interleukin-2 in patients with human immunodeficiency virus infection," *New England Journal of Medicine* 332(1995):567–575.

4. J. E. Gallant, R. D. Moore, and R. E. Chaisson, "Prophylaxis for opportunistic infections in patients with HIV infection: A review," *Annals of Internal Medicine* 120(1994):932–944.

5. A. J. Saah, D. R. Hoover, Y. He, et al., "Factors influencing survival after AIDS: Report from the Multicenter AIDS Cohort Study (MACS)," *Journal of Acquired Immune Deficiency Syndromes* 7(1994):287–295.

6. G. O. Coodley, M. O. Loveless, and T. M. Merrill, "The HIV wasting syndrome: A review," *Journal of Acquired Immune Deficiency Syndromes* 7(1994):681–694.

7. Concorde Coordinating Committee, "Concorde: MRC/ANRS randomised double-blind controlled trial of immediate and deferred zidovudine in symptom-free HIV infection," *Lancet* 343(1994):871–881.

8. P. A. Volberding, S. W. Lagakos, M. A. Koch, et al., "Zidovudine in asymptomatic human immunodeficiency virus infection: A controlled trial in persons with fewer than 500 CD4-positive cells per cubic millimeter," *New England Journal of Medicine* 322(1990):941–949.

9. J. P. Ioannidis, J. C. Cappelleri, J. Lau, et al., "Early or deferred zidovudine therapy in HIV-infected patients without an AIDS-defining illness: A meta-analysis," *Annals of Internal Medicine* 122(1995):856–866.

10. S. Hammer, D. Katzenstein, M. Hughes, et al. for the ACTG 175 Study Team, "Nucleoside monotherapy vs. combination therapy in HIV infected adults: A randomized, double-blind, placebo-controlled trial in persons with CD4 counts 200–500/mm3," Abstract No. LB-1, presented at the 35th Interscience Conference on Antimicrobial Agents and Chemotherapy, San Francisco, CA (1995) and the ACTG 175 Executive Summary, September 14, 1995.

11. B. Gazzard, J. Darbyshire, et al. for the International Coordinating Committee of the Delta Trial, "New HIV/AIDS trial shows two drugs better than one: Preliminary results of a European/Australian trial for people with HIV infection and AIDS," *MRC Press Release*, September 26, 1995.

12. B. A. Larder, S. D. Kemp, and P. R. Harrigan, "Potential mechanism for sustained antiretroviral efficacy of AZT-3TC combination therapy," *Science* 269(1995):696–699.

13. T. Robins and J. Plattner, "HIV protease inhibitors: Their anti-HIV activity and potential role in treatment," *Journal of Acquired Immune Deficiency Syndromes* 6(1993):162–170.

14. S. H. Cheeseman, D. Havlir, and M. M. McLaughlin, "Phase I/II evaluation of nevirapine alone and in combination with zidovudine for infection with human immunodeficiency virus," *Journal of Acquired Immune Deficiency Syndromes and Human Retrovirology* 8(1995):141–151.

11

Long-time Survivors: What Can We Learn from Them?

ROBERT COLEBUNDERS

As the AIDS pandemic grows older, increasing numbers of long-term survivors have been identified. Scientific interest in HIV-infected individuals who have remained healthy for many years is growing rapidly, for they may help discover characteristics related to survival.

The median time between HIV infection and AIDS is estimated at about 10 years, and median progression from AIDS to death is about 2 years.[1-5] In the industrialized world, the incubation period of AIDS has apparently lengthened, perhaps as a result of better patient care, including prophylactic antiviral and antibiotic treatment.[6,7] In developing countries, however, patients generally die considerably sooner.[8] Progression rates towards AIDS also differ considerably among individuals; some develop AIDS within 2–4 months after infection, while others can and do remain healthy for more than 16 years.[9,10,11]

Seven to 12 years after infection, approximately 10 percent of persons with HIV infection maintain a stable number of CD4 lymphocytes.[12,13] However, even among these "non-progressors," immune system abnormalities have been observed. This suggests that over time, all HIV-infected individuals may eventually develop AIDS.[14] (HIV-2 infection progresses much more slowly towards disease than HIV-1 infection [Chapter 12]).[15]

Thus far, of the relatively few published studies of long-term survivors, most involve homosexual men (Table 11-1).[16-26] In nearly all studies only small numbers of persons were included. Several common virological and immunological characteristics have been observed among long-time survivors: a low infectious virus load; infection with a less cytopathic HIV strain or a genetically defective HIV strain; absences of enhancing antibodies; Th1 cell response > Th2 cell response; a strong CD8 positive cell HIV suppressive activity; strong HIV-specific CTL responses; the absence of p24 antigen and presence of p24 antibodies; and intact lymph-node architecture.[27-38] The interpretation of these findings is difficult, as long-term survivors are a heterogeneous group of people, including slow-progressors and nonprogressors. Non-progressors seem to maintain high levels of CD4 lymphocytes and to control viral replication without increased CD8 positive cell activity.[39]

Table 11-1 Cohort studies of HIV-infected people initiated in the early-to-mid-1980s

Cohort study	Date started	Cohort size at onset of study
Homosexual men		
San Francisco men's health study[1,2]	1984	290
San Francisco city clinic cohort[3]	1978–83	583
Multicenter AIDS cohort study (U.S.)[4,5]	1984–85	2,168
Atlanta cohort[6]	1982–83	75
Vancouver lymphadenopathy AIDS study[4]	1982–84	348
Amsterdam cohort[7,8]	1984–85	273
London cohort[9]	1982–84	173
Stockholm cohort[10]	1982–83	115
Persons with hemophilia		
Edinburgh hemophiliac cohort[11]	1984	18
London hemophiliac cohort[12,13]	1979–85	111
Italian hemophiliac cohort[14]	1981–86	119
Heterosexuals		
Prostitutes, Kigali, Rwanda[15]	1984	29

[1]H. W. Sheppard, W. Lang, M. S. Ascher, et al., "Characterization of non-progressors: Long-term HIV-1 infection with stable CD4+ T-cell levels," *AIDS* 7(1993):1159–1166.

[2]H. W. Jaffe, W. W. Darrow, D. F. Echenberg, et al., "Acquired immunodeficiency syndrome in a cohort of homosexual men," *Annals of Internal Medicine* 103(1985):210–214.

[3]S. Buchbinder, M. Feinberg, B. Walker, P. O. Malley, and M. Katz, "Factors associated with long-term non-progression in HIV-infected men," Abstract 454, presented at the VI International Congress for Infectious Diseases, Prague, Czechoslovakia, April 1994.

[4]M. T. Schecter, K. J. B. Craib, N. L. Thinh, et al., "Progression to AIDS in seroprevalent and seroincident cohorts of homosexual men," *AIDS* 3(1989):347–353.

[5]C. G. Lyketsos, D. R. Hoover, M. Guccione, et al., "Depressive symptoms as predictors of medical outcomes in HIV infection," *Journal of the American Medical Association* 270(1993):2563–2567.

[6]J. E. Kaplan, T. J. Spira, D. B. Fiscbein, et al., "Six-year follow-up of HIV-infected homosexual men with lymphadenopathy," *Journal of the American Medical Association* 260(1988):2694–2697.

[7]I. P. M. Keet, A. Krol, M. Klein, et al., "Characteristics of long-term survival early and late in HIV infection," Abstract WS-C03-3, presented at the IX International Conference on AIDS, Berlin, Germany, June 1993.

[8]M. Koot, I. P. M. Keet, A. H. V. Vos, et al., "Prognostic value of HIV-1 syncytium-inducing phenotype of rate of CD4+ cell depletion and progression to AIDS," *Annals of Internal Medicine* 118(1993):681–688.

[9]G. E. Kelly, B. S. Stanley, and I. V. D. Weller, "Natural history of human immunodeficiency virus infection: A five-year study in a London cohort of homosexual men," *Genitourinary Medicine* 66(1990):238–243.

[10]A. Karlsonn, G. Bratt, G. Van Krogh, et al., "Prospective study of 115 initially asymptomatic HIV-infected gay men in Stockholm, Sweden," *Scandinavian Journal of Infectious Diseases* 23(1991):431–441.

[11]R. J. G. Cuthbert, C. A. Ludlam, J. Tucker, et al., "Five year prospective study of HIV infection in the Edinburgh haemophiliac cohort," *British Medical Journal* 301(1990):956–961.

[12]C. A. Lee, A. N. Phillips, J. Elford, et al., "Progression of HIV disease in a haemophilic cohort followed for 11 years and the effect of treatment," *British Medical Journal* 303(1991)1093–1096.

[13]A. N. Phillips, C. A. Sabin, J. Elford, et al., "Prospects for long-term AIDS-free survival after HIV infection," Abstract 22, presented at the IV European Conference on Clinical Aspects and Treatment of HIV Infection, Milan, Italy, 1994.

[14]E. Santagostino, A. Gringeri, D. Cultraro, et al., "Slow progression of HIV disease in a cohort of Italian hemophiliacs with normal CD4 cell counts for at least 7 years," Abstract 28, presented at the IV European Conference on Clinical Aspects and Treatment of HIV Infection, Milan, Italy, 1994.

[15]E. Bulterys, E. Nzabihimana, A. Chao, et al., "Long-term survival among HIV-1-infected prostitutes," *AIDS* 7(1993):1269–1285.

Much less is known about long-term survivors' lifestyle and other personal characteristics. While it has been proposed that re-exposure to HIV and other sexually transmitted infections may be a cofactor for disease progression, most studies have not found an association between the practice of safer sex and long-term asymptomatic HIV infection.[40-43] The role of other infections (e.g., cytomegalovirus, herpes, HTLV-1, and mycoplasma) as cofactors for disease progression also remains unclear.[44,45] Cigarette smoking may alter the immune response to HIV-1 infection but appears to have no marked effect on clinical outcome.[46] Finally, in cohorts of persons who acquired HIV infection through injecting drug use, abstaining from drugs was not associated with long-term asymptomatic HIV infection.[47,48]

People with HIV infection often state that long survival is associated with a better psychological response and a positive attitude towards HIV infection.[49] However, this has been very difficult to assess. A positive attitude may also be characteristic of people who are motivated to recognize infectious complications earlier and who comply with treatment, thus increasing survival time. In a small study among homosexual men in San Francisco, symptoms of depression did predict a more rapid decline in CD4 lymphocyte counts.[50] However, this finding was not confirmed in the larger multicenter AIDS cohort study.[51]

Age also influences the rate of progression to AIDS. In general, HIV infection progresses more rapidly in infants, while children with hemophilia develop AIDS more slowly than adults.[52] After childhood, the influence of age on progression rates is less clear. Among men with hemophilia, older men develop AIDS more rapidly than younger men; among homosexual men, however, the opposite is true.[53]

Recently it has been suggested that genetic factors may help explain differences in disease progression, and an association has been declared between certain HLA haplotypes and progression of HIV infection.[54,55]

To identify factors associated with long-time survival, further study of "non-progressors" must be compared with people progressing rapidly to AIDS. Such studies should also include people from developing countries. Thus far, only a few natural history studies have been performed in the developing world, and long-term follow-up was not obtained in any of them.[56] Also, dates of HIV infection are generally not known in developing countries, and HIV diagnosis is often made only when patients are hospitalized in an advanced stage of their disease.

Also, since clinical and immunological non-progression over a period of at least 7 years is exceptional in HIV infection, studies require multicenter collaboration. Cohort studies initiated more than 10 years ago are particularly useful for investigating long-term survival (Table 11-1). Individuals infected with HIV are enthusiastic about participating in such studies. The current absence of good hypotheses to explain the differences in progression rates suggests that it is unlikely that a single factor will be identified to explain long-term survival. A large number of factors are probably involved, and their discovery should be an urgent scientific priority.

REFERENCES

1. R. L. Colebunders and A. S. Latif, "Natural history and clinical presentation of HIV-1 infection in adults," *AIDS* 5(suppl.1)(1991):s103–s112.
2. R. J. Biggar and the International Registry of Seroconverters, "AIDS incubation in 1891 HIV seroconverters from different exposure groups," *AIDS* 4(1990):1059–1066.
3. M. T. Schechter, K. J. P. Craib, N. L. Thinh, et al., "Progression to AIDS in seroprevalent and seroincident cohorts of homosexual men," *AIDS* 3(1989):347–353.
4. C. A. Lee, A. N. Phillips, J. Elford, et al., "Progression of HIV disease in a hemophilic cohort followed for 11 years and the effect of treatment," *British Medical Journal* 303(1991):1093–1096.
5. A. Karlsonn, G. Bratt, G. Van Krogh, et al., "Prospective study of 115 initially asymptomatic HIV infected gay men in Stokholm, Sweden," *Scandinavian Journal of Infectious Diseases* 23(1991):431–441.
6. G. F. Lemp, S. F. Payne, D. Neald, et al., "Survival trends for patients with AIDS," *Journal of the American Medical Association* 263(1990):402–406.
7. J. M. G. Taylor, J. M. Kuo, and R. Detels, "Is the incubation period of AIDS lengthening?" *Journal of Acquired Immune Deficiency Syndromes* 4(1991):69–75.
8. Colebunders, "Natural history."
9. J. A. Levy, "HIV pathogenesis and long-term survival," *AIDS* 7(1993):1401–1410.
10. H. W. Sheppard, W. Lang, M. S. Ascher, et al., "Characterization of non-progressors: Long-term HIV-1 infection with stable CD4+ T-cell levels," *AIDS* 7(1993):1159–1166.
11. S. Buchbinder, M. Feinberg, B. Walker, P. O. Malley, and M. Katz, "Factors associated with long-term non-progression in HIV-infected men," Abstract 454, presented at the VI International Congress for Infectious Diseases, Prague, Czechoslovakia, April 1994.
12. Sheppard, "Characterization of non-progressors."
13. Buchbinder, "Factors associated."
14. Taylor, "Is the incubation period of AIDS lengthening?"
15. K. M. De Cock, G. Adjorlolo, E. Ekpini, et al., "Epidemiology and transmission of HIV-2," *Journal of the American Medical Association* 270(1993):2083–2086.
16. Sheppard, "Characterization of non-progressors."
17. Buchbinder, "Factors associated."
18. L. Katoff, J. Rabkin, and R. Remien, "Psychological study of long term survivors of AIDS," Abstract TU.D.105, presented at the VII International Conference on AIDS, Florence, Italy, June 1991.
19. I. P. M. Keet, A. Krol, M. Klein, et al., "Characteristics of long-term survival early and late in HIV infection," Abstract WS-C03-3, presented at the IX International Conference on AIDS, Berlin, Germany, June 1993.
20. A. R. Lifson, S. P. Buchbinder, H. W. Sheppard, et al., "Long-term human immunodeficiency virus infection in asymptomatic homosexual and bisexual men with normal CD4+ lymphocyte counts: Immunologic and virologic characteristics," *Journal of Infectious Diseases* 163(1991):959–965.
21. A. N. Phillips, C. A. Sabin, J. Elford, et al., "Prospects for long-term AIDS-free survival after HIV infection," Abstract 22, presented at the IV European Conference on Clinical Aspects and Treatment of HIV Infection, Milan, Italy, 1994.
22. E. Santagostino, A. Gringeri, D. Cultraro, et al., "Slow progression of HIV disease in a cohort of Italian hemophiliacs with normal CD4 cell counts for at least 7 years," Abstract 28, presented at the IV European Conference on Clinical Aspects and Treatment of HIV Infection, Milan, Italy, 1994.
23. E. Harrer, T. Harrer, S. Buchbinder, et al., "HIV-1-specific CTL response in healthy

long-term non-progressing seropositive persons," presented at the First National Conference on Human Retroviruses, Washington D.C., 1994.

24. M. Bulterys, E. Nzabihimana, A. Chao, et al., "Long-term survival among HIV-1-infected prostitutes," *AIDS* 7(1993):1269–1285.

25. P. Van de Perre, P. Lepage, A. Simonon, et al., "Biological markers associated with prolonged survival in African children maternally infected by the human immunodeficiency virus type 1," *AIDS Research and Human Retroviruses* 8(1992):435–437.

26. M. Koot, I. P. M. Keet, A. H. V. Vos, et al., "Prognostic value of HIV-1 syncytium-inducing phenotype for rate of CD4+ cell depletion and progression to AIDS," *Annals of Internal Medicine* 118(1993):681–688.

27. J. A. Levy, "HIV pathogenesis and long-term survival," *AIDS* 7(1993):1401–1410.

28. Sheppard, "Characterization of non-progressors."

29. Buchbinder, "Factors associated."

30. Harrer, "HIV-1-specific CTL response."

31. Van de Perre, "Biological markers."

32. Koot, "Prognostic value of HIV-1."

33. C. Rinaldi, X.-L. Huang, Z. Fan, M. Ding, L. Beltz, A. Logar, D. Panicali, G. Mazzara, J. Liebmann, M. Cottrill, and P. Gupta, "High levels of anti-human immunodeficiency virus type 1 (HIV-1) memory cytotoxic T-lymphocyte activity and low viral load are associated with lack of disease in HIV-1-infected long-term nonprogressors," *Journal of Virology* 9(1995):5838–5842.

34. M. R. Klein, C. A. van Baalen, A. M. Holwerda, S. R. Kerkhof Garde, R. J. Bende, I. P. M. Keet, J. K. M. Eeftinck-Schattenkerk, A. D. M. E. Osterhaus, H. Schuitemaker, and F. Medema, "Kinetics of Gag-specific cytotoxic T lymphocyte responses during the clinical course of HIV-1 infection: A longitudinal analysis of rapid progressors and long-term asymptomatics," *Journal of Experimental Medicine* 181(1995):1365–1372.

35. Y. Cao, L. Qin, L. Zhang, J. Safrit, and D. D. Ho, "Virologic and immunologic characterization of long-term survivors of human immunodeficiency virus type 1 infection," *New England Journal of Medicine* 332(1995):201–208.

36. G. Pantaleo, S. Menzo, M. Vaccarezza, C. Graziosi, O. J. Cohen, J. F. Demarest, D. Montefiori, J. M. Orenstein, C. Fox, L. K. Schrager, J. B. Margolick, S. Buchbinder, J. V. Giorgi, and A. S. Fauci, "Studies in subjects with long-term nonprogressive human immunodeficiency virus infection," *New England Journal of Medicine*, 332(1995):209–216.

37. F. Kirchhoff, T. C. Greenough, D. B. Brettler, J. L. Sullivan, and R. C. Desrosiers, "Brief report: absence of intact *nef* sequences in a long-term survivor with nonprogressive HIV-1 infection," *New England Journal of Medicine*, 332(1995):228–232.

38. N. L. Michael, G. Chang, L. Z. D'Arcy, P. K. Ehrenberg, R. Mariani, M. P. Busch, D. L. Birx, and D. H. Schwartz, "Defective accessory genes in a human immunodeficiency virus type 1-infected long-term survivor lacking recoverable virus," *Journal of Virology*, 7(1995):4228–4236.

39. J. Ferbas, A. H. Kaplan, M. A. Hausner, L. E. Hultin, J. L. Matud, Z. Liu, D. L. Panicali, H. Nerng-Ho, R. Detels, and J. V. Giorgi, "Virus burden in long-term survivors of human immunodeficiency virus (HIV) infection is a determinant of anti-HIV CD8 lymphocyte activity," *Journal of Infectious Diseases* 172(1995):329–339.

40. Colebunders, "Natural history."

41. A. O. Anzala, F. A. Plummer, P. Wambugu, N. J. Nagelkerke, J. O. Ndinya-Achola, J. Bwayo, and E. N. Ngugi, "Incubation time to symptomatic disease (SD) and AIDS in women with a known duration of infection," Abstract TU.C.103, presented at the VII International Conference on AIDS, Florence, Italy, June 1991.

42. Buchbinder, "Factors associated."

43. Keet, "Characteristics of long term survival."

44. A. R. Moss and P. Bacchetti, "Natural history of HIV infection," *AIDS* 3(1989):55–61.

45. V. L. Katseni, C. B. Gilroy, B. K. Ryait, K. Ariyoshi, P. D. Bieniasz, J. N. Weber, and D. Taylor-Robinson, "*Mycoplasma fermentans* in individuals seropositive and seronegative for HIV-1," *Lancet* 341(1993):271–273.

46. D. N. Burns, A. Kramer, F. Yellin, D. Fuchs, H. Wachter, R. A. DiGioia, W. C. Sanchez, R. J. Grossman, F. M. Gordin, R. J. Biggar, and J. J. Goedert, "Cigarette smoking: A modifier of human immunodeficiency virus type 1 infection," *Journal of Acquired Immune Deficiency Syndromes* 4(1991):76–83.

47. P. Selwyn, P. Alcabes, D. Hartel, et al., "Clinical manifestations and predictors of disease progression in drug users with human immunodeficiency virus infection," *New England Journal of Medicine* 327(1992):1697–1703.

48. Italian Seroconversion Study, "Disease progression and early predictors of AIDS in HIV-seroconverted injecting drug users," *AIDS* 6(1992):421–426.

49. Katoff, "Psychological study."

50. J. H. Burack, D. C. Barrett, R. D. Stall, M. A. Chesney, M. L. Ekstrand, and T. J. Coates, "Depressive symptoms and CD4 lymphocyte decline among HIV-infected men," *Journal of the American Medical Association* 270(1993):2568–2573.

51. C. G. Lyketsos, D. R. Hoover, M. Guccione, W. Senterfitt, M. A. Dew, J. Wesch, M. J. Van Raden, G. J. Treisman, and H. Morgenstern, "Depressive symptoms as predictors of medical outcomes in HIV infection," *Journal of the American Medical Association* 270(1993):2563–2567.

52. Biggar, "AIDS incubation."

53. *Ibid.*

54. Buchbinder, "Factors associated."

55. S. Itescu, U. Mathur-Wagh, M. L. Skovron, et al., "HLA-B35 is associated with accelerated progression to AIDS," *Journal of Acquired Immune Deficiency Syndromes* 5(1991):37–45.

56. Colebunders, "Natural history."

12

HIV-2 Infection: Current Knowledge and Uncertainties

KEVIN M. DE COCK AND FRANÇOISE BRUN-VÉZINET

In contrast to the extensive spread of HIV-1 on all continents, dissemination of HIV-2 has been relatively limited. This review examines the geographic distribution of HIV-2 infection, its modes of transmission, disease associations, and natural history, and concludes with a consideration of dual serologic reactivity and future research needs.

Geographic distribution of HIV-2

Overall, the most striking feature about the global epidemiology of HIV-2 infection is its lack of epidemic spread internationally.[1] While the spread of HIV-1 in sub-Saharan Africa has been very rapid, HIV-2 is largely restricted to West Africa.[2-5] In Guinea Bissau, Senegal, and The Gambia, rates of HIV-2 infection exceed those for HIV-1. The highest HIV-2 seroprevalence has been reported from Guinea Bissau, where in 1992, 13.4 percent of a group of asymptomatic men were found to be infected. As with HIV-1 infection elsewhere, the highest rates of infection with HIV-2 in these three countries have been found among sex workers. Although the prevalence of HIV-2 infection is higher than for HIV-1 in these countries, the incidence of the latter is disproportionately high, so that the predominance of HIV-2 is unlikely to persist.

Although HIV-2 infection exists in most West African countries, and in some, was probably present first, HIV-1 has become the predominant virus in most countries of West Africa. Several reports have documented increasing levels of HIV-1 infection while the prevalence of infection with HIV-2 has remained stable. Dual reactivity, i.e., simultaneous serologic reactivity to both viruses, is especially prevalent in Côte d'Ivoire, Mali, and Burkina Faso, countries geographically located between areas of almost pure HIV-2 infection to the west and HIV-1 infection to the east.

Outside of West Africa, the greatest numbers of HIV-2 infections have been reported from Angola, Mozambique, France, and Portugal. In Portugal, 10 percent of cases of AIDS have been attributed to HIV-2, and a substantial proportion of HIV-2-infected persons are thought to have acquired their infections in West Africa. The spread of HIV-2 in Angola and Mozambique is also likely to have been influenced by social change and population movement during the Portuguese colonial period. In France, most HIV-2 infections have been in persons originating from West Africa.

HIV-2 infection has recently been documented in India, but the published data do not allow assessment of its prevalence. Sporadic cases of HIV-2 infection have also been described in several African and most European countries other than those already mentioned, as well as in North and South America, and the Caribbean.

Heterosexual transmission

Mathematical models and epidemiologic studies have suggested that transmission of HIV-1 by heterosexual intercourse is considerably more efficient than for HIV-2.[6,7] Laboratory evidence indicates that persons infected with HIV-2 have a lower viral burden than those infected with HIV-1, and this difference persists until late in the course of infection.[8] However, with advanced immunodeficiency, viral burden in both infections is high. It is likely that these laboratory differences indicate lower transmissibility for HIV-2 throughout most of the course of infection, with infectiousness increasing during a relatively short period late in the course of infection.

The lower incidence of infection with HIV-2 compared with HIV-1 throughout West Africa further suggests its lower transmissibility. However, efficient transmission does occur from persons with long-standing infections, as witnessed by similar rates of serologic concordance in the spouses of men with HIV-1 and HIV-2-associated disease.[9]

Perinatal transmission

Although HIV-2 perinatal transmission can occur, it is much less frequent than mother-to-child transmission of HIV-1, and HIV-2-infected children have far better survival rates. The results of three prospective studies examining the perinatal transmission of HIV-2 are now available, from Côte d'Ivoire, France, and Guinea Bissau.[10,11,12] The Côte d'Ivoire study reported an HIV-2 perinatal transmission rate of 1 percent, approximately 21 times lower than the mother-to-child transmission rate for HIV-1.[13] In the studies in France and Guinea Bissau, no perinatal transmission of HIV-2 was documented. Dually reactive (i.e., serologic reactivity to both HIV-1 and HIV-2) women in Côte d'Ivoire transmitted to their offspring in a similar proportion of cases as women infected with HIV-1 only; of 11 dually reactive women who transmitted to their infants, 10 transmitted HIV-1 alone, and 1 transmitted both viruses.[14] The results of these recently completed prospective studies complement earlier cross-sectional data showing low rates of serologic concordance between HIV-2-infected mothers and their living children.[15,16,17]

Differences in perinatal transmission rates for HIV-1 and HIV-2 are also associated with differences in child survival. A retrospective cohort study in Côte d'Ivoire found that children of HIV-2-infected mothers had survival rates similar to children of HIV-negative mothers and therefore significantly better rates than children of HIV-1-positive mothers.[18] Prospective data showed that infants born to women with HIV-2 infection had a higher mortality than the children of seronegative women, but still had a much more favorable survival than the children of HIV-1-infected mothers.

Disease associations and natural history

Abundant cross-sectional data show that similar diseases are associated with HIV-2 as with HIV-1, including tuberculosis. A study in Côte d'Ivoire compared autopsy findings in 174 HIV-1-positive and 40 HIV-2-positive persons who had died of complications relating to their HIV infection.[19] The pathologies described were similar, but cholangitis, HIV encephalitis, and severe cytomegalovirus disease were significantly more frequent among the HIV-2-infected patients. In HIV-1 disease in industrialized countries, these lesions are usually associated with prolonged, advanced immunodeficiency; these observations suggest that the HIV-2-infected patients in Côte d'Ivoire had survived longer than those infected with HIV-1. Cross-sectional studies of HIV-1- and HIV-2-infected persons have generally shown less severe impairment in immunologic function in HIV-2-infected people as compared with HIV-1-infected people.[20,21]

A prospective cohort study of commercial sex workers in Senegal showed that women with incident HIV-2 infections were significantly less likely than those with incident HIV-1 infections to develop AIDS or CD4 + lymphocyte depletion. After 5 years of follow-up, 100 percent of HIV-2-infected women remained AIDS-free, compared with 67 percent of women with incident HIV-1 infections.[22]

Virology of HIV-2 infection and dual reactivity

Quantitative studies of viral load in persons infected with HIV-1 and HIV-2 have shown important differences over the course of the two infections.[23] In HIV-2-infected persons with CD4 + counts of less than $200/\mu l$, the cellular HIV-2 viral load was similar to that in persons with HIV-1 infection, but the rate of HIV-2 isolation from plasma was significantly lower (40 percent and 83 percent, respectively). In persons with higher CD4 + counts, viral load was significantly lower in those infected with HIV-2. Single polymerase chain reaction (PCR) technique using HIV-2-specific primers was less sensitive than expected from experience with HIV-1 infection (although sensitivity was improved using nested PCR technique). The reasons for these differences in viral load over the course of infection in HIV-1 and HIV-2 are unclear but are of potential clinical and epidemiological importance.

Biologic differences and genomic variability within strains of HIV-2 are of comparable magnitude as found for HIV-1. The HIV-2 prototype strain, HIV-2$_{ROD}$, isolated from a patient from Cape Verde, exhibited 49 percent amino acid homology with HIV-1 and 72 percent with SIV$_{mac}$/SIV$_{sm}$. A divergent HIV-2 strain from a Liberian patient has been characterized as very closely related to SIV$_{mac}$/SIV$_{sm}$.[24] The V3 regions (as described in Chapter 13) of HIV-2 and HIV-1 seem to vary to a similar degree. The variability of

HIV-2 over several years in the same individual has not been studied. The regulatory genes of HIV-1 and HIV-2 are highly divergent and the differences in regulation and transactivation merit investigation.

Serologic reactivity to both HIV-1 and HIV-2 (dual reactivity) has received little attention recently. Earlier PCR studies in Côte d'Ivoire involving relatively few persons had shown that between one-third and two-thirds of individuals with this serologic profile were infected with both viruses; the others were thought to be infected with only one virus, with cross-reactivity to the other.[25,26] Serologic studies of female commercial sex workers in Côte d'Ivoire showed that dual reactivity was associated with increased sexual exposure and duration of prostitution, suggesting a substantial proportion of the women had been exposed to both viruses. Overall, 30 percent of these women were dually reactive, and dual reactivity represented 38 percent of all seropositive profiles; these absolute and proportional rates are the highest reported in any population.[27]

As mentioned above, dually reactive mothers can transmit both agents to their offspring, but in most instances where transmission occurs, it involves only HIV-1. Serologic testing of female sex partners of dually reactive men with advanced disease in Côte d'Ivoire showed that 44 percent of the partners were infected with HIV-1, 8 percent with HIV-2, and 20 percent were themselves dually reactive.[28]

It was recently reported that HIV-2-positive female sex workers in Senegal had a significantly lower incidence of HIV-1 infection than seronegative women.[29] Although women with HIV-2 infection had higher rates of other sexually transmitted infections than seronegative women, their HIV-1 incidence rate was 1.06 per 100 person years, compared with 2.45 per 100 person years in HIV-negative women, for an adjusted relative risk of 0.32. No reduction in HIV-2 incidence was found in women infected with HIV-1. The authors speculated that HIV-2 infection gives partial protection against subsequent HIV-1 infection, which has obvious implications for future efforts at vaccine development.

Future research

Better understanding of the natural history of HIV-2 infection and its transmission dynamics is required. Studies of natural history, progression of immune deficiency, and transmission should be combined with assessment of viral load. Transmission to sex partners should be examined in relation to viral burden in the infected index person. The extent of HIV-2 strain variation is largely unstudied, and it is unknown whether strain differences have clinical implications. Further studies of the virology and biology of HIV-2 may give insight into the mechanisms of the apparent different natural history of HIV-2 from that of HIV-1, with potential implications for understanding HIV pathogenesis in general. Such research will involve various disciplines and will require collaboration between West African field workers and laboratory workers in the industrialized world.

REFERENCES

1. K. M. De Cock, G. Adjorlolo, E. Ekpini, et al., "Epidemiology and transmission of HIV-2—why there is no HIV-2 pandemic," *Journal of the American Medical Association* 270(1993):2083–2086 [erratum corrected in 27(1994):903–904].

2. K. M. De Cock and F. Brun-Vezinet, "Epidemiology of HIV-2 infection," *AIDS* 3(suppl.1)(1989):s89–s95.

3. K. M. De Cock, F. Brun-Vezinet, and B. Soro, "HIV-1 and HIV-2 infection and AIDS in West Africa," *AIDS* 5(suppl.1)(1991):s21–s28.

4. De Cock,"Epidemiology and transmission of HIV-2."

5. P. J. Kanki and K. M. De Cock, "Epidemiology and natural history of HIV-2," *AIDS* 8(suppl.1)(1994):s85–s93.

6. C. Donnelly, W. Leisenring, P. Kanki, T. A. Awerbuch, and S. Sandberg, "Comparison of transmission rates of HIV-1 and HIV-2 in a cohort of prostitutes in Senegal," *Bulletin of Mathematical Biology* 55(1993):731–743.

7. P. Kanki, K. Travers, S. M'Boup et al., "Slower heterosexual spread of HIV-2 than HIV-1," *Lancet* 343(1994):943–946.

8. F. Simon, S. Matheron, C. Tamalet, et al., "Cellular and plasma viral load in patients infected with HIV-2," *AIDS* 7(1993):1411–1417.

9. J. M. N'Gbichi, K. M. De Cock, V. Batter, et al. "HIV status of female sex partners of men reactive to HIV-1, HIV-2 or both viruses in Abidjan, Côte d'Ivoire," *AIDS* 9(1995):951–954.

10. G. Adjorlolo-Johnson, K. M. De Cock, E. Ekpini, et al., "Prospective comparison of mother-to-child transmission of HIV-1 and HIV-2 in Abidjan, Côte d'Ivoire," *Journal of the American Medical Association* 272(1994):462–466.

11. Y. Moudoub, "Rate of mother-to-child transmission of HIV-2 in the French National Prospective Study," Abstract PO-C16–2981, presented at the IX International Conference on AIDS, Berlin, June 1993.

12. P. A. Andreasson, F. Dias, A. Naucler, S. Andersson, and G. Biberfeld, "Prospective study of vertical transmission of HIV-2 in Bissau, Guinea-Bissau," *AIDS* 7(1993):989–993.

13. Adjorlolo-Johnson, "Prospective comparison."

14. *Ibid.*

15. H. D. Gayle, E. Gnaore, G. Adjorlolo, et al., "HIV-1 and HIV-2 infection in children in Abidjan, Côte d'Ivoire," *Journal of Acquired Immune Deficiency Syndromes* 5(1992):513–517.

16. A. Del Mistro, J. Chotard, A. J. Hall, H. Whittle, A. De Rossi, and L. Chieco-Bianchi, "HIV-1 and HIV-2 seroprevalence rates in mother-child pairs living in The Gambia (West Africa)," *Journal of Acquired Immune Deficiency Syndromes* 5(1992):19–24.

17. A. G. Poulsen, B. B. Kvinesdal, P. Aaby, et al., "Lack of evidence of vertical transmission of human immunodeficiency virus type 2 in a sample of the general population in Bissau," *Journal of Acquired Immune Deficiency Syndromes* 5(1992):25–30.

18. K. M. De Cock, F. Zadi, G. Adjorlolo, et al., "Retrospective study of maternal HIV-1 and HIV-2 infections and child survival in Abidjan, Côte d'Ivoire," *British Medical Journal* 308(1994):441–443.

19. S. B. Lucas, A. Hounnou, C. Peacock, et al., "Mortality and pathology of HIV infection in a West African city," *AIDS* 7(1993):1569–1579.

20. Kanki, "Epidemiology and natural history."

21. L. Kestens, K. Brattegaard, G. Adjorlolo, et al., "Immunological comparison of HIV-1-, HIV-2-, and dually-reactive women delivering in Abidjan, Côte d'Ivoire," *AIDS* 6(1992):803–807.

22. R. Marlink, P. Kanki, I. Thior, et al., "Reduced rate of disease development after HIV-2 infection as compared to HIV-1," *Science* 265(1994):1587–1590.

23. Simon, "Cellular and plasma viral load."

24. F. Gao, L. Yue, A. T. White, et al., "Human infection by genetically diverse SIV$_{sm}$ related HIV-2 in West Africa," *Nature* 358(1992):495–499.

25. J. R. George, C.-Y. Ou, B. Parekh, et al., "Prevalence of HIV-1 and HIV-2 mixed infections in Côte d'Ivoire," *Lancet* 340(1992):339–340.

26. M. Peeters, G.-M. Gershy-Damet, K. Fransen, et al., "Virological and polymerase chain reaction studies of HIV-1/HIV-2 dual infection in Côte d'Ivoire," *Lancet* 340(1992):339–340.

27. P. D. Ghys, M. O. Diallo, V. Ettiegne-Traore, et al., "Dual seroreactivity to HIV-1 and HIV-2 in female sex workers in Abidjan, Côte d'Ivoire." *AIDS* 9(1995):951–954.

28. J. M. N'Gbichi, "HIV status of female sex partners."

29. K. Travers, S. Mboup, R. Marlink, et al., "Natural protection against HIV-1 infection provided by HIV-2," *Science* 268(1995):1612–1615.

13

HIV Heterogeneity in Transmission and Pathogenesis

JAY A. LEVY

Since the discovery of the human immunodeficiency virus (HIV) in 1983, a variety of procedures have been developed to identify viral subtypes. This important aspect of AIDS research has defined the existence of the two major virus types—HIV-1 and HIV-2—and can provide information relevant to disease transmission, evolution of HIV strains, epidemiologic spread, and pathogenesis. It also raises key questions for development of effective therapies and vaccines. Distinct viral properties can be identified by biologic, serologic, and molecular features.

Biologic features

Viruses isolated from different individuals vary according to five major biologic properties: (1) cellular host range; (2) kinetics of virus replication; (3) extent of virus production; (4) ability to kill the infected cell; and (5) induction of latency. Thus, HIV isolates may be distinguished according to their ability to grow in T-cell lines versus macrophages, their kinetics of replication (fast or slow) and extent of replication (high or low), their ability to form syncytia (multinucleated cells) in established T-cell lines, and other properties.

Researchers use these biologic properties to categorize HIV isolates. For example, one isolate may be a macrophage-tropic nonsyncytia-inducing (NSI) virus. Another may be a fast-replicating syncytia-inducing (SI) virus that replicates well in T-cell lines. The transmission and pathologic effects of viruses with differing biologic profiles is then examined.

The host range (cell type targeted by an HIV strain) reflects the intracellular environment for the virus and can influence the extent to which its biologic properties will be expressed. Viral genetic factors also are involved, and biological characteristics of viruses (e.g., extent of HIV entry, the speed of viral replication, and the quantity of virus produced) result from interactions between intracellular factors and viral genetic material. For example, peripheral blood mononuclear cells (PBMC) from a variety of normal donors will show differences in their ability to grow either the same or different viral isolates.[1]

Some biologic features of HIV can be influenced by HIV accessory genes. Viral kinetics, for example, appears to be determined by regulatory genes, particularly *tat*.

The ability of HIV to kill cells may require a variety of viral genetic determinants and biologic processes, such as changes in membrane permeability and apoptosis (i.e., programmed cell death).[2,3,4] The factors involved in cell killing are most likely influenced by both the extent of virus replication (e.g., amount of viral proteins made) and the structure of the viral envelope proteins (e.g., conformation and glycosylation pattern).[5,6,7]

The establishment of a latent state (i.e., infection without production of progeny viruses) also reflects the interplay of both viral and cellular factors. Differences in latency among viral strains can be seen in cell culture.[8,9] In the host, salient virus infection can be recognized in blood and lymphoid tissue and probably mirrors anti-HIV immune responses.[10,11]

Role of biologic features in viral transmission

Certain biologic viral phenotypes have been associated with transmission at specific stages in HIV pathogenesis. Some researchers believe macrophage-tropic NSI viruses are preferentially transmitted perhaps secondary to infected macrophages in genital fluids, or to macrophages serving as targets in the rectum, vagina, or lymph node.[12] This observed predominance of NSI strains in primary infection has several exceptions however (for example, SI viruses are also recovered in acute infection) and needs further evaluation.[13]

Role of biologic features in pathogenesis

Many viruses isolated in asymptomatic individuals have been of the NSI type, and several of these are macrophage-tropic. When disease develops, fast-replicating, highly cytopathic SI-type viruses are often identified. These viruses are related genetically to the NSI types and thus appear to be derived from them in the host. The SI viruses are able to replicate well in PBMC and T-cell lines, but they often do not productively infect macrophages.[14,15] As noted earlier, the extent of replication may depend on both the cells and the particular virus.

The relationship of viral biologic properties to pathogenesis has been evaluated in the SCID-hu mouse system. In these studies using immunodeficient animals reconstituted with human PBMC, NSI strains appeared to lead to a faster loss of CD4+ cells than SI viruses.[16] In other studies using fetal thymus and liver implants, SI viruses that rapidly destroy CD4+ cells in culture appeared to have the same effect in animals.[17] In the first instance, apoptosis is probably a major cause of this cell death, in the latter, both apoptosis and direct cytopathicity may have been involved.

These findings indicate that it is still not known if particular HIV virus subtypes are directly linked to the loss of CD4+ cells in human hosts. It is possible that the virulent cytopathic strains may result from the prior loss in immune responses, rather than being the cause of this immune deficiency. For example, over time, reduction in CD4+ cells induced by NSI viruses could bring about the gradual destruction of the immune defense against

HIV. With the release of more virions and increased HIV replication in the host, viral mutations can take place, leading to the more cytopathic, fast-replicating strains that may contribute to advancement to disease. Thus, the more virulent virus would not necessarily be the major determinant of disease progression. The observation of AIDS developing in some children infected by NSI viruses supports this hypothesis.[18]

Serologic features

Just as biologic properties can determine the extent of virus spread in the host and the amount of CD4+ cell destruction, the ability of the individual infected to suppress virus through antibody or cellular immune responses can influence the extent of HIV pathogenesis. The sensitivity of virus strains to this immune response represents an additional parameter for distinguishing viral subtypes. A few reports have suggested a classification of HIV by serologic studies. One group subclassified HIV-1 strains by their ability to be neutralized by three HIV seropositive sera.[19] Other studies have dealt with the ability of viruses to be neutralized by a variety of polyclonal and monoclonal antibodies directed particularly at the variable (V3) loop in the HIV envelope gp120.[20,21] A definitive classification by antigenic subtype is not yet available, but viruses sharing regions in the V3 loop, particularly the "signature" sequence GPGR, can be cross-neutralized by several polyclonal and monoclonal antibodies.[22] Apparently, some of the broadly reactive antibodies respond to a conformational (versus linear) epitope in the envelope region. Also, some anti-envelope antibodies can kill virus-infected cells by antibody-directed cellular cytotoxicity (ADCC).[23] Variations in this response, depending on the HIV strain and the antibody species, have been described.[24]

Some data suggest that cross-reacting antibodies may reflect an immune response against the CD4 binding site of HIV which by necessity is highly conserved. The CD4 molecule is the major attachment site for HIV.[25,26] Nevertheless, because this binding site on the viral envelope is a discontinuous epitope formed from a folding conformational structure, multiple antibodies may be required to completely neutralize viruses at this region.[27] For this reason, recent evidence suggests that many broadly reacting antibodies are directed at the V3 loop rather than the CD4 binding site.[28]

Serologic studies have also indicated that some sera that neutralize certain isolates may not neutralize others (resistant strains) and may in fact enhance infection by other virus isolates. This antibody-dependent enhancement (ADE) is defined by a two- to fourfold increase in virus replication in cell culture after prior exposure of the virus to the antibody. Most importantly, it has been shown that some viral strains can change over time within an individual and lose sensitivity to neutralization and become sensitive to antibody enhancement.[29] In some cases, the same antibodies in the serum of a subject at a given time in the course of infection may have different effects against other autologous isolates, depending on when the viruses were recovered from the same subject. Whether these observations have relevance to the clinical state needs further evaluation, but it is known that over time, viruses in the host are not well-neutralized by the concomitant serum specimen. HIV, through envelope mutations, can "escape" antiviral immune responses.

The genetic changes correlating with serologic differences have been approached through studies of selective viral isolates and monoclonal antibodies. Using human monoclonal antibodies to a discrete epitope in the V3 loop, Kliks et al. found that only one amino acid difference could determine whether an HIV strain is sensitive to or resistant to neutralization or enhancement.[30] Several amino acid changes in this viral envelope (V3) domain were needed to change a virus into being sensitive to neutralization or enhancement. Nevertheless, the results suggest that viruses can escape the immune system by only a few alterations in their envelope structure.

Resistance of virus strains to neutralization has also been demonstrated by alterations outside of the epitope recognized by the particular antibody. Changes in gp41, for example, can make previously sensitive viruses resistant to anti-gp120 or anti-V3 antibodies.[31] Obviously, modifications in certain regions of the viral envelope can alter the conformation of the antigenic site in another region of the envelope. This change can influence sensitivity to antibody-mediated neutralization or enhancement.

Molecular features

The molecular heterogeneity among isolates was first recognized when restriction enzyme studies were performed on various HIV molecular clones. When genetic sequencing on these clones was completed, it became evident that viruses could be distinguished from one another in a variety of different genomic regions. The greatest variability in amino acids was found in the envelope *(env)* and regulatory genes (e.g., *tat*).[32] Although the viral reverse transcriptase can cause mutations throughout the viral RNA, many of these mutations are "synonymous" changes that do not affect amino acid expression. Only "nonsynonymous" mutations that cause amino acid changes would be selected during immune surveillance, and these alterations are most prominent in the *env* regions of HIV. HIV's ability to mutate and establish new envelope subtypes over time may be due to attempts to escape host immune responses.

Using molecular procedures such as polymerase chain reaction (PCR) and DNA sequencing, various domains of the virus (primarily *env* and *gag*) have been used to classify subtypes (or clades) of the HIV-1 strains recovered from many parts of the world (Box 13-1).[33]

BOX 13-1

The global distribution of HIV-1 genotypes

FRANCINE E. McCUTCHAN AND GERALD MYERS

How are HIV variants analyzed?

To organize and interpret HIV-1 genetic data, DNA and protein sequences from virus isolates are aligned, inspected for regions of similarity and difference (nucleotide distance measurement), and

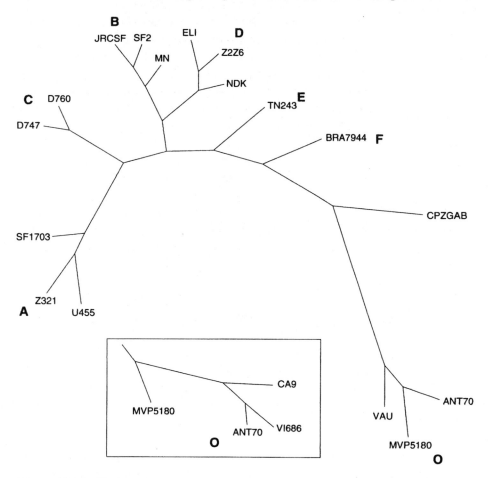

Figure 13-1.1   Phylogenetic tree analysis of HIV-1 envelope gene sequences.

classified. Two of HIV's structural genes have provided most of the raw material for analysis: *gag* (encoding the internal core proteins of the virion) and *env* (which specifies the envelope glycoprotein); together these genes encompass about 40 percent of the viral genome. In addition to complete gene sequences, considerable data have also been gathered on select subfragments of genes; in particular, there are more than 1,000 sequences for the third hypervariable (V3) region of the HIV-1 envelope.

These nucleotide distance measurements and phylogenetic tree analyses have both been used to investigate genetic relationships among virus isolates. (Tree analysis attempts to reconstruct the series of mutational changes that gave rise to present forms.) Regardless of the analytical approach or the gene sequence analyzed, a highly consistent family tree of HIV-1 has emerged.

The criteria for separating variants into clades

HIV-1 virus prevalent in major centers of the pandemic can be subdivided into at least six genetic subtypes called *clades* (A–F). Each sequence subtype is virtually equidistant from the others. The distance separating the subtypes encompasses about 30 percent of the *env* gene and about 14 percent of the gag gene. For comparison, viruses of different types, such as HIV-1 and HIV-2, differ by at least 50 percent in both genes. Within clades, the genetic distance can be half or greater of what is seen between clades. As HIV-1 sequences are determined and analyzed, they can usually be assigned to one of the six clades (A–F). Viral forms intermediate between clades have thus far not been found. On the other hand, rare samples with sequences falling outside the six clusters (tentatively designated G, H, and I) are being discovered.[1] HIV-1 variation may be accelerated in part by the dynamics of AIDS transmission, a phenomenon of "epidemic-driven variation."[2]

Recently, analysis of a second group of HIV-1 subtypes, called the *O group* (for "outlying"), has provided a startling glimpse into the rise of AIDS in the world.[3,4,5] These HIV-1s are also approximately 30 percent apart from one another in their *env* gene sequences—arms of a second star phylogeny— and they are at least 50 percent apart in *env* from the main group of the six subtypes A through F (Figure 13-1.1). While O forms seem to be minor contributors to the epidemic, they suggest a second, independent HIV-1 evolutionary radiation event. Fortunately, it appears to be the case with such diverse forms that they are detectable by standard serological tests.

It is still unclear whether some clades are more virulent. There is no evidence of host genetic specificity related to the clades, nor have cases of infection of one person by two or more HIV-1 clades been encountered in countries having co-circulating viruses. Identification of a small number of distinct genetic clades does allow a limited number of prototype viruses that represent the full range of pathogens to be selected. However, these genetic groupings may not have a direct relationship with the viral properties that are most important for therapy and prevention.

The regional prevalence of HIV clades

Most continents harbor mixtures of genetic subtypes in differing proportions that undoubtedly reflect viral trafficking patterns (Figure 13-1.2). HIV-1 isolates from North America have been of the B clade. This suggests that of all viruses that *could* have been introduced, only one form was introduced and rapidly amplified through homosexual transmission in the mid-70s. In South America and Europe, clade B viruses have also been predominant, yet clades A, C, D, and F (and group O) have also been recovered, in smaller numbers. The recent fulminating epidemic in Asia has been associated with B,

Figure 13-1.2 Global distribution of HIV-1 subtypes. The prevalence of genetic subtypes A through F varies by locale. The apparent proportion of subtype isolates that are most closely matched to current candidate vaccines, is shown relative to other subtypes. In sites where field trials are planned or are under way, the proportion of subtype B isolates varies significantly.

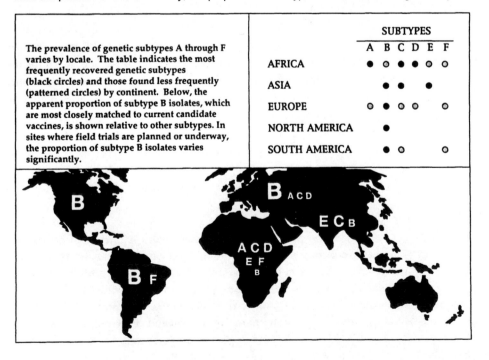

The prevalence of genetic subtypes A through F varies by locale. The table indicates the most frequently recovered genetic subtypes (black circles) and those found less frequently (patterned circles) by continent. Below, the apparent proportion of subtype B isolates, which are most closely matched to current candidate vaccines, is shown relative to other subtypes. In sites where field trials are planned or underway, the proportion of subtype B isolates varies significantly.

	A	B	C	D	E	F
AFRICA	●	○	●	●	○	○
ASIA		●	●		●	
EUROPE	○	●	○	○		○
NORTH AMERICA		●				
SOUTH AMERICA		●	○			○

C, and E clades, with E and C clades appearing to predominate. Clades A, C, and D are most frequently found in African countries, but here again, all other clades, along with the group O forms, have been recorded.

References

1. W. Janssens, L. Heyndrickx, K. Fransen, J. Motte, M. Peeters, J. N. Nkengasong, P. M. Ndumbe, E. Deleporte, J.-L. Perret, C. Atende, P. Piot, and G. van der Groen, "Genetic and phylogenetic analysis of *env* subtypes G and H in central Africa," *AIDS Research and Human Retroviruses* 10(1994):600–650.
2. G. Myers and B. Korber, "Future of human immunodeficiency virus," in *Evolutionary Biology of Viruses,* S. S. Morse, ed. (New York: Raven, 1994).
3. M. Vanden Haesevelde, J.-L. Decourt, R. De Leys, B. Vanderborght, G. van der Groen, H. van Heuverswijn, and E. Saman, "Genomic cloning and complete sequence analysis of a highly divergent African human immunodeficiency virus isolate," *Journal of Virology* 68(1994):1586–1596.
4. L. G. Gurtler, P. H. Hauser, J. Eberle, A. von Braun, S. Knapp, L. Zekeng, J. M. Tsague, and L. Kaptue, "New subtype of human immunodeficiency virus type 1 (MVP-5180) from Cameroon," *Journal of Virology* 68(1994):1581–1585.
5. W. Janssens, N. Nkengasong, L. Heyndrickx, K. Fransen, P. M Ndumbe, E. Delaporte, M. Peeters, J.-L. Perret, A. Ndoumou, P. Piot, and G. van der Groen, "Further evidence of the presence of genetically very aberrant strains in Cameroon and Gabon," *AIDS* 8(1994):1012–1013.

The epidemiology of clade distribution and evolution worldwide will be critical for vaccine development. If sufficiently broad (cross-clade) protection cannot be achieved with vaccine, limited geographic useful and eventual "viral escape" with reduced vaccine efficacy can be anticipated.

The ability to distinguish viruses by their molecular sequences can also be helpful in tracing transmission among individuals and the spread of viruses throughout various countries. It has already proven valuable for demonstrating the transfer of virus from mother to child, among sexual partners, and from a dentist to his patients.[34] Increased understanding of HIV heterogeneity may make it possible to predict new clades that might arise through continual alterations in amino acid sequences in the envelope region. This knowledge will be important for vaccine development. For the same reason, it is important to determine the correlation of sequence subtypes to sensitivity to serum neutralization. Other issues needing further evaluation include susceptibility to suppression by cellular immune response (e.g., $CD8^+$ cells), whether the present clade separation indicates antigenic subtypes, and whether given clades are excluded from parts of the world because of serologic cross-reactivity.[35]

In conclusion, biologic, serologic, and molecular analyses can identify subtypes of HIV that help further our understanding of HIV transmission and epidemiologic spread, and of the pathologic course of disease. Knowledge of biologic subtypes may provide information on whether an infected person will experience a rapid or slow progression of AIDS, whether "virulent" strains are evolving in populations, and other important implications. Understanding serologic subtypes could help identify the pathogenic course in terms of host immune response. In this regard, strong CD8+ cell antiviral activity correlates directly with long-term survival in HIV infection.[36] Molecular differences among HIV strains define the genetic diversity that determines properties of viral replication and pathogenesis, as well as sensitivity to host immune responses.

Research on AIDS over the past 10 years has increased the understanding of how HIV can undergo high mutability and selection within the host. Further research that clarifies the effects and transmission of viral subtypes, identifies distinguishing criteria, and examines how subtypes correlate with genetic variations in the viral genome may provide information that can lead to effective therapies and antiviral vaccines.

REFERENCES

1. L. A. Evans, T. M. McHugh, D. P. Stites, and J. A. Levy, "Differential ability of human immunodeficiency virus isolates to productively infect human cells," *Journal of Immunology* 138(1987):3415–3418.

2. J. A. Levy, "Pathogenesis of human immunodeficiency virus infection," *Microbiological Reviews* 57(1993):183–289.

3. M. L. Gougeon, S. Garcia, J. Heeney, et al., "Programmed cell death in AIDS-related HIV and SIV infections," *AIDS Research and Human Retroviruses* 9(1993):553–563.

4. R. F. Garry, "Potential mechanisms for the cytopathic properties of HIV," *AIDS* 3(1989):683–694.

5. Levy, "Pathogenesis."

6. Garry, "Potential mechanisms."

7. M. Stevenson, C. Meier, A. M. Mann, et al., "Envelope glycoprotein of HIV induces interference and cytolysis resistance in CD4+ cells: Mechanism for persistence in AIDS," *Cell* 53(1988):483–496.

8. Levy, "Pathogenesis."

9. T. M. Folks and D. P. Bednarik, "Mechanisms of HIV-1 latency," *AIDS* 6(1992):3–16.

10. J. A. Levy, "Pathogenesis of human immunodeficiency virus infection," *Microbiological Reviews* 57(1993):183–289.

11. J. Embretson, M. Zupancic, J. Beneke, et al., "Analysis of human immunodeficiency virus-infected tissues by amplification and *in situ* hybridization reveals latent and permissive infections at single-cell resolution," *Proceedings of the National Academy of Sciences USA* 90(1993):357–361.

12. T. Zhu, H. Mo, N. Wang, et al., "Genotypic and phenotypic characterization of HIV-1 in patients with primary infection," *Science* 261(1993):1179–1181.

13. J. A. Levy, "Pathogenesis of human immunodeficiency virus infection," *Microbiological Reviews* 57(1993):183–289.

14. M. Tersmette, R. A. Gruters, F. de Wolf, et al., "Evidence for a role of virulent human immunodeficiency virus (HIV) variants in the pathogenesis of acquired immunodeficiency syndrome," *Journal of Virology* 63(1989):2118–2125.

15. C. Cheng-Mayer, D. Seto, M. Tateno, and J. A. Levy, "Biologic features of HIV-1 that correlate with virulence in the host," *Science* 240(1988):80–82.

16. D. E. Mosier, R. J. Guliza, P. D. MacIsaac, et al., "Rapid loss of CD4+ T cells in human-PBL-SCID mice by noncytopathic HIV isolates," *Science* 260(1993):689–692.

17. D. Camerini, B. D. Jamieson, J. A. Zack, et al., "Pathogenesis of syncytium-inducing and non-syncytium inducing HIV-1 isolates and molecular clones in SCID-hu mice," *Journal of Cellular Biochemistry* 18B(1994):155.

18. S. Wolinsky, personal communication (1994).

19. C. Cheng-Mayer, J. M. Homsy, L. A. Evans, et al., "Identification of HIV subtypes with distinct patterns of sensitivity to serum neutralization," *Proceedings of the National Academy of Sciences USA* 85(1988):2815–2819.

20. Levy, "Pathogenesis."

21. K. Javaherian, A. J. Langlois, G. J. LaRosa, et al., "Broadly neutralizing antibodies elicited by the hypervariable neutralizing determinant of HIV-1," *Science* 250(1990):1590–1593.

22. *Ibid.*

23. Levy, "Pathogenesis."

24. A. von Gegerfelt, C. Diaz-Pohl, E. M. Fenyo, and K. Broliden, "Specificity of antibody-dependent cellular cytotoxicity in sera from human immunodeficiency virus type 1-infected individuals," *AIDS Research and Human Retroviruses* 9(1993):883–889.

25. Levy, "Pathogenesis."

26. J. P. Moore and R. W. Sweet, "HIV gp120-CD4 interaction: A target for pharmacological or immunological intervention?" *Perspectives in Drug Discovery and Design* 1(1993):235–250.

27. *Ibid.*

28. M. K. Gorny, A. J. Conley, S. Karwowska, et al., "Neutralization of diverse human immunodeficiency virus type 1 variants by an anti-V3 human monoclonal antibody," *Journal of Virology* 66(1992):7538–7542.

29. J. Homsy, M. Meyer, and J. A. Levy, "Serum enhancement of human immunodeficiency virus (HIV) correlates with disease in HIV-infected individuals," *Journal of Virology* 64(1990):1437–1440.

30. S. C. Kliks, T. Shioda, N. L. Haigwood, et al., "V3 variability can influence the ability of an antibody to neutralize or enhance infection by diverse strains of human immunodeficiency virus type 1," *Proceedings of the National Academy of Sciences USA* 90(1993):11518–11522.

31. M. Thali, M. Charles, C. Furman, et al., "Resistance to neutralization by broadly reactive antibodies to the human immunodeficiency virus type 1 gp120 glycoprotein conferred by a gp41 amino acid change," *Journal of Virology* 68(1994):674–680.

32. Levy, "Pathogenesis."

33. G. Myers, B. Korber, S. Wain-Hobson, et al., *Human retroviruses and AIDS I–V. A Compilation and Analysis of Nucleic Acid and Amino Acid Sequences*" (Los Alamos, New Mexico: Los Alamos National Laboratory, 1989).

34. Levy, "Pathogenesis."

35. *Ibid.*

36. C. Mackewicz and J. A. Levy, "CD8+ cell anti-HIV activity: Non-lytic suppression of virus replication," *AIDS Research and Human Retroviruses* 8(1992):1039–1050.

14

HIV Vaccine Development—Progress and Problems

DONALD P. FRANCIS

Vaccines offer enormous potential to protect individuals and society against AIDS. Efforts are underway to develop a vaccine, but scientific challenges, combined with limited resources and incentives, have resulted in a significant gap between current efforts and potential approaches to solving this problem. The scientific progress and other factors that must be addressed to improve the prospects for successful vaccine development are examined below.

Scientific progress

The principle of vaccination is well understood. In theory, development of a vaccine requires an understanding of the immune response that induces protection from infectious diseases and a laboratory marker that reflects this state of protection after recovery from infection. For example, for hepatitis B virus, it is known that an antibody specific to the surface protein of the virus confers protection against subsequent infection.[1] Even passive administration of this antibody from people who have recovered from hepatitis B infection protects against infection.[2]

Unfortunately, for HIV-1 the story is more complex. In contrast to almost all other viral infections in humans, HIV-1 appears to be almost universally progressive. In other words, there is no group of patients who have recovered from HIV infection. Without this group, researchers have been unable to uncover a specific immune response towards which vaccine-induced immunity should be targeted.

In the absence of a correlate of protection, vaccine researchers have been forced to proceed more or less blindly, guided only by knowledge of other virus models. Research has been based on the presumption that, as for hepatitis B virus, antibodies directed against surface proteins of HIV-1 should neutralize the virus, render it inactive, and protect against subsequent infection.

In addition, the major guidepost for vaccine development has traditionally been the successful immunization of animals with a prototype vaccine. In this regard, since HIV-1 will not infect lower animals, researchers have been forced to experiment on rare and expensive chimpanzees.[3]

Yet HIV-1 vaccine development has progressed despite both our limited understanding of a correlate of protection and the complex difficulties involving animal models. Initial studies showed that, in the laboratory, as predicted, antibodies directed towards envelope proteins of HIV-1 neutralized the virus.[4] Later it was demonstrated that passive administration of antibodies that produced high levels of neutralization antibodies could protect chimpanzees from virus challenge.[5]

These experiments led vaccine developers to the next step: making a prototype vaccine, immunizing a chimpanzee, and then challenging the animal with live virus. Two chimpanzees were protected with such a prototype vaccine (an LAI-derived vaccine consisting of gp120 expressed in Chinese hamster ovary cells).[6] Soon after, two other chimpanzees were protected after immunization with a combination of envelope proteins.[7] Both of these procedures used the same cell-free virus for challenge that was used to make the vaccine. Later, it was shown that chimpanzees could be protected from both cell-associated virus and from virus more distantly related to the vaccine strain.[8]

These successes encouraged some manufacturers to initiate human vaccine trials. The earliest trials used products made by recombinant technology utilizing nonmammalian cell culture systems (bacterial or yeast). Unfortunately, these antigens failed to produce neutralizing antibodies in humans.[9-11] Later studies used recombinant technology which utilized mammalian cells to produce surface proteins, and these have been much more successful.[12] The difference is assumed to be the close resemblance of mammalian cell–produced proteins to those found in humans.

Two prototype vaccines, one manufactured by Biocine, Inc. (Emeryville, California, U.S.) and another by Genentech, Inc. (South San Francisco, California, U.S.) have progressed through phase I and phase II clinical trials.[13] In addition, several other vaccines have entered phase I trials. One vaccine, developed by Pasteur Vaccins (France), utilizes a combination approach of primary immunization by a poxvirus recombinant "vector" carrying HIV-1 gp120, followed by booster doses of either pure gp120 or subunit peptides of gp120.[14,15] Another prototype vaccine, produced by Immuno AG (Vienna, Austria), consists of a recombinant gp160 protein. A variety of other approaches, developed by other companies, are still in earlier stages of development.

Considerable information is available on the two prototype vaccines that have completed phase II testing. Hundreds of people have received the Biocine or Genentech vaccine. The vaccines appear to be safe and immunogenic, but placebo-controlled testing among high-risk populations will be required to determine whether they are able to protect humans from HIV infection.

Scientific concerns

Two major scientific issues will determine whether HIV vaccines will be effective. The first involves variations in the virus subtypes that exist around the world (Chapter 13). The nucleic acid sequence of HIV-1 envelopes can vary by as much as 30 percent among subtypes. Virus neutralization assays indicate that some of this variation may not be important, but it is likely that a vaccine capable of protecting against all HIV strains may have to be a mixture of antigens. Will this "cocktail" have to include seven viral subtypes, or 70? Obviously, including seven is possible, but 70 may not be.

The second critical issue is whether antibodies will protect against infection and disease. Some investigators have suggested that cell-mediated immunity can be important in eliminating infected cells once HIV has established itself.[16,17,18] For example, in the SIV model in macaque monkeys, immunization that failed to protect against infection still induced some protection against disease.[19] If cell-mediated immunity was the mechanism of this protection, then antigens and antigen presentation formulations that maximize cell-mediated immunity may prove valuable.

The answers to these two questions will have to await clinical trials that test a variety of vaccine approaches in populations infected with a variety of virus types.

Social concerns

Considering the immensity of the threat posed by HIV-1, an equally immense vaccine development effort should be underway to meet this threat. Has this happened? Clearly, the answer is no.

Although several companies have attempted to develop HIV vaccines, their approaches have been rather narrow and have centered on the virus strains circulating primarily in the industrialized world. Given the empirical nature of vaccine development, multiple parallel approaches using a variety of antigens should be undertaken. However, a matrix that shows the approaches vaccinologists could take in developing an HIV-1 vaccine and the subtypes of HIV-1 that may need a vaccine (Table 14-1) demonstrates a considerable gap between current efforts and potential avenues that could be taken to maximize the chances of success.

One reason for this gap is the way vaccines are developed. Although some governmental and non-profit organizations may participate in vaccine development, the predominant developers of vaccines have been private pharmaceutical firms in the industrialized world.[20] The motive that drives these firms is profit. One might assume that the profits resulting from a successful HIV vaccine would be immense but, if this were true, multiple competitors would be trying all possible approaches to win the race to develop it. Early on, several large vaccine manufacturers invested considerable resources in work to develop an HIV vaccine, but most of them have either abandoned or markedly decreased their programs.

Why has this happened? There are several reasons. First, the development of an HIV vaccine has not been easy. In the absence of a clear correlate of protection and an inexpensive animal model, the scientific challenge has been considerable. Second, vaccines—particularly for the developing world—are not viewed by the pharmaceutical business as very profitable products, especially when compared with therapeutic drugs. Finally, in

Table 14-1 Investment in preventive vaccine product development by approach and virus subtype (vaccine approaches from left to right according to perceived safety)

Subtype	Peptides	Protein subunits	Virus-like particles and other particles	DNA	Live recombinant vectors	Whole killed	Live attenuated
B[a]	+	+	+	+/−	+	0	0
A	+/−	0	0	0	0	0	0
C	+/−	0	0	0	0	0	0
D	+/−	0	0	0	0	0	0
E	+/−	0	0	0	0	0	0
F	0	0	0	0	0	0	0
G	0	0	0	0	0	0	0

0 = no product in development; +/− = product currently in development but not yet in human trials; + = product currently in phase I/II trials in humans.
[a]Virus subtype B predominates in North America and Europe.

practice the world does not highly value prevention. Of course, each of these reasons for the relative lack of interest in HIV-1 vaccine development is related.

Scientific challenges have not necessarily hampered the pursuit of pharmaceutical products. Immense investments have been made attacking monumental scientific obstacles. Vaccines, however, pose unique problems. Unlike other pharmaceuticals, the guideposts used to determine the likelihood of success are often absent in vaccine development, especially for HIV. Although a prototype HIV vaccine may induce certain immune responses in animals or humans, not knowing if these responses will create immunity from disease can cause company decision makers to lose interest in investing further resources. In addition, while animal experiments could serve as indicators of progress, few such experiments are possible because chimpanzees are the sole susceptible animal. This limitation has been further compounded by the unavailability of chimpanzee challenge stocks of virus needed to ensure consistent infection rates.[21]

Despite these scientific limitations, companies would probably invest in HIV vaccine development if the potential rewards were great enough to justify the gamble. But although vaccines can be profitable, most are only marginally so. They must be produced in large volume, and offer relatively low profit per dose. When weighing options for financial success, industry decision makers often favor low volume/high profit items such as therapeutic drugs over high volume/low profit items like vaccines.

Profit could motivate development of HIV vaccines targeted for sales in industrialized countries. However, little profit will result from selling vaccines to impoverished developing countries, where the public health need is so great, yet where resources to purchase vaccines are so limited. No existing program guarantees purchase of a vaccine for developing countries. Even companies with a strong social conscience say they forsee AIDS vaccine development as a possible route to bankruptcy.

Ultimately the issue is value. If the world valued an HIV vaccine, business would respond to make one. Although it is rare to hear anyone speak against an HIV vaccine, no organized group actively encourages its development. This silence is related to a broader social attitude that does not value prevention and results in the continued occurrence of many problems beyond AIDS, that are clearly preventable.

Solutions

An imbalance exists between great social need for an HIV vaccine and the limited incentives for the private sector to develop one. This situation will not change unless, by good fortune, one of the prototype vaccines currently in development proves successful. While this is possible, an alternative approach for accelerating and ensuring development of an HIV vaccine is needed.

Some historical models and precedents exist. For example, polio vaccine development was spurred by an immense public demand, which resulted in the establishment in the United States of the National Foundation for Infantile Paralysis and substantial funding for vaccine development. In other situations as well, governments have intervened and provided support for vaccine development and manufacturing.

In many countries, government resources support much of the basic research upon which HIV vaccine development is based. The actual development of vaccine is usually left to the private sector, but government and nongovernment organizations can do many things to encourage the private sector to expand its role. For example, when the California State Legislature learned that the immense power of its biotechnology industry was not being directed toward HIV vaccine development, several steps were taken. After investigations revealed that the large costs of developmental and clinical research were a deterrent, funds were set aside to support some of these costs. The absence of social demand for an HIV vaccine was addressed by establishing a purchase order to procure HIV vaccine for California. Finally, to alleviate fear of litigation against a newly developed AIDS vaccine, protection against non-negligent litigation was offered.[22,23] These incentives had an important impact; both of the prototype HIV vaccines in phase II trials have come from California.

A much greater effort is needed at a global level. Substantial funding will be required—first to stimulate vaccine development, and then to purchase vaccine for use in the developing world.[24] Without an appropriate fund to drive development, it is unlikely that an HIV vaccine will be developed or delivered, and without significant public pressure, appropriate funding may never materialize.

REFERENCES

1. S. Krugman, L. R. Overby, I. K. Mushahwar, et al., "Viral hepatitis, type B. Studies on natural history and prevention reexamined," *New England Journal of Medicine* 300(1979):101–106.

2. A. G. Redeker, J. W. Mosley, D. J. Gocke, et al., "Hepatitis B immune globulin as a propylactic measure for spouses exposed to acute type B hepatitis," *New England Journal of Medicine* 293(1975):1055–1059.

3. P. N. Fultz, H. M. McClure, R. B. Swenson, et al., "Persistent infection of chimpanzees with human T-lymphotropic virus type III/lyphadenopathy-associated virus: A potential for acquired immunodeficiency syndrome," *Journal of Virology* 56(1986):116–124.

4. L. A. Lasky, J. E. Groopman, C. W. Fennie, et al., "Neutralization of AIDS retrovirus by antibodies to a recombinant envelope glycoprotein," *Science* 233(1986):209–212.

5. A. M. Prince, H. Reesink, D. Pascual, et al., "Prevention of HIV infection by passive immunization with HIV immunoglobulin," *AIDS Research and Human Retroviruses* 7(1991):971–973.

6. P. W. Berman, T. J. Gregory, L. Riddle, et al., "Protection of chimpanzees from infection by HIV-1 after vaccination with recombinant glycoprotein gp120 but not gp160," *Nature* 345(1990):622–625.

7. M. Girard, M. P. Kieny, A. Pinter, et al., "Immunization of chimpanzees confers protection against challenge with human immunodeficiency virus," *Proceedings of the National Academy of Sciences USA* 88(1991):542–546.

8. P. H. Fultz, P. Nara, F. Barre-Sinoussi, et al., "Vaccine protection of chimpanzees against challenge with HIV-1 infected peripheral blood mononuclear cells," *Science* 256(1992):1687–1690.

9. P. W. Berman, K. K. Murthy, T. Wrin, et. al., "Protection of MN-rgp 120-immunized chimpanzees from heterologous infection with a primary isolate of human immunodeficiency virus Type I," *Journal of Infectious Diseases* 173(1996):52–59.

10. P. E. Fast and M. C. Walker, "Human trials for experimental AIDS vaccines," *AIDS* 7(suppl.1)(1993):s147–s149.

11. R. B. Belshe, B. S. Graham, M. C. Keefer, et al., "Neutralizating antibodies to HIV-1 in seronegative volunteers immunized with recombinant gp120 from the MN strain of HIV-1. NIAID AIDS Vaccine Clinical Trials Network," *Journal of the American Medical Association* 272(1994):475–480.

12. M. Girard, M. P. Kieny, A. Pinter, et al., "Immunization of chimpanzees confers protection against challenge with human immunodeficiency virus," *Proceedings of the National Academy of Sciences USA* 88(1991):542–546.

13. Rockefeller Foundation, *HIV-Vaccines—Accelerating the Development of Preventive HIV Vaccines for the World*, summary report and recommendations of an international meeting held in Bellagio, Italy, March 7–11, 1994 (New York: Rockefeller Foundation, 1994).

14. Girard, "Immunization of chimpanzees."

15. Fast, "Human trials."

16. W. C. Koff and D. F. Hoth, "Development and testing of AIDS vaccines," *Science* 241(1988):426–432.

17. Z. F. Rosenberg and A. S. Francis, "The immunopathogenesis of HIV infection, *Advances in Immunology* 47(1989):377–431.

18. P. H. Fultz, P. Nara, F. Barre-Sinoussi, et al., "Vaccine protection of chimpanzees against challenge with HIV-1 infected peripheral blood mononuclear cells," *Science* 256(1992):1687–1690.

19. J. Cohen, "AIDS vaccine research. A new goal: preventing disease, not infection," *Science* 262(1993):1820–1821.

20. Fast, "Human trials."

21. J. Palca, "Errant HIV strain renders test virus stock useless," *Science* 256(1992):1387–1388.

22. J. Vacsoncellos, *AIDS: Vaccine Research and Development Grant Program*, Assembly Bill 2404, California Health and Safety Code (Sacramento, CA: State Legislature, 1986):chaptered 1462, 199.5–199.60.

23. Vasconcellos, *AIDS: Immunization*, Assembly Bill 2404, California Health and Safety Code (Sacramento, Calif.: State Legislature, 1986):chapters 1463, 199.5–199.60.

24. Rockefeller Foundation, *HIV-Vaccines*.

15

Preparing for HIV Vaccine Efficacy Trials in Developing Countries

WILLIAM L. HEYWARD, SALADIN OSMANOV, AND
JOSÉ ESPARZA

Despite intense national and international efforts, the HIV epidemic continues to spread to new areas and to worsen in areas previously affected.[1] A safe, effective and affordable HIV vaccine would complement current prevention efforts and play a crucial role in future global prevention strategies. Although it may be years before such a vaccine is available, the groundwork must be established now for conducting vaccine efficacy trials in both industrialized and developing countries.[2]

Why conduct HIV vaccine trials in developing countries?

It would be impractical and unethical to exclude developing countries from the HIV vaccine development process. Just as the HIV epidemic is global, so too must the strategy for HIV vaccine development. International HIV vaccine trials will require extensive collaboration and coordination among the host countries and their research institutions, the pharmaceutical manufacturers, regulatory agencies, the World Health Organization (WHO), and other national and international institutions. While it is necessary to conduct all phases of vaccine trials in industrialized countries, it is of paramount importance that the vaccines also be tested in developing countries. There are several reasons for this: (1) the large majority of HIV infections occur in developing countries, where an effective vaccine would eventually be used and have the most benefit; (2) phase III vaccine efficacy trials will need to be conducted in populations with a high incidence of HIV infection in order to produce valid and timely results; (3) the genetic/antigenic variability of HIV may require testing candidate vaccines in different areas of the world; and (4) it may be necessary to evaluate how different routes and/ or cofactors for HIV transmission influence vaccine protection.

Immediate issues in preparing for field trials

Before field trials of HIV vaccines can be conducted in developing countries, several critical issues must be addressed, such as strengthening research infrastructure, monitoring HIV variability, and ethical and social–behavioral matters.

Research infrastructure

Unfortunately, the research infrastructure needed to conduct vaccine trials in most developing countries is limited. In 1992, the WHO Steering Committee on Vaccine Development identified four countries (Brazil, Rwanda, Thailand, and Uganda) for collaboration with national authorities and scientists to implement comprehensive plans for HIV vaccine research, development, and evaluation. In conjunction with this effort, the U.S. National Institutes of Health (NIH) has established the HIV Vaccine Efficacy Trials Network (HIVNET) in nine countries to strengthen field sites for future vaccine trials.

Currently, WHO and institutions in the U.S. and Europe are also collaborating to strengthen capacity in epidemiology and data management, and are supporting cohort studies on HIV incidence to identify potential groups for future HIV vaccine trials. These efforts are helping developing countries face some specific challenges. For example, before trials can begin, accurate estimates of HIV incidence in the target populations are needed to determine sample sizes. These estimates must consider the likely protective effect of nonvaccine interventions (pre- and post-test counseling, education, promotion of condoms, and perhaps STI treatment) which would be made available during a vaccine trial. In addition, if vaccines do not protect against infection, they may still protect against disease. Trial sites must be prepared to evaluate prevention of disease (AIDS) as the end point of a vaccine trial. Finally, laboratory capability will be required to assess a variety of laboratory markers which may predict progression from HIV infection to disease, evaluate unexpected clinical events, and assess immunologic mechanisms for vaccine-induced protection.

HIV variability

The significance of HIV variability for vaccine protection or the immunologic correlates of protection is not yet known. Therefore, genetic and antigenic characterization of HIV in the trial populations is being done in preparation for efficacy trials. This will help ensure that the most appropriate vaccines are selected, and will make it possible to evaluate subtype-specific vaccine efficacy during the trial. WHO has established a Global Network for HIV Isolation and Characterization to monitor HIV genetic and antigenic variability worldwide. The WHO Network is composed of primary laboratories in the vaccine evaluation sites and 13 secondary laboratories in the U.S. and Europe. These laboratories will collaborate to ensure better understanding of the significance of HIV variability, and they will interact with vaccine manufacturers to disseminate relevant results and provide viral strains and other vaccine-related reagents (Chapter 13).

Repeat phase I/II trials

In order to assess the safety and immunogenicity of HIV vaccines in developing country populations with different endemic diseases and immunologic responses, it will be necessary to repeat phase I/II trials locally before initiating a large-scale phase III trial. WHO is working with vaccine manufacturers, national authorities, local scientists, and other institutions to develop the capacity to conduct these trials with appropriate vaccines. As of late 1995, repeat phase I/II trials have been or are being conducted in Brazil and Thailand using three different HIV vaccine candidates.

Ethical and social–behavioral issues

All HIV vaccine trials must be conducted according to the highest ethical standards, and systems must be in place to ensure the protection of human rights. In the cultural context of many developing countries, however, concepts and procedures such as randomization, blinding, placebo, informed consent, and risk/benefit may be largely unknown. To ensure truly informed consent, methods are being developed to communicate these concepts effectively to potential trial participants. To ensure community support, the population at large must be informed as well. In addition, vaccine-related social and behavioral research is needed to determine ethical and logistically feasible incentives for recruiting trial volunteers and ensuring their cooperation in long-term follow-up. Finally, new methods which are applicable to developing country populations are being developed to assess and monitor risk behaviors.

Additional challenges for the future

Availability of an effective vaccine

Even the most effective HIV vaccine will not have an impact on the global HIV/AIDS epidemic unless it is accessible and affordable to all.

Multiple HIV vaccine trials

It is likely that multi-arm and/or multiple trials will be necessary to identify and develop the optimal HIV vaccines. It will be important to coordinate these trials so that results from different geographic locations and populations can be compared. In addition, after an HIV vaccine is developed which is at least minimally effective, it might become difficult to conduct placebo-controlled trials. This means that later efficacy trials may compare a new vaccine to a previous vaccine known to have limited effect. This will require even larger study populations and will also raise difficult ethical issues.

Post-licensure phase IV evaluation of HIV vaccine(s)

Even once an effective HIV vaccine is generally available, innovative strategies must be developed to study HIV incidence and vaccine usage so that the overall public health effectiveness of the vaccine can be evaluated.

REFERENCES

1. M. Merson, "Slowing the spread of HIV: Agenda for the 1990s," *Science* 260(1993):1266–1268.

2. J. Esparza, S. Osmanov, L. Kallings, and H. Wigzell, "Planning for HIV vaccine trials: The World Health Organization perspective," *AIDS* 5(suppl.2)(1991):s159–s163.

16

Women-Controlled HIV Prevention Methods

CHRISTOPHER J. ELIAS, LORI L. HEISE, AND ERICA GOLLUB

The development of new methods of HIV prevention that women can control is an essential part of a comprehensive strategy for limiting the further spread of the AIDS pandemic. Long-standing inequities in gender-based power relations often limit women's ability to avoid sexual partnerships that put them at risk of HIV and other sexually transmitted infections. These same dynamics also restrict many women's ability to successfully negotiate condom use.[1,2] A method of HIV prevention that a woman could employ without requiring the knowledge or consent of her male partner would help many women who are not currently able to protect themselves adequately against HIV infection.[3] Unfortunately, the identification and testing of woman-controlled prevention methods has only recently received attention (Table 16-1).[4]

There are three promising approaches:

- Further development and evaluation of vaginal barrier devices applied by women—including the diaphragm (used with and without spermicide), the cervical cap, and the vaginal pouch ("female condom")
- Clarification of the safety and efficacy of currently available over-the-counter spermicidal products containing nonoxynol-9 or other biodetergent ingredients
- Evaluation of new microbicidal vaginal products based on chemical protection provided by novel ingredients or innovative formulations

In 1993 the U.S. Food and Drug Administration approved the Reality® female condom for marketing. The package insert for this product indicates, "Reality® is intended to be worn by women during sex. It can help prevent pregnancy and sexually transmitted diseases, including HIV infection" (Wisconsin Pharmacal, Jackson, WI). Reality® thus became the first physical barrier device applied by women to be approved for use in the prevention of STIs. There is hope that other vaginal contraceptive methods, such as the cervical cap and diaphragm, may also provide a measure of protection against some STIs.[5]

Based on a review of ten observational studies, Rosenberg and Gollub

Table 16-1   Women-controlled STI/HIV prevention methods

Prevention method, legal status in United States, and cost per vaginal intercourse	Contraceptive effectiveness	Estimated STI effectiveness	Advantages	Disadvantages	Use w/other available methods	Distribution worldwide
BARRIERS						
Female condom; approved May 1993; $1.50–$3.00[a]	79%–95%[b]	79%–95%[c]	Continuous barrier; used by woman; soft feel	Visible to partner; one-time use only	Can be used with spermicide; concurrent condom use not tested	Mainly Europe, U.S.; research protocols in Africa, Asia
Diaphragm; approved; $0.80[d]	82%–98%[e]	50%–75%[f]	Not seen by partner; repeated use	Must currently be fitted; requires spermicide	Use with spermicide for maximum benefit; can be used with male condom	Mostly industrialized countries
Cervical cap; approved 1988; $0.50	82%–94%[e]	50%–75%[f]	Not seen by partner; 2 days wear; less dependent on spermicide for protection; refitting and replacement less frequent than diaphragm	Available models must be fitted	Use with vaginal spermicide for maximum benefit; can be used with male condom	U.K., Germany, U.S., South Africa, Canada
MARKETED SPERMICIDES						
Nonoxynol-9, octoxynol-9; approved; $0.50	79%–100%	50%	Not seen by partner; woman applies; no fitting required	Allergies or irritation possible, especially with higher doses; may require water or disposal facilities; some require waiting time before sex and reinsertion every hour	Use with vaginal barrier or male/female condom for maximum benefit	Both industrialized and developing countries but very variable
Benzalkonium chloride; unapproved; unknown	Similar to N-9	May be superior to nonoxynol-9 in vivo but requires further study; effective against all organisms in vitro	Not seen by partner; woman applies; no fitting required	Possible allergies or sensitivities with long-term use; probable waiting time required between insertion and intercourse	Use with vaginal barrier or male condom for maximum benefit	Canada, France
Menfegol; unapproved; unknown	Similar to N-9	—	Not seen by partner; woman applies; no fitting required	Possible allergies or sensitivities with long-term use; warming action disliked by some; probable waiting time required between insertion and intercourse	Use with vaginal barrier or male condom for maximum benefit	Many developing countries

(continued)

Table 16-1   Women-controlled STI/HIV prevention methods—continued

Prevention method, legal status in United States, and cost per vaginal intercourse	Contraceptive effectiveness	Estimated STI effectiveness	Advantages	Disadvantages	Use w/other available methods	Distribution worldwide
Chlorhexidine; unapproved; unknown	—	Shown to be effective against HIV, gonorrhea, and chlamydia, in vitro	Not seen by partner; woman applies; no fitting required	Possible allergies or sensitivities with long-term use	Use with vaginal barrier or male condom for maximum benefit	Widely available as an antiseptic but limited use in disease prophylaxis
MICROBICIDES UNDER DEVELOPMENT						
Sulfated polysaccharides; other sulfated polymers, reverse transcriptase inhibitors, defensins, synthetic breast milk lipids, monoclonal antibodies, and other surfactants initial stages of research (animal testing); unknown	—	—	Not seen by partner; woman applies; potential for noncontraceptive effect	—	Could be used with vaginal barrier or male condom	Not yet available

[a]Price range reflects difference between public and private sector pricing. Public assistance funds support this product in many U.S. states.

[b]From U.S. trial of Reality® female condom.

[c]Estimate for female condom based on contraceptive efficacy rate. U.S. Food and Drug Administration used contraceptive efficacy as a proxy for anti-STI efficacy in accordance with the Premarket Testing Guidelines for Female Barrier Contraceptive Devices Also Intended to Prevent Sexually Transmitted Diseases (Washington, D.C., USFDA, April 4, 1990).

[d]Assumes initial fitting cost ($125 diaphragm/$200 cap), purchase of device ($30 diaphragm/$50 cap); 2-year average lifetime for diaphragm and 5-year average lifetime for cap; intercourse frequency of twice a week. Figures given are computed over the average lifetime of the device.

[e]Lower boundary represents use-effectiveness, or the effectiveness experienced by women who did not use the product perfectly (some call this "typical use"). Upper boundary is highest effectiveness rate found in any U.S. study of the product. R. A. Hatcher, J. Trussell, F. Stewart, G. K. Stewart, D. Kowal, F. Guest, W. Cates, and M. Policar, *Contraceptive Technology* (New York: Irvington Publishers, 1994): Ch. 8, 9, 27.

[f]Estimate for diaphragms, cervical caps, and spermicides based on review of literature for diaphragms and spermicides (see Rosenberg and Gollub, 1992; Rosenberg, Holmes, and WHO Working Group, 1993). The cervical cap is assumed to be equivalent in STI protection to that of a diaphragm.

Additional references

R. Chalker, *Complete Cervical Cap Guide* (New York: Harper & Row, 1987):175–176.

R. A. Hatcher, J. Trussell, F. Stewart, G. K. Stewart, D. Kowal, F. Guest, W. Cates, and M. Policar, *Contraceptive Technology* (New York: Irvington Publishers, 1994): Ch. 8, 9, 27.

F. Mendez, A. Castro, and A. Ortega, "Use-effectiveness of a spermicidal suppository containing benzalkonium chloride," *Contraception* 34(1986):353–363. Population Information Programme, Spermicides—simplicity and safety are major assets. *Population Reports Series H* 5(1979):H78–118.

M. J. Rosenberg, R. S. Phillips, and the WHO Working Group on Virucides, "Virucides in prevention of HIV infection," *Sexually Transmitted Diseases* 20(1993):41–44.

J. Trussell, J. Strickler, and B. Vaughan, "Contraceptive efficacy of the diaphragm, the sponge and the cervical cap," *Family Planning Perspectives* 25(1993):100–105.

J. Trussell, R. A. Hatcher, W. Cates, F. H. Stewart, and K. Kost, "Contraceptive failure in the U.S.: An update," *Studies in Family Planning* 21(1990):51–54.

N. J. Alexander, H. L. Gabelnick, J. M. Spieler, eds., *Heterosexual Transmission of AIDS* (New York: Wiley-Liss, 1990).

estimate that use of existing female barrier methods reduces transmission of conventional STIs (gonorrhea, chlamydia) by roughly 50 to 75 percent.[6] (Significantly, 9 of 10 observational studies that compared the effect of condoms, diaphragms, or spermicides on the risk of sexually transmitted infections found lower risk among users of female-controlled devices than among condom users. This finding suggests that couples frequently fail to use, or they misuse, male condoms, greatly compromising their effectiveness.) No research at all is available measuring the effect of these barriers against HIV infection, even though their ability to protect the cervix could offer some protection. This should be a high priority area for future investigation.

Tragically, the research community has neglected to explore adequately the safety and efficacy of existing over-the-counter spermicidal products for use as vaginal microbicides. There is considerable evidence that in vitro, nonoxynol-9 and other biodetergent compounds rapidly inactivate HIV, as well as several other STI pathogens.[7,8] Data from clinical studies convincingly suggest that spermicidal products containing nonoxynol-9 provide some protection against cervical infection with gonorrhea and chlamydia under conditions of typical use.[9]

The published studies regarding HIV, however, are conflicting.[10,11] One study of sex workers in the Cameroon demonstrated substantial protection from HIV infection with the vaginal contraceptive film.[12] Another study in Nairobi was discontinued because of concerns that, by causing irritation and microlesions in the vaginal wall, the nonoxynol-9 containing Today® sponge might be augmenting HIV infection rates in a group of sex workers.[13] More recent data suggest that the irritant effects of nonoxynol-9–containing products may be related to both dose and frequency of application.[14] This suggests that under more typical use conditions, existing vaginal spermicides might be recommended for use with a diaphragm or alone as secondary forms of protection when condom use is not possible.[15]

Clarifying the safety and efficacy of various dosages and formulations of nonoxynol-9 is an urgent matter for clinical research. Since these products are already licensed and currently marketed and have a considerable record of consumer safety, they have the potential to play a vital role in expanding women's options for HIV prevention during the relatively long time that will be required until more innovative microbicidal agents become available.

The principle challenges involved in the development of new vaginal microbicidal products have recently been summarized.[16] There are several promising leads being explored, all of which exploit one of two basic strategies: killing or inactivating the virus as soon as it enters the vagina or interfering with the virus' ability to infect epithelial cells.[17] Several investigators are attempting to develop a new generation of surfactants that, like nonoxynol-9, work by disrupting cell membranes. Others are trying to harness the vagina's natural ability to fend off pathogens by developing a gel that will help maintain the naturally acidic environment of the vagina, even in the presence of the strong buffering capacity of semen. (Many scientists believe that the normally low pH of the vagina impairs or inactivates HIV.)

Another promising class of compounds is sulphated polysaccharides, which appear to form a protective chemical barrier blocking HIV transmission in vitro at concentrations significantly below that associated with significant cellular toxicity.[18] Their less irritating nature may allow these products to be safe and effective even under conditions of frequent use. As with other HIV prevention technologies (e.g., vaccines), fully exploring the potential for this approach to HIV prevention will require considerable governmental and nonprofit leadership in collaboration with private industry.[19]

It must be remembered, however, that the spread of HIV will not be stopped with a simple technological fix. The complex issues of human rights, public policy, and social betrayal that have been crystallized by the AIDS pandemic belie such a simplistic approach. We must be prepared to make the long-term, strategic investments necessary to change society, in particular with regard to giving women the power they need to define intimate relationships. The development of woman-controlled prevention approaches, however, is an important incremental step along this road to more fundamental change.

REFERENCES

1. D. Worth, "Sexual decision-making and AIDS: Why condom promotion among vulnerable women is likely to fail," *Studies in Family Planning* 20(1989):297–307.
2. G. R. Gupta and E. Weiss, *Women and AIDS: Developing a New Health Strategy*, policy series 1 (Washington, DC: International Center for Research on Women, 1993).
3. L. L. Heise and C. J. Elias, "Transforming AIDS prevention to meet women's needs: A focus on developing countries," *Social Science and Medicine* 40(1995):931–943.
4. Z. A. Stein, "HIV prevention: The need for methods women can use," *American Journal of Public Health* 80(1990):460–462.
5. M. J. Rosenberg et al., "Barrier contraceptives and sexually transmitted diseases in women: A comparison of female-dependent methods and condoms," *American Journal of Public Health* 82(1992):669–674.
6. M. J. Rosenberg and E. Gollub, "Methods women can use that may prevent sexually transmitted disease, including HIV," *American Journal of Public Health* 82(1992):1473–1478.
7. N. J. Alexander, H. L. Gabelnick, and J. M. Spieler, eds., *Heterosexual Transmission of AIDS* (New York: Alan R. Liss, 1990).
8. M. Malkovsky, A. Newell, and A. G. Dalgleish, "Inactivation of HIV by nonoxynol-9," *Lancet* 1(1988):645.
9. Rosenberg, "Methods women can use."
10. W. Cates, F. H. Stewart, and J. Trussell, "Quest for women's prophylactic methods—hopes vs. science," *American Journal of Public Health* 82(1992):1479–1482.
11. Z. A. Stein, "Double bind in science policy and the protection of women from HIV infection," *American Journal of Public Health* 82:(1992)1471–1472.
12. L. Zekeng, P. J. Feldblum, R. M. Oliver, and L. Kaptue, "Barrier contraceptive use and HIV infection among high-risk women in Cameroon," *AIDS* 7(1993):725–731.
13. J. Kreiss et al., "Efficacy of nonoxynol-9 contraceptive sponge use in preventing heterosexual acquisition of HIV in Nairobi prostitutes," *Journal of the American Medical Association* 268(1992):477–482.
14. S. Niruthisard, R. E. Roddy, and S. Chutivungse, "Effects of frequent nonoxynol-9 use on the vaginal and cervical mucosa," *Sexually Transmitted Diseases* 18(1991):176–179.
15. New York State Health Department, *Methods of Personal Protection for Women to Reduce Transmission of HIV Through Vaginal Intercourse*, policy statement (New York: AIDS Institute, January 1992).

16. C. J. Elias and L. L. Heise, "Challenges for the development of female-controlled vaginal microbicides," *AIDS* 8(1994):1–9.

17. J. Cohen, "Fighting transmission of HIV to women," *Science* 269(1995):778.

18. R. Pearce-Pratt and D. M. Phillips, "Studies on adhesion on lyphocytic cells: Implications for sexual transmission of HIV," *Biology of Reproduction* 48(1993):431–445.

19. C. J. Elias, "Critical issues concerning the accessibility of essential AIDS related health technologies for the developing world," in *AIDS, Health and Human Rights*, J. Mann and C. Dupuy, eds. (Lake Annecy, France: Fondation Marcel Mérieux, 1993):195–200.

17

Who Sets the Global Research Agenda for Biomedical Science?

ROY WIDDUS

Worldwide, when research agendas in biomedical science are set, the dominant influence involves what can loosely be termed "economic" factors. Because research resources are disproportionately available in the industrialized countries, their scientists and policymakers set the research agendas. This is true in both the public and private sectors, although the driving mechanisms differ. Even the small fraction of biomedical research funding allocated to HIV/AIDS in developing countries goes primarily to research areas determined by industrialized countries. This reality highlights the industrialized world's responsibility to ensure that the research agenda will help people everywhere—and as soon as possible.

It is not clear whether the agenda(s) would be completely different if developing country scientists and policymakers were in charge. If developing countries did have more representation in shaping research, however, it is likely that: (1) their priorities would be addressed more directly; (2) the practicality of implementing certain interventions in developing countries would receive more consideration; and (3) the urgency of vaccine development would be heightened.

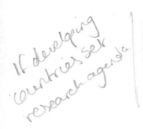

The decision-making process is very similar in most industrialized countries. This article focuses on the U.S., however, because more than 80 percent of the research money is spent by U.S. agencies (Table 17-1).

Public sector (government) biomedical research funds are justified largely on the basis of which benefits will accrue in the U.S. The "constituency" most likely to lobby for increased research budgets is the one that will most immediately benefit—the community of biomedical researchers. Also likely to lobby for generous research budgets are AIDS activist and advocacy groups, often composed of individuals infected with or affected by HIV. The success of activism in influencing research funding is not new to AIDS, although the degree of influence may be unprecedented. Other effective lobbying and activism focusing on research resources have targeted diabetes and hemophilia, the "war on cancer," and more recently, Alzheimer's disease, breast cancer, and women's health. A tension exists in this relationship, however. Although academic biomedical researchers ulti-

Table 17-1 Estimates of the global annual expenditure in 1993 on HIV/AIDS research and development (in U.S. $ million)

	Total expenditure on HIV/AIDS research and development	
	Biomedical & behavioral	Preventive HIV vaccines
INTERGOVERNMENTAL		
WHO	10.0	2.7
European Union	8.2	1.3
Other	N/A	<1.0
GOVERNMENTAL		
France	36.0	6.9
Germany	11.7	2.1
Japan	4.8	0.7
Sweden	6.5	1.0
United Kingdom	23.0	2.5
United States	1,362.0	111.0
Other	4.0	25.0
COMMERCIAL	N/A	<5.0
PHILANTHROPIC	N/A	<2.0
TOTAL	>1,476.2	<160.0

Source: Rockefeller Foundation, *HIV Vaccines—Accelerating the Development of Preventive HIV Vaccines for the World,* summary report and recommendations of an international meeting held in Bellagio, Italy, March 7–11, 1994 (New York: Rockefeller Foundation, 1994).
   Note: N/A, data not available.

mately want drugs or vaccines to come from their work, they lean (perhaps sometimes unconsciously) more towards research that will expand knowledge. AIDS activists, on the other hand, are most likely to press for whatever research they perceive will develop satisfactory treatments most rapidly. The debate on the U.S. agenda for biomedical research shows clear evidence of this "creative" but sometimes heated tension.[1,2]

Broad proposals for research budgets are developed by agency scientists 2, 3 or more years in advance of when funds will be spent. This anticipatory prioritization of research areas may be shaped by proposal developers alone or in consultation with advisory committees or agencies. In fact, the early budget process is predominantly in the hands of government scientists, and advice comes mostly from the academic biomedical community. Although community representatives (e.g., from AIDS advocacy groups) have been added to research advisory committees, their influence at this stage has not been large. Their more visible roles have included lobbying for increased appropriations for research; promoting legislation to change the mechanisms for managing AIDS research (such as the National Institutes of Health's Office of AIDS Research); stimulating expansion of treatment research opportunities in the community rather than in academic centers; and, in some cases, influencing legislators to earmark considerable funds for particular facets of biomedical research, such as pediatric AIDS. Finally, although pharmaceutical companies are in a sense "consumers" of the basic research funded by the public sector, they have little visible role in influencing its priorities or utility to their work.

In both the public and the private sectors, the nature of the budget cycle makes it difficult for research agendas to respond flexibly to change. The budget cycle (including commitment to multi-year projects that will obligate funds in future budgets) for government research funding and the product development "pipeline" in industry are both many years long. This makes it hard to make rapid major revisions in research and development priorities. Establishing flexible discretionary funds has sometimes been proposed as one way to respond quickly to emerging opportunities.

In general, the influence of politics on the research agenda has been to raise or lower the overall emphasis on the issue of AIDS. In the U.S., the Democrat-controlled Congress regularly increased the funding for AIDS research above the amount requested by the former Republican administration. Politicians generally have much more influence over the total *amount* of the research budget than they do over the substantive *content* of the research. However, even this area has seen changes recently—for example, when Congress withheld federal money for sexual/behavioral research. Under the current administration, responsibility for decision-making on the research agenda is once again mainly in the hands of the researchers.

Deciding which specific project proposals to fund within broadly defined research areas is usually left to the peer review process. Peer review panels are drawn predominantly from the academic research community, and they usually focus primarily on scientific quality rather than on whether the results are likely to be applicable.

Translating basic research into products such as drugs, diagnostic tools, and vaccines has traditionally been the province of the research-based pharmaceutical companies. These are, of course, also overwhelmingly located in industrialized countries. Investment in private sector biomedical research and development is largely shaped by the market place. Pharmaceutical companies develop products that they believe will sell at a profit, reward their shareholders for their investment, and provide revenues to support future research and development. This means that the products they consider most attractive are generally for industrialized country markets, and therapeutic agents are usually favored over vaccines, since they normally generate more revenue.

New ways need to be found to focus the industrialized world's immense capacity for research more intensely on the needs of countries heavily affected by HIV. It is to be hoped that such innovations will serve as a model for addressing therapeutic needs in AIDS and other emerging problems in developing countries.

REFERENCES

1. B. N. Fields, "AIDS: Time to turn to basic science," *Nature* 369(1994):95–96.
2. G. Kolata, "AIDS research chief takes conciliatory stance," *New York Times* (May 31, 1994):C3.

18

AIDS Research: Solidarity?
Rivalry? Fraternity?

ANTHONY J. PINCHING

People looking at AIDS research from the outside—whether they are from the media, from advocacy groups, or are researchers in other fields—have often failed to grasp the nature of the research process in general and how it has been applied to AIDS. They have tended instead to focus on a few big issues, which have not been representative of the bulk of research being done and which often have been caricatured beyond all recognition.

The scientific process

Research advances by the creative interaction of data and hypotheses. Hypotheses are framed in an attempt to explain existing data and form the basis of seeking more data to support or, more challengingly, to refute or falsify the hypotheses. As data emerge, hypotheses are modified or rejected, and new ones take their place. One fundamental precept of research is that data have supremacy over hypotheses. Scientists, however, often have a strong personal and emotional investment in their hypotheses (though not in data), and it requires formidable humility to abandon any of them. Of course, this process is not unique to science, indeed it is a basic means by which we come to understand the world around us. Much of the framing of hypotheses is derived from pattern recognition. Our minds connect fragments of information by filling in the gaps, then determine whether the implied picture is valid. An object with four legs could be a dog or a chair. We hypothesize that it is a dog, but closer investigation shows that it is solid, cold, and inanimate. Rejecting the dog hypothesis, we note that it has a seat, and, supposing that it could be a chair, sit down comfortably. We accept, provisionally, that it is indeed a chair, until or unless contradictory data emerge. But if we insist this is a dog, because we desperately need it to be a dog, we deceive ourselves and may deceive others. We become emotionally driven advocates of an untenable hypothesis, and sooner or later, our credibility will be damaged.

Scientific inquiry requires an important question and the methodology with which to test it. The hypothesis may be interesting and important, but

205

if we lack the techniques to investigate it, it cannot advance our ideas. Testability is crucial. If we can control the variables that would inform other hypotheses, then we can put our own hypotheses to a more robust test that uniquely challenges our view. A positive result would more strongly support our hypothesis and might allow us to proceed to a more rigorous test, and so on.

To test a hypothesis, we need to simplify both the system being tested and our conceptual framework. This is essential to scientific process, but we risk oversimplifying and losing sight of the original issue under investigation or, worse, of a valid test of our perspective. At one level, we simplify to help to explain complex phenomena, to give our conception of the world some order so we can control it or at least be able to live with it. To investigate complex phenomena we must take them apart into small controllable and conceptually containable fragments. Sometimes, however, the conviction with which we observe changes that seem meaningful blinds us to the intrinsic limitations of our experimental systems.

A clean and clear-cut observation is seductive. We are driven by our desperate need for answers to big and very human problems—such as how HIV wreaks its destructive effects. When this drive is laced with whatever constitutes personal ambition, it can lead us to look for the mythical "magic bullet."

Our culture in general, and scientific culture in particular, tends to reward individuals for achieving big breakthroughs. This leads to a simplistic view of the scientific process and its protagonists as fairy-tale heroes (and, inevitably, villains) whose discoveries change history. Such discoveries do indeed occur, but the bulk of scientific progress is more like a giant jigsaw puzzle. Each piece added is modest, yet essential to the whole and vital to placing the adjacent pieces. Unless we stand back, we will not see how we have contributed to the big picture or recognize the crucial role the other piece-fitters play. This model of science gives teamwork its due.

Clinical research is a form of scientific inquiry in which observation of patients is the source of ideas, issues, and questions for scientific testing and a wealth of relevant data to apply to the hypotheses. Changes induced by disease can offer insights into normal function and unusual and potent tools with which to study it.

Basic and clinical science are mutually supportive. They can be seen as a double-sided jigsaw where both sides constitute the "big picture." As the pictures take shape, a piece entered on the clinical side can clarify where pieces go on the basic side, and vice versa. (Data from one domain generate new hypotheses to test on the other.) Similarly, when the basic side adds a plausible piece, the clinical side may see that it doesn't fit the clinically derived picture, and vice versa. (Data from one domain falsify the hypothesis in another domain.)

Researchers identify the special opportunities they have to frame and test hypotheses, and use their training and knowledge of their research environment to determine their best potential contribution to the puzzle. They may decide they can be more effective by collaborating with colleagues, a process requiring an understanding and respect for the knowledge and techniques of others, and a willingness to be changed by them. Nowhere has this process been more crucial than in AIDS research.

Early observations on AIDS

AIDS was recognized as an immunodeficiency disease by pattern recognition of the constellation of opportunistic infections associated with it. These revealed the underlying defect in host defense, specifically, in cell-mediated immunity.

The first clinical observations included laboratory data on patients showing severely reduced levels of CD4 cells (recently made readily identifiable by monoclonal antibody labeling) and other defects in cell-mediated immune function. These supported the clinically derived view about the nature of the process and identified a likely target for the causative agent of the disease.

Initially, AIDS was seen to affect a particular group, homosexual men, and this led to a series of hypotheses on causation that might apply to gay men—including recreational drug use, immunosuppression due to allogenic semen exposure, and infective causes. When, shortly thereafter, the disease was seen to affect others—injecting drug users, people with hemophilia, transfusion recipients, and heterosexual contacts and children of these groups, many previously valid hypotheses were immediately rejected (or should have been). The focus shifted to a common, underlying sexually transmitted, blood-borne and vertically transmitted agent that was probably viral and of a type that could survive the processing of blood factor VIII. In this case, pattern recognition was derived from experience with hepatitis B, non-A non-B hepatitis, and other such sexually transmissible agents. The tools of clinical epidemiology were essential to this understanding.

Pursuing a causative agent required combining the techniques of clinical virology with epidemiology to sift and test the possibilities. Testing plausible causative agents against the full epidemiological range of disease sharpened the critical faculties of those in the field. When HIV-1 was proposed and tested, it had a different ring about it than any of the earlier candidates. Further tests were increasingly convincing.

Observations in Africa provided further clues. A new variant of Kaposi's sarcoma (KS) was noted in increasing numbers of patients showing other signs of immunosuppression, such as multidermatomal shingles. Patients with the new variant of KS, but not those with the endemic form, were seropositive for HIV, as were those with the new severe forms of shingles.

These early studies illustrate some key features of the scientific process as applied to AIDS: the origin of questions in new, recognizable but different forms of disease; the synergistic interactions between clinical observation, epidemiology, and laboratory investigation; the ability, indeed the necessity, to encompass all the different populations in whom the new disease was emerging; and above all, the essentially multidisciplinary nature of the work. People had to understand the strengths and limitations of their own and neighboring specialties.

Within a short time, people working in the field started meeting in international and multidisciplinary fora to present their observations and test their ideas on colleagues. Many were strongly motivated by the depth and scale of the unfolding tragedy and were driven by a sense of urgency transmitted by their patients and the wider community. Few have adequately described the extraordinary collegiality of the early years and the openness with ideas and observations that characterized that time. This stood out in marked contrast to previous high-profile and pioneering research. Perhaps it was due to the clinical role that many investigators played, as well as to their relative youth, idealism, and willingness to be challenged.

Of course, not everything went smoothly. Some enthusiastic advocates of particular views were blind to the fact that even the early data offered no support. Theories from scientists working on other types of immunosuppression confused matters by using common words for different things. A misunderstanding about the nature of the clinical disease process spawned many theories. Nonetheless, this early exchange of ideas and data was highly creative, and a vector of all these processes rapidly emerged to establish a common view.

Early researchers faced several hurdles outside the conferences and laboratories. In many countries, official research bodies were slow to understand the importance of AIDS and to establish funding for the range of work that was required. This innate conservatism, plus a certain bias against clinical research in favor of pure biomedical research, proved to be a significant hurdle. Outsiders also failed to recognize that the few initially reported cases represented the beginning of a pandemic. Still others did not appreciate that work on AIDS was likely to facilitate studies in other areas of biomedical research. On the other hand, many scientific journals were quick to recognize the pace of development and streamlined their procedures to help get ideas and data published promptly.

Early on, the necessary eclecticism of the task ran counter to the individualist approach to scientific inquiry. But inevitably, scientists began to champion their own sphere, even though their work depended critically on the framework of ideas being built by the whole group. As the subject area diversified, there was a tendency over time to narrow one's focus to one's own sphere. The majority of researchers, however, retained the fraternal ethos that ensured that competition and ambition enhanced rather than impeded progress. The widely publicized and discussed exceptions have tended to obscure the prevailing tone of cooperation and sharing that we all experienced.

Features of AIDS research

AIDS research illustrates many of the key issues common to all research, but it has also been affected by a number of special features, some of which heightened certain tensions implicit in the research process. First has been the imperative to respond to the human tragedy of AIDS. Directly and indirectly, the patients have given research the means and the motivation to find longer-term solutions to complement the immediate care needs. The general impact of this has been favorable, keeping the focus on the main goals; but the desire for immediate solutions has created an unrealistic impatience with the scientific process. In some cases, notably in areas of clinical trials of new therapies, it has also delayed or diverted progress.

Similarly, while the high media profile of AIDS has helped to draw needed attention to AIDS issues, it has created its own problems. In the early years, considerable misinformation stemmed from the media's mixture of scare tactics and reassurance on the one hand, and unrealistic and uncomprehending reporting on the other—particularly in stories looking for breakthroughs and cures. (The lack of differentiation between a test-tube effect and a clinically proven therapy comes to mind.) Impatience for results has led to false hopes and dashed expectations and to the creation of pseudo-heroes and -villains. Over time, the media's search for novelty has also placed undue emphasis on the fringes of knowledge, and beyond. Patients, the public, and politicians have all been victims of distorted media images.

As AIDS and people working on it continued to make headlines, jealousies were created. Some scientists in other fields felt that AIDS' eventual success in attracting funding and attention diverted resources and interest from their own areas. Eventually, once much of the mainstream thinking on AIDS had been adopted by governments and statutory bodies, some media turned their attention to fostering new mythologies based on increasingly bizarre and scientifically unsustainable heterodoxies. This provided an opportunity to set the "establishment" up for attack. In addition, a few highly publicized issues, whether real or misconstrued, have been used to attack the integrity and motivation of specific AIDS researchers and, by extension, of all AIDS research, casting them as ambitious and callous villains.

Most productive scientists will have made some mistakes and errors of judgment in their work or in the presentation of their results. These can be grossly distorted under the media spotlight, often because of a failure to understand that science moves forward specifically by proposing new ideas or interpretations of data. By necessity, some of them may prove incorrect. No scientist claims infallibility, but the glare of media attention creates a dangerously unforgiving atmosphere. None of this, of course, excuses naïveté, self-promotion, or arrogance—all of which are seen in AIDS research, as in any other area of life. But in the final analysis, few organs of the media have given the public a sound basis for understanding the research process and its outcomes, let alone for exploring its limitations and time course.

AIDS work is by nature multidisciplinary, running the gamut from molecular biology to education psychology, and this has been something of a two-edged sword. Although it has been a creative tool in field work, it has also led to some confusions of concept and misreadings of data because researchers have had to branch out into disciplines they know less well.

Perhaps nowhere else have the dangers of a little bit of knowledge been so evident. Immunological and virological concepts have been oversimplified and misunderstood in translation to other contexts. Some scientists have not always understood the nature of clinical diagnosis or how epidemiology describes what actually happens (as opposed to what might happen). Clinical and basic scientists have ventured into the hazardous terrain of the social sciences, where it is all too easy to get lost, despite seemingly familiar landmarks. And tools designed and validated for one purpose have been transferred unthinkingly to quite different applications, such as using surveillance criteria for AIDS clinical diagnosis, or changing CD4 from prognostic markers to markers for response to therapy, with inevitable confusion.

Probably the most difficult AIDS issues have been in the area of treatment and therapeutic research. The fact that legions of patients need treatment decisions now has led researchers to try to take short-cuts in evaluating new therapies. This has spawned spurious certainties, either based more on hope than on data or extrapolated beyond what the preliminary findings show. Promising treatments are offered as certain solutions, making it harder to determine their real role. If the early promise is not sustained, the reaction may be to deny what has been established. Nowhere is this more evident than in the changing perceptions about using zidovudine (AZT) to treat asymptomatic and symptomatic HIV infection. It is hard to explain and sustain the uncertainty principles essential to conducting clinical trials, when these have been bypassed to meet current patient needs. These problems often result from a genuine and understandable desire to bring today's patients better news; sadly, the result may be to deny future patients the knowledge that would have resulted from a more cautious and modest approach.

Disappointments such as the results of the Concorde trial are a learning process for all concerned, and lead to more realistic goal setting.[1] Concorde has provided a better understanding of why clinical trials follow certain rules. It has also caused a re-thinking of the limitations of current approaches and knowledge, and above all, of the inherently provisional nature of any current therapy. It has brought home to all concerned that wanting something to be true because we need an answer now, is no substitute for the slow hard slog of testing and proving these approaches through the formal scientific process. Reinventing the wheel, however painful it may be, reminds one of why it is round!

Another inherent tension that has characterized therapeutic research in AIDS is that between the evident human tragedy and the imperatives of the pharmaceutical industry. Most therapies are developed by industry and can only become available if that industry is financially secure. Yet the profit motive is seen as distasteful when set against human need. A compound's early promise in the test tube may be promoted, for example, in the financial media, to gain financing for clinical trials, yet such promotion creates high expectations among those affected. Without some publicity, however, companies, especially small ones, may be unable to proceed with the costly, high-risk process of clinical evaluation of new agents.

If there is evidence of clinical promise, it is hard for commercial enterprises to assess their data dispassionately, and they may present an overly positive gloss. Bad news about possible toxicity or limited efficacy may seem to be stifled, but the company needs to get the product licensed in order to recoup development costs before patent protection runs out. Without these funds, industry cannot survive and no drugs would ever reach the patients. Yet there is a strong perception that people's needs are being exploited. It serves no one, however, if industry's involvement is deterred by mindless attacks that are rooted in a failure to understand the essential symbiosis between pharmaceutical companies and front-line work with patients.

The international and multicultural nature of AIDS is another area where misunderstanding has bedeviled scientific research. In the early years, researchers from industrialized countries traveled worldwide to map HIV's spread. Naiveté and cultural insensitivity, combined with the use of poorly validated research tools, sometimes made their motives suspect. Thoughtless pursuit of the "origins" of the epidemic fueled the perception that certain peoples, notably in Africa, were being blamed for the emergence of AIDS.

Such concerns were exacerbated by the fact that foreign investigators did research and published the results without reference to or the involvement of local workers. Not only did this lead to the exclusion of many *bona fide* workers, it also fueled the political and social denial of the epidemic in some regions. Alienated groups in societies throughout the world have had similar experiences, and are often legitimately concerned that HIV is being used to enhance preexisting discrimination. Such painful experiences highlight the fact that knowledge is neither neutral nor abstract. Whether being acquired or disseminated, it is interlocked with human rights.

AIDS research has reminded us not only that the public needs to understand the process, methods, and limitations of science, but also that researchers need to understand the social and human context in which their work is conducted. These first years of AIDS research have taught us all many lessons that should facilitate our work in this and other areas. Greater mutuality of respect and understanding, with more humility and openness, should provide the platform for more effective collaborative research in the future.

REFERENCES

1. Concorde Coordinating Committee, "Concorde: MRC/ANRS randomised double-blind controlled trial of immediate and deferred zidovudine in symptom-free HIV infection," *Lancet* 343(1994):870–881.

PART III

RESPONSE: INDIVIDUALS AND POPULATIONS

When a new problem arises in science, public health, or any other domain, there are two general and distinct ways of perceiving the new situation and responding to it. The first is to use existing tools, methods, and conceptual frameworks; the second is to recognize that previous approaches are inadequate, and so the situation requires new ideas and methods.

The initial response to HIV/AIDS was to apply already existing tools and concepts. This early work led to many important programs and useful discoveries. Yet now, more than a decade later, it is becoming clear that the yield from continued application of these initial approaches is rapidly diminishing.

Pioneering work is increasingly underway. This part of the book examines the transition from earlier to newer frameworks and methods in the context of HIV prevention and care efforts involving different population groups. In each area—including youth, homosexual men, heterosexual men and women, injecting drug users, prisoners, and young children—a similar pattern can be observed.

In each instance, recent work has identified a social dimension that is the critical missing element in prevention programs. In various ways, depending upon the group being considered, society seems to be interfering with more effective HIV prevention. Thus, for youth, social ambivalence about autonomy and responsibility is highlighted; among homosexual men, social stigma still constitutes a formidable barrier to effective prevention; among heterosexuals, the social role and status of women seems vital to future progress; and for blood recipients in the developing world and prisoners in most countries, a lack of social will impedes progress. Current approaches have demonstrated both their usefulness and their limits, and can now be seen as clearly inadequate. Future success in HIV/AIDS prevention will hinge upon the development of a capacity to understand and respond to the missing social dimensions.

19

HIV/AIDS among Women

Three facts are clear: women are increasingly affected in direct, indirect, and complex ways by the HIV/AIDS pandemic; research, prevention, and care activities for women have been slow to develop; and the attention–action gap for women and HIV/AIDS remains large. This chapter provides some details on the scope and impact of what might be called the "acquired attention deficit disorder" towards women in the context of HIV/AIDS.

Analysis of women and HIV/AIDS has also led to insights that have become critical to understanding the entire pandemic. Each of the issues mentioned above shares a common denominator: the unequal role and status of women worldwide. As described further in Part V, this is the heart of the problem of HIV/AIDS and women, whether considering research on HIV infection and clinical AIDS in women, design of HIV prevention programs, or studies on counseling, support, and treatment for women with HIV disease.

Thankfully, awareness of the inextricable linkage between gender inequality and vulnerability to HIV/AIDS is now becoming common knowledge. Yet the challenge that this knowledge presents remains virtually unheeded. What must be done to reduce the "gender gap," as is clearly needed for control of this pandemic? This chapter outlines some of the issues; later chapters on vulnerability and human rights explore the way forward.

Women and AIDS: building a new HIV prevention strategy

Geeta Rao Gupta, Ellen Weiss, and Daniel Whelan

Gender roles and relations

Biological and physiological realities only partially explain gender differences regarding risk of HIV infection. This is because "people, and specifically individual and collective human behavior, constitute the key dimension . . . in the HIV equation."[1] A comprehensive understanding of gender differences in HIV risk must go beyond biological factors to analyze male and female behavior and the ways in which behavior is influenced by gender roles and relations.

Gender relations have been defined as "the processes, structures, and institutions by means of which societies order sex differences and invest them with cultural meanings for the people who act them out in daily life."[2] In most societies, gender relations are characterized by an unequal balance of power, with women having less access than men to education, credit, and formal employment.[3] Women experience great difficulty obtaining access to institutional credit, often because they lack title to land which is often required as collateral.[4] In addition, women farmers receive a far smaller percentage of the credit available through banks and agricultural cooperatives.[5,6,7] Only 30 percent of women in Africa are employed in salaried or wage-earning jobs; in some African countries, fewer than 10 percent of all economically active women are formally employed. Even in Latin America, where women's participation in the formal labor force has been higher, economic crises and adjustment programs are threatening women's wage employment.[8] Throughout the world there are increasingly more poor women than poor men.[9] Also, women are now the sole economic providers in up to one-third of households in the developing world, and these households are disproportionately poor.[10]

These gender inequalities are also reflected in sexual relations between men and women. Men are more likely than women to initiate, dominate, and control sexual interactions and reproductive decision-making. Several studies show that women frequently are denied the right to decide when to have sex and with whom.[11] Evidence now reveals the extent to which women experience forced sex, sexual assault, and physical violence, both within and outside of consensual unions. Decision-making on the use of contraceptives is often also controlled by men, although women generally bear the responsibility for using contraceptives.[12,13]

Assumptions underlying AIDS prevention strategies

Currently, four basic recommendations form the core of most programs for preventing sexual transmission of HIV: abstain from sexual intercourse; practice mutual monogamy; use condoms consistently and correctly; and access appropriate treatment for other sexually transmitted infections. These recommendations assume that people are able to exercise control over the conduct of their sexual relations, and that to reduce the risk of HIV infection, individuals must decide to adopt and sustain HIV-preventive behaviors. In examining the portrait of women's risk of HIV infection, however, it is essential to consider the economic and sociocultural determinants of sexual behavior and the ways in which women are put at risk both by their *own* behavior and by the behavior of their *male partners*, which, in many instances, is currently beyond women's control.

For many women around the world, sociocultural constructions of sexuality and male–female sexual interactions create formidable barriers to adopting HIV risk–reducing behaviors—a reality which directly places women at risk for infection. The economic context of women's lives further complicates the situation. The daily assessment of what must be done to survive in the short-term compromises women's ability to adopt strategies that would reduce the risk of HIV infection in the long-term. Therefore, in order to reduce women's risk, it is necessary to reexamine the assumptions upon which current risk reduction strategies are based. A new set of assumptions must take account of the economic and sociocultural context within which many women live and the realities of their interactions with men.

Economic risk factors

The worldwide economic recession of the 1980s severely affected developing countries. For the 75 percent of the world's women who live in countries with falling or nominally increasing gross domestic products (GDPs), that impact was even more profound.[14] Coupled with already limited access to education, formal sector employment, credit, training, and support for agricultural work, economic recession resulted in even greater economic vulnerability for women.

In this context, for many women worldwide, sexual networking has become an important survival strategy. In Bombay, India, interviews with poor, widowed, divorced, and abandoned women have revealed that they have sex with slum lords in order to guarantee their physical safety and access to resources.[15] In order to meet immediate economic needs, women in Zaire seek occasional sexual partners known as *pneus de rechange* or "spare tires."[16] In Uganda, it has been reported that girls from low-income families are particularly vulnerable to the enticements of older men or "sugar daddies" who offer money or gifts in exchange for sex.[17] In a study from Zimbabwe, high school girls acknowledged the sugar daddy phenomenon and reported that having sex with these men was largely motivated by economic factors.[18] These women are unlikely to adopt HIV prevention messages that encourage reducing the number of sexual partners.

While sexual networking places women at risk for HIV infection, more commonly, adult women are vulnerable to HIV infection as a result of the nonmonogamous sexual activity of their sole male partner. Women perceive the economic consequences of leaving such a relationship to be far more serious than the health risks associated with staying in the relationship. According to a low-income, married woman living in Bombay:

> A woman needs some support. How long will her parents support her. A single woman just can't stay alone, 'isn't it'? So, a woman like me will say, if I've got to have clothes to wear and food to eat, then you do whatever you want (with my body) but keep me as a wife.[19]

For women who lack economic independence and therefore must remain in situations in which they are at risk, the only option is to attempt to negotiate changes in the behavior of their male partners. However, data from research projects conducted in South Africa, Brazil, Guatemala, Papua New Guinea, and India reveal that many women who are aware of their partner's infidelity feel helpless in their ability to change their partner's sexual behavior, since raising the issue of infidelity can disrupt the partnership and even jeopardize the physical safety of the woman.[20-24] For example, a 53-year-old woman from a rural area of Papua New Guinea reported, "I don't get angry or even fight with my husband if he goes out with other ladies because he used to belt me like pigs and dogs."[25] Likewise, an Indian woman from Bombay stated, "When I asked my husband why he had married again, he beat me very badly that night."[26]

Raising the issue of condom use also can lead to conflict, loss of support, and violent repercussions.[27,28] A study conducted in Rio de Janeiro and São Paulo, Brazil, found that women from low-income communities believed that if they were to ask their partners to use a condom, they would implicate themselves as unfaithful and have to bear the repercussions of anger and violence.[29]

Of course, not all women are powerless in sexual relations. A study of African American and Latino women from New Jersey (U.S.) found that the women were able to exert considerable power by withholding sex if the partner did not agree to use a condom.[30] Similarly, Yoruba women from southwest Nigeria were able to refuse sex without violent consequences if their partner had a sexually transmitted infection.[31] In these instances, the women were financially independent, highlighting the importance of economic factors in sexual negotiation.[32]

For women at risk of HIV infection either as a result of sexual networking or as a result of their inability to leave nonmonogamous male partners, economic dependence diminishes their ability to carry out HIV-preventive measures. Economic factors—at both the macroeconomic and household levels—compromise women's ability to protect themselves from HIV infection by forcing them to choose between two competing imperatives: individual HIV risk reduction and economic survival.

Sociocultural risk factors

Beyond the economic determinants of HIV risk is the much broader and complex framework of sociocultural attitudes and norms which shape gender relations. These sociocultural determinants place women at risk by promoting behaviors which favor the sexual transmission of HIV and constraining women's ability to adopt HIV-preventive behaviors.

Feminine ideals and HIV risk

Societal constructions of ideal feminine attributes and roles typically emphasize sexual innocence, virginity, and motherhood. Cultures in many parts of the world consider female ignorance of sexual matters a sign of purity and, conversely, knowledge of sexual matters and reproductive physiology as evidence of diminished virtue.[33,34,35] Recent studies carried out in Brazil, India, Mauritius, and Thailand found that young women knew little about their bodies, pregnancy, contraception, and sexually transmitted infections

(STIs).[36,37,38] Poor, married women from Bombay said they had received no information about sex prior to their own experience.[39]

These cultural norms do not generally apply to men. In Brazil, for example, both men and women believe that men should be more knowledgeable and experienced in sexual matters and that they should be women's teachers.[40] Results from focus group discussions with both men and women in Guatemala also support this finding: one man stated that "It's better that [the husband] is the one to open her eyes. It should be him." One woman said: "It is the man that should orient us."[41]

Such cultural attitudes inhibit women from becoming knowledgeable about their bodies, sexuality, and STI/HIV prevention, thereby constraining their ability to make informed decisions about their sexual behavior and reproductive health. Studies carried out in Latin America among youth without formal sex education showed that adolescent boys were more likely than adolescent girls to know how to use a condom properly, and to recognize the symptoms of STIs.[42,43] Researchers at a STI clinic in Guatemala also reported that one of the women they interviewed had no idea why she was at the clinic nor the purpose of the health service—reportedly she was told to go there by her husband.[44]

Lack of information about their bodies limits women's ability to identify gynecological symptoms that could signify a STI. In many cultures, women accept the itching, burning, discharge, discomfort, and abdominal and back pain of STIs as an inevitable part of their womanhood.[45] Not recognizing these symptoms as evidence of an STI prevents proper diagnosis and treatment.

Lack of information about reproductive physiology contributes to fears among women about condom use. In studies from India, Jamaica, and Brazil, some women reported not liking condoms because they feared that if the condom fell off inside the vagina, it could get lost or travel to the throat.[46,47,48] In South Africa, rural women were particularly concerned about condoms becoming lodged in the vagina during intercourse. Some feared that the woman's reproductive organs would come out when the condom was removed.[49]

Strong cultural norms that emphasize the value of virginity limit young women's ability to seek information or to talk about sex. Young women fear that seeking information on sex or condoms will label them as sexually active regardless of the true extent of their sexual activity. Talking about sexual matters clearly conflicts with the need to preserve the outward appearance of virginity.[50] Low-income adolescents from Recife, Brazil, for example, feared that if their families found out that they had sought gynecological services, their virginity would be questioned.[51]

In cultures where virginity is highly valued, some young women practice alternative sexual behaviors in order to preserve their virginity, although these behaviors may place them at risk for HIV. Anecdotal reports from Latin America suggest that anal sex is practiced among unmarried couples to prevent pregnancy and safeguard virginity.[52,53] Young, unmarried women working in export processing zones in Mauritius report a practice referred

to as "light sex," which is not construed as being sexual intercourse. However, "light sex" involves rubbing the penis against the female genitalia and
vaginal penetration up to the point of pain. Women who practiced "light
sex" felt they were protecting their virginity, and did not perceive themselves to be at risk for pregnancy or HIV infection.[54]

Female virginity symbolizes an innocence and passivity which some men
find erotic. According to one Brazilian man, "I am going to be honest here;
every man likes to have a virgin. To be first is to be the best; to not be
forgotten. I am the first man in her life and she never forgets that, never."[55]
In the age of HIV/AIDS, virginity also signifies cleanliness and purity, and
thus, freedom from disease. In some areas with high prevalence of HIV
infection, it has been reported that older men are seeking out ever younger
girls in the belief that, as virgins, they are free from HIV. In Thailand, the
price men pay for having sex with a virgin at commercial sex establishments is often higher than for sexually active women. In some societies,
men believe that having sex with a virgin will actually cure them of an STI
or HIV infection.[56,57]

The practice of female genital mutilation represents the high price that an
estimated 84 to 114 million women and girls pay as a result of societal
efforts to safeguard virginity and regulate female sexual activity.[58] Female
genital mutilation contributes to subsequent increased trauma during intercourse, which may increase the risk for HIV transmission from an infected
male partner.[59]

Motherhood, like virginity, is generally considered a feminine ideal. Having children defines self-worth and social identity for many women around
the world.[60,61] Economic realities and social pressures also reinforce the
value of motherhood for women, contributing to high fertility rates. Children are viewed as sources of labor for the family and security for parents
in old age.

Given that motherhood is a deeply valued life goal, women remain at risk
for HIV infection during their reproductive years.[62,63] Other than mutual monogamy, HIV preventive behaviors—abstinence, nonpenetrative sex, and
condom use—prevent conception. Without alternative technologies for HIV
prevention, women face a serious dilemma, forcing them to choose between
disease prevention and fulfillment of their highly cherished reproductive
role. Thus, "to provide women exclusively with HIV prevention methods
that contradict the fertility norms of most societies is to provide many
women with no options at all."[64]

Masculine ideals and HIV risk

An understanding of both women's vulnerability to HIV and their options for
HIV prevention also requires examining cultural norms and attitudes about
men's sexual behavior. Cultural norms often condone multiple partnerships
for men and put the emphasis on male pleasure and control in sexual relations.[65-68]

Results from sexual behavior studies around the world indicate that men,
both single and married, have higher reported rates of partner change than

women.[69,70,71] Both men and women in many cultures believe that variety in sexual partners is an essential part of men's nature.[72,73,74] "What happens (having multiple partners) is instinctual," said one Guatemalan man interviewed at a STI clinic. "There is nothing like variation." Another male STI patient from Guatemala remarked, "A man can't be like a woodpecker, always pecking in the same hole."[75] In South Africa, men from rural and periurban communities felt they needed to maintain the tradition of their fathers and grandfathers by having more than one sexual partner. Young men in particular equated having many relationships with being popular and important in the community.[76]

The recognition and condoning of multiple partner relationships for men but not for women begins during adolescence. As a Zimbabwean high school boy remarked, "It feels o.k. about boys having more than one partner. But girls should be faithful to one boy." Another said: "It's not nice for a girl to have many boyfriends but for men it's allowed."[77] In such cultures, therefore, expecting women to discuss mutual monogamy with their partners directly conflicts with the definition of masculinity. Focus group discussions with Jamaican working women revealed that they were very concerned about infidelity by their male partners, but felt that male monogamy was a "pie-in-the-sky" notion.[78]

The emphasis on male sexual pleasure also interferes with HIV prevention by women. In cultures where women are socialized to please men and defer to male authority—particularly in sexual interactions—women feel they cannot refuse to engage in high-risk sexual behavior which they believe is pleasurable for their male partners. For example, in parts of west, central, and southern Africa, many women insert external agents to dry the vagina because of the belief that increased friction is sexually more satisfying for men. These agents include herbs and roots as well as scouring powders which may cause inflammation, lacerations, and abrasions that could increase the efficiency of HIV transmission.[79,80,81] In South Africa, women have reportedly used such drying agents not only to increase their partners' pleasure, but because they believed their partners could construe their vaginal secretions as a sign of an STI, which would suggest infidelity.[82]

Anal sex, practiced to varying degrees by women around the world, is another sexual behavior which places women at risk of infection in an effort to please their male partners.[83] Women factory workers in Rio de Janeiro and São Paulo reported that their partners pressure them to engage in anal sex. According to one married female factory worker:

> My husband wants to have anal sex with me. . . . He thinks it is pleasurable, but I don't. He gets angry. He says that I am his woman and I have to accept these things. . . . I think that my husband possibly looks outside for this.[84]

For some Brazilian men, anal sex implies the conquering of a second virginity and symbolizes their power and control over women:

> [Anal sex] is a conquest because women never want to give there. One must be careful because it is an intimate part of her. When you do it there, he did her over again like a virgin. Anal sex is the ultimate, the final barrier. Many

people feel this way. Many women feel that it shows a lack of respect on the part of the man. (São Paulo, male factory worker, age 24).[85]

Nonconsensual sex, the most extreme form of male control, is a pervasive reality in adolescent girls' and women's lives and is increasingly being recognized as a barrier to reducing women's risk of HIV infection. Many women are forced to have intercourse against their will, both within and outside of consensual unions.[86] In these circumstances, partner reduction and condom use may be impossible preventive options for women (Box 19-1).

BOX 19-1

Relationship between women's status and HIV risk

DANIEL WHELAN

Evidence from around the world suggests that women's risk of HIV is closely related to their social and economic status. To explore this relationship, the author measured the association between HIV seroprevalence among pregnant women in 19 countries[1] and two indicators of women's status.[2] The women's status indicator was developed from a compilation of several statistics measuring women's health, family status, education, employment, and social equality. The gender equality indicator is based on the level of gender equality within the following areas: life expectancy; marital status (widowed, divorced, separated); literacy; share of paid employment; and societal equality. A high score for both indicators of women's condition represents a high rating, whether overall or in comparison to men. As Figures 19-1.1 and 19-1.2 show, there is a negative association between each of the indica-

Figure 19-1.1 Correlation between Women's Status Indicators and HIV Seroprevalence among Pregnant Women in 19 Countries. (Sources: U.S. Bureau of the Census and Population Crisis Committee)

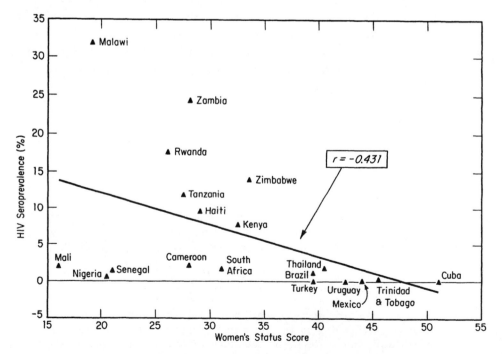

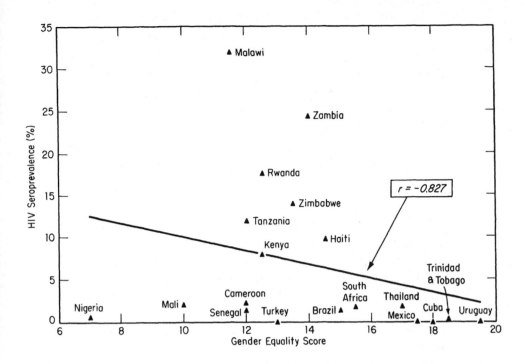

Figure 19-1.2 Correlation between Gender Equality Indicators and HIV Seroprevalence among Pregnant Women in 19 Countries. (Sources: U.S. Bureau of the Census and Population Crisis Committee)

6:03:22rs and HIV seroprevalence. In other words, the higher the level of women's status or gender equality, the lower the HIV seroprevalence among pregnant women. Whereas this analysis is only suggestive, it does lend support to the qualitative data presented above.[3]

References

1. U.S. Bureau of the Census, Center for International Research, *HIV/AIDS Surveillance Database* (Washington, DC: U.S. Bureau of the Census, 1994).
2. Population Crisis Committee, *Country Rankings of the Status of Women: Poor, Powerless, and Pregnant* (Washington, DC: Population Crisis Committee, 1988).
3. Regarding the sample size of 19 countries, the following should be noted: not all developing countries were ranked by the Poor, Powerless, and Pregnant (PPP) index, most notably countries that have the most reliable seroprevalence data on pregnant women, such as Uganda, Zaire, Burundi, and Botswana. In preparing this analysis, the following criteria were used to choose and calculate national seroprevalence data for each country in the analysis. First, the authors chose data that met "high scientific standards," as defined by the Center for International Research of the U.S. Bureau of the Census. Second, neither HIV-2 nor dual HIV-1/HIV-2 infection seroprevalence data was used. Third, all sample sizes from individual seroprevalence studies with sample sizes <100 were eliminated. Finally, although developed countries in North America and Europe were indexed by the PPP study, they were not included because corresponding data for pregnant women were not available from the Center for International Research.

Building a new HIV prevention strategy

During the formulation of many of the current HIV risk reduction strategies in the mid-to-late 1980s, very little was known about the risks that women, other than sex workers, faced in the age of HIV/AIDS. However, recent research illuminates many of the realities of women's sexual lives, including ways in which economic and sociocultural realities and norms directly influence women's vulnerability to HIV infection. These analyses highlight the inadequacy of current risk reduction approaches for many women around the world. Failure to recognize economic and sociocultural factors in any examination of women's vulnerability to HIV will be devastating in terms of HIV-related morbidity and mortality for millions of women around the world.[87]

New policies and programs to reduce women's vulnerability to HIV infection are urgently required. The following recommendations target the societal context of women's lives:

- Focus resources on structural changes to improve the status of women by increasing women's access to education, credit, skills training, and employment. AIDS has exposed the damaging consequences to society of women's powerlessness. Improving women's economic status would also contribute to a more equitable power balance in gender relations.
- Support biomedical research for the development of a female-controlled preventive technology that women can use without the knowledge of their partner (Chapter 19).
- Make STI services more available and accessible to women by integrating them with family planning and maternal health services. This integration would help remove the social stigma attached to seeking STI services and would make diagnosis and treatment of STIs more likely, thus reducing women's vulnerability to HIV infection as well as their risk of serious gynecological complications.
- Help to empower adolescent girls and women by (1) increasing their knowledge about their bodies and sexuality, as well as about HIV and other STIs, and (2) improving their skills in using condoms and negotiating safe sexual behaviors with their partners. Provide girls and women with opportunities for group interactions to model new behaviors, share personal experiences, and develop a critical consciousness about their sexual roles. Such efforts can facilitate individual behavior change as well as possibly lead to collective action to change sociocultural norms in the community.
- Design programs for adolescent boys and men that promote sexual and family responsibility. Educating men and boys on the consequences of multiple partnerships and high-risk sexual behavior is clearly essential to reducing both their own risk of HIV infection and that of their female partners.
- Fund participatory action research that (1) examines the cultural, economic, and social factors related to sexuality and gender relations; and (2) ensures a strong focus on the realities of women's lives. In many countries, data are limited regarding the sexual attitudes of men and women, the cultural and socioeconomic factors that put women at risk, and the options available to women for AIDS prevention. Such

information is critical for designing appropriate and effective interventions for women and for initiating a policy dialogue on women's needs and vulnerability.

REFERENCES

1. J. Mann, D. Tarantola, and T. Netter, eds., *AIDS in the World* (Cambridge, MA: Harvard University Press, 1992).
2. B. G. Schoepf, "Gender, development, and AIDS: A Political Economy and Culture Framework," in *Women in Development Annual*, Vol. 3, R. S. Gallin, A. Ferguson, and J. Harper, eds. (Boulder, CO: Westview Press, 1993):53–85.
3. M. Buvinic and S. W. Yudelman, *Women, Poverty and Progress in the Third World*, Headline Series 289 (New York: Foreign Policy Association, 1989).
4. M. Lycette, *Improving Women's Access to Credit in the Third World: Policy and Program Recommendations* (Washington, DC: International Center for Research on Women, 1984).
5. L. Fortmann, "Women's work in a communal setting: The Tanzanian policy of Ujamaa" in *Women and Work in Africa*, E. Bay, ed. (Boulder, CO: Westview Press, 1982):191–205.
6. K. Staudt, "Bureaucratic resistance to women's programs: The case of women in development," in *Women, Power and Politics*, E. Bonepart, ed. (New York: Pergamon Press, 1982):263–279.
7. B. Knudson and B. A. Yates, *Economic Role of Women in Small Scale Agriculture in the Eastern Caribbean—St. Lucia* (Barbados: University of the West Indies, 1981).
8. UN, *World's Women 1970–1990: Trends and Statistics*, Social Statistics and Indicators, Series K No. 8 (New York: UN, 1991).
9. R. L. Sivard, *Women, A World Survey* (Washington, DC: World Priorities, 1985).
10. Buvinic, *Women, Poverty*.
11. C. J. Elias and L. Heise, *Development of Microbicides: A New Method of HIV Prevention for Women*, working paper 6 (New York: Programs Division, Population Council, 1993).
12. M. L. Boulos, R. Boulos, and D. J. Nichols, "Perceptions and practices relating to condom use among urban men in Haiti," *Studies in Family Planning* 22(1991):318–325.
13. A. K. Boye, K. Hill, S. Isaacs, et al., "Marriage law and practice in the Sahel," *Studies in Family Planning* 22(1991):343–349.
14. UN, *World's Women*.
15. A. George and S. Jaswal, *Understanding Sexuality: Ethnographic Study of Poor Women in Bombay*, Women and AIDS Program Research Report Series (Washington, DC: International Center for Research on Women, 1994).
16. B. G. Schoepf, E. Walu, W. N. Rukarangira, et al., "Gender, power and risk of AIDS in Zaire," in *Women and Health in Africa*, M. Turshen, ed. (Trenton: Africa World Press, 1991):187–203.
17. Panos Institute, *AIDS and Children: A Family Disease* (London: Panos Institute, 1989).
18. M. T. Bassett and J. Sherman, *Adolescent Sexual Behavior and HIV Prevention*, Women and AIDS Program Research Report Series (Washington, DC: International Center for Research on Women, 1994).
19. George, *Understanding Sexuality*.
20. Q. Abdool Karim, et al., *Determinants of a Woman's Ability to Adopt HIV Protective Behaviour in Natal/Kwazulu, South Africa: A Community Based Approach*, Women

and AIDS Program Research Report Series (Washington, DC: International Center for Research on Women, 1994).

21. D. Goldstein, *Culture, Class, and Gender Politics of a Modern Disease: Women and AIDS in Brazil*, Women and AIDS Program Research Report Series (Washington, DC: International Center for Research on Women, 1994).

22. B. Bezmalinovic, W. Skidmore DuFlon, and A. Hirschmann, *Guatemala City Women: Empowering a Hidden Risk Group to Prevent HIV Transmission*, Women and AIDS Program Research Report Series (Washington, DC: International Center for Research on Women, 1994).

23. National Sex and Reproduction Research Team and C. Jenkins, *National Study of Sexual and Reproductive Knowledge and Behaviour in Papua New Guinea*, monograph 10 (Goroka, Papua New Guinea: Papua New Guinea Institute of Research, 1994).

24. George, *Understanding Sexuality*.

25. National Sex Research Team, *National Study*.

26. George, *Understanding Sexuality*.

27. Schoepf, "Gender, power and risk."

28. D. Richardson, *Women and AIDS* (New York: Methuen Books, 1988).

29. Goldstein, *Culture, Class, and Gender*.

30. A. Kline, E. Kline, and E. Oken, "Minority women and sexual choice in the age of AIDS," *Social Science and Medicine* 34(1992):447–457.

31. I. O. Orubuloye, J. C. Caldwell, and P. Caldwell, "African women's control over their sexuality in an era of AIDS—a study of the Yoruba of Nigeria," *Social Science and Medicine* 37(1993):859–872.

32. Elias, *Development of Microbicides*.

33. A. Ankomah, "Premarital sexual relationships in Ghana in the era of AIDS," *Health Policy and Planning* 7(1992):135–143.

34. J. C. Caldwell, P. Caldwell, and P. Quiggin, "Social context of AIDS in sub-Saharan Africa," *Population and Development Review* 15(1989):185–234.

35. K. Carovano, "More than mothers and whores: Redefining the AIDS prevention needs of women," *International Journal of Health Services* 21(1992):131–142.

36. A. Vasconcelos, A. Neto, A. Valença, et al., *AIDS and Sexuality among Low-Income Adolescent Women in Recife, Brazil*, Women and AIDS Program Research Report Series (Washington, DC: International Center for Research on Women, 1994).

37. A. Bhende, *Evolving a Model for AIDS Prevention Education among Underprivileged Adolescent Girls in Urban India*, Women and AIDS Program Research Report Series (Washington, DC: International Center for Research on Women, 1994).

38. K. Cash and B. Anasuchatkul, *Experimental Educational Interventions for AIDS Prevention Among Northern Thai Single Migratory Female Factory Workers*, Women and AIDS Program Research Report Series (Washington, DC: International Center for Research on Women, 1994).

39. George, *Understanding Sexuality*.

40. Goldstein, *Culture, Class, and Gender*.

41. Bezmalinovic, *Guatemala City Women*.

42. L. Morris, P. Bailey, and L. Nunez, *Young Adult Reproductive Health Survey in Two Delegations of Mexico City: English Language Report* (Mexico City: Centro de Orientación para Adultos Jovenes, 1987).

43. G. Castellanos, A. Conde, and E. Monterroso, *Encuesta Sobre Salud y Educación Sexual de Jovenes, Departamento de Guatemala, Areas Urbanas, Reporte Final* (Guatemala City: Asociación Guatemalteca de Educación Sexual [AGES], 1989).

44. Bezmalinovic, *Guatemala City Women*.

45. George, *Understanding Sexuality.*
46. *Ibid.*
47. Bezmalinovic, *Guatemala City Women.*
48. Goldstein, *Culture, Class, and Gender.*
49. Abdool Karim, *Determinants.*
50. S. Schensul, G. Oodit, J. Schensul, et al., *Young Women, Work, and AIDS-Related Risk Behavior in Mauritius,* Women and AIDS Program Research Report Series (Washington, DC: International Center for Research on Women, 1994).
51. Vasconcelos, *AIDS and Sexuality.*
52. *Ibid.*
53. Bezmalinovic, *Guatemala City Women.*
54. S. Schensul, *Young Women, Work.*
55. Goldstein, *Culture, Class, and Gender.*
56. Bezmalinovic, *Guatemala City Women.*
57. R. Dixon-Mueller and J. Wasserheit, *Culture of Silence* (New York: International Women's Health Coalition, 1991).
58. N. Toubia, *Female Genital Mutilation: A Call for Global Action* (New York: Women, Ink., 1993).
59. Bezmalinovic, *Guatemala City Women.*
60. Carovano, "More than mothers."
61. P. Mane and S. A. A. Maitra, *AIDS Prevention—The Sociocultural Context in India* (Bombay: Tata Institute of Social Sciences, 1992).
62. F. A. Mahmoud, B. O. de Zalduondo, D. Zewdie, et al., "Women and AIDS in Africa: Issues old and new," presented at the Annual Meeting of the African Studies Association, Atlanta, Georgia, November 1989.
63. Mane, *AIDS Prevention.*
64. Carovano, "More than mothers."
65. J. W. McGrath, C. B. Rwabukwali, D. A. Schumann, et al., "Anthropology and AIDS: The cultural context of sexual risk behavior among urban Baganda women in Kampala, Uganda," *Social Science and Medicine* 36(1993):429–439.
66. Orubuloye, "African women's control."
67. Mane, *AIDS Prevention.*
68. E. Weiss and G. Rao Gupta, "AIDS prevention for women: Issues and challenges," in *Women at the Center: Development Issues and Practices for the 1990s,* G. Young, V. Samarasinghe, and K. Kusterer, eds. (West Hartford: Kumarian Press, 1993): 168–181.
69. National Sex Research Team, *National Study.*
70. Orubuloye "African women's control."
71. W. Sittitrai, T. Brown, P. Ohanuphak, et al., "Survey of partner relations and risk of HIV infection in Thailand," Abstract M.D.4113, presented at the VII International Conference on AIDS, Florence, Italy, June 1991.
72. Orubuloye, "African women's control."
73. Goldstein, *Culture, Class, and Gender.*
74. Mane, *AIDS Prevention.*
75. Bezmalinovic, *Guatemala City Women.*
76. Abdool Karim, *Determinants.*
77. Bassett, *Adolescent Sexual Behavior.*
78. G. E. Wyatt, M. B. Tucker, D. Eldemire, et al., *Female Low Income Workers and AIDS in Jamaica,* Women and AIDS Program Research Report Series (Washington, DC: International Center for Research on Women, 1994).
79. Abdool Karim, *Determinants.*
80. C. I. Niang, *Sociocultural Factors Favoring HIV Infection, and Integration of Tradi-*

tional Women's Associations in AIDS Prevention Strategies in Kolda, Senegal, Women and AIDS Program Research Report Series (Washington, DC: International Center for Research on Women, 1994).

81. A. Runganga, M. Pitts, and J. McMaster, "Use of herbal and other agents to enhance sexual experience," *Social Science and Medicine* 35(1992):1037–1042.

82. Abdool Karim, *Determinants.*

83. M. deBruyn, "Women and AIDS in developing countries," *Social Science and Medicine* 34(1992):249–262.

84. Goldstein, *Culture, Class, and Gender.*

85. *Ibid.*

86. J. Elias, *Development of Microbicides.*

87. *Ibid.*

20

HIV in Women: What Are the Gaps in Knowledge?

ZENA A. STEIN AND LOUISE KUHN

There are two reasons why research on the HIV epidemic in women has been slow to develop. First, the gay rights movement was a driving force behind much initial activism and AIDS research in the United States and Western Europe, thus research has focused on HIV in men. The HIV epidemic has since spread to women in these countries, but it has predominantly affected women with particularly limited power to challenge or influence the medical and research establishment. Second, as shown in Figure 20-1, although women in developing countries, particularly in sub-Saharan Africa, have been infected with HIV in equal or greater numbers than men since the start of the epidemic, AIDS research has been driven primarily by the concerns of industrialized nations. As a result, issues of considerable importance to women have been generally neglected. By definition, the knowledge gap regarding HIV/AIDS and women means that research has not been sufficiently focused on problems that are specific to women. What are these major outstanding questions?

HIV transmission

In heterosexual transmission, the major source of new infections worldwide, the vulnerability of women is related to both biological and social factors (Box 20-1). High rates of HIV infection among adolescent women have been demonstrated in many developing countries.[1,2] Young women appear to be biologically more susceptible to HIV infection than older women, and HIV is more efficiently transmitted from men to women than from women to men. Considerable study is needed to establish the reasons for these differences in susceptibility.

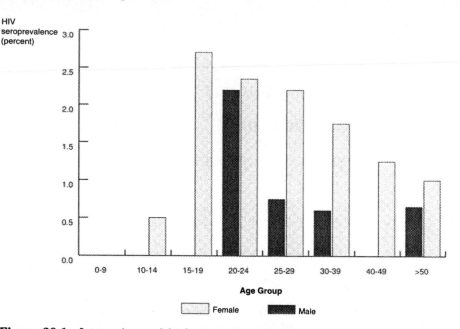

Figure 20-1 Interaction and biologic and social risk: HIV seroprevalence by age and sex in Natal/KwaZulu, South Africa, 1990. Adapted from Obdool Karim, et al., *AIDS* 6 (1992):1535–1539.

BOX 20-1

Gynecologic disease among women with HIV/AIDS

CAROLA MARTE

Gynecological and other women-specific issues are only now entering the HIV/AIDS agenda. As an example, since the beginning of the epidemic, oral candidiasis (thrush) has played a prominent role in disease staging in both clinical care and research (and has been a benchmark for service-related entitlements in the United States). However, there is still no definitive research on persistent vaginal candidiasis, the most common problem among HIV-infected women.

Vaginal candidiasis can be used to illustrate certain general issues of diagnosis and treatment. After the acute retroviral syndrome, vaginal candidiasis is likely to occur at an earlier stage in HIV disease progression than is oral candidiasis[1] (Figure 20-1.1). Effective treatment is available, but left untreated, vaginal candidiasis can cause painful and disabling ulceration. Women with frequent recurrences benefit from a regimen of suppressive therapy. While these are strong arguments for diligence about diagnosis and treatment, most women and often their providers still regard any genital infection as shameful. As a result, many women suffer silently and unnecessarily with candidiasis.

Treatment for vaginal candidiasis, as for oral thrush, can be topical or systemic. Recently, systemic therapy for more severely immune-suppressed individuals has gained favor, for it offers convenient and effective treatment for oral and vaginal candidiasis simultaneously and also provides prophylaxis against opportunistic fungal infections like esophageal candidiasis or cryptococcal meningitis in severely immune-suppressed individuals.[2] Unfortunately, systemic drugs are expensive and drug-resistant candidiasis has also been reported. Most clinical trials on candidiasis do not address vaginitis; it is obviously important for women that future clinical trials include this problem.

The relationship between HIV infection and cervical cancer is the gynecologic issue that has re-

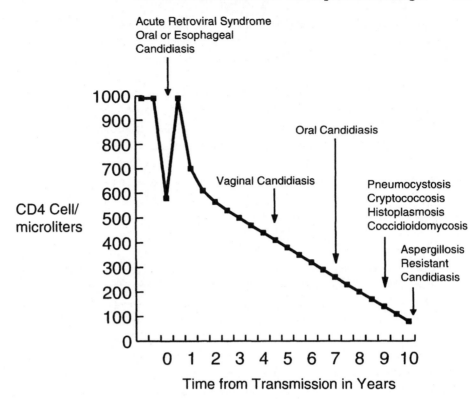

Figure 20-1.1 Occurrence of fungal infections during the course of progressive HIV infection. Adapted from *Clinical Care* 6 (1994).

ceived the most attention. Most cervical cancer arises in women with prior human papillomavirus (HPV) infection, the most common STI worldwide. The cervical dysplasia triggered by HPV is a pre-malignant lesion, the end stage of which is invasive cervical carcinoma (ICC). ICC rates vary greatly worldwide; ICC is the most common female cancer in sub-Saharan Africa, Southeast Asia, Latin America, and the Caribbean, regions disadvantaged by insufficient screening and treatment for cervical disease or STIs. Therefore, women in countries with rates of HIV in women such as Thailand, India, and Uganda will bear the full impact of ICC-HIV comorbidity and mortality.

Women with HIV infection are at a much higher risk—five- to eightfold higher—for cervical dysplasia, the precursor for ICC.[3] Both prevalence and severity of cervical dysplasia correlate with CD4 lymphocyte depletion and degree of immunosuppression.[4-8] The large majority of cases of mild dysplasia progress slowly, if at all; most do not advance to cancer in women with normal immune function. It is not yet known whether dysplasia is more likely to become cancerous or to progress more rapidly in immunodeficient women.

Much less is known about HIV and ICC. Clinical reports suggest that ICC is more aggressive in HIV-infected women; in these women, recurrences and multifocal and high-grade lesions are unusually common.[9] Therefore, an urgent research question is whether current therapies are adequate to treat cervical disease and prevent the development of carcinoma in HIV-infected women. As always, the cost of therapy will be a critical issue for developing countries.

The 1994 revision of the U.S. Centers for Disease Control and Prevention (CDC) AIDS Case Definition includes ICC as an AIDS indicator disease.[10] ICC has also been proposed for inclusion in a revised AIDS definition for resource-poor countries.[11] Naming ICC as an AIDS indicator disease was an unusual step because few reports so far have demonstrated increased ICC in HIV-infected women.

The rationale, however, is that HIV-infected women's increased susceptibility to cervical dysplasia, the precursor lesion to ICC, has been well documented. The relationship of cervical cancer's frequency and severity to degree of immunosuppression in HIV-infected women and its viral etiology (analogous to EBV-related lymphoma) increases the likelihood that HPV-related disease is an opportunistic infection and that HIV-infected women are highly vulnerable to ICC.

A very large or very long study would be needed to document increased ICC rates among HIV-infected women. In contrast to HPV infection and cervical dysplasia, background rates of ICC are low in the more affluent countries which have the resources both to treat dysplasia before it progresses to ICC and to undertake large clinical studies. In addition, the latency period prior to development of ICC (20 years in women with normal immune function) is about twice as long as the average for developing life-threatening opportunistic infections in HIV-infected people. Thus HIV-related death would often precede mortality from ICC. Further, HPV and HIV have the same socioeconomic and STI risk factors, making it difficult to sort out the epidemiological relationship between HIV disease and HPV disease in smaller study populations.

Research is also markedly inadequate for other women-specific HIV-related conditions. Developing topical virucides will require much more research on the role of vaginal mucosa in either inhibiting or facilitating HIV transmission. Also, little is known about the interrelation of immunosuppression and hormonal changes that may be due to HIV itself or to antiretroviral and other agents used to treat HIV-infected women. Widespread use of oral contraceptives and increasing use of implanted or injectable hormonal contraceptive agents worldwide make this an urgent gynecologic question.

Finally, even when gynecologic issues achieve some priority on the HIV agenda, research will be of little benefit unless the social context in which research findings could be effectively applied is also considered. Sexual behavior and the impact of cultural attitudes on sexual choices must come to the center of the discussion.[12] If these issues are granted the attention they deserve, much information of great importance to the lives and well-being of women and girls could be gathered in the next few years.

References

1. N. Imam, C. Carpenter, K. H. Mayer, et al., "Hierarchical pattern of mucosal candida infections in HIV-seropositive women," *American Journal of Medicine* 89(1990):142–146.

2. S. D. Nightingale, S. X. Cal, D. M. Peterson, et al., "Primary prophylaxis with fluconazole against systemic fungal infections in HIV-positive patients," *AIDS* 6(1992):191–194.

3. T. Wright, T. Ellerbrock, M. Chiasson, et al., "Cervical intraephithelial neoplasia in women infected with human immunodeficiency virus: Prevalence, risk factors and validity of Pap Smears," *American Journal of Obstetrics and Gynecology* 84(1994):591–597.

4. S. H. Vermund, K. F. Kelley, R. S. Klein, et al., "High risk of human papillomavirus infection and cervical squamous intraepithelial lesions among women with symptomatic human immunodeficiency virus infection," *American Journal of Obstetrics and Gynecology* 165(1991):392–400.

5. A. Shafer, W. Friedmann, M. Mielke, et al., "Increased frequency of cervical dysplasia-neoplasia in women infected with the human immunodeficiency virus is related to the degree of immunosuppression," *American Journal of Obstetrics and Gynecology* 164(1991):593–599.

6. C. Marte, P. Kelly, M. Cohen, et al., "Papanicolaou smear abnormalities in ambulatory care sites for women infected with human immunodeficiency virus," *American Journal of Obstetrics and Gynecology* 166(1992):1232–1237.

7. M. Laga, J. P. Icenogle, R. Marsella, et al., "Genital papillomavirus infection and cervical dysplasia—opportunistic complications of HIV infection," *International Journal of Cancer* 50(1992):45–48.

8. M. Conti, A. Agarossi, F. Parazzini, et al., "HPV, HIV infection, and risk of cervical intraepithelial neoplasia in former intravenous drug abusers," *Gynecologic Oncology* 49(1993):344–348.

9. M. Maiman, R. G. Fruchter, L. Guy, et al., "Human immunodeficiency virus infection and invasive cervical carcinoma," *Cancer* 71(1993):402–406.

10. Centers for Disease Control, "1993 revised classification system for HIV infection and expanded surveillance case definition for AIDS among adolescents and adults," *Morbidity and Mortality Weekly Review* 41(1992):1–19.

11. K. De Cock, S. Lucas, D. Coulibaly, et al., "Expansion of surveillance case definition for AIDS in resource-poor countries," letter, *Lancet* 342(1993):437–438.

12. E. Reid, "Changing the focus," *IAS Newsletter* 9(1994):11–13.

It is now well established that infection with other sexually transmitted infections (STIs) increases the transmission of and susceptibility to HIV infection.[3,4] Barriers which hinder the prompt identification and appropriate treatment of STIs in women need to be determined (Chapter 6). Several other factors which may increase women's susceptibility to HIV infection also need to be investigated further. Vaginal drying agents and dry sex may lead to inflammation or abrasion of the vagina and cervix, which is a plausible mechanism to increase the efficiency of HIV transmission. Hormonal contraceptives may increase the risk of HIV infection through their effect on cervical ectropion.[5] This raises further questions about the risk of HIV infection throughout stages of the menstrual cycle. Finally, there is still no information on sexual practices that might permit transmission of HIV from woman to woman.

Prevention programs

Thus far, HIV prevention programs that focus on sexual behavior change among heterosexuals have had only limited success. Prevention programs need to address gender differences in the ability to negotiate and ensure safer sex practices; thus far, it has been difficult to incorporate this focus in prevention programs.

Women-controlled prevention technologies

The issue of woman-controlled methods of HIV prevention has recently received greater recognition and impetus.[6] The introduction of the female condom into industrialized country markets and increasing interest in currently available barrier methods (cervical cap, diaphragm, spermicides) are important recent advances. Further research is needed to determine the effectiveness of these methods in preventing HIV infection. However, since preliminary evidence supports a protective benefit, these methods should be promoted as alternatives, especially for women whose male partners are unwilling to use traditional condoms.[7,8]

For some women, the fact that condoms (and other barriers used for HIV prevention) also prevent conception is a major impediment to their use. It is possible that a microbicide could have viricidal but not spermicidal properties; it has not yet been established whether sperm itself is a source of virus. HIV prevention programs need to include approaches that allow the possibility of becoming pregnant, for example, by limiting unprotected sex to fertile days of the menstrual cycle. Although such a message is complex, programs promoting natural family planning have found that even women with little education can successfully learn these methods.[9] Increasing women's knowledge of their bodies is both necessary for such an approach and beneficial for prevention in general.

Societal dimensions

Both economic dependence on men and male violence (and/or the threat of violence) may also interfere with risk reduction for many women. Therefore, prevention programs need to take into consideration existing gender inequality and continue to devise innovative strategies for rapid empowerment of individual women. Yet in the long term, societal changes are crucial to improving the position of women. The social position of women, while universally disadvantaged relative to men of similar class and racial backgrounds, is different around the world. More understanding of the specific forms of this inequality of power relations in different countries and cultural and social settings is needed.[10–13]

Enormously high rates of HIV infection among sex workers have been reported in some studies which have also highlighted sex workers' extreme vulnerability to HIV infection and their need for support to protect themselves from infection. In some societies, men traditionally frequent brothels; sex workers may play an important part in sexual relations in circumstances where job demands remove men from home for long periods of time, for example, members of the military, migrant workers, truck drivers, and sailors.[14] Most research has focused on women self-identifying as sex workers or working within brothels or other establishments. There is little understanding of the range of contexts in which sex is exchanged for money, goods, services, or accommodation—circumstances not necessarily perceived as direct sex work.[15]

Injection drug use among women and their male partners has made the major contribution to HIV infection in women in the United States and Western Europe. It has seemed easier to focus on unsafe drug-using practices than on sexual risk behavior. Yet injection drug use may actually be overshadowed by sexual transmission, even in the United States and Europe. High-risk sexual encounters and sex for drugs have also been associated with the use of crack cocaine in cities in the United States, thus contributing to sexual transmission of HIV.[16] Finally, the role of alcohol in HIV transmission has not been well researched; alcohol may impede safer sex practices or lead to abusive and violent behavior in male partners of women.

Urbanization and migration have long been recognized as important factors in the spread of STIs.[17] Studies in Africa have consistently reported an urban–rural gradient (higher to lower) in HIV prevalence and have also demonstrated an increased risk of HIV infection associated with migration.[18,19] In circumstances in which mainly the men move, the behavior of a male partner may be more important in determining the HIV risk for a woman than her own sexual behavior.

Care and support

Finally, women undertake most of the care of people with HIV disease and the care of surviving children of other HIV-infected women. Long-term societal impacts of these burdens on women must be documented.

There are clearly important, unresolved questions about HIV/AIDS and women. The existence and persistence of an "attention–action gap" with regard to women and HIV/AIDS provides additional evidence that a societal approach is needed to complement current research and action in prevention and care.

REFERENCES

1. E. Reid and M. Bailey, *Young Women: Silence, Susceptibility and the HIV Epidemic.* United Nations Development Program (New York: United Nations, 1992).

2. Q. Abdool Karim, S. S. Abdool Karim, B. Singh, R. Short, and S. Ngxongo, "Seroprevalence of HIV infection in rural South Africa," *AIDS* 6(1992):1535–1539.

3. M. Laga, M. Alary, N. Nzila, et al. "Condom promotion, sexually transmitted diseases treatment, and declining incidence of HIV-1 infection in female Zairian sex workers," *Lancet*, 344(1994):246–248.

4. H. Grosskurth, F. Mosha, J. Todd, et al., "Impact of improved treatment of sexually transmitted diseases on HIV infection in rural Tanzania: Randomised control trial." *Lancet* 346(1995):530–536.

5. G. B. Moss, D. B. A. Clemetson, L. D'Costa, et al., "Association of cervical ectopy with heterosexual transmission of HIV: results of a study of couples in Nairobi, Kenya," *Journal of Infectious Diseases* 164(1991):588–591.

6. J. M. A. Lange, M. Karam, and P. Pilot, "Boost for vaginal microbicides against HIV," *Lancet* 341(1993):1356.

7. C. Elias and L. Heise, *Development of Microbicides: A New Method of HIV Prevention in Women*, working paper 6 (New York: Programs Division, Population Council, 1993).

8. Z. Stein, "HIV Prevention: An update on the status of methods women can use," *American Journal of Public Health* 83(1993):1379–1382.

9. WHO, "Prospective multicentre trial of the ovulation method of natural family planning. II. The effectiveness phase," *Fertilization and Sterility* 36(1981):591–598.

10. K. Jochelson, M. Mothibeli, and J. P. Leger, "Human immunodeficiency virus and migrant labor in South Africa," *International Journal of Health Services* 21(1991):157–173.

11. G. R. Gupta and E. Weiss, *Women and AIDS: Developing a New Health Strategy*, policy series 1 (Washington, DC: International Center for Research on Women, 1993).

12. H. Amaro, "Love, sex and power," *American Psychologist* 50(1995):437–447.

13. M. T. Bassett and M. Mhloyi, "Women and AIDS in Zimbabwe: The making of an epidemic," *International Journal of Health Services*, 21(1995):143–156.

14. M. Ramphele, "Dynamics of gender politics in the hostels of Cape town: Another legacy of the South African migrant labor system," *Journal of South African Studies* 15(1989):393–414.

15. Jochelson, "Human immunodeficiency virus."

16. M. A. Chiasson, R. L. Stonegumer, D. S. Hildebrandt, et al., "Heterosexual transmission of HIV-1 associated with the use of smokable freebase cocaine (crack)," *AIDS* 5(1991):1121–1126.

17. S. L. Kark, "Social pathology of syphilis in Africans," *South African Medical Journal* 23(1949):77–84.

18. Abdool Karim, "Seroprevalence of HIV."

19. M. J. Wawer, D. Serwadda, S. D. Musgrave, J. K. Konde-Lule, M. Musagara, and N. K. Sewankambo, "Dynamics of spread of HIV-1 infection in a rural district of Uganda," *British Medical Journal* 303(1991):1303–1306.

Youth and HIV/AIDS

Societies around the world have great difficulty promoting and protecting the health of young people (which we will consider here as 13–24 years old) against HIV infection as well as other hazards. Yet the HIV/AIDS pandemic will have a growing impact on their health and their lives.

It is appropriate to focus on young people as they fall between children and adults, two well-established demographic and social categories. Children are generally considered to be in need of protection against HIV, to which they may be exposed through their relation to and the actions of others: through HIV-infected mothers, unsterile medical injections, contaminated blood products, or sexual abuse by adults. In contrast, adults are assumed to be capable of protecting themselves; they are seen as independent and autonomous, as making informed choices and using appropriate health and social services. Within this framework, the concept of childhood virtually denies personal choice or preference, while personal responsibility for actions and outcomes is the defining principle of adulthood.

However, since young people are caught in a period of transition from "helpless" childhood to "responsible" adult status, they exist in a "no person's land" in both social and public health terms. Societies around the world have ambivalent attitudes towards youth, seeing them simultaneously as small adults and as immature, inexperienced, and untrustworthy children (large children). Consequently, it is not surprising that public health is conflicted and confused in its approach to young people and HIV prevention.

This chapter illustrates and explores the consequences for HIV prevention of profound social ambivalence regarding young people. The main expression of this ambivalence is a pervasive unwillingness to consider and respect the real lives of young people. This constitutes a special form of socially derived vulnerability that handicaps and constrains efforts to prevent HIV infection among young people. These realities have not generally been taken into account in designing and implementing prevention strategies for young people.

HIV/AIDS in young people

Neal D. Hoffman and Donna Futterman

According to available data, young people worldwide can be estimated to account for less than 10 percent of total AIDS cases. However, this low percentage is misleading as an indication of the impact of AIDS on young people. In the United States, for example, by 1988 AIDS was already the sixth leading cause of death for youth.[1] Information on the broader extent of HIV infection among young people worldwide has generally been limited to studies of specific subpopulations. For example, in 1990, among young people entering the U.S. Job Corps (a federally funded training program for disadvantaged young men and women aged 16 to 21), 3 per 1,000 were HIV positive, and in a shelter for homeless and runaway youth in New York City, the seroprevalence between 1987 and 1990 was more than ten times higher (50 per 1,000).[2,3] Among street youth in Toronto, the HIV seroprevalence rate was 2 per 1,000 in the early 1990s[4] and the median seroprevalence at five sites serving homeless youth (less than age 25) between 1989 and 1992 was 23 per 1,000 (range: 0–73 per 1,000).[5] The HIV seroprevalence among secondary school students 15–24 years of age in Mwanza, Tanzania, was 16 per 1,000.[6]

In the absence of population-based seroprevalence data, other indicators may be necessary to suggest the extent of HIV infection among young people.[7,8] In the U.S., by using back-calculation to link data on the incidence of AIDS to the incidence of HIV infection, an overall decline in the estimated mean age at the time of HIV infection has been noted: before 1986 the mean age at HIV infection was 29 years and during the late 1980s it declined to 21 years.[9] Alarmingly, in the U.S. between 1987 and 1991, one of every four persons newly infected with HIV was under the age of 22.[10]

A youth-centered approach to HIV/AIDS prevention

All HIV prevention programs must address the central realities of the target population. The identification of these realities is difficult for any group, for two reasons. First, the issues of highest importance for HIV risk and prevention will likely be sensitive, potentially threatening, or embarassing to reveal. Second, to identify, acknowledge, and address these realities, the full, voluntary, and informed participation of the target group is absolutely necessary. In addition to these generic difficulties, genuine concern and respect for, and partnership with, young people may be hampered by the extent to which parental roles, desires, or fears intervene.

Research and experience in different cultural and social settings suggest that four realities are vital to thinking about and developing HIV prevention strategies for young people:

1. youth are marginalized and disempowered within society
2. youth are actively developing their personal behaviors and values
3. the familial and intrafamilial roles of young people are changing

4. youth are confronting important barriers to making and effecting free and informed choices

Youth marginalization and disempowerment

In general, youth are simultaneously prized (as "the future of our country") and treated with a lack of respect for their individual capacity and competence. For example, while AIDS prevention strategies all recognize the vital importance of information, education, and health services, young people's access to health information and services is often severely restricted. Two reasons for this limitation include a lack of resources and adult censorship. Information may be withheld intentionally or omitted as a result of adult fears, inexperience, or lack of knowledge. Adults have difficulty acknowledging the actual extent of adolescent sexual activity and often express common, ill-informed prejudices against sex education, such as the belief that it will encourage early experimentation with sex. (Box 21-1 reviews sex education studies that contradict such fears).

BOX 21-1

Sex education: adolescents' future versus adults' fears

MARIELLA BALDO

For an HIV/STI prevention program to be effective for youth, educators and young people must be able to talk together openly about sex and sexuality. This requirement often conflicts, however, with two common prejudices held by many adults: that sex education encourages young people to experiment with sex prematurely, and that teaching about contraception and condom use means condoning sexual activity. Adults and policymakers who hold such beliefs can put up powerful barriers to the introduction of school-based HIV prevention programs. The impact of these prejudices is reinforced by the fact that planners, teachers, parents, community leaders, and the media all tend to underestimate the extent of sexual activity and STI in adolescents, despite clear trends toward earlier age at first intercourse.[1,2]

To address these objections to discussing sex in health education programs, the WHO Global Programme on AIDS commissioned three reviews of studies on the effects of sex education.[3,4,5] Most published studies are from industrialized countries.[6] While they generally report increased levels of knowledge and some attitude change among students who have attended a sex education course, it has been established that this does not necessarily translate into safe sexual practices.[7,8] Therefore, one of the three WHO-sponsored reviews focused on the behavioral impact of sex education programs as measured by rates of teenage pregnancy, abortion, birth, sexually transmitted infections (STIs), and self-reported sexual activity.[9] The studies in this review showed that:

- sex education programs did not lead to earlier or increased sexual activity in young people, even when contraceptives were made available
- sex education programs may delay initiation of sexual intercourse, decrease sexual activity, and increase the adoption of safer sexual practices in sexually active young people

One study was particularly relevant to adult fears that young people's access to and use of condoms will increase promiscuity. It found that a fourfold increase in condom use among 17 to 20 year olds (during 5 years of systematic campaigns) did not increase casual sexual activity, nor did it result in earlier sexual activity or an increase in the number of sexual partners.[10]

A separate study of U.S. high school students showed a decline in sexual activity and number of partners and an increase in condom use among sexually active youths under 15 years of age, the vast majority of whom reported having received information and education on HIV.

The nature and content of school-based sex education programs are crucial to their success.[11] Programs which tend to be most effective are attended before the onset of sexual activity;[12] combine participatory methods, parents' involvement, and access to health services;[13] and use a social-influence approach.[14] The latest sex education curricula have adopted a social-influence approach and have been more effective than their predecessors. The new curricula focus on the context of sexual relationships, and insist on the creation of social norms conducive to safer practices; develop specific life skills necessary to resist pressures for unwanted and unprotected intercourse; and often use peer leaders. Sex education programs which tend to be less effective are those which offer abstinence as the only prevention method,[15] are limited to short presentations[16] and stand against a set of strong determinants of early intercourse.[17]

Parents and other adults must be informed of these findings about sex education and sexual behavior. Like fears that needle availability or exchange will increase injection drug use, fears that sex education will lead to increased sexual activity are seriously interfering with effective HIV prevention. Planners need to work with the users of their programs: adolescents are seldom asked to articulate their needs and aspirations in life, from which their views on prevention will develop. This flaw in the planning process often translates into programs that focus on sex-related problems as perceived by adults, rather than on young people's experience, motivation and strengths.[18]

References

1. M. Leslie-Harwit and A. Meheus, "STD in young people: The importance of health education," *Sexually Transmitted Diseases* 16(1989):15–20.
2. E. R. Allgeier, "HIV/AIDS and sex education strategies," unpublished review (Geneva: WHO, Global Programme on AIDS, 1993).
3. E. R. Allgeier, "HIV/AIDS and sex education."
4. N. Ford, A. Ankomah, A. Fort D'Auriol, E. Davies, and E. Mathie, *Review of Literature on the Health and Behavioural Outcomes of Population and Family Planning Education Programmes in School Settings in Developing Countries* (Geneva: WHO, Global Programme on AIDS, 1992).
5. A. Grunseit and S. Kippax, *Effects of Sex Education on Young People's Sexual Behaviour* (Geneva: WHO, Global Programme on AIDS, 1993).
6. M. Baldo, P. Aggleton, and G. Slutkin, "Does sex education lead to earlier or increased sexual activity in youth?", Abstract PO-D02-3444, presented at the IX International Conference on AIDS, Berlin, Germany, June 1993.
7. J. D. Fisher, S. J. Misovich, and W. A. Fisher, "Impact of perceived social norms on adolescents' AIDS-risk behavior and prevention," in *Adolescents and AIDS*, R. J. DiClemente, ed. (Newbury Park, CA: Sage Publications, 1992).
8. D. Kirby, "Sexuality education: A more realistic view of its effects," *Journal of School Health* 55(1985):421–424.
9. Grunseit, *Effects of Sex Education.*
10. M. Blanchard, F. Narring, and P. A. Michaud, "Effects of the Swiss Stop-AIDS campaigns 1987–1992: Increase in condom use without promotion of sexual promiscuity," Abstract PO-D02-3474, presented at the IX International Conference on AIDS, Berlin, Germany, June 1993.
11. A. Grunseit, S. Kippax, P. Aggleton, M. Baldo, and G. Slutkin, "Sex education and its effects on young people's sexual behaviour: A review of studies," submitted for publication.
12. M. Howard and H. B. McCabe, "Helping teenagers postpone sexual involvement," *Family Planning Perspectives* 22(1990):21–26.
13. L. S. Zabin, M. B. Hirsch, E. A. Smith, R. Streett, and J. B. Hardy, "Evaluation of a pregnancy prevention program for urban teenagers," *Family Planning Perspectives* 18(1986):119–126.
14. D. Kirby, "School-based prevention programs: Design, evaluation and effectiveness," in *Adolescents and AIDS*, R. J. DiClemente, ed. (Newbury Park, CA: Sage Publications, 1992).

15. F. S. Christopher and M. W. Roosa, "Evaluation of an adolescent pregnancy prevention program: Is 'just say no' enough?" *Family Relations* 39(1990):68–72.

16. C. Newman, R. H. DuRant, C. S. Ashworth, and G. Gaillard, "Evaluation of a school-based AIDS/HIV education program for young adolescents," *AIDS Education and Prevention* 5(1993):327–339.

17. W. Marsiglio and F. L. Mott, "The impact of sex education on sexual activity, contraceptive use, and pre-marital pregnancy, among American teenagers," *Family Planning Perspectives* 18(1986):151–162.

18. World Health Organization, United Nations Educational, Scientific and Cultural Organization, School Health Education to Prevent AIDS and Sexually Transmitted Diseases: A Resource Package for Curriculum Planners (WHO, Geneva, and UNESCO, Paris: WHO/UNESCO/GPA 1994 1/2/3).

Adult attitudes towards young people, even if they are well intentioned, generally violate the basic criteria for partnership. The power imbalance between youth and adults exacerbates this difficulty, which adults (as the powerful agent) may not perceive. However, to the extent that young people are not considered and treated as genuine partners in dialogue and decision-making, programs for youth are unlikely to be well designed or effective.

Development of personal behaviors

Physical maturity and both physical and intellectual competence are by definition in a state of quite rapid development during this time of life. In addition, young people are engaged in serious personal and social development tasks unique to this age-group, specifically including sexuality and drug use. Given young people's psychological state of perceived invulnerability, the concept of risk-taking has different meanings for young people than for adults.

Both entertainment and advertising media play a significant role in the lives of youth, particularly with respect to messages about sexuality. One review of the entertainment media in the U.S. found that young people watching television for 3–5 hours after school see about 57 acts of sexual behavior weekly; in the evening hours they can see nearly three times that number in a week. Two-thirds of music videos portray sexual feelings and three-fourths of popular songs are about love and sex. In addition, the typical R-rated* film in the United States shows from one to two dozen sexual acts. Yet this explicit depiction of sexual intimacy is rarely accompanied by references to STIs and pregnancy.[11] For example, in the U.S., none of the major television networks allows condoms to be advertised. As a result, young people receive little practical information from the media about sexuality, intimacy, and protection. They are not helped in developing the skills necessary to negotiate intimacy with their peers and to protect themselves from adverse consequences of their sexual experiences.

Risk-taking and experimentation are characteristic of adolescent development. Adolescence is a series of stages with associated development issues.

*In the U.S., an "R" rating allows people under the age of 17 to view a movie in a public theater only when accompanied by an adult.

For HIV prevention programs to help modify risk-taking behaviors they must take these stages into account. Theories about how health-related behavior is modified generally identify certain prerequisites for making and maintaining positive changes. However, in working with adolescents, it is necessary to link these general prerequisites with youth-specific, personal development issues.[12] For example, physical, mental, and emotional development occur at different and uneven rates in adolescence.[13] During adolescence social skills improve and the ability to think in abstract terms, understand and identify with others, show empathy, and be secure in beliefs and values increases. In many cases, however, physical maturity occurs before youth have developed the intellectual, emotional, and social skills necessary to behave in ways that will limit their risk of exposure to HIV.[14]

Risk-taking is an outgrowth of the development of individual identity and the testing of social conventions, combined with feelings of invulnerability.[15] As their intellectual abilities develop, youth will often learn through trial and error, and their ability to link actions with consequences increases. As they move through adolescence, their feelings of omnipotence and immortality tend to resolve and they develop a greater ability to compromise and set limits on their behavior. As part of the maturation process, youth often question established social norms, for they are in the process of forming lasting attitudes and behaviors.[16]

Young people are also engaged in the process of separating from family and identifying with peer groups. In early adolescence, youth strive to become independent by intensifying peer relationships and initiating activities separate from parents and family. Parental conflicts and peer involvement and conformity peak during middle adolescence, as youth increasingly identify with peer group values and behavior. At this stage, youth may use group norms to justify particular behaviors, and risk reduction programs must recognize and try to influence such pressures. Usually, during late adolescence, there is a redirection from peer to more intimate relationships and a refinement of one's value system, often reintegrating parental values.[17]

For homosexual men and women, the development of a positive sexual identity will be influenced both by the youth's ability to cope with social stigma and by whether he or she finds adult role models. This may be especially difficult in the many societies where the concept of a gay identity does not exist.[18] School-based education about sexuality is often limited to the experience of heterosexual young people. This disregards both the range of sexual experience among youth and the unique social and developmental issues facing homosexual minority youth.

Opposite-sex experiences are also common for lesbian and gay youth, both as a part of self-discovery and as a way to conceal their homosexuality from themselves, their peers, family, or larger community.[19-22]

Finally, the use of alcohol, marijuana, and other substances can impair judgment and is associated with potentially unsafe sexual behaviors, although the precise temporal relationship between exposure to drugs and decisions regarding unsafe sexual practices is unclear. Among a cohort of young male conscripts in the Royal Thai Army, frequent contact with female sex workers was associated with sexual debut before age 17 and with both alcohol and marijuana use.[23] In the northwestern U.S., a study of 241 pregnant young women under age 17 significantly correlated alcohol use in general and alcohol use during sexual intercourse with unsafe sexual behaviors.[24]

Changing roles of young people

The role of youth in societies and families throughout the world is rapidly changing. Particularly in developing countries, this is a period of transition in which youth are assuming new, nontraditional roles, often involving more responsibility and more authority over their lives. Contributing to this transition is an ongoing erosion of traditional family structures and intrafamilial relations. Traditional cultural values have come into conflict with imported values, and young people have become increasingly skeptical about the relevance of received cultural values, particularly in the context of societal tensions, unemployment, violence, political instability, corruption, economic recession and, perhaps, the HIV/AIDS pandemic. Reducing youth's vulnerability to HIV infection requires understanding that young people's role in the balance of power within familial and intrafamilial relations has already changed and will likely change further.

Barriers to making choices

Together, these realities create substantial barriers against young people's capacity to make and effect free and informed choices. Many adults harbor distorted ideas and myths about their own personal histories and the social realities of sexual behavior. Many adults simply did not encounter similar situations when they were young and may not be able to understand the challenges and issues faced by young people today.

Health care and HIV prevention

Health care systems do not generally serve the best interests and the needs of young people. Although many models of health care for youth exist, few provide a comprehensive approach to pregnancy, or STI and HIV education, prevention, testing, and treatment. Integration of young people into the health care system is important for prevention education, as youth report that they generally view health care providers as a useful and preferred source of health information (Table 21-1).[25]

In the United States, acute care rather than prevention is often the focus of health professionals' interaction with youth. The U.S. Centers for Disease Prevention and Control's National Ambulatory Medical Care Survey found that preventive health screening procedures, such as Papanicolaou (Pap) smears, breast and vision examinations, and cholesterol measurements, were performed in less than 5 percent of office visits to physicians by youth. Further, in 66 percent of these visits, no counseling or advice was pro-

Table 21-1   Models of STI/HIV care services for youth

	Advantages	Disadvantages
Adolescent health clinic	Integration of STI with primary care; HIV counseling and testing available; appealing environment for youth	Hours and location often not convenient
STI clinic	STI expertise; HIV counseling available; more convenient hours and locations	Unable to provide primary care; not appealing to youth
School-based clinic	Able to offer primary care; convenient for youth	Does not reach out-of-school youth; STI care, HIV counseling and testing, and contraceptive services not always available
Office-based	Widely available	Limited STI expertise; expensive; unable to offer time needed for HIV counseling; not youth-specific

vided, and HIV transmission issues were discussed in fewer than 1 percent of visits.[26]

Health care visits by youth are also frequently quite brief. U.S. data on office visits by youth with a health care provider indicate that nearly half the visits are shorter than 10 minutes, and 30 percent last only 10 to 15 minutes.[27] Thus youth may not interact with the health care system long enough for providers to communicate risk reduction messages adequately, despite the young person's potential receptivity to information presented in this setting.

The U.S. Society of Adolescent Medicine has identified several factors that have contributed to youths' lack of integration into comprehensive health care programs, including availability, visibility, quality, confidentiality, affordability, flexibility, and coordination.[28]

While school-based initiatives are a potentially valuable source of health care for youth, further progress in providing services will conflict with societal prejudices and will likely encounter political resistance. Societies around the world will likely resist efforts to provide youth with additional freedom and services that are perceived as being outside parental or other adult control.

Partnerships and programs

Genuine partnerships between young people and education or health authorities are needed. One such partnership is the HIV/AIDS Education Program which reaches one million children and youth in the New York City school system. The program's designers produced developmentally appropriate curricula for different age-groups, and from the beginning, both students and parents were encouraged to provide input. HIV/AIDS education teams are composed of students, parents, and teachers who have completed a three-and-a-half day training program designed and taught by both local and national experts.[29]

Another innovative program involves one-third of the state schools in São Paulo, Brazil. Developed by the Work and Research Group for Sex Education, this program requires its sexuality educators to attend a preliminary, 16-hour workshop on learning methodology and to receive ongoing weekly supervision. They learn how to be a catalyst for open discussion and debate and how to create a safe space where students can discuss their sexual values, beliefs, or fears. Both parents and students are invited to an introductory meeting, although a youth's participation in the program is not contingent upon his or her parent's attendance. On the first day, students choose which areas they want to explore. Preliminary reports by both educators and youth indicate that students who participated in the curriculum were more able to articulate opinions and question issues, and felt more solidarity and companionship with their classmates.[30]

Yet if prevention initiatives for youth were limited to schools, a large number of young people would be neglected. In developing countries in 1985 there were 277 million out-of-school youth between the ages of 12 and 17.[31] In Latin America more than half of all 15-year-olds have already left school.[32] These young people must be reached.

Worldwide, an estimated 100 million youth live on the street.[33] Particularly in Latin America and certain cities in industrialized countries, the concept of disenfranchised youth includes two categories: youth who live on the streets by day but who can go home at night (*niños en la calle*, or "youth on the street"), and youth who live and sleep on the streets (*niños de la calle, meninos and meninas de rua*, "youth of the street").[34] Many of these young people are runaways who have left home without parental consent, others are "throwaways" forced out by parental rejection, and still others are homeless because they have been orphaned or as a result of poverty or war. Regardless of the circumstances, this early separation from home and family often disrupts adolescent development.[35]

Since many of these youths engage in survival sex in exchange for food, clothing, shelter, and protection, as well as have sex to obtain companionship and affection, they are at substantial risk for HIV infection. In addition, several surveys indicate that many street youth engage in commercial sex for money and/or drugs, often with adults and injection drug users who are more likely to be infected with HIV and other STIs. Few of these young people report that they use condoms consistently.[36] Among street youth who smoke crack cocaine, high rates of HIV infection, syphilis, and gonorrhea have already been reported.[37-40]

Often sexual abuse at home may be the factor that leads youths to leave and to live on the streets.[41] But whether it drives them from home or not, sexual victimization not only places them at immediate risk for HIV infection, but also increases their future risk by affecting their psychosocial development with regard to sexual self-esteem, self-concept, and overall adaptive functioning (Box 21-2). Within a cohort of pregnant youth, those who had been sexually victimized had initiated sexual activity 1 year earlier, were less likely to use contraception at first intercourse, and were more likely to have used drug or alcohol during their first intercourse.[42] Over half of females and about a quarter of males in a cohort of HIV-positive youth in New York City reported a history of sexual abuse as minors.[43]

BOX 21-2

Sexual abuse of children and HIV/AIDS

GEORGE A. GELLERT

Sexual abuse illustrates the linkage between approaches to HIV/AIDS in children and larger societal issues affecting children's health. First, HIV may be transmitted to children through sexual abuse. Sexually transmitted infections (STIs) are already recognized as serious sequelae of child sexual abuse. Over 300,000 cases of child sexual abuse are reported each year in the United States,[1] and 5 to 6 percent of adults recall sexual victimization during childhood.[2] Two to 10 percent of children examined after they had been sexually abused were diagnosed with an STI.[3,4] Gonorrhea, condylomata acuminata (human papilloma virus), and chlamydial and herpes infections have been documented in sexually abused children.[5,6,7,8,9] While these data suggest a need for concern about HIV infection as a result of child sexual abuse, prevalence and trends remain unknown.[10] Nevertheless, as the incidence of both HIV infection and reported sexual abuse rises, transmission of HIV to abused children may increase.

However, some information about HIV and sexual abuse is available. A practitioner survey in the U.S. identified 18 abused children with HIV infection.[11] A U.S. national study identified 28 children with a history of sexual abuse who were infected in the absence of any other risk factor for infection.[12] Among these 28 children, 64 percent were female, 71 percent were African-American, and the mean age was 9 years.[13] Co-infection with another STI occurred in 9 (33 percent) cases. The basis for HIV antibody testing included physical findings suggestive of HIV infection (9; 32 percent); identification of an HIV seropositive or high-risk perpetrator (8; 28 percent); and the presence of another STI in the victim (4; 14 percent). In this study, perpetrators involved a child's parent in 10 (42 percent) cases, and another relative in 6 (25 percent) cases. Only 16 (50 percent) of perpetrators had known behavioral risk factors or signs/symptoms of HIV infection. Six children were reported to have been infected through five or fewer abusive episodes, which suggests that sexual abuse was a relatively efficient setting for HIV transmission, perhaps owing to trauma associated with sexual abuse and immaturity of the child's genital tract.

In a study in Zimbabwe, 12 of 54 children who were sexually abused were tested for HIV: four were seropositive, six were negative, and the results for two were unavailable.[14]

Child sexual abuse and subsequent risk of HIV acquisition

Not surprisingly, psychosocial difficulties are common among adults who were abused as children. Several studies have suggested that adults with a prior history of having been sexually abused may have an increased likelihood of having high-risk sexual behavior.[62,63] Thus sexual abuse of children, even when not resulting in HIV transmission, may contribute to the victim's later, eventual risk of becoming HIV infected.

Toward a better response

Among HIV-infected children, perinatal transmission should not be automatically assumed. Situational and sociodemographic factors may increase the likelihood of both maternal HIV infection and child sexual abuse. Sexual abuse should be considered as a potential mode of transmission of HIV infection, and certainly of other STIs, to children. Children who have been abused should be evaluated for

STIs and selectively for HIV infection, particularly if the perpetrator is known to be seropositive or to engage in high risk behaviors, if abuse occurred in a geographic area of high disease prevalence, or if the child has symptoms of HIV infection or another STI. Children found to have an STI or to be infected with HIV (and lacking a clear history of prior transfusion or maternal-perinatal infection) should be evaluated for sexual abuse. Physicians and health and social service providers for children require education about the risk of HIV infection resulting from sexual abuse and they need guidelines on how to respond to situations where sexual abuse possibly occurred.[15]

References

1. Council on Scientific Affairs, "AMA diagnostic and treatment guidelines concerning child abuse and neglect," *Journal of the American Medical Association* 254(1985):769–800.
2. D. Finkelhor, "Sexual abuse of children: Current research reviewed," *Psychiatric Annual* 17(1987):233–241.
3. S. T. White, F. A. Loda, D. Ingram, et al., "Sexually transmitted disease in sexually abused children," *Pediatrics* 72(1983):16–21.
4. A. R. DeJong, "Sexually transmitted diseases in sexually abused children," *Sexually Transmitted Diseases* 13(1986):123–127.
5. D. L. Ingram, S. T. White, M. F. Durfee, et al., "Sexual contact in children with gonorrhea," *American Journal of Diseases of Children* 136(1982):994–996.
6. J. Seidel, J. Zonata, and E. Totten, "*Condylomata acuminata* as a sign of sexual abuse in children," *Journal of Pediatrics* 95(1979):553–554.
7. T. S. Keskey, M. Suarez, N. Gleicher, et al., "*Chlamydia trachomatis* infection in sexually abused children," *Mount Sinai Journal of Medicine* 5(1987):129–134.
8. M. Gardner and J. G. Jones, "Genital herpes acquired by sexual abuse of children," *Journal of Pediatrics* 104(1984):243–244.
9. G. A. Gellert and M. J. Durfee, "HIV infection and child abuse," letter, *New England Journal of Medicine* 321(1989):685.
10. *Ibid.*
11. G. A. Gellert, M. J. Durfee, and C. D. Berkowitz, "Developing guidelines for HIV antibody testing among pediatric victims of sexual abuse," *Child Abuse and Neglect: The International Journal* 14(1990):9–17.
12. G. A. Gellert, M. J. Durfee, C. D. Berkowitz, et al., "Situational and sociodemographic characteristics of children infected with HIV from child sexual abuse," *Pediatrics* 91(1993):39–44.
13. *Ibid.*
14. O. Oneko, K. Meursing, O. Coutinho, et al., "Child sexual abuse in relation to STD/HIV transmission, Bulawayo, Zimbabwe," Abstract T.P.C 087, presented at the VIII International Conference on AIDS in Africa, Marrakech, Morocco, December 1993.
15. G. A. Gellert "Developing guidelines."

One out-of-school initiative developed by the WHO Adolescent Health Programme brought together youth leaders from 11 African countries affiliated with the World Assembly of Youth and the World Organization of the Scout Movement. Using role play, these young people created a scenario between two adolescents that might lead to pregnancy. They also developed a questionnaire designed to let respondents modify the story as it was being enacted. They then conducted surveys among more than 13,000 youth in both urban and rural areas. The project documented poor communication among youth about relationships and about sexuality. Using this premise, the youth leaders were brought together again to meet with representatives of their ministries of health to plan community projects to teach other youth about sexuality and communication, STIs and pregnancy.[44]

Summary

Increased prevention efforts and improved diagnostic and treatment services for youth are important, especially given that STIs account for significant morbidity and, in the case of HIV, increasing mortality among youth. Health care services for youth should be accessible, age appropriate, and comprehensive, providing reproductive and mental health services and substance abuse treatment. This is essential not only for the early identification and treatment of HIV infection among youth, but also to help youth incorporate HIV/STI risk reduction into a broader range of healthful behaviors. Moreover, youth around the world, so often disenfranchised and without skills, need safe havens in which to have time to develop their own coping and survival strategies to protect themselves against exposure to HIV. Finally, resources should be invested in developmentally appropriate risk-reduction programs that address sexual behavior and sexuality in a positive manner and that acknowledge a wider range of experience for youth. Innovating and improving the quality of the HIV/AIDS informational programs for youth in and out of school will have major health and social benefits (Box 21-3). HIV prevention programs for young people will also create an opportunity for young people to become more knowledgeable, compassionate, and involved in the ethical and social dimensions of growing up in a world with AIDS.

BOX 21-3

Young people, AIDS, and STIs: peer approaches in developing countries

NANCY FEE AND MAYADA YOUSSEF

Many HIV prevention programs for youth now use youth-to-youth or peer approaches as a key interpersonal strategy. In a peer-based approach, members of a social group or network communicate with, educate, or counsel members of their own group. Some of the theoretical and practical issues leading to this new focus on peer approaches include:

- *Young people's participation:* Youth have a wealth of commitment, energy, and enthusiasm—all of which are needed in AIDS prevention programs.
- *Adults' discomfort and difficulties with adolescent sexuality and providing explicit information on HIV/AIDS:* It may be difficult or controversial for adults to provide youth with such information. There is usually less objection to having young people do so.
- *The value of youth networks:* As compared to adults, young people may be able to more easily contact their peers (especially hard-to-reach youth) through their social networks, and to communicate information in effective and appropriate terms.
- *Peer credibility:* Young people often identify their peers as frequent, reliable, and preferred sources of information on sexuality-related topics, including AIDS and STIs.[1]

Youth as a resource in program development and implementation

When motivated for HIV/STI prevention, and when provided with appropriate support, young people usually want to share this information with other youth. When peer approaches are well conceived and implemented, young people can reach large numbers of their peers in a cost-effective, efficient, and effective manner.

HIV prevention programs have used peer approaches to reach youth in a wide range of settings including schools, venues in the community, and with high-risk groups (e.g., street youth).[2] Generally such programs have three interrelated approaches, based on the function, the intensity, and the objective of the peer activity. The first is the peer information approach, which undertakes specific informa-

Table 21-3.1   Typology of peer approaches: objective, coverage, intensity, focus, and examples

	Peer information	Peer education	Peer counseling
Objectives	Information building; some attitude change	Information and skill building; attitude change; may also include social support	Information and skill building; attitude change; problem-solving and social support
Coverage	High	Medium	Low
Intensity	Low	Medium/high	High
Focus	Community/group	Small groups	Individual
Relative Cost	Low	Medium	High
Examples	Drama, community meetings, leaflet distribution by young people to other young people	Peer-led group education activities	School, health facility, or community-based peer counselors

tion and education activities for large audiences. In Jamaica, for example, a youth theater group has developed a drama and a video on young people's sexual health, AIDS, and STIs. The troupe has performed this drama, *Vibes in a World of Sexuality,* to impart information and to foster the development of social norms that support healthy lifestyles and preventive behaviors.

A more structured and targeted approach, the peer education approach, helps smaller groups of young people build their knowledge, attitudes, and safer sex skills through educational activities carried out by members of their peer group who are trained as peer educators. In Ghana, for example, trained Red Cross youth volunteers have implemented educational activities with groups of out-of-school, working class youth.

Perhaps the most structured, most focused, and most intensive approach, the peer counseling approach, focuses on training young people as sexual health, HIV, and STI counselors to discuss personal problems and problem-solving strategies with other youth on an individual basis. In Indonesia, the Friends of Youth project uses university students to counsel young people on a range of sexual health issues, including HIV prevention. This counseling is available by post, by telephone, and in person.

The objectives, coverage, intensity, focus, and examples of these peer approaches are summarized below in Table 21-3.1.

References

1. C. L. Perry and R. Sieving, *Peer Involvement in Global AIDS Prevention among Adolescents* (Geneva: WHO, Global Programme on AIDS, December 1991).
2. M. Connolly and C.N. Franchet, "Manila street children face many sexual risks," *Network: Family Health International* 14(1993):24–25.

REFERENCES

1. A. Novello, *Final Report of the Secretary's Work Group on Pediatric HIV Infection and Disease* (Washington, DC: U.S. Department of Health and Human Services, 1988).
2. M. E. St. Louis, G. A. Conway, C. R. Hayman, et al., "HIV infection in disadvantaged adolescents: Findings from the U.S. Job Corps," *Journal of the American Medical Association* 266(1991):2387–2391.

3. R. L. Stricof, J. T. Kennedy, T. C. Nattel, et al., "HIV seroprevalence in a facility for runaway and homeless adolescents," *American Journal of Public Health* 81(1991):50–53.

4. D. DeMatteo, S. Read, B. Bock, et al., "HIV seroprevalence in Toronto street youth," Abstract PoC 4315, presented at the VIII International Conference on AIDS, Amsterdam, The Netherlands, July 1992.

5. D. A. Allen, J. S. Lehman, T. A. Green, et al., "HIV infection among homeless adults and runaway youth, United States, 1989–1992," *AIDS* 8(1994):1593–1598.

6. B. Jacobs, J. Miwe, A. H. Klokke, et al., "Secondary school students: A safer blood donor population in an urban settlement with high HIV seroprevalence in Africa," Abstract Th.P.A.019 presented at the VIIIth International Conference on AIDS in Africa & VIIIth African Conference on Sexually Transmitted Diseases, Marrakech, Morocco, 12–16 December 1993.

7. Centers for Disease Control, "Estimates of HIV prevalence and projected AIDS cases: Summary of a workshop, October 31–November 1, 1989," *Mortality and Morbidity Weekly Report* 39(1990):110–112, 117–119.

8. *Ibid.*

9. P. S. Rosenberg, J. J. Goedert, and R. J. Biggar, "Back calculation models of age-specific HIV incidence," Abstract PO-C05–2689, presented at the IX International Conference on AIDS, Berlin, Germany, June 1993.

10. P. S. Rosenberg, M. H. Gail, and R. J. Carroll, "Estimating HIV prevalence and projecting AIDS incidence in the United States: A model that accounts for therapy and changes in the surveillance definition of AIDS," *Statistics in Medicine* 11(1992):1633–1655.

11. J. D. Brown, B. S. Greenberg, and N. L. Buerkel-Rothfuss, "Mass media, sex, and sexuality," in *Adolescents in the Media, Adolescent Medicine: State of the Art Reviews*, V. C. Strasburger and G. A. Comstock, eds. (Philadelphia, PA: Hanley & Belfus, 1993).

12. N. Fee and M. Youssef, personal communication.

13. J. C. Coleman and L. Hendry, *Nature of Adolescence* (London: Routledge, 1990).

14. H. L. Friedman, "Changing patterns of adolescent sexual behavior: Consequences for health and development," paper presented at the Fifth Congress of the International Association for Adolescent Behavior, Montreux, Switzerland, July 1991.

15. N. J. Bell and R. W. Bell, eds., *Adolescent Risk Taking* (London: Sage Publications, 1993).

16. J. D. Fisher, S. J. Mosovitch, and W. A. Fisher, "Impact of perceived social norms on adolescents' AIDS-risk behavior and prevention," in *Adolescents and AIDS: A Generation in Jeopardy*, R. J. DiClemente, ed. (London: Sage Publications, 1992).

17. N. Fee and M. Youssef, personal communication.

18. M. Horton, "Homosexually active men and the evolving global epidemic of HIV," Abstract PS-08-2, presented at the IX International Conference on AIDS, Berlin, Germany, June 1993.

19. P. A. Paroski, "Health care delivery and the concerns of gay and lesbian adolescents," *Journal of Adolescent Health Care* 8(1987):188–192.

20. M. J. Rotheram-Borus, H. F. L. Meyer-Bahlburg, M. Rosario, et al., "Lifetime sexual behaviors among predominantly minority male runaways and gay/bisexual adolescents in New York City," *AIDS Education and Prevention* (special suppl.)(1992):34–42.

21. J. Hunter, M. Rosario, and M. J. Rotheram-Borus, "Sexual and substance abuse acts that place adolescent lesbians at risk for HIV," Abstract PO-D02-3432, presented at the IX International Conference on AIDS, Berlin, Germany, June 1993.

22. T. Myers, G. Godin, L. Calzavara, J. Lambert, D. Locker, and The Canadian AIDS Soci-

ety, *The Canadian Survey of Gay and Bisexual Men and HIV Infection: Men's Survey* (Ottawa: Canadian AIDS Society, 1993).

23. D. D. Celentano, K. E. Nelson, S. Suprasert, et al., "Behavioral risk factors for frequent prostitute use among northern Thai men and association with HIV infection," Abstract PO-C08-2775, presented at the IX International Conference on AIDS, Berlin, Germany, June 1993.

24. M. R. Gillmore, S. S. Butler, M. J. Lohr, and L. Gilchrist, "Substance use and other factors associated with risk sexual behavior among pregnant adolescents," *Family Planning Perspectives* 24(1992):255–261, 268.

25. P. M. Levenson, J. R. Morrow, W. C. Morgan, and B. Pfefferbaum, "Health information sources and preferences as perceived by adolescents, pediatricians, teachers, and school nurses," *Journal of Early Adolescence* 6(1986):183–195.

26. V. Igra and S. G. Millstein, "Current status and approaches to improving preventive services for adolescents," *Journal of the American Medical Association* 269(1993): 1408–1412.

27. C. Nelson, "Office visits by adolescents," *Advance Data from Vital and Health Statistics* 196 (Washington, DC: U.S. Department of Health and Human Services, 1991).

28. J. D. Klein, G. B. Slap, A. B. Elster, and S. K. Schonberg, "Access to health care for adolescents," *Journal of Adolescent Health* 13 (1992): 162–170.

29. J. Blair and K. Hein, "Public policy implications of HIV/AIDS in adolescents," *Future of Children* 4 (Los Altos, CA: David and Lucile Packard Foundation, 1994): 73–94.

30. M. Suplicy, "Sexuality education in Brazil," *Sex Information and Education Council of the U.S. Report* 22(1994):1–6.

31. B. J. Ferguson, "Youth at the threshold of the 21st century: The demographic situation," *Journal of Adolescent Health* 14(1993):638–644.

32. M. Maddaleno and T. J. Silber, "Epidemiological view of adolescent health in Latin America," *Journal of Adolescent Health* 13(1993):595–604.

33. UNICEF, *Primera aproximacion de analisis de situaciones de menores en circumstancias especialmente dificiles* (First attempt at an analysis of state of youth in very difficult situations) (San José, Costa Rica: UNICEF, 1990).

34. L. S. Bond, R. Mazin, and M. V. Jiminez, "Street youth and AIDS," *AIDS Education and Prevention* (special suppl.)(1992):14–23.

35. G. C. Luna and M. J. Rotheram-Borus, "Street youth and the AIDS pandemic," *AIDS Education and Prevention* (special suppl.)(1992):1–13.

36. Rotheram-Borus, "Lifetime sexual behaviors."

37. M. Chaisson, R. Stoneburner, A. Lifson, et al., "Risk factors for HIV infection in patients at a sexually transmitted disease clinic in NYC," *American Journal of Epidemiology* 131(1990):208–220.

38. R. Fullilove, M. Fullilove, B. Bowser, et al., "Risk of sexually transmitted disease among black adolescent crack users in Oakland and San Francisco, CA," *Journal of the American Medical Association* 263(1990):851–855.

39. R. J. Rice, P. L. Robert, H. H. Handsfield, and K. K. Holmes, "Sociodemographic distribution of gonorrhea incidence: Implications for prevention and behavioral research," *American Journal of Public Health* 81(1991):1252–1258.

40. J. E. Anderson, T. E. Freese, and J. N. Pennbridge, "Sexual risk behavior and condom use among street youth in Hollywood," *American Journal of Public Health* 26(1994): 22–25.

41. L. S. Bond, R. Mazin, and M. V. Jiminez, "Street youth and AIDS," *AIDS Education and Prevention* (special suppl.)(1992):14–23.

42. D. Boyer and D. Fine, "Sexual abuse as a factor in adolescent pregnancy and child maltreatment," *Family Planning Perspectives* 24(1992):4–11, 19.

43. D. Futterman, K. Hein, N. Reuben, et al., "HIV-infected adolescents: The first 50 patients in a New York City program," *Pediatrics* 91(1993):730–735.

44. H. L. Friedman, "Overcoming obstacles to good adolescent health," *Network: Family Health International* 14(1993):4–6.

22

Male Homosexuality and HIV

Behavior changes among homosexual men

Anthony P. M. Coxon

State of knowledge

In those epicenters of AIDS where homosexual transmission has predominated, sexual behavior and HIV-1 incidence have been monitored closely since the onset of the pandemic. North America has the greatest number of extensive research sites, followed by Europe and Australia.[1-5] Several major cross-sectional national investigations have been conducted, including studies in France and the seven-nation WHO Homosexual Response Studies.[6,7] However, there is virtually no comparable information available from Islamic countries, India, China, or many areas of Africa.

The main problems in obtaining reliable and valid data on homosexual behavior have been cultural and methodological. Since homosexual behavior is illegal, proscribed, or stigmatized in most societies, obtaining information is subject to numerous biasing factors. In addition, international comparisons have often been difficult due to the absence of consistent definitions and methods of data collection. Nonetheless, although the available studies all suffer to varying degrees from selection bias (toward the urban, younger, better-educated, and gay-identified males), there is considerable convergence in their findings:

- The vast majority of gay men's sexual activity involves three behaviors: masturbation, fellatio, and anal intercourse.
- An important fraction (between 10 and 20 percent) of gay-identifying men currently have sex with women.
- A significant proportion of men who have sex with men do not identify in any way with the gay community.
- Anal intercourse remains unequivocally the most risky homosexual activity, yet most studies show that about one-third of gay men engaged in unprotected receptive anal intercourse during the past month.

Around 9 percent of gay men are engaging exclusively in receptive anal intercourse; this group is at highest risk of HIV infection.

- The role pattern of involvement in anal intercourse differs internationally, but the most common pattern is to participate in both insertive *and* receptive intercourse. Among other patterns, twice as many men are insertive (only) versus receptive (only), and the proportion of those who engage in anal intercourse is higher in Latin and Mediterranean countries than in the Northern countries.

- The median number of sexual partners in the last year is about seven (plus or minus two), but the number of *penetrative* partners is usually considerably less, and often only averages about one a year.

Changes in sexual behavior

In the industrialized world, accurate knowledge of risk factors is almost universal among homosexual men. The main source of information about risk is typically the gay community itself. The evidence from *reported* changes in gay men's sexual risk behavior is generally encouraging. Most trends are in the direction of reducing high-risk sexual behavior, discriminating between the more risky (receptive) and less dangerous sexual activities, and adopting condom use. The behaviors most reduced are fellatio with ejaculation and anal intercourse (especially receptive), plus a dramatic reduction in anal intercourse with casual partners. The United States and the Netherlands have reported the highest rates of behavior change, with reductions in anal intercourse and increases in condom use. In Europe, condoms are rarely used in oral intercourse, which reflects disagreement about the riskiness of this activity. Unfortunately, relatively little is known about current practices and changes in sexual behavior among gay men in the developing world.

Critical issues

The understanding of sexual behavior among gay men is limited by three converging factors: difficulties in defining homosexual behavior; problems in accessing a broader and more representative sample of gay men; and current conceptual and methodological limits in sexual behavior research itself. These limitations should be considered when evaluating the effectiveness of HIV prevention programs directed at gay men. A simple "cause-and-effect" relationship between HIV education and services and falling HIV seroincidence (as was observed in the San Francisco cohort) cannot be accepted uncritically.

Several additional issues should be recognized. First, the persistence of the HIV/AIDS epidemic leads to important behavior changes over time. For example, in several well-studied cohorts of gay men (e.g., San Francisco, Britain, Amsterdam), HIV incidence and rates of unprotected anal intercourse have recently started to rise. Since these findings are from studies of cohorts of gay men who have been followed over time, they cannot be explained by the entry of younger and perhaps less cautious gay men. Some U.S. researchers have described this phenomenon as "relapse," perhaps implying that a major motivation is fatigue, hopelessness, or frustration with safer sex practices.[8,9] In contrast, British and Australian researchers have stressed the interpersonal context within which changes to unprotected sex occurs; they argue that changes represent "negotiated safety" or a rational choice within a relationship.[10,11,12] In any event, behavior change and its maintenance cannot be assumed to be permanent.

Another consideration related to the duration of the pandemic is the response of young gay men to safe sex messages. Evidence regarding the sexual behavior of young gay men is conflicting. In addition, information on this group is limited because younger gay men are more resistant to investigation than older gay men.

Finally, data from San Francisco and elsewhere suggest that the idea of a homogeneous "gay response" to HIV is a myth. Available seroincidence data demonstrate that the responses of gay men of color in the United States differ from the responses of white, middle-class gay men. In addition, gay men who do not identify with the gay community may, like other people who are isolated, have greater difficulty learning about and applying their knowledge about HIV and its prevention. Similarly, the responses of gay men from ethnic minorities may be influenced by cycles of deprivation, greater reliance on heterosexual activity, and relative invisibility to researchers and policy-makers. More broadly, this problem of invisibility and marginalization applies to most gay men in the developing world, who may still lack basic information about HIV/AIDS and have little in the way of services or social support.

In summary, it would be a tragic mistake to consider the challenge of HIV prevention among gay men to be resolved. Despite some favorable data on HIV seroincidence and changes in reported behaviors, too little is known about gay male sexuality and the epidemic is too new to draw widespread conclusions—or to declare victory.

HIV, homosexuality, and vulnerability in the developing world

Dennis Altman

The fact that AIDS was first conceptualized as a new "disease" among American gay men and was even known for a short time as "Gay Related Immune Deficiency Syndrome" has had a continuing effect upon the way it is perceived internationally. In many developing countries, including Thailand, the Philippines, and much of South and Central America, the first AIDS cases reported were also due to homosexual transmission.

Cumulative figures between 1983 and 1994 show that over 40 percent of AIDS cases in Mexico and most of South America resulted from homosexual transmission of HIV, as is true of over half of known AIDS cases to date in Indonesia (though not of reported HIV).[13] While some countries do compile data on AIDS cases or even HIV infections by transmission category, this does not allow meaningful estimation of the extent of homosexual transmission of HIV; in many countries there is also very uneven access to testing and powerful incentives to lie about sexual orientation.[14]

The early emphasis on AIDS and homosexuality may have allowed many people to distance themselves from the epidemic and to deny their own vulnerability to HIV infection.[15] Today, however, the emphasis of official programs in the developing world is overwhelmingly on heterosexual transmission. Unfortunately, while this emphasis is largely justified, it may lead to the neglect of homosexual transmission, especially given the reluctance of many governments to acknowledge homosexual behavior within their societies. In many developing countries there is virtually no specific outreach directed at men who have sex with men, and the emphasis on heterosexual transmission has led some men to assume that homosexual contact is safe. Comparatively few projects in developing countries involved with sex work have targeted men, even though male sex workers were estimated to comprise at least 5 percent of sex workers in Colombia, the Czech Republic, Egypt, Nigeria, Senegal, and Thailand.[16] Antihomosexual attacks in countries as different as Mexico, Iran, and Zimbabwe claim to combat foreign-inspired "degeneracy," ignoring traditions which predate Western influence. In much of the Middle East and Africa there is considerable denial and even draconian persecution of homosexuality, which makes any genuine assessment of its extent very difficult. In addition, the combination of different conceptions of sex and gender, and widespread prudery on the part of governments and health officials, means that it is very difficult to gain a meaningful picture of homosexual behaviors and identities in developing countries.

Anthropological evidence suggests that homosexual behavior is probably universal, but that identities defined by sexuality are far less common. In many societies homosexuality is linked to particular gender orders, so that some men and less commonly, women, are conceived as a "third sex" that combines particular ways of acting out gender and sexuality.[17] In many cases, homosexual behavior is an accepted part of the male sexual repertoire, and men are defined as "homosexual" only if they adopt the "passive" role in such behavior.[18]

"Homosexual" is also a blanket term that includes ritualized male-to-male sex in traditional societies, such as Papua New Guinea, commercial same-gender sex in which the worker may have no self-image as homosexual, and groups with strong commitments to gay, lesbian, even "queer" identities.[19] It has been suggested that in Peru there is a "taxonomy of seven homosexually active male characters," and in Thailand a study identified at least 29 terms used to describe male and female homosexuals.[20,21,22]

While figures range widely, these are no accurate estimates of the number of people who engage in homosexual sex or how they define themselves. A recent American study concluded that the oft-misquoted Kinsey figure of 10 percent of men is almost certainly an overestimate.[23] In most societies, probably many more men engage in homosexual sex than is generally acknowledged. In turn, this compounds their vulnerability to HIV; some people are at high risk through homosexual sex yet may have no contact with a homosexual subculture.

At the same time, an assertive gay and lesbian movement in the United States and other Western countries has emerged, starting at the end of the 1960s; this movement has been well chronicled. Parallel developments in some developing countries have also taken place, most particularly in South America and more recently in Eastern Europe and some Southeast Asian countries such as the Philippines.[24-30] Thus in some countries, gay movements were already in place when AIDS brought new demands and new urgencies to mobilizing and reaching homosexual communities.[31] AIDS also provided the impetus to develop such organizations, and in some cases provided resources with which this could be accomplished.[32] In Southeast Asia, for example, groups such as FACT (Fraternity for AIDS Cessation in Thailand), Pink Triangle in Malaysia, and the Library Foundation in the Philippines all emerged as essentially gay responses to the epidemic.

In Manila, the Library Foundation has organized workshops that give men who have sex with men better knowledge and capabilities to negotiate safe sex. In Thailand, FACT has presented AIDS information shows in bars, aimed at both commercial sex workers and their clients. Pink Triangle was the first activist HIV/AIDS organization in Malaysia. The activities of these groups and others like them (e.g., Action for AIDS, Singapore, or the Hong Kong AIDS Foundation) have helped the growth of self-conscious gay communities in Asia.[33] Issues of community affiliation which have proved important in developed countries appear to influence homosexual men in other parts of the world as well.

New images and identities that are part of a relentless economic and cultural globalization have contributed to the ways in which non-Western homosexuals understand themselves and HIV. Pressure from international gay groups, from Western governments aware of their own gay constituencies, and from the large number of gay men in international HIV/AIDS work are all contributing to shifts in sexual paradigms. For example, the Naz project, based in London, has simultaneously worked with southern Asians in Britain and among vulnerable populations in India, helping to support emerging gay movements. In China and Vietnam, despite official hostility to any acknowledgment of homosexuality, AIDS has caused some recognition of the epidemic, resulting in semiofficial outreach programs targeting men who have sex with men. In South Africa, the new government has recognized the rights of homosexuals.

There is also a political economy of sex, symbolized by the appearance of young Polish hustlers in the saunas of Berlin and of gay sex tourism in most countries of Southeast Asia, the Caribbean, and parts of West Africa. Greater movements of populations, due to tourism, immigration, study, migrant labor, and international development, are helping to link people, including gay and lesbian people, into global networks.

It is nonetheless easy to misjudge the vulnerability of homosexual men in much of the world. The fragility of gay organizations and existing hostility towards homosexuals creates an atmosphere of considerable risk and vulberablity to HIV for most men engaging in homosexual sex outside the middle-class, urban enclaves of the developed world.

REFERENCES

1. R. Stall, M. Ekstrand, L. Pollack, L. McKusick, and T. J. Coates, "Relapse from safer sex: The next challenge for AIDS prevention efforts," *Journal of Acquired Immune Deficiency Syndromes* 3(1990):1181–1187.

2. J. G. Joseph, S. M. Adib, J. S. Koopman, and D. G. Ostrow, "Behavioral change in longitudinal studies: Adoption of condom use by homosexual/bisexual men,"*American Journal of Public Health* 80(1990):1513–1514.

3. P. M. Davies, F. C. I. Hickson, P. Weatherburn, A. Hunt, P. J. Broderick, A. P. M. Coxon, T. J. McManus, and M. J. Stephens, *Sex, Gay Men and AIDS* (London: Falmer Press, 1993).

4. G. J. P. van Griensven, E. M. M. de Vroome, J. Goudsmit, and R. A. Coutinho, "Changes in sexual behaviour and fall in incidence of HIV infection among homosexual men," *British Medical Journal* 298(1989):218–221.

5. S. Kippax, R. W. Connell, G. W. Dowsett, and J. Crawford, *Sustaining Safer Sex* (London: Falmer Press, 1993).

6. M. Pollack, "Assessing AIDS prevention among male homo- and bisexuals," in *Sociologie d'une Epidémie*, F. Paccaud, J. P. Vader, and F. Gutzwiller, eds. (Paris: AM Métailié, 1992):137–157.

7. A. P. M. Coxon, *International Homosexual Response Studies of WHO*, working paper (Colchester, U.K.: Department of Sociology, University of Essex, June 1992).

8. S. M. Adib, J. G. Joseph, D. G. Ostrow, and A. J. Sherman, "Predictors of relapse in sexual practices among homosexual men," *AIDS Education and Prevention* 3(1991):293–304.

9. Stall, "Relapse."

10. SIGMA, *Final Report to the Department of Health* (London: Project SIGMA [Socio Sexual Investigations of Gay Men and AIDS], 1990).

11. P. M. Davies, "Safer sex maintenance among gay men: Are we moving in the right direction?" *AIDS* 7(1993):279–280.

12. Kippax, *Sustaining Safer Sex*.

13. Pan American Health Organisation, Regional Program on AIDS/STDs, *Quarterly Report*, March 18, 1995.

14. M. Tan, "Recent HIV/AIDS trends among men who have sex with men," Plenary address, presented at the Tenth International Conference on AIDS, Yokohama, Japan, August 1994.

15. Interview with Dr. Nkosazana Zuma, Health Minister of South Africa, *Global AIDS News* 1995:2.

16. J. Mann, D. Tarantola, and T. Netter, eds., *AIDS in the World* (Cambridge, MA: Harvard University Press, 1992).

17. G. Herdt, *Third Sex, Third Gender* (New York: Zone, 1994).

18. Peter Aggleton, ed., *Bisexualities and HIV/AIDS* (London: Taylor & Francis, 1995).

19. G. Herdt, *Third Sex, Third Gender* (New York: Zone, 1994).

20. C. Cárceres, "New representations of male bisexuality in Latin America and the prevention of AIDS," paper presented at the Tenth International Conference on AIDS, Yokohama, Japan, August 1994, Abstract 170D.

21. P. Jackson, "Kathoey><Gay><Man: the historical emergence of gay male identity in Thailand" in *Sites of Desire/Economies of Pleasure*, L. Manderson and M. Jolly, eds. (Chicago: University of Chicago Press, 1995).

22. J. W. de Lind van Wijngaarden, "A social geography of male homosexual desire," *Ninth International Conference on AIDS in Asia and the Pacific Newsletter,* Chiang Mai, Thailand 2 (4), July–September 1994.

23. E. Lautmann, J. Gagnon, R. Michael, and S. Michaels, eds., *The Social Organization of Sexuality* (Chicago: University of Chicago Press, 1995).

24. B. Adam, *The Rise of a Gay and Lesbian Movement* (Boston: GK Hall, 1986).

25. D. Altman, *The Homosexualization of America* (New York: St. Martin's Press, 1981).

26. H. Daniel and R. Parker, *Sexuality, Politics and AIDS in Brazil* (London: Falmer, 1993).

27. S. O'Murray, "The 'underdevelopment' of modern gay/homosexuality in Mesoamerica," in K. Plummer, ed., *Modern Homosexualities* (London: Routledge, 1992).

28. J. Trevisan, *Perverts in Paradise* (London: GMP, 1986).

29. D. Remoto, *Seduction and Solitude* (Manila: Anvil, 1995).

30. R. Parker, *Bodies, Pleasures and Passions* (Boston: Beacon Press, 1991).

31. D. Altman, *Power and Community: Organisational and Cultural Responses to AIDS* (London and Philadelphia: Taylor and Francis, 1994).

32. M. Roberts, "Emergence of gay identity and gay social movements in developing countries: The AIDS crisis as catalyst," *Alternatives* 20(1995):243–264.

33. D. Altman, *The New World of Gay Asia* (Melbourne: Meridien, 1995).

23

Sexual Behavior among Heterosexuals

ANKE A. EHRHARDT

Worldwide, over 70 percent of HIV infections result from heterosexual behavior. This chapter briefly summarizes available knowledge about heterosexual behavior, highlights deficiencies in understanding, and identifies critical prevention needs.

Patterns of sexual behavior and hierarchy of risk

Our knowledge of patterns of sexual behavior is quite limited. Few countries have conducted national sexual behavior surveys.[1-5] The vast majority of people in all cultures engage in sexual intercourse throughout their adult lives. Typically, men in their 20s and 30s have the highest number of partners and tend to have more partners than women.[6]

The hierarchy of risk for HIV infection is well understood. Receptive anal penetrative sex is the most risky sexual practice. Several surveys have found that a substantial number of heterosexual women (around 25 percent) and men occasionally or regularly engage in anal intercourse.[7] Anal intercourse is almost always omitted from prevention programs for heterosexuals. This is clearly a serious shortcoming that needs correction.

Unprotected vaginal intercourse is at the next level of risk for HIV infection, with significantly greater risk of infection to the woman than to the man.[8] The risk is dramatically increased when one or both partners have other sexually transmitted infections.

The risk of becoming infected through receptive oral sex appears much lower than through anal and vaginal sex, but it is not zero. A small number of cases, mainly involving gay men, have documented this transmission route.[9] Oral sex is also a common practice. For example, in a 1991 survey of men in the United States, 75 percent had performed oral sex and 79 percent of them had received oral sex.[10] Woman-to-woman transmission through oral sex has not been sufficiently studied; however, based on existing reports, the risk appears to be relatively low.

Social context

Partner frequency increases when people do not live in a coupled relationship. In many countries, young people start to have sexual intercourse, often with a number of partners, until they begin a relationship of cohabitation or marriage. At the same time, age of first marriage has increased in many societies, which prolongs this "uncoupled" phase. In areas where the divorce rate is high, many people have uncoupled phases between marriages. Thus, many people have uncoupled periods at several points in their lives, and during these times they tend to have more than one partner. Women are often expected to be monogamous, while men have frequent outside relationships.

Barriers to condom use

Condom use is not a popular method of birth control. A focused and concerted effort is required if it is ever to become a norm for disease prevention.[11] Even after a decade of AIDS awareness, condom use is still low, especially for consistent and long-term use. In surveys of women of reproductive age in the U.S., about 20 percent of currently sexually active women reported condom use, but one in five women did not have condom-protected sexual intercourse at their last occasion.[12] The 1991 Study of American Men, involving several thousand African-American and white American men, ages 20 to 39, found that 27 percent of sexually active men had used a condom in the 4 weeks before interview. African-American men reported more condom use than white men (38 percent and 25 percent, respectively), and men younger than 30 were more likely to use a condom than older men (36 percent and 19 percent, respectively).[13]

The same survey assessed perceptions regarding consequences of condom use.[14,15] From a psychological and interpersonal perspective, men most frequently stated that a condom "shows that you are a concerned and caring person." This was more true for African-American than for white men, for younger than older men, and for men of lower educational status. However, the same men usually agreed that using a condom sends unwanted messages to the sexual partner, such as it "makes your partner think that you have AIDS" or "shows that you think that your partner has AIDS."

The barriers for condom use for white men and for those who are more highly educated tended to focus on embarrassment when buying condoms. Other important obstacles included concerns that condom use results in reduced sexual sensation, that care must be taken during sex to prevent condom breakage, and that quick withdrawal after sex is required or the condom may come off.

If condoms are to be successfully promoted as a global strategy to decrease risk of HIV infection, the major barriers to condom use must be understood. These barriers vary by age, community norms, the social context of a relationship, and most of all, by gender. Heterosexual men have been neglected in research on condom use. This is a critical gap, since men have much greater control over condom use than women.

Prevention

To move ahead, several approaches are needed:

- Heterosexual men must have a central role in programs designed to increase condom use.
- Programs for women need a different focus. Women around the world do not control condom use and have considerably less power than men in sexual relations. Thus, for women prevention strategies need to focus on their ability to negotiate and refuse. In many societies, women's lower status is reflected in a double standard about sexuality and partner frequency. This obviously requires a broader strategy than simply seeking to change sexual behavior.[16]
- New methods for HIV prevention that are under women's control are needed. These new methods of prevention must be developed with the same urgency as new drugs for the treatment of HIV infections.
- Prevention efforts must take into account age and stage of personal development. For example, a recent report suggests that young adolescent women are disproportionately at risk for HIV.[17] Young women who became HIV infected from sexual intercourse are infected 5 to 10 years earlier than young men. Explanations include: greater physiological vulnerability of the young female genital tract; hurried, nonconsensual, and inexperienced sexual intercourse, which increases the likelihood of physical trauma; and a lack of access to health services, thus leaving other sexually transmitted infections untreated. Therefore, programs to help prevent HIV acquisition by adolescent women must address these factors.

BOX 23-1

Sexuality in women with HIV infection

CATHERINE HANKINS

Preliminary results from small studies are beginning to shed light on the sexuality of women living with HIV infection. Findings from industrialized countries suggest that the majority of HIV-positive women experience significant disruptions in sexual desire, arousal, and orgasmic functioning. In comparison with noninfected women, they have fewer sexual thoughts and tend to desire sex less frequently.[1] This lowered sexual drive is accompanied by a decreased frequency of sexual activity, which while usually transient, may become chronic in up to one-third of HIV-infected women.[2,3] Even when these women appear physically healthy, they commonly express feelings of loss of physical and sexual appeal, as well as anxiety and confusion about their options for sexual activity.[4] The majority of HIV-infected women either continue or resume sexual activity, but their enjoyment of sex may be lowered due to fears of transmitting HIV.[5,6] It is unclear whether male dominance in sexual decision-making affects the period of sexual adjustment.

Women with HIV infection are counseled to avoid exposure to sexually transmitted diseases because of their potential impact on disease progression. Even when extensive counseling services are available and knowledge levels are high, a majority of sexually active HIV-infected women in both industrialized and nonindustrialized countries are unable to get their partners to always use protection.

The reasons are likely complex, culture-specific, and multifactorial. Safer sex practices seem to be adopted more frequently when the male partner is known not to be infected.[7] This is consistent with studies that have found that couples where the woman is the infected partner are more likely to use condoms than couples where the man is infected.[8,9,10]

Counseling that places value on the safe and satisfying aspects of sexual intimacy will help women with HIV infection to choose between abstinence, self-pleasuring, or interpersonal sex. Assisting HIV-infected women to become self-supporting from activities that are unrelated to risk of HIV transmission will reduce the influence of socioeconomic factors on sexual choices. Finally, the rapid development and field trials of safe, effective, accessible, acceptable, woman-controlled methods for preventing HIV transmission are critical if women with HIV infection are to have a full range of options available to them.[11]

References

1. H. Meyer-Bahlburg, C. Nostlinger, T. Exner, et al., "Sexual functioning in HIV+ and HIV- injected drug-using women," *Journal of Sex and Marital Therapy* 19(1993):56–68.

2. G. Brown and J. Rundell, "Prospective study of psychiatric morbidity in HIV-seropositive women without AIDS," *General Hospital Psychiatry* 12(1990):30–35.

3. G. Brown, J. Rundell, J. Pace, et al., Psychiatric morbidity in early HIV infection in women: Results of a 4 year prospective study, presented at the First International Conference on Biopsychosocial Aspects of HIV Infection, Amsterdam, The Netherlands, September 1991.

4. J. Chung and M. Magraw, "Group approach to psychosocial issues faced by HIV-positive women," *Hospital and Community Psychiatry* 43(1992):891–894.

5. Meyer-Bahlburg, "Sexual functioning."

6. C. Hankins, S. Gendron, D. Lamping, et al., "Does an HIV positive test result improve a woman's sex life?" Abstract PO-D20-3974, presented at the IX International Conference on AIDS, Berlin, Germany, June 1993.

7. S. Lo Caputo, P. Congedo, G. Angarano, et al., "Changes in sexual behaviour of women come to knowledge of HIV positivity," Abstract M.D.4224, presented at the VII International Conference on AIDS, Florence, Italy, June 1991.

8. S. Allen, J. Tice, P. Van de Perre, et al., "Effect of serotesting with counselling on condom use and seroconversion among HIV discordant couples in Africa," *British Medical Journal* 304(1992):1605–1609.

9. M. Kamenga, R. W. Ryder, M. Jingu, et al., "Evidence of marked sexual behavior change associated with low HIV-1 seroconversion in 149 married couples with discordant HIV-1 serostatus: Experience at an HIV counseling center in Zaire," *AIDS* 5(1991):61–67.

10. D. Serwadda, R. Gray, N. Sewankambo, et. al., "Gender specific HIV transmission/prevention in discordant couples in Rural Uganda," Abstract 107C, presented at the Xth International Conference on AIDS, Yokohama, Japan, August 1994.

11. Z. Stein, "HIV prevention: The need for methods women can use," *American Journal of Public Health* 80(1990):460–462.

REFERENCES

1. ACSF Principal Investigators and their associates, "Analysis of sexual behavior in France (ACSF). A comparison between two modes of investigation: telephone survey and face-to-face survey," *AIDS* 6(1992):315–323.

2. H. Leridon, "Number, sex, and type of partners," in *Sexual Behaviour and AIDS* A. Spira, N. Bajos, and the ACSF Group, eds. (Aldershot: Anebury, 1994):104–116.

3. J. Wadsworth, J. Field, A. M. Johnson, S. Bradshaw, and K. Wellings, "Methodology of the National Survey of Sexual Attitudes and Lifestyles," *Journal of the Royal Statistical Society* 156(1993):407–421.

4. N. Bajos, J. Wadsworth, B. Ducot, A. Johnson, F. LePont, K. Wellings, A. Spira, J. Field, and the ACSF Group, "Sexual behaviour and HIV epidemiology: comparative analysis in France and Britain," *AIDS* 9(1995):735–743.

5. J. Gagnon, G. Kolata, E. Laumann, and R. Michael, *Sex in America: a Definitive Survey* (Boston: Little, Brown and Company, 1994).

6. J. O. G. Billy, K. Tanfer, W. R. Grady, and D. H. Klepinger, "Sexual behavior of men in the United States," *Family Planning Perspectives* 25(1993):52–60.

7. B. Voeller, "AIDS and heterosexual anal intercourse," *Archives of Sexual Behavior* 20(1991):233–276.

8. A. A. Ehrhardt and J. N. Wasserheit, "Age, gender, and sexual risk behaviors for sexually transmitted diseases in the United States," in *Research Issues in Human Behavior and Sexually Transmitted Diseases in the AIDS Era*, J. N. Wasserheit, S. O. Aral, K. Holmes, and P. J. Hitchcock, eds. (Washington, DC: American Society for Microbiology, 1991).

9. A. R. Lifson, P. M. O'Malley, N. A. Hessol, S. P. Buchbinder, L. Cannon, and G. W. Rutherford, "HIV seroconversion in two homosexual men after receptive oral intercourse with ejaculation: Implications for counseling concerning safe sexual practices," *American Journal of Public Health* 80(1990):1509–1511.

10. J. O. G. Billy, K. Tanfer, W. R. Grady, and D. H. Klepinger, "Sexual behavior of men in the United States," *Family Planning Perspectives* 25(1993):52–60.

11. W. D. Mosher, "Contraceptive practice in the United States, 1982–1988," *Family Planning Perspectives* 22(1990):198–205.

12. K. Kost and J. D. Forrest, "American women's sexual behavior and exposure to risk of sexually transmitted diseases," *Family Planning Perspectives* 24(1992):244–254.

13. K. Tanfer, W. R. Grady, D. H. Klepinger, and J. O. G. Billy, "Condom use among U.S. men, 1991," *Family Planning Perspectives* 25(1993):61–66.

14. K. Tanfer, "National survey of men: Design and execution," *Family Planning Perspectives* 25(1993):83–86.

15. W. R. Grady, D. H. Klepinger, J. O. G. Billy, and K. Tanfer, "Condom characteristics: The perceptions and preferences of men in the United States," *Family Planning Perspectives* 25(1993):67–73.

16. E. Reid, "Gender knowledge and responsibility," in *AIDS in the World*, J. Mann, D. Tarantola, and T. Netter, eds. (Cambridge, MA: Harvard University Press, 1992):657–667.

17. HIV and Development Programme, *Young Women: Silence, Susceptibility and the HIV Epidemic* (New York: United Nations Development Programme, 1993).

24

Risk Reduction among Injecting Drug Users

DON C. DES JARLAIS AND SAMUEL R. FRIEDMAN

HIV infection among injecting drug users (IDUs) has been reported from more than 80 countries and could conceivably spread to at least 40 other countries in which people inject illicit drugs.[1,2] In some localities, such as Edinburgh (U.K.), Bangkok (Thailand), Bologna (Italy), and Manipur (India), the spread of HIV among IDUs has been as rapid as that among any at-risk population.[3] In many industrialized countries, moreover, the local population of HIV-infected IDUs has been the predominant source for both heterosexual and perinatal transmission of HIV.[4]

However, contrary to initial pessimistic expectations regarding the ability of IDUs to change their behavior in response to AIDS, evidence now exists that IDUs have reduced their HIV risk behavior in response to a wide variety of interventions. Evidence also indicates that after learning about AIDS through mass media and/or their own oral communication networks, IDUs have reduced their risk behaviors even in the absence of formal prevention programs.[5,6] Indeed, in many areas drug users have formed their own organizations to combat the epidemic.[7]

Effective risk-reduction programs to date have included educational programs, drug abuse treatment, syringe exchange, over-the-counter syringe sale, and community outreach and bleach distribution programs.[8,9] In many areas, large-scale risk reduction among IDUs (i.e., 50 percent or more reporting that they have changed their risk behavior) has been followed by reduced rates of HIV seroconversion and stabilization of HIV seroprevalence among the local IDU population. However, no single type of prevention program has been shown to be superior to all others, particularly given the complexity and range of problems to be addressed in various localities and among differing sectors of the IDU population. There is a developing consensus that effective AIDS prevention programs for IDUs must combine multiple approaches for reducing HIV risk, including the promotion of treatment for reducing illicit drug use, providing means for safer injection, and promoting safer sex. For reasons that have yet to be fully determined, changing the sexual risk behavior of IDUs has proven to be much more difficult than changing drug injection risk behavior.[10]

Two general "types" of HIV epidemics among IDUs have been identified. In some areas, HIV has been introduced into the local population of IDUs, but seroprevalence has remained low (less than 5 percent) and stable over time.[11] In these places, potentially large-scale HIV epidemics appear to have been averted largely because AIDS prevention efforts were begun relatively early, and because these efforts included both community outreach to IDUs and good access to sterile injection equipment.

The other type of HIV epidemic among IDUs involves a period of rapid transmission following the introduction of HIV, followed by large-scale behavior change and stabilization of seroprevalence. Stabilization of HIV seroprevalence in these situations does *not* mean that new HIV infections are not occurring. Rather, stable seroprevalence is a balance between loss of HIV seropositives from the group and the occurrence of new HIV infections. For example, in Amsterdam, which has many AIDS prevention programs for IDUs, seroprevalence has stabilized at approximately 30 percent, and HIV seroincidence is approximately four new infections per 100 person-years at risk.[12] However, in New York City, seroprevalence has stabilized at approximately 50 percent, and HIV seroincidence is estimated at between four to six new infections per 100 person-years at risk.[13]

A number of fundamental questions about the spread of HIV among IDUs require additional research. First, more knowledge is needed on the spread of illicit drug injection in both industrialized and developing countries (Box 24-1). A second critical question involves how HIV is introduced into local populations—through travel by IDUs and/or by "bridge populations"—and how the international spread of HIV could be reduced. While there is compelling evidence that IDUs will reduce their risk behaviors, relatively little is known about the processes through which these changes occur or how risk reduction can be sustained over extended periods of time. Social processes, including the development of new social norms—for example, IDUs themselves expressing disapproval of sharing injection equipment or approving of condom use—may be extremely important.[14,15] Also, as noted above, more knowledge is required about how to change the sexual behavior of IDUs.

BOX 24-1

Injecting drug use in India: transition from heroin to semisynthetic narcotic analgesic

S. SUNDARARAMAN

Injecting drug use has recently increased in Madras, India. Two important factors help explain the upsurge in injecting drug use. First, the early 1980s witnessed the beginning of ethnic conflict in the neighboring island country of Sri Lanka, where indigenous Tamils constituted the largest ethnic minority population. The advent of a militant movement led to drug running, associated with financing operations. Consequently, drugs were channeled into India through the state of Tamilnadu. Heroin ("brown sugar") began to be increasingly used in Tamilnadu, particularly in Madras. However, in general this was "chased" and not injected. However, the assassination of Prime Minister Rajiv Gandhi near Madras in 1991 led to major changes. Militant influx through the Indian coastline was severely restricted and thus movement of drugs into Tamilnadu was limited. The sudden depletion in "brown sugar" supplies resulted in most drug users shifting to the locally available, injectable drug, Tedigesic (bupreo norphine). This widespread change was strengthened by its easy availability and low cost.

Second, many IDUs have recently migrated to Madras from the northeastern Indian state of Manipur. When HIV was first detected in Manipur among IDUs, public opinion bordered on paranoia. IDUs were tested forcibly and if found HIV-infected, they were confined in isolation homes. This forced many IDUs underground, or they migrated to safer areas, and Madras was a favored destination. This migration has led to the increase in injecting drug use in Madras.

The history of injecting drug use in Madras illustrates the range of factors that can create rapid changes in the vulnerability of drug users to injection drug use and HIV infection.

No prevention program to date has led to complete risk elimination among IDUs. The daunting problem of reversing well-established, high HIV-seroprevalence epidemics among IDUs may thus require a second (or even a third) generation of prevention programs. However, resources are often limited (some developing countries lack the resources to provide sterile injection equipment for medical care purposes and are unable to support sterile injection of illicit drugs) and the effectiveness of some practices (such as the use of bleach for disinfecting used injection equipment) has recently been questioned.[16]

Finally, despite the spread of HIV among IDUs, political and public health leaders in many countries continue to deny that significant injecting drug use even exists. Other leaders, while acknowledging an injecting drug use problem, have responded only with intensified law enforcement—without recognition of the public health aspects of the problem or support for AIDS prevention programs. Reducing the transmission of HIV among IDUs is thus at least as much a question of how to change the behavior of political and public health leaders as it is of changing the behavior of IDUs.

REFERENCES

1. G. V. Stimson, "The health and social costs of drug injecting: The challenge to developing countries," presented at the VI International Conference on the Reduction of Drug-Related Harm, Florence, Italy, March, 1995.
2. D. C. Des Jarlais, S. R. Friedman, K. Choopanya, et al., "International epidemiology of HIV and AIDS among injecting drug users," *AIDS* 6(1992):1053–1068.
3. S. R. Friedman and D. C. Des Jarlais, "HIV among drug injectors: The epidemic and the response," *AIDS Care* 3(1991):239–250.
4. S. R. Friedman, D. C. Des Jarlais, T. P. Ward, et al., "Drug injectors and heterosexual AIDS," in *AIDS and the Heterosexual Population*, L. Sherr, ed. (Chur, Switzerland: Harwood Academic Publishers, 1994):41–65.
5. D. C. Des Jarlais, S. R. Friedman, and W. Hopkins, "Risk reduction for the acquired immunodeficiency syndrome among intravenous drug users," *Annals of Internal Medicine* 103(1985):55–59.
6. S. R. Friedman, D. C. Des Jarlais, J. L. Sotheran, et al., "AIDS and self-organization among intravenous drug users," *International Journal of the Addictions* 22(1987): 201–219.

7. S. R. Friedman, W. de Jong, and A. Wodak, "Community development as a response to HIV among drug injectors," *AIDS* 7(suppl. 1)(1993):s263–s269.

8. D. C. Des Jarlais and S. R. Friedman, "AIDS prevention programs—for injecting drug users," in *AIDS and Other Manifestations of HIV Infection*, G. P. Wormser, ed. (New York: Raven Press, 1992):645–658.

9. D. C. Des Jarlais, S. R. Friedman, J. Woods, and J. Milliken, "HIV infection among intravenous drug users: Epidemiology and emerging public health perspectives," in *Substance Abuse: A Comprehensive Textbook*. Second Ed. J. H. Lowinson, et al., eds. (Baltimore, MD: Williams & Wilkins, 1992):734–743.

10. Friedman, "Drug injectors."

11. D. C. Des Jarlais, H. Hagan, S. R. Friedman, et al., "Maintaining low HIV seroprevalence in populations of injecting drug users," *Journal of the American Medical Association* 274(1995):1226–1231.

12. E. J. C. van Ameijden, A. van den Hoek, and R. A. Coutinho, "Risk factors for HIV seroconversion in injecting drug users in Amsterdam, The Netherlands," Abstract TH.C.104, presented at the VII International Conference on AIDS, Florence, Italy, June 1991.

13. D. C. Des Jarlais, S. R. Friedman, J. L. Sotheran, et al., "Continuity and change within an HIV epidemic: Injecting drug users in New York City, 1984 through 1992," *Journal of the American Medical Association* 271(1994):121–127.

14. A. Neaigus, S. R. Friedman, R. Curtis, et al., "Relevance of drug injectors' social networks and risk networks for understanding and preventing HIV infection," *Social Science and Medicine* 38(1993):67–78.

15. S. R. Friedman, B. Jose, A. Neaigus, et al. "Consistent condom use in relationships between seropositive injecting drug users and sex partners who do not inject drugs," *AIDS* 8(1994):357–361.

16. J. W. Curran, L. W. Scheckel, and R. A. Millstein, *HIV/AIDS Prevention Bulletin*, letter (Atlanta, GA: U.S. Department of Health and Human Services, April 1993):1–4.

25

HIV/AIDS in Prisons

T. W. HARDING

The prison environment plays an important role in the overall epidemiology of HIV/AIDS. Data on HIV infection in prison systems of industrialized countries continue to show both a close relation to the proportion of injecting drug users (IDUs) in the prison population and to the prevalence of HIV infection among IDUs in the community.[1] For example, while Spain's prison population has shown a significant decrease in HIV prevalence (28 percent in 1987; 20 percent in 1992), prevalence nonetheless remains high, reflecting the high proportion of IDUs in the Spanish prison population.[2] In industrialized countries, prevalence among women prisoners is consistently higher than for men, reflecting the high proportion of IDUs among women inmates. For example, 21 percent of women in a New York City jail were HIV seropositive.[3,4] In addition, 168 known cases of HIV infection were reported among prisoners in Dublin's main prison; this represents 17 percent of all known cases of HIV infection in the Republic of Ireland, which underlines the importance of the prison environment in the overall epidemiology of HIV/AIDS.[5]

In developing countries as well, HIV infection in prison populations reflects high HIV prevalence among young, urban adults in the community. Although data are limited, supporting examples include Botswana, Tanzania, Mozambique, Côte d'Ivoire, and Uganda, where virtually no prisoners are IDUs.[6] Finally, and not surprisingly, the epidemiological profile in prisons of Brazil and Thailand shows HIV infection both among IDUs and non-IDUs.[7]

Clinical AIDS in prison

As the pandemic matures, a growing number of countries report a problem of symptomatic AIDS in prisoners. For example, 21 percent of the known HIV-infected prisoners in Ireland were classified in Centers for Disease Control (CDC) group IV.[8] In the state prison systems of California and New York several hundred such prisoners die each year while in detention.[9] Unfortunately, around the world, treatment resources in prison systems are strained and psychosocial support is inadequate. In prisons in Africa and

Latin America no adequate prophylaxis or treatment for opportunistic infection is available for HIV-infected prisoners.

HIV/AIDS and tuberculosis in prison

The association of HIV disease and tuberculosis (TB) is of particular importance in prisons where overcrowding, poor ventilation, frequent changes in human contacts, and poor general health status all favor rapid spread of airborne infections.[10] In the decade of 1980 to 1990 the incidence of TB among New York State prison inmates rose fivefold to 134 per 100,000.[11] Despite routine isoniazid prescription, high rates of tuberculin skin test conversion during incarceration are also reported. Multidrug-resistant TB, previously reported in New York State prisons, has since emerged in California prisons, likely implicating intraprison transmission.[12,13] The identified risk factors for multidrug-resistant TB include high prevalence of HIV infection among inmates, delayed TB diagnosis, delayed and inadequate isolation precautions, and frequent transfers of inmates. Public health authorities have emphasized the need for regular TB screening of both staff and inmates, but this is rarely carried out effectively. However, the potential for TB case detection by skin tuberculin testing is also limited. This was illustrated by a study in an urban U.S. jail. Of 1,314 entrants to the jail's opiate detoxification unit, 73 (5.6 percent) had chest X-ray abnormalities associated with TB, but 17 of the 26 most serious cases would have been missed on skin testing alone.[14] In Barcelona, Spain, the prevalence of pulmonary tuberculosis among entering prisoners with a high prevalence of injecting drug use (48 percent) and of HIV infection (36 percent) was estimated to be 2.7 percent.[15]

The need for environmental control measures in prisons has also been stressed.[16] Tuberculosis associated with HIV disease is a major problem in African prisons, where treatment is often unavailable. Reports from prisons in Uganda, Tanzania, and Zambia have revealed high mortality rates that are probably due to HIV-associated TB.[17] In the first 9 months of 1995, 819 prisoners died in Kenya's prisons, from a prison population of 40,000.[18]

Injecting drug use and prison

Several studies indicate that IDUs continue to inject while in prison. Although they use drugs at a lower rate than outside prison, HIV transmission risks may be increased by needle/syringe sharing in an environment where needle exchange and disinfectants are unavailable.[19,20] In a Scottish prison, for example, several prisoners seroconverted for both hepatitis B virus and HIV after sharing a syringe.[21] In a 1992 WHO survey, 16 of 55 prison systems reported having introduced some form of disinfectant distribution to prisoners, usually in the form of diluted bleach.[22] Recently, however, concern has been expressed that diluted bleach is an ineffective virucidal agent for dried blood in syringes and is therefore inadequate for use in prisons.[23] But until more effective measures can be introduced, diluted bleach should remain available, and prisoners should be warned that protection is incomplete. Alternative methods of disinfecting injection equipment include powdered hypochlorite, as distributed in prisons in the State of Victoria, Australia, or iodized disinfectants. Meanwhile, there has been virtually no progress in making needle/syringe exchange available in prisons. A sole exception involves several experimental programs in Swiss prisons under the auspices of the Swiss Federal Bureau of Health. Early results from these programs are encouraging.

International guidelines

In 1993 WHO and the Council of Europe published two new sets of international guidelines in the field of HIV/AIDS in prisons.[24,25] Both stress that principles adopted in national AIDS programs should be applied in prison settings; measures undertaken in prison must be complementary and compatible with those in the community. Thus, the guidelines condemn any form of obligatory HIV antibody testing in prison and emphasize the need for strictly protecting the confidentiality of health information, including HIV status, from the prison administration and the judiciary. Care available to prisoners with HIV disease should be equivalent to that in the general community, and release for prisoners with advanced AIDS should be facilitated on humanitarian grounds to allow them to be closer to family and friends and to die with dignity. Both WHO and the Council of Europe guidelines reaffirm the need for condoms to be freely available in prisons, both for use within the institutions and on release. The guidelines also assume that drugs are available in virtually every prison that has significant numbers of IDUs. Therefore, it is not sensible, in public health terms, to base a prevention policy on keeping drugs out of prisons. The reports advocate a realistic approach based on:

- making treatment programs leading to abstinence available for motivated IDUs in prison (for example, drug-free sections, organized as a therapeutic community)
- encouraging IDUs to take drugs by less dangerous means (e.g., smoking or sniffing)
- making methadone maintenance available
- providing bleach solution or powder to prisoners, with instructions on how to disinfect needles and syringes
- considering clean needle and syringe distribution within prison

The European Committee for the Prevention of Torture and Inhuman or Degrading Treatment or Punishment (CPT) also recently addressed the problem of HIV/AIDS in prison.[26] The Committee, which has visited prisons in 23 European countries, stressed the need for an HIV/AIDS policy based on nondiscrimination and confidentiality and affirmed that there is no medical justification for the segregation of HIV-infected prisoners. The CPT's outspoken comments on this issue indicate that it considers it a violation of these principles to constitute inhuman or degrading treatment, and therefore represents a serious violation of human rights. Given CPT's official, intergovernmental status, this position is of considerable importance.

The Canadian prison system has adopted a clear policy based on confidentiality, noncoercive measures, and condom availability, but in general, few countries fully apply the international guidelines in their prison system. Systematic HIV antibody testing is commonly carried out in U.S. prisons and results are regularly communicated to the prison administration.[27] Segregation of HIV-infected prisoners is also widespread, and an official report from Ireland illustrates how difficult it is to end segregation once it has been adopted.[28] Only 5 percent of U.S. prison systems make condoms available. The 1991 comment by the U.S. National Commission on AIDS that "only a handful of prison systems distribute condoms" remains valid in 1994.[29] In Europe, however, considerable progress has been made to increase condom distribution; 22 of 32 prison systems surveyed in late 1992 now make condoms available.

In conclusion, HIV/AIDS issues in prisons remain unresolved, particularly in the field of discrimination, segregation, and coercive approaches. A review of the global situation in prisons in 1994 highlights the general failure to apply effective, health-oriented public preventive measures to the problems of HIV/AIDS.

REFERENCES

1. WHO, Global Programme on AIDS, *HIV/AIDS and Prisons: A Survey Covering 55 Prison Systems in 31 Countries* (Geneva: University Institute of Legal Medicine, 1992).
2. M. Diez, L. Martin, and A. Granados, "Programme for the prevention and control of HIV/AIDS in Spanish prisons," Abstract MO 0037, presented at the VIII International Conference on AIDS, Amsterdam, The Netherlands, July 1992.
3. D. Borne, A. Ivanoff, N. El-Bassel, R. Schilling, B. Grodd, and B. Heller, "Sexual risk behaviour among sentenced drug using inmates in a New York City jail," Abstract PoD 5053, presented at the VIII International Conference on AIDS, Amsterdam, The Netherlands, July 1992.
4. R. L. Gido, "Invisible women: The status of incarcerated women with HIV/AIDS," *Justice Professional* 7(1992):25–33.
5. M. Murphy, K. Gaffney, O. Carey, E. Dooley, and F. Mulcahy, "Impact of HIV disease on an Irish prison population," *International Journal of STD and AIDS* 3(1992):426–429.
6. D. Bertrand, "African prison officials worried," *World AIDS Briefing* 19(1992):5–6.
7. WHO, *HIV/AIDS and Prisons.*
8. Murphy, "Impact of HIV disease."
9. Correctional Association of New York, "AIDS in prison and jail fact sheet," document prepared for the First National Roundtable on AIDS in Prison, San Francisco, CA: November 1993.
10. WHO, "HIV/AIDS and Prisons."
11. J. B. Glaser, J. K. Aboujaoude, and R. Greifinger, "Tuberculin skin test conversion among HIV-infected prison inmates," *Journal of Acquired Immune Deficiency Syndromes* 5(1992):430–431.
12. Centers for Disease Control, "Transmission of multidrug-resistant tuberculosis among immunocompromised persons in a correctional system, New York," *Mortality and Morbidity Weekly Report* 41(1991):507–508.
13. Centers for Disease Control, "Probable transmission of multidrug-resistant tuberculosis in a correctional facility, California," *Mortality and Morbidity Weekly Report* 42(1993):48–51.

14. E. Bellin, D. Fletcher, and S. Safyer, "Abnormal chest X-rays in intravenous drug users: Implications for tuberculosis screening programmes," *American Journal of Public Health* 83(1993):698–700.

15. V. Martin, P. Gonzalez, J. A. Cayla, J. Mirabeut, J. Canellas, J. M. Pina, and P. Miret, "Casefinding of pulmonary tuberculosis on admission to a penitentiary centre," *Tubercle and Lung Disease* 75(1994):49–53.

16. W. W. Stead, "Control of tuberculosis in crowded public places in the HIV/AIDS era," *Journal of Prison and Jail Health* 12(1993):13–31.

17. University Institute of Legal Medicine, *Network and HIV/AIDS in Prison*, update survey (Geneva: University Institute of Legal Medicine, 1993).

18. Reply by Minister of Justice in the parliament of Kenya, October 9, 1995.

19. J. Strang, "Sexual and injecting behaviours in prison: From disciplinary problem to public health conundrum," *Criminal Behaviour and Mental Health* 3(1993):393–402.

20. M. Gaughwin and D. Vlahov, "Assessing the risk of HIV-1 transmission in correctional centres," in *Psychoactive Drugs and Harm Reduction*, N. Heather, A. Wodak, et al., eds. (London: Whurr Publications, 1993):310–319.

21. B. Christie, "HIV outbreak investigated in Scottish jail," *British Medical Journal* 307(1993):151.

22. WHO, *HIV/AIDS and Prisons*.

23. National Institute on Drug Abuse, *Community Alert Bulletin: Proposed Recommendation to Prevent HIV Transmission by Sharing Drug Injection Equipment* (Washington, DC: National Institute on Drug Abuse, March 25, 1993).

24. WHO, *World Health Organization Guidelines on HIV Infection and AIDS in Prison* (Geneva: WHO, 1993).

25. Council of Europe, *Recommendation No. R(93)6 of the Committee of Ministers of Member States* (Strasbourg, France: Council of Europe, 1993).

26. Council of Europe, *Third Annual Report of the CPT* (Strasbourg, France: Council of Europe, 1993).

27. J. Lillis, "Dealing with HIV/AIDS-positive inmates," *Corrections Compendium* 18(1993):1–3.

28. Advisory Committee, *Report of the Advisory Committee on Communicable Disease in Prison* (Dublin, Ireland: Ministry of Justice, 1993).

29. U.S. National Commission on AIDS, *Report: HIV Disease in Correctional Facilities* (Washington, DC: National Institute of Justice, 1990).

26

Pediatric HIV/AIDS

In 1995, worldwide, 500,000 children were born with HIV infection (Chapter 1). The majority of these children (345,000; 69 percent) were in sub-Saharan Africa where HIV transmits predominantly heterosexually, resulting in the infection of large numbers of women in their reproductive age. In Southeast Asia, where the number of young women becoming HIV infected began to rise more recently, a subsequent spread of infection from mother to off-spring is anticipated.

The rapid and dynamic evolution of knowledge and experience during the pandemic is clearly illustrated when considering children and HIV/AIDS. From the initial image of a young child with AIDS, the picture of pediatric HIV/AIDS has broadened enormously to include a more complete under-standing of routes of infection, diversity of clinical expression, influence of social context, and the world of infected children as they survive and grow towards adolescence.

Breast-feeding and HIV/AIDS

Sophie Le Coeur and Marc Lallemant

There is now increased awareness that HIV is transmitted through breast-feeding and greater understanding about the extent and range of circum-stances in which this occurs. The two major settings of HIV transmission are breast-feeding by a mother who was HIV infected during pregnancy, and breast-feeding by a mother who became HIV infected after delivery.

The most frequent context involves mothers who are both pregnant and HIV infected. In this setting, it has been particularly difficult to distinguish the added contribution of HIV transmission through breast-feeding from the risk of HIV acquisition in utero or during childbirth. For example, while cohort studies from France and Europe reported substantially lower HIV infection rates among children when their HIV-infected mothers did not breast-feed (14 percent and 17 percent, respectively), compared with rates when mothers breast-fed their infants (28 percent and 44 percent, respectively),[1,2] and a study from Kinshasa, Zaire, reported a higher prevalence of HIV infection among infants when women did not breast-feed, other studies have found no difference in HIV infection rates between breast-fed and non–breast-fed infants.[3,4] Nevertheless, taking all available studies into account, a meta-analysis estimated the additional risk of postnatal transmission through breast-feeding to be 14 percent (95 percent confidence interval: 7–22 percent).[5]

That HIV can be transmitted through breast milk and breast-feeding is now widely accepted. This section considers factors that may influence the rate of HIV transmission via breast-feeding and the translation of scientific information into policies on breast-feeding, particularly in the developing world. Data suggests a dose-response relationship between transmission and duration of breast-feeding; and characteristics of the breast milk, such as high viral load and/or low specific anti-HIV IgM and IgA, have been associated with increased transmission, independent of the mother's immune status.[6,7] Second, the timing of breast-feeding may also be important. The frequency of detection of HIV-1 DNA in colostrum is high, decreasing sharply in breast milk after a few days.[8,9] Therefore, breast-feeding with colostrum, which is particularly rich in lymphocytes, may be associated with an increased risk of HIV transmission. Nevertheless, transmission through breast milk can occur later in the postpartum period. Evidence for later transmission includes a report of several breast-fed infants born to HIV-infected mothers. The infants were seronegative at birth and at 12 months of age, yet became seropositive by 18 months of age.[10,11,12] Since other risk factors for postnatal HIV infection were absent, breast milk ingested later in infancy was considered to be the most likely mode of infection for these children.

In the second scenario, maternal HIV infection occurs after delivery and breast-feeding therefore occurs when maternal viremia as well as virus load in breast milk are high.[13] Moreover, in this situation, maternal infection usually goes undetected since conventional serological tests are negative. Indeed, this is the setting in which postnatal transmission of HIV was first described—among infants whose mothers were infected by blood transfusion during or immediately after delivery.[14-17] Children breast-fed during this period are exposed to a large quantity of virus without the benefit of any passively transmitted maternal anti-HIV immunity. Thus, in a prospective study in Kigali, Rwanda, 36 percent of breast-fed children of mothers for whom postnatal infection was carefully documented, became HIV infected, compared to 25 percent of breast-fed children born to women who were infected prior to pregnancy in the same study.[18] A meta-analysis of all available data has yielded an overall transmission risk of 29 percent (CI 95 percent: 16–42 percent) among breast-fed children born to mothers themselves HIV-infected after delivery.[19,20,21] Therefore, postnatal transmission can be important in regions of very high HIV incidence. In Kigali, for example, about 13 percent of all perinatally infected children are thought to have been infected during the postpartum period as a consequence of HIV transmission through breast-feeding by their newly HIV-infected mother.[22]

How have these data on HIV and breast-feeding been translated into policy and practice?

In the late 1980s, when case reports suggested that HIV was transmissible through breast milk, public health officials in industrialized countries advocated that HIV-infected women refrain from breast-feeding.[23] In developing countries, however, the initially hypothetical risk of this form of transmission was balanced against the reality of excess infant mortality associated with bottle-feeding. In these countries, bottle-feeding had been shown to substantially increase the risk of diarrheal diseases and malnutrition, while breast-feeding protected against the most common infectious diseases, ensured optimal nutrition, and strengthened interaction with the mother.[24-27] Breast-feeding also has other advantages: it is low cost and prolongs postpartum amenorrhea, thus favoring increased birth spacing.[28] For all these reasons, during the past three decades, breast-feeding has been heavily promoted to combat infant morbidity and mortality in developing countries. Thus, new doubts about the safety of breast-feeding related to HIV infection were seen by many public health agencies as a threat to years of prevention efforts. Accordingly, the position initially adopted in 1987 by the World Health Organization for developing countries was conservative: despite the expansion of the HIV epidemic among women of child-bearing age, breast-feeding was still recommended.[29]

Models were then developed to analyze the impact of breast-feeding transmission on diverse populations in the developing world, taking into account a range of issues, including the local HIV epidemic, levels of risk behaviors, accessibility of voluntary testing and counseling, and rates and prevalent causes of infant and childhood mortality.[30,31,32] The central question was whether and under what circumstances the increase of HIV transmission associated with breast-feeding would outweigh the protective effect of breast-feeding. Using one such model, one concludes that where HIV testing is not available, all mothers, unless they have clinical AIDS, should be advised to breast-feed their infants, even if the risk of transmission through breast-feeding is as high as 25 percent and the childhood mortality rate (CMR) less than 100 per 1,000 live births. Conversely, where HIV testing is available, three possibilities arise: (1) HIV-positive mothers should be advised to breast-feed except where CMR is under 100 per 1,000; (2) HIV-negative mothers with low-risk behavior can breast-feed safely; and (3) HIV-negative mothers with high-risk behavior should breast-feed and should also be counseled about the risk of postnatal transmission if they become infected.

In reality, however, situations in which a decision has to be made on breast-feeding are much more diverse and complex than what these models can assimilate. In addition, new information about the substantial potential risk of HIV transmission via breast-feeding must be taken into account. Accordingly, in 1992 WHO and UNICEF issued new recommendations which sought to respond to new data and to resolve these tensions. The new recommendations emphasize the importance of services for breast-feeding women (such as availability of confidential testing, counseling, and support). Yet until or unless those needs are met, the guidance on breast-feed-ing remains vague; the new guidelines reflect the pervasive difficulty in seeking to harmonize AIDS-specific policy recommendations with other, preexisting health policies.[33]

Now that prevention of mother-to-child transmission is envisioned in de-veloping countries, alternatives to breast-feeding should also be considered a "medical" intervention to prevent HIV transmission.[34] In this context, there is an urgent need to launch operational research protocols to evaluate its feasibility, effectiveness, and cost, in addition to other methods to reduce mother-to-child transmission.

References

1. S. Blanche, C. Rouzioux, M. L. Guihard Moscato, et al., and the HIV Infection in New-borns French Collaborative Study Group, "Prospective study of infants born to women seropositive for human immunodeficiency virus type 1," *New England Journal of Medicine* 320(1989):1643–1648.

2. European Collaborative Study, "Children born to women with HIV-1 infection: Natural history and risk of transmission," *Lancet* 337(1991):253–260.

3. C. Hutto, W. P. Parks, S. Lai, et al., "Hospital-based prospective study of perinatal infection with human immunodeficiency virus type 1," *Journal of Pediatrics* 118(1991):347–353.

4. C. Kind, B. Brändle, C. A. Wyler, et al., "Epidemiology of vertically transmitted HIV-1 infection in Switzerland: Results of a nationwide prospective study," *European Journal of Pediatrics* 151(1992):442–448.

5. D. T. Dunn, M. L. Newell, A. E. Ades, and C. S. Peckham, "Risk of human immunodefi-ciency virus type 1 transmission through breastfeeding," *Lancet* 340(1992):585–588.

6. M. de Martino, P. A. Tovo, A. E. Tozzi, et al., "HIV-1 transmission through breast-milk: Appraisal of risk according to duration of feeding," *AIDS* 6(1992):991–997.

7. P. Van de Perre, A. Simono, D. G. Hitimana, F. Dabis, P. Msellati, B. Mukamabano, J. B. Butera, C. Van Goethem, E. Karita, and P. Lepage, "Infective and anti-infective proper-ties of breastmilk from HIV-1-infected women," *Lancet* 341(1993):914–918.

8. *Ibid.*

9. A. J. Ruff, J. Coberly, N. A. Halsey, et al., "Prevalence of HIV-1 DNA and p24 antigen in breast milk and correlation with maternal factors," *Journal of Acquired Immune De-ficiency Syndromes* 7(1994):68–73.

10. P. Lepage, P. Van de Perre, A. Simono, P. Msellati, D. G. Hitimana, and F. Dabis, "Tran-sient seroreversion in children born to human immunodeficiency virus 1-infected mothers," *Pediatric Infectious Disease Journal* 11(1992):892–894.

11. M. Lallemant, S. Le Coeur, L. Samba, D. Cheynier, P. M'Pelé, S. Nzingoula, and M. Essex, "Mother-to-child transmission of HIV-1 in Congo, central Africa," *AIDS* 8(1994):1429–1436.

12. P. Datta, J. E. Embree, J. Kreiss, J. O. Ndinya-Achola, J. Muriithi, K. K. Holmes, and F. A. Plummer, "Resumption of breast-feeding in later childhood: A risk factor for mother to child human immunodeficiency virus type 1 transmission," *Pediatric Infec-tious Disease Journal* 11(1992):974–976.

13. E. S. Daar, T. Moudgil, R. D. Meyer, and D. D. Ho, "Transient high levels of viremia in patients with primary human immunodeficiency virus type 1 infection," *New England Journal of Medicine* 334(1991):961–964.

14. J. B. Zeigler, D. A. Cooper, R. O. Johnson, and J. Gold, "Postnatal transmission of AIDS-associated retrovirus from mother to infant," *Lancet* 1(1985):896–898.

15. P. Lepage, P. Van de Perre, M. Caraël, et al., "Postnatal transmission of HIV from mother to child," letter, *Lancet* 2(1987):400.

16. R. Colebunders, B. Kapita, W. Nekwei, Y. Bahwe, I. Lebughe, M. Oxtoby, and R. Ryder, "Breast-feeding and transmission of HIV," letter, *Lancet* 2(1988):1487.

17. P. Weinbreck, V. Loustaud, F. Denis, B. Vidal, M. Mounier, and P. De Lumbreck, "Postnatal transmission of HIV infection," *Lancet* 1(1988):482.

18. P. Lepage, P. Van De Perre, P. Msellati, et al., "Mother-to-child transmission of human immunodeficiency virus type 1 (HIV-1) and its determinants: A cohort study in Kigali, Rwanda," *American Journal of Epidemiology* 137(1993):589–599.

19. S. K. Hira, U. G. Mangola, C. Mwale, C. Chintu, W. E. Tambo, and P. L. Perine, "Apparent vertical transmission of human immunodeficiency virus type 1 by breast-feeding in Zambia," *Journal of Pediatrics* 117(1992):421–424.

20. P. Palasanthiran, J. B. Ziegler, G. J. Stewart, M. Stuckey, J. A. Armstrong, D. A. Coopere, R. Penny, and J. Gold, "Breast-feeding during primary maternal human immunodeficiency virus infection and risk of transmission from mother to infant," *Journal of Infectious Diseases* 167(1993):441–444.

21. D. T. Dunn, M. L. Newell, A. E. Ades, and C. S. Peckham, "Risk of human immunodeficiency virus type 1 transmission through breastfeeding," *Lancet* 340(1992):585–588.

22. P. Van de Perre, D. G. Hitimana, F. Dabis, E. Karita, and P. Lepage, "Postnatal transmission of HIV-1 (reply)," *New England Journal of Medicine* 326(1992):643–644.

23. Centers for Disease Control, "Recommendations for assisting in the prevention of perinatal transmission of human T-lymphotropic virus type III/lymphadenopathy-associated virus and acquired immunodeficiency syndrome," *Mortality and Morbidity Weekly Report* 341(1985):721–732.

24. M. Minchin, "Infant Formula: A mass, uncontrolled trial in perinatal care," *Birth* 14(1987):25–34.

25. C. G. Victora, P. G. Smith, J. P. Vaughan, et al., "Evidence for protection by breast-feeding against infant deaths from infectious diseases in Brazil," *Lancet* 329(1987):319–322.

26. A. S. Goldman, "Immune system of human milk: Antimicrobial, antiinflammatory and immunomodulating properties," *Pediatric Infectious Disease Journal* 12(1993):664–671.

27. A. Lucas, R. Morley, T. J. Cole, G. Lister, and C. Leeson-Payne, "Breast milk and subsequent intelligence quotient in children born preterm," *Lancet* 339(1992):261–264.

28. A. Perez, M. H. Labbok, and J. T. Queenan, "Clinical study of the lactational amenorrhoea method for family planning," *Lancet* 339(1992):968–970.

29. "Breast-feeding/breast milk and human immunodeficiency virus (HIV)," *Weekly Epidemiological Record* 33(1987):245–246.

30. S. J. Heymann, "Is breast feeding at risk? The challenge of AIDS," *AIDS in the World*, J. Mann, D. Tarantola, and T. Netter, eds. (Cambridge, MA: Harvard University Press, 1992):616–629.

31. S. A. Lederman, "Estimating infant mortality from human immunodeficiency virus and other causes in breast-feeding and bottle-feeding populations," *Pediatrics* 89(1992):290–296.

32. D. J. Hu, W. L. Heyward, R. H. Byers, B. M. Nkowane, M. J. Oxtoby, S. E. Holck, and D. L. Heymann, "HIV infection and breast-feeding: Policy implications through a decision analysis model," *AIDS* 6(1992):1505–1513.

33. A. Nicoll, M. L. Newell, E. Van Praag, P. Van de Perre, and C. Peckham, "Infant feeding policy and practice in the presence of HIV-1 infection," *AIDS* (1995), 9:107–119.

34. M. Lallemant, S. Le Coeur, D. Tarantola, J. Mann, M. Essex, "Preventing perinatal transmission," *Lancet* 343(1994):1429–1430.

27

Orphans of the HIV/AIDS Pandemic

CAROL LEVINE, DAVID MICHAELS, AND SARA D. BACK

In one Ugandan dialect a child whose parents have died is called *efuuzi*, or "one who regrets all the time." Local terms for orphans vary from poetic to prosaic, and definitions vary by age and whether one or both parents have died. Grief and vulnerability, however, are universal characteristics of orphans.

A great deal of information—both quantitative and qualitative—is now available about AIDS orphans. The global scope and extent of the AIDS orphan situation is now better appreciated (Box 27-1). Many of the countries in which the effects of HIV/AIDS have been most severe also have high adult mortality rates from many other causes, including civil conflict and war. As a result, these countries already had many orphans even in the absence of HIV/AIDS. For example, before the onset of the HIV/AIDS pandemic, it was estimated that between 5.5 and 7 percent of children below the age of 15 in four East African countries (Kenya, Malawi, Tanzania, and Uganda) had lost one or both parents. Yet, since HIV/AIDS affects mainly young and middle-aged adults, AIDS will cause a marked increase in the risk of being orphaned. In some areas, the increase may be as much as 50 percent.[1]

BOX 27-1

Projections of numbers of AIDS orphans

D. MICHAELS AND S. BACK

The estimates displayed in Table 27-1.1 involve children who have lost their mothers to AIDS in selected countries. While the loss of large numbers of fathers to HIV/AIDS is likely to be devastating for both the children and society as a whole, it is far more difficult to study. Few data exist on the male equivalent of female fertility rates, making it difficult to construct mathematical projections of the number of children who lose their fathers to HIV/AIDS. However, the magnitude of the tragedy resulting from the loss of fathers to the epidemic is enormous, and must not be overlooked.

To develop these projections, HIV prevalence estimates for rural and urban areas of each country were selected from the HIV/AIDS Surveillance Data Base, compiled by the Center for International

Table 27-1.1 Estimated numbers of children orphaned by AIDS (children having lost their mothers to AIDS) in selected countries and approximate proportion of AIDS orphans in entire population <15 years old, 1995 and 2000[a,b]

Country	Year 1995: No. of AIDS orphans (percent of <15 year-old population)	Year 2000: No. of AIDS orphans (percent of <15-year-old population)
Argentina	5,000–20,000 (0.04%–0.2%)	8,000–50,000 (0.05%–0.3%)
Cote D'Ivoire	110,000–140,000 (1.2%–1.7%)	220,000–300,000 (1.9%–2.7%)
Dominican Republic[c]	5,000–16,000 (0.15%–0.4%)	12,000–40,000 (0.27%–0.9%)
Ethiopia	120,000–230,000 (0.4%–0.7%)	340,000–650,000 (0.8%–1.5%)
Honduras	1,000–12,000 (0.03%–0.4%)	2,000–30,000 (0.06%–0.9%)
Kenya[c]	210,000–310,000 (1.1%–1.7%)	380,000–580,000 (1.5%–2.4%)
Tanzania	260,000–360,000 (1.3%–1.8%)	490,000–680,000 (1.7%–2.5%)
Thailand[c]	15,000–30,000 (0.06%–0.14%)	30,000–100,000 (0.1%–0.4%)
Uganda[c]	220,000–460,000 (1.5%–3.3%)	410,000–880,000 (2.1%–4.9%)
United States[d]	40,000–60,000 (0.05%–0.07%)	70,000–125,000 (0.07%–0.13%)
Zambia[c]	180,000–300,000 (2.9%–4.6%)	320,000–490,000 (4.0%–7.1%)

[a]Except for the United States, estimates were derived using the *Demographic Projection Model (DemProj)* and *AIDS Impact Model (AIM)* software programs. These programs employ demographic data (population size and age distribution, total fertility rates, infant mortality rates, life expectancy) obtained from the Population Council Databank System, which compiled country-specific information from the Population Division of The United Nations Department of International and Economic and Social Affairs; and from N. Keyfitz and W. Flieger, *World Population Growth and Aging: Demographic Trends in the Late Twentieth Century* (Chicago: University of Chicago Press, 1990). Estimates on the rate at which people who are infected with HIV develop AIDS, and progression to death among people with AIDS were supplied by the Global AIDS Policy Coalition.

[b]For the years 1995 and 2000, this table contains range estimates of the cumulative number of children whose mothers have died of HIV/AIDS before the child reaches the age of 15, and (in parentheses) the estimated proportion of all children in the population age-group 0–14 who are AIDS orphans.

[c]Projections for the Dominican Republic, Kenya, Thailand, Uganda, and Zambia were originally calculated for publication in WHO and UNICEF, *Action for Children Affected by AIDS* (Geneva and New York: WHO and UNICEF, 1994).

[d]The estimated numbers and proportions for the United States were calculated for children and youth younger than 18 years old.

Research, U.S. Bureau of the Census, and from prevalence data reported in WHO and UNICEF, *Action for Children Affected by AIDS.*[1] Only prevalence estimates obtained from relatively large population-based samples (e.g., pregnant women and blood donors) were used. Separate prevalence curves were then constructed for each country's rural and urban regions, using high and low prevalence figures estimated for the years 1995 and 2000 by the Global AIDS Policy Coalition. The rural and urban curves were combined in a proportionately weighted manner, reflecting the population distribution in each country, to generate overall prevalence figures for the model. In general, the lower bound of the reported range represents application of the most conservative data and assumptions, including the assumption that HIV prevalence will not continue to increase after 1996.

For the United States a mathematical model was constructed in which cumulative fertility rates were applied to the number of reported AIDS deaths of adult women younger than 50 years old. The results were adjusted for underreporting of HIV-related mortality, pediatric AIDS deaths, infant mortality, ethnic and racial variation in fertility, and decreased fertility associated with late-stage HIV disease.[2]

References

1. WHO and UNICEF, *Action for Children Affected by AIDS* (Geneva: WHO and New York: UNICEF, 1994).
2. D. Michaels and C. Levine, "Estimates of the number of motherless youth orphaned by AIDS in the United States," *Journal of the American Medical Association* 268(1992):3456–3461.

The number of children who will have been orphaned by HIV/AIDS by the year 2000 has been estimated to range from five to 10 million.[2-5] This large range reflects variations in the parameters and assumptions used in the prediction models, as well as the different definitions of "orphan" (children without mothers, or children who have lost either or both parents). Estimates from models constructed for specific countries are likely to have somewhat smaller ranges; for policy and program planning, national projections are essential.

Estimates of numbers and distribution of orphans of the HIV/AIDS pandemic provide a quantitative measure of impact. Yet considerable information is now also available on the problems faced by these children and by families, communities, and organizations seeking to help them. Three general observations about these orphans provide a basis for analysis and planning:

- First, most orphaned children are not HIV infected.
- Second, whether infected or affected, the orphans of the HIV/AIDS pandemic create special stress on family and community resources and are highly vulnerable because families affected by HIV/AIDS usually have more than one ill or dying member.
- Third, while in many African countries the HIV/AIDS pandemic has added a new group of orphans to the already serious problem of children who are parentless, in industrialized Western countries the phenomenon of large numbers of children left parentless from a single disease is unprecedented. In Asia the rapid spread of HIV infection, especially among young women, presages a crisis around orphans.

To gather information and impressions of the social impact of this aspect of the HIV/AIDS pandemic, governmental and nongovernmental agencies and individuals identified with the issue in over 50 countries were sent a 20-page survey questionnaire. Twenty-nine responses were received. The main headings of the questionnaires were definitions of orphans, enumerations and estimates, cultural and legal norms, quality of life, organizations and services, orphanages, social attitudes, finances, and future directions and needs. Because the survey was intended to provide background for a broad overview, there was no attempt to make the sample statistically valid. Furthermore, as expected, most of the information came from sub-Saharan Africa, which has had the most experience in dealing with orphans. Recent analyses from the United Kingdom and Thailand have contributed to the growing body of knowledge.[6,7] The information collected through the survey was supplemented by a literature review and discussions with people having direct field experience.*

By necessity, the trends reported here are suggested rather than conclusive; in addition, many findings are specific to the culture and circumstances of the respondent.

First, many organizations and individuals strongly believe that orphans of the HIV/AIDS pandemic should not receive or be identified for special attention and benefits; the focus of intervention should be on all orphans, along with all other vulnerable children.[8] On the other hand, participants in a meeting examining the unmet needs in six U.S. cities could not reach a consensus on whether the needs of children orphaned by HIV/AIDS should be addressed through categorical programs and funding or through reform of existing systems that affect families, such as child welfare, education, the judiciary, and health care.[9]

Some survey respondents reported no difference in the quality of life experienced by orphans in general and orphans of the HIV/AIDS pandemic. A Romanian respondent noted that a significant distinction is not between orphans and non-orphans but between children living in institutions, some of whom are HIV infected, and those living in the community. However, some respondents stated that orphans of the HIV/AIDS pandemic had a poorer quality of life, were more stigmatized, and in general, suffered more deprivation and rejection than other orphans. For instance, over half of survey respondents felt that orphans of the HIV/AIDS pandemic were subjected to "much more" or "more" social rejection than those orphaned from other causes. These differences were particularly apparent in severely affected regions. According to one African respondent, a family may have spent so much money on the parent's illness that they are unwilling or unable to provide any more resources to care for the children. Funerals are a major cost that depletes the family's resources. Intrafamily jealousies and disagreements may also bear on the treatment accorded surviving children.

When parents die of AIDS, where do the children go?

When a parent dies, the children most often stay with the surviving parent. However, in Africa, when the mother dies of AIDS, the children are less likely to stay with the father, perhaps because he is ill or otherwise unable to care for them. When the father dies, the children tend to stay with their mother. Sometimes the father's family blames the mother for bringing HIV into the home and sends her and her children away, even though it may often be the man who first contracted HIV infection.

In both industrialized and developing countries, when both parents have

*Among the many individuals who provided advice on the survey and information about orphans were Martha Ainsworth, Maxine Ankrah, Susan Hunter, Aklilu Lemma, Elizabeth Preble, Jan Williamson, and John Williamson. The staff of the Global AIDS Policy Coalition provided invaluable assistance in the design and conduct of the survey. The authors of this chapter alone are responsible for the data and interpretations.

died of AIDS, the children are most often taken in by some members of the extended family—grandparents, aunts and uncles, and, less frequently, older siblings.

From the African survey responses a clear pattern of power and decision-making emerged, favoring the paternal family. In most instances the paternal family decides the future of the orphaned children. For instance, two-thirds of survey respondents stated that when both parents have died, the paternal extended family controls the orphan's property. In Africa orphaned children have relatively few legal or customary rights to property or to decision-making about their future, unless the father has made specific provisions for them in a will. Although many orphans are cared for by loving families who share their resources willingly, these dependent children are at risk for exploitation, deprivation of property rights, abuse, and neglect. Orphaned girls may be even less welcome in families than boys because they must be provided with a marriage dowry. However, girls may also be considered valuable as household help or concubines. In cultures that value women primarily as economic or sexual objects, orphaned girls are particularly vulnerable to exploitation.

Acceptance of orphaned children also depends on the age of the orphan. Young infants and toddlers in the developing world are often seen as particularly burdensome because of the level of care required, while older children can work alongside other family members. In contrast, in the industrialized world, it is usually easier to find a home for babies than for older children, particularly teenagers, who are seen as presenting potential behavior problems.

What are the burdens for families related to AIDS orphans?

Traditional family structures, already stressed by poverty, poor health, and increased burdens of care, are in many instances reaching the breaking point.[10] Many of the conditions that promote social dislocation and family stress preceded the HIV/AIDS pandemic; this is as true in the United States as in Africa.[11] A study of the care of people with AIDS in a rural population in southwest Uganda found evidence of limited care by family members because of poverty, other responsibilities, and stigma. Some adult patients were cared for by children because there were no other adults in the home.[12] A review of the impact of AIDS on the urban Ugandan family also found that although "material assistance, such as food, bedding, medicine, and school fees, is needed to make up for lost income, more than money is needed to overcome the burden of AIDS on families. There must be a change in the climate of fear . . . and ways that families can adapt to the loss of mobility that prevents normal patterns of family interaction in the dispersed kin network."[13]

If the general "safety net" for people with AIDS has gaps, the net for dependent orphaned children after the death of a parent is even looser. While many families have absorbed orphaned children out of love, custom, or moral obligation, they may not be able to do so indefinitely. Nevertheless, an independent assessment is needed to determine the level of assistance required to promote family function. As stated in *Action for Children Affected by AIDS*, "ultimately it will be the affected families and communities that find ways to cope with AIDS and with the social and economic damage that the illness inflicts. . . . Wherever possible, resources should be directed to enabling families and communities to establish and maintain a sufficient economic base to provide for children's needs."[14]

Organizational support for orphans

Governmental and nongovernmental organizations are attempting to support and supplement existing family structures. In Uganda alone, over 300 organizations are providing direct services to orphans of the HIV/AIDS pandemic, including medical care, housing, food, education (school fees), a family environment, legal assistance, emotional support, clothing, recreation, skills training, and financial assistance. In New York City, The Orphan Project identified over 70 organizations that provide services appropriate for children and families affected by HIV/AIDS.[15]

Despite the variety of services and the growing number of involved organizations, the needs of orphaned children are still not being met. A broad distinction has emerged between organizations' adequacy in providing short-term assistance and often more complex, long-term support. For example, needs for clothing, medical care, legal assistance, food and housing were generally better met than needs for education and skills training. Additional gaps were noted in several areas: reaching orphans in rural villages (where many are sent from cities after the parent's death); bereavement planning and counseling; and providing caregivers, who are mostly women, with emotional and financial support.

Orphanages have traditionally been a solution of last resort. More recently, although orphanages in industrialized countries have largely been replaced by nonrelative foster care, congregate care institutions continue to exist in other parts of the world. Survey respondents were generally opposed to creating new orphanages, as these would isolate children from their communities and make it difficult, if not impossible, for them to return and be accepted as full community participants (see Box 27-2). Orphanages are also expensive to build and maintain, yet some have been created as a response to the HIV/AIDS pandemic.

BOX 27-2

A community-based program for orphans and vulnerable children, Luwero District, Uganda: strategies for implementation

DEAN SHUEY, HENRY BAGARUKAYO, SAMUEL SENKUSU, AND KIM RYAN

Uganda has a population of almost 17 million, 55 percent of whom are under the age of 18. There are an estimated 1.5 million HIV-infected people in Uganda, and the HIV seroprevalence in antenatal clinics ranges from 5 to 30 percent.[1]

The Ugandan government has defined an orphan as any child under the age of 18 years with one missing parent. The 1991 census showed that 1.48 million Ugandan children, 16.2 percent of the age-cohort, met this definition. The main causes of orphaning are AIDS and civil disturbance.

The magnitude of the orphan situation has made standard institutional approaches unfeasible. The government is encouraging community-based approaches, hoping to keep children in their communities and within extended families. Since 1994, the Association François-Xavier Bagnoud (AFXB) has extended support to the African Medical and Research Foundation (AMREF) in designing and implementing a program in two subcounties of Luwero district. This central Ugandan district with a population of 450,000 was severely affected by civil war in the early 1980s. It has also reported the sixth highest number of AIDS cases, even though it is only the sixteenth most populous district in Uganda. Overall, 20.8 percent of children in Luwero district are orphaned. In two subcounties, Semuto (population, 15,000) and Butuntumula (24,000), AMREF has ongoing community-based health activities. The orphan-related work started with sensitization through community meetings to emphasize the community-based nature of the program. To avoid the development of dependency, great care was taken to avoid the labeling of "AMREF" or "AFXB" orphans.

Next, a needs assessment was conducted among political leaders, civil servants, religious leaders, guardians, and orphans themselves. The highest priority needs, in descending order, were:

1. School fees
2. Scholastic materials
3. Feeding
4. Bedding
5. Clothing
6. Medical care
7. Skills development for older orphans

The community level political structures (Resistance Councils Level I) were then mobilized to compile a list of orphans. Consistent with census data, 3,160 orphans were identified in Butuntumula and 2,200 in Semuto. A wide variety of circumstances, necessitating flexibility in response, was found. No children were living completely without adult supervision. The number of orphans in households varied from one to 17, and mothers were the most common guardians. Careful assessment was necessary, as less needy children or relatives of leaders were occasionally placed on the orphan list in anticipation of assistance. A district steering committee and subcounty working committees met regularly, and parish committees were formed to monitor program activities. The program strategies include:

- Primary level schooling
- Assistance to guardian groups and individual guardians
- Emergency humanitarian assistance
- Ad hoc vocational training
- Counseling on the rights of children and widows.

As of late 1995, sixteen primary schools in Semuto and 14 in Butuntumula had been assisted with materials and income-generating supplies, and a total of 1,183 children had been admitted to school without fees for two years. Only three cases of possible misappropriation of supplies had occurred, and each had been pursued by the local groups, with satisfactory results.

Thirty-five guardian groups caring for a total of 717 orphans and 26 individual guardians caring for 278 orphans had been given assistance with income-generating projects. Assistance included agricultural supplies, plowing fees, bee-keeping equipment, and sewing machines. Early experience suggests that individual projects may be more successful than group projects.

Finally, 35 orphans received ad hoc apprenticeship training, and emergency humanitarian assistance had been given to 127 orphans, mainly in the form of food, bedding, or medical care.

The following lessons were learned through this project:

- Community sensitization is crucial.
- Community ownership must be emphasized and dependency must be prevented.
- Widespread dissemination of information and programmatic transparency are vital.
- Income-generating is difficult in distressed economies.
- A steady, long-term response is better than projects with intensive inputs for short periods of time.
- Community-based work is labor and time intensive.
- Multisectoral approaches are needed.

In conclusion, a community-based approach, while difficult, is both feasible and necessary to face the enormous problem of AIDS orphans in Uganda and in many other parts of the world. The sharing of experiences is essential for this learning process.

References

1. AIDS Control Programme Surveillance Report, Ministry of Health, Uganda (June 1993).

Meeting current and future needs

Current efforts are failing to keep pace with the epidemic in both industrialized and developing countries. Key indicators include increases in malnutrition, children living on the streets, child-headed households, and child prostitution.

The future impact of the HIV/AIDS pandemic will include the loss of many productive workers (of the parents' generation); the potential loss of the children's future contribution through their lack of education and training; unmet basic needs for shelter, nutrition, and medical care; and exposure to HIV and other life-threatening diseases.[16] Orphans live in a volatile and threatening world, and the HIV/AIDS pandemic exposes and exacerbates their vulnerability. This is especially true in urban areas, where orphaned youngsters are "prime targets for HIV infection . . . emotionally vulnerable and economically hard-up, such children are easily drawn into selling sexual favors."[17]

A short- and long-term perspective is needed

Assistance to orphans should not be viewed a short-term project but rather as a long-term commitment to support local, sustainable initiatives.[18] HIV/AIDS is a disease that is linked to social, cultural, and economic conditions. Only a broad approach can alter the course of the epidemic. The well-being of children orphaned by the epidemic, like children in distress from other causes, is the test of our future commitment to social stability, economic development, and human rights.

REFERENCES

1. M. Ainsworth and M. Over, "The economic impact of AIDS: Shocks, responses, and outcomes," Africa Technical Department, Population, Health and Nutrition Division, The World Bank, Washington, DC, Technical Working Paper No. 1, June 1992.
2. WHO and UNICEF, *Action for Children Affected by AIDS* (Geneva: WHO and New York: UN, 1994).
3. UNICEF, *AIDS and Orphans in Africa* (New York: UN, 1991).
4. J. Chin, "Growing impact of the HIV/AIDS pandemic in children born to HIV-infected women," *Clinics in Perinatology* 21(1994):1–14.
5. Estimate of the Global AIDS Policy Coalition, Cambridge, Massachusetts, 1994.
6. J. Imrie and Y. Coombes, *No Time to Waste: The Scale and Dimensions of the Problem of Children Affected by HIV/AIDS in the United Kingdom* (Essex, UK: Barnardos, 1995).
7. T. Brown and W. Sittitrai, "The HIV/AIDS epidemic in Thailand: Addressing the impact on children," *Asia-Pacific Population and Policy* no. 35 (1995).
8. UNICEF, *Report on a Meeting about AIDS and Orphans in Africa* (New York: UN, 1991).
9. C. Levine and G. L. Stein, *Orphans of the HIV Epidemic: Unmet Needs in Six U.S. Cities* (New York: Orphan Project, 1994):5.
10. T. Barnett and P. Blaikie, *AIDS in Africa: Its Present and Future Impact* (New York and London: Guilford Press, 1992):110–126.
11. Levine, *Orphans*.
12. J. Seeley, E. Kajura, C. Bachengana, et al., "Extended family and support for people with AIDS in a rural population in south west Uganda: A safety net with holes?" *AIDS Care* 5(1993):117–122.
13. J. W. McGrath, E. Maxine Ankrah, D. A. Schumann, et al., "AIDS and the urban family: Its impact in Kampala, Uganda," *AIDS Care* 5(1993):55–69.
14. WHO and UNICEF, *Action for Children Affected by AIDS*.
15. C. Levine, ed., *Death in the Family: Orphans of the HIV Epidemic* (New York: United Hospital Fund, 1993):124–153.
16. S. Hunter, "Orphans as a window on the AIDS epidemic in sub-Saharan Africa: Initial results and implications of a study in Uganda," *Social Science and Medicine* 31(1990):681–690.
17. UNICEF, *Children and AIDS: An Impending Calamity* (New York: UN, 1990):17.
18. S. Poonawala and R. Cantor, *Children Orphaned by AIDS: A Call for Action for NGOs and Donors* (Washington, DC: National Council for International Health, March 31, 1991).

28

Blood and Blood Product Safety

NORBERT GILMORE

Despite its life-saving potential, treatment with blood and blood products has never been without risk, including the potential for transmission of infections such as HIV, hepatitis, syphilis, malaria, and trypanosomiasis. Indeed, it has been estimated that as many as 10 percent of people infected with HIV have been infected through treatment with blood or blood products.[1] This risk can be nearly eliminated by HIV screening of blood donations, preventing HIV-infected people from donating blood, reducing the need for treatment with blood, and in the case of blood products (e.g., Factor VIII), ensuring conformity with certain production standards. In industrialized countries, these measures are all in place. However, concern remains about their quality and, in some countries, about whether these measures were implemented as soon and as thoroughly as possible.* (Box 28.1) In contrast, being able to afford and implement these measures in developing countries still represents a formidable challenge.[2,3]

BOX 28-1

The growing aftermath of HIV infection from blood and blood component treatment: compensation, litigation, and public inquiries

By the end of the 1980s, it was becoming clear that many people, treated with blood or blood components, might have escaped being infected with HIV had governments, blood transfusion services, and manufacturers of blood components responded sooner or more decisively to protect the blood supply from HIV. The media, the public, and many of those who were infected soon described this situation as a "tragedy" or a "scandal," and those infected were referred to as its "victims."[1] Many of those who were infected, perceiving themselves to have been wronged, sought compensation, redress in the

---

*Allegations about avoidable delays in or the inconsistent implementation of laboratory screening have been reported from Canada (R. Mickleburgh, "Delay in testing for AIDS costs lives," *Globe and Mail* [Toronto: November 19, 1992]:A1); France (J. Kramer, "Bad blood: Why people are dying of AIDS for France's 'honor,'" *New Yorker* [New York: October 11, 1993]:74–95); Germany (I. Traynor, E. Vulliamy, D. Gow, and C. Mihill, "HIV blood scare grips Europe," *Guardian* [Manchester: November 6, 1993]:1); and Switzerland (A. MacGregor, "Another blood scandal," *Lancet* 342[1993]:429).

courts, and a public accounting of why this situation occurred. Governments, in turn, sought to determine why so many people were infected with HIV through treatment with blood and blood components, why this was not prevented, and who or what institutions may have contributed to the problem, and, perhaps, been culpable for not preventing it.

As a result, governments in many industrialized countries began to compensate recipients of infected blood and blood components. Many governments, along with blood transfusion services and blood component manufactures, found themselves responding to lawsuits brought by people whose HIV infection was acquired medically. Several governments brought criminal charges against officials responsible for blood safety at the time when many recipients of blood and blood components became infected with HIV. And, some governments have conducted formal, often judicial and sometimes public, inquiries in order to define and understand the events that led so many recipients of blood or blood components to become infected with HIV, as well as to discover what can be done to prevent such a situation from happening again.

Compensation

More than 22 countries have compensated people whose HIV infection was attributable to blood or blood component treatment. Compensation is paid by the government directly in seven countries (Denmark, the United Kingdom, Eire, Hungary, the Netherlands, Thailand, and initially by Canada); in nine countries it is funded jointly by governments and other organizations such as insurance, pharmaceutical, or national blood organizations (Australia, Austria, France, Italy, Japan, Portugal, Spain, Switzerland, and more recently by Canada); and, existing legislation in six countries authorizes this compensation (Bulgaria, Finland, New Zealand, Norway, and Sweden).[2]

Compensation varies from a lump-sum settlement of $145,000 in Denmark to a life-long $22,000 annual payment in Canada.[3] Several Australian states award a one-time payment and free lifetime health care to people who acquired their HIV infection medically.[4] In 1989, the Canadian federal government compensated eligible claimants for four years. Thereafter, they were compensated jointly by provincial governments, pharmaceutical and insurance companies, and the Canadian Red Cross Society, receiving life-long compensation which continued after the claimant's death with a smaller five-year amount given to the claimant's spouse or offspring. To be eligible for compensation, claimants have had to waive legal claims against the compensation funders.[5] Following the 1993 discovery of a German plasma collection and processing company that failed to screen its blood donors adequately, the German government instituted a more comprehensive compensation programme for people infected through treatment with blood or blood components.[6-9] In Japan, 1,800 of that nation's 5,000 hemophiliacs have been infected with HIV, and the courts have recommended they be compensated jointly by the federal government and by pharmaceutical companies who manufactured blood components which transmitted HIV.[10] A national compensation programme has not been established in the U.S., where more than 15,000 recipients of blood or blood components are infected. Recently, a public inquiry recommended that a no-fault compensation programme be established there.[11]

Civil litigation

AIDS has been reported to be the most litigated infectious disease in U.S. legal history, and many of these suits have been brought by, or on behalf of, recipients of infected blood or blood components.[12] Often, plaintiffs have claimed their infection could have been avoided had government authorities, blood collection agencies, and manufactures of blood components acted sooner, by questioning and excluding potentially infected donors, by screening them or their donations for HIV itself or, prior to that, by screening them for surrogate markers of HIV infection such as hepatitis B virus infection, and by making heat-treated factor VIII concentrate available earlier. Armour Pharmaceutical Company, for example, reported in 1995 that it was responding to 321 lawsuits brought by HIV-infected hemophiliacs or their survivors.[13] The economic implications of this litigation can be staggering. In 1989, the Canadian federal government estimated that awards arising from lawsuits brought against it could each cost in excess of $2 million, and $100,000 in legal costs.[14] In one recent case, legal costs exceeded $750,000.[15]

Criminal charges

Criminal charges have been laid against some public officials, scientists, staff of blood transfusion services, and blood processing or pharmaceutical industry employees. Perhaps, the most notorious situation is in France where a former Prime Minister and several government ministers and their advisers are being investigated, and at least one prominent epidemiologist has been indicted on charges of "collusion in posioning."[16,17] Earlier, four officials of France's National Blood Transfusion Service were convicted for their part in the transmission of HIV by blood components obtained in France. Two of them have received prison sentences.[18,19,20] The Director of the Swiss Red Cross Central Laboratory was charged recently with inflicting grievous bodily harm for allowing the use of possibly infected blood.[21] And, the director and four staff members of a German company found to have knowingly sold HIV-infected blood products have been charged with inflicting grievous bodily harm.[22]

Public inquiries

Several governments have established inquiries into events before 1986 that led to HIV transmission by treatment with blood and blood components. These inquiries have focused on delays or impediments to the implementation of procedures and practices aimed at ensuring blood safety in general, and at preventing HIV transmission in particular. The inquiries have addressed such issues as the availability of heat-treated factor VIII, the use and stringency of donor questioning and self-deferral practices, and implementation of laboratory screening of donors. Implicit in these inquiries has been a concern that protective measures could have been implemented more quickly so that fewer people would have been exposed to HIV through treatment with blood or blood components.

In France, an internal government inquiry into the infection of almost 5,000 recipients of blood and blood products has led to the laying of criminal charges in 1991, with more charges expected. In 1992, the U.S. Secretary of Health asked the National Academy of Sciences Institute of Medicine to examine responses of the U.S. public health system with regard to HIV transmission through blood and blood components.[23] This inquiry did not find any individuals culpable, but it found that public health responses were often the least aggressive ones that could be justified. Among the problems contributing to this situation were a lack of government leadership, poor communication, and conflicts arising from a failure to dissociate the analysis of HIV transmission risks from their subsequent management.[24] In Canada, a Royal Commission is examining the events that led to the infection of more than 1,000 recipients of blood or blood components.[25] An interim report has been released suggesting ways to improve blood safety, but the final report is not expected before the autumn of 1996.[26,27] A German parliamentary investigation concluded that HIV infection of about 60 percent of Germany's 2,000 hemophiliacs could have been avoided had protective measures been implemented sooner. It also recommmended the establishment of a compensation programme, jointly funded by federal and state governments, the pharmaceutical industry, and hospitals, and that the German government should publicly apologize to those who were infected.[28] The Ombudsman of the Netherlands government recently found government authorities were too passive, ill-informed, and slow to react to the dangers of HIV transmission by treatment with blood and blood components that infected 170 of the 1,500

Dutch hemophiliacs.[29] In 1994, the Swiss federal government established a Blood and AIDS Task Force whose report has yet to be released. In the meantime, the government has brought criminal charges against at least one official.[30]

A decade's wisdom

The responses to events that occurred more than a decade ago point out that the infection of many of the people treated with blood or blood components could have been avoided. Unfortunately, at the time, governments and their public health systems, blood transfusion services, manufacturers of blood components, and the medical profession were often ill-prepared to respond to the threats posed by HIV. Many of the impediments to protecting the blood supply, then as now, were complex, sometimes difficult to overcome, and were all too often to some extent the result of uncertainty, inertia, denial, under-recognition of the risks involved, poor communication, and a lack of leadership and political will to act quickly and decisively. These responses also point out that delays in protecting the blood supply from HIV were far more costly than protecting it quickly, not only in terms of illness, suffering, premature mortality, and health care costs but also in terms of compensation, legal costs, and lost opportunities.

The new wisdom has also led to a safer blood supply by improving the recruitment of donors and the collection, processing, distribution, and use of blood. As a result, the risk of HIV transmission from treatment with blood or blood components has diminished. Fewer HIV-infected individuals donate blood and the sensitivity of ELISA screening methods has improved, resulting in a risk that is extremely small.[31,32] In the U.S., for example, only one donation in every 450,000 to 660,000 is estimated to be from a donor who is HIV infected but undetected by the safety procedures and practices now in place.[33] Nevertheless, there is continuing pressure on governments, blood transfusion services, and manufacturers of blood components to reduce this risk even more.[34]

Problems again: p24 antigen screening

One example of this seemingly relentless pursuit of safer blood and blood component treatment is the recent U.S. government decision requiring blood donors to be screened by a p24 antigen test, in addition to the ELISA test in use since 1985.[35] This decision has been a controversial one, partly because p24 antigen screening will produce only a small reduction in an already small risk, and because the price of obtaining this benefit will be extremely high.[36,37] To discover one infected donor now undetectable by ELISA screening, as many as a million donors will have to be screened.[38] That means millions of dollars will be spent to discover each previously undetected, infected donor—a cost far in excess of other health interventions.[39]

The p24 antigen screening test is also relatively insensitive, with as many as three donors remaining undetected for every one that is discovered.[40] This raises the worrisome concern that p24 antigen screening could worsen the situation it is designed to improve, by attracting recently infected individuals to donate blood and then failing to detect them. In one U.S. study, 6 percent of blood donors reported that they had donated blood in order to obtain HIV testing, and less than 1 percent of them subsequently directed that their blood not be used.[41] In another study, 14 percent of ELISA seropositive infected individuals reported that they had donated blood in order to be tested.[42] If newly infected individuals were to donate in order to be tested for p24 antigen, they would be doing so when they are most infectious and when the infection is undetectable by ELISA screening.[43]

Since no more than one-fourth to one-half of donors recently infected by HIV are likely to be detected by p24 antigen screening, two or three of them could end up donating blood for every one who is detected, thereby adding more HIV-contaminated donations to the blood supply than if donors were not screened with the p24 antigen test.[44]

For p24 antigen screening to strengthen the safety of the blood supply, other procedures and practices that protect that supply have to be in place. Among them are the following: (1) recruiting donors who are healthy while encouraging potentially infected individuals to refrain from donating; (2) thoroughly questioning and excluding potential donors who may have been exposed to blood-transmissible diseases; (3) ensuring that donors who may have been exposed to blood-transmissible diseases will confidentially indicate their donation is not to be used for treatment; (4) meticulously following testing protocols and good manufacturing practices; (5) having strong public health support whereby the public is educated not to donate in order to be tested and by making testing readily and easily accessible at sites unrelated to where blood is collected; and (6) reducing the demand for treatment with blood and blood components by preventing clinical situations when such treatment would be needed and by use of substitutes for blood or blood components.[45,46]

New threats, old solutions

As the introduction of ELISA screening a decade ago has shown, and as the introduction of p24 antigen screening is showing, once again, safety procedures and practices are essential responses if the blood supply is to be protected from blood-transmissible infections in general, and from HIV in particular.[47] As other possibly blood-transmissible agents, such as that of Creutzfeld-Jakob disease and hepatitis G, threaten the safety of the blood supply, and as new, and often more expensive, methods to detect blood-transmissible agents become available, such as the polymerase chain reaction (PCR) assay, screening procedures and practices will nevertheless remain the first and foremost protection of the blood supply.[48,49,50,51]

References

1. Associated Press, "AIDS suit accuses companies of selling bad blood products," *New York Times* (October 4, 1993):18.
2. Testimony of Mr. B. O'Mahoney, President of the World Federation of Hemophilia to The National Academy of Sciences Institute of Medicine, Division of Health Promotion and Disease Prevention, Committee to Study HIV Transmission through Blood Products Public Meeting, Washington, DC, September 12, 1994. (accessed via the Internet at HTTP://WWW.Nmia.com /~mdibbl/hiv/hiv1.htm1)
3. A. Picard, "Tainted blood around the world: how Canada stacks up," *Globe and Mail* (Toronto, 7 September 7, 1993):A4 (quoting the World Federation of Hemophilia and the International Society of Blood Transfusion).
4. M. Ragg, "Australia: compensation for medically acquired AIDS," *Lancet* 339 (1992):419.
5. W. Kondro, "Curtailed Canadian HIV compensation," *Lancet* 343 (1994):783–784.
6. Editorial, "Europe's HIV-contaminated blood," *Nature* 366 (1993):95.
7. P. Aldhous, "German HIV-blood scandal reveals flaws in the system," *Science* 262 (1993):1205.
8. S. Kinzer, "Fear of HIV-infected blood spread past German borders," *New York Times* (November 5, 1993):A1.
9. C. R. Whitney, "Germany to pay victims in AIDS blood scandal," *New York Times* (November 13, 1995):A1.
10. D. Swinbanks, "Japan faces new questions on HIV in blood . . . ," *Nature* 367 (1994):584.
11. National Academy of Sciences Institute of Medicine, "Recommendation 3," in *Institute of Medicine Report: HIV and the Blood Supply. An Analysis of Crisis Decision Making* (Washington, DC: National Academy Press, 1995).
12. Most litigated.
13. Associated Press, "Drug maker turned aside alert on AIDS," *New York Times* (October 6, 1995):A17.
14. A. Picard, "Blood liability put at $1-billion," *Globe and Mail* (Toronto, January 29, 1996):A1.
15. *Pittman Estate v Bain et al* (1994) 112 DLR (4th) 257; 19 CCLT (2d) Ont Ct Gen Div, as reported in A. Picard, "Blood liability put at $1-billion," *Globe and Mail* (Toronto, January 29, 1996):A1.
16. A. Riding, "French AIDS scandal inquiry widens to former Premier," *New York Times* (October 1, 1994):1.
17. D. Butler, "Uproar greets new blood scandal indictment," *Nature* 375 (1995):526.
18. J-M. Bader, "France: Prison sentences for doctors," *Lancet* 340 (1992):1087.
19. Editorial, "France's blood scandal draws blood," *Nature* 359 (1992):759.
20. D. Butler, "Verdict in French blood trial shames science," *Nature* 359 (1992):764.
21. M. Simons, "Swiss Red Cross faces AIDS probe," *New York Times* (May 22, 1995):1 (Sec. 1).

22. A. Abbott, ". . . as German executives are charged," *Nature* 367 (1994):584.

23. L. K. Altman, "Report urges new steps to protect blood supply," *New York Times* (July 14, 1995):A15.

24. P. M. Rowe, "IOM criticises U.S. blood product safety measures," *Lancet* 346 (1995):243.

25. W. Kondro, "Canada: blood transfusion inquiry," *Lancet* 341 (1993):1465–1466.

26. Commission of Inquiry on the Blood System in Canada: Interim Report. Ottawa, Canada Communication Group—Publishing, 1995 [Cat. No. CP32-62/1-1995].

27. W. Kondro, "Improving safety of Canada's blood," *Lancet* 345 (1995):641.

28. H. Karcher, "German parliament investigates HIV infections," *British Medical Journal* 309 (1994):1389–1390.

29. T. Sheldon, "Dutch face up to blood scandal," *British Medical Journal* 311 (1995):347.

30. A. McGregor, "Swiss law for safer blood," *Lancet* 345 (1995): 640.

31. M. P. Busch, L. L. Lee, G. A. Satten, et al., "Time course of detection of viral and serological markers preceding human immunodeficiency virus type 1 seroconversion: Implications for screening of blood and tissue donors," *Transfusion* 35 (1995):91–97.

32. F. Le Pont, D. Costagliola, C. Rouzioux, et al., "How much would the safety of blood transfusion be improved by including p24 antigen in the battery of tests?" *Transfusion* 35 (1995):542–547.

33. E. M. Lackritz, G. A. Satten, J. Aberle-Grasse, et al., "Estimated risk of transmission of the human immunodeficiency virus by screened blood in the United States," *The New England Journal of Medicine* 333 (1995):1721–1725.

34. M. P. Busch, H. J. Alter, "Will human immunodeficiency virus p24 antigen screening increase the safety of the blood supply, and, if so, at what cost?" *Transfusion* 35 (1995):536–539.

35. K. C. Zoon, *Recommendations for Donor Screening with a Licensed Test for HIV-1 Antigen,* Washington DC Center of Biologics Evaluation and Research, Food and Drug Administration, Department of Health and Human Services, U.S. Government, 8 August 1995 (Memorandum) [accessed via the Internet at http://www.fda.gov/cber/cberftp.html, and at ftp://ftp.fda.gtove./CBER/bld_mem/hiv-ag (either as a WordPerfect 5.1 file (.WP51) or an ASCII text file (.TXT))]

36. *Ibid.*

37. Busch, "p24 anitgen screening."

38. H. J. Alter, J. S. Epstein, S. G. Swenson, HIV Antigen Study Group, et al., "Prevalence of human immunodeficiency virus type 1 p24 antigen in U.S. blood donors—an assessment of the efficacy of testing in donor screening," *The New England Journal of Medicine* 323 (1990):1312–1317.

39. J. P. Au Bouchon, J. D. Birkmeyer, M. P. Busch, "Cost-effectiveness of expanded HIV test protocols for donated blood," *Transfusion* 35 (1995) [supplement]:43S (Abstract S169).

40. Busch, "p24 antigen screening."

41. A. E. Williams, R. A. Thomson, J. A. Horton, S. H. Kleinman, "Characterization of active blood donors who recently donated blood primarily to receive an HIV test," *Transfusion* 35 (1995) [supplement]:42S Abstract S166).

42. E. M. Lackritz, M. B. Kennedy, L. S. Doll, et al., "Risk behaviors and test seeking among HIV-positive blood donors," *Transfusion* 35 (1995) [supplement]:42S (Abstract S167).

43. L. R. Peterson, G. A. Satten, R. Y. Dodd, HIV Seroconversion Study Group, et al., "Duration of time from onset of human immunodeficiency virus type 1 infectiousness to development of detectable antibody," *Transfusion* 34 (1994):283–284.

44. Busch, "p24 antigen screening."

45. American College of Physicians, "Practice strategies for elective red blood cell transfusion," *Annals Internal Medicine* 116 (1992): 403–406.

46. Global Blood Safety Initiative, *Use of Plasma Substitutes and Plasma in Developing Countries,* Geneva, World Health Organization, 1989 [Document: WHO/GPA/INF/89.17].

47. Le Pont, "How much?"

48. K. C. Zoon, *Precautionary Measures to Further Reduce the Possible Risk of Transmission of Creutzfeldt-Jakob Disease by Blood and Blood Products,* Center of Biologics Evaluation and Research, Food and Drug Administration, Department of Health and Human Services, U.S. Government, Washington, DC, 8 August 1995 (Memorandum) [accessed via the Internet at thttp://www.fda.gov/cber/cberftp.html, and at ftp://ftp.fda.gtove./CBER/bld_mem/hiv-ag (either as a WordPerfect 5.1 file (.WP51) or an ASCII text file (.TXT))]

49. L. K. Altman, "Three newly discovered viruses may cause unexplained hepatitis," *New York Times* (April 11, 1995):C3.

50. J. N. Simons, T. J. Pilot-Matias, T. P. Leary, et al., "Identification of two flavivirus-like genomes in the GB hepatitis agent," *Proceedings of the National Academy of Sciences USA* 92 (1995):3401–3405.

51. Busch, "p24 antigen screening."

Screening blood donations

The most efficient measures to reduce the risk of HIV transmission are laboratory screening of blood donations, so that infected blood will not be transfused, and the use of heat treatment to inactivate HIV if present in blood products.[4-7] These measures have dramatically reduced the risk of HIV infection from blood transfusion and from treatment with factor VIII and IX concentrates.[8,9] Screening can identify more than 99 percent of infected donations, and its efficacy is limited only by the sensitivity of the screening method used and by the prevalence of donors who have recently been HIV infected but have not yet produced antibodies against HIV, that is, people in the "window period" of HIV infection.[10,11] In the U.S. it is estimated that for every 225,000 blood donations, one donation will be HIV infected but undetectable by screening; this risk for HIV transmission is lower than for hepatitis B (1 in 200,000) or hepatitis C (1 in 3,300) virus transmission.[12,13] For blood products that can be heat treated, the risk of HIV transmission has virtually been eliminated through this treatment. By 1987 the incidence of HIV among people with hemophilia plummeted to essentially zero, a protection attributable to the introduction of heat-treated factor VIII concentrate.[14]

The impact of laboratory screening for HIV infection can be illustrated dramatically in countries with a high HIV prevalence among potential donors. For example, blood screening in Zimbabwe (starting in July 1985) identified (and discarded) 3.4 percent of the donations collected between 1986 and 1989; had this blood been used, more than 10,000 people could have become HIV infected.[15,16] Of the blood donations collected in Rwanda between 1986 and 1990, 5.6 percent would have been from infected donors, while in Uganda between 1988 and 1990, 15.6 percent of blood donors were seropositive, including 42 percent of 20–25-year-old women donors without secondary school education.[17,18]

The spread of HIV-2 and other HIV variants can jeopardize this success when screening methods are used that may not detect these viruses.[19-23] To address this problem countries are modifying their screening methods. For example, while 69 of 70 countries surveyed in 1992 reported screening all blood donations for HIV-1 infection, 56 percent also reported screening for HIV-2 infection.[24]

Current practice regarding HIV testing of blood donations in developing countries varies.[25] Estimates in 1989, 1990, and 1991 suggest that as much as one-third of donated blood may be unscreened for HIV in some regions and countries.[26,27,28] In addition, heat-treated blood products are commercial products and their availability is limited by their affordability. The reasons for partial or inconsistent screening vary from country to country. Screening may be considered unaffordable despite being cost-beneficial.[29,30] It has been estimated that blood screening would require less than 5 percent of total HIV prevention resources in developing countries.[31] Nevertheless, screening may not have been implemented because blood safety is undervalued as a national health priority.[32] Other problems may include excessive demands for screened blood combined with a scarcity of blood donations, un availability of screened blood in rural or sparsely populated areas in some countries, or interference with access to screened blood due to geography, climate, natural catastrophes such as drought and floods, and wars.[33-36] Technical problems such as the intermittent or persistent unavailability of equipment, reagents, and proficient personnel, and processing, storage, or distribution breakdowns can also interfere with screening.[37] Organizational and management problems often aggravate these situations, reflecting the marginal sustainability of laboratory screening in some countries.

Excluding infected donors

Preventing donors who may be HIV infected from donating is another strategy to improve blood safety.[38] Since 1983 many countries have requested potential donors with illnesses suggestive of AIDS or who are from populations or regions with a high prevalence of HIV not to donate, and have excluded them as donors.[39] At times this has been divisive and controversial,* but it is a first-line defense to prevent the donation of infected blood and an important adjunct to screening.[40,41] It has the advantage of reducing costs because fewer infected donations will need to be replaced by uninfected ones, fewer screening tests will need to be repeated, and the risk of false negative screening results (including the "window period") will be reduced.[42,43] A 1992 survey found that 97 percent of responding countries reported excluding one or more categories of potential donors.[44] However, there are at least two situations in which the efficacy of donor exclusion may be jeopardized. First, infected donors are unable to self-exclude if they do not know they are HIV infected. Second, the efficacy of donor self-exclusion may be jeopardized when HIV testing is not readily available except when donating blood. In this situation, people who may be infected may donate for the purpose of being tested for HIV infection rather than exclude themselves from donating. Despite these potential problems, questioning and counseling of potential donors remains helpful.[45,46] In Rwanda, for example, this strategy decreased donor HIV seroprevalence from 13.5 percent to 2.1 percent, and in Uganda HIV donor seroprevalence was reduced by 50 percent from 1989 to 1992.[47,48] The sensitivity and specificity of this approach was assessed in Côte d'Ivoire, where excluding 31 percent of donors would have eliminated 73 percent of HIV-infected donations.[49]

Another strategy to improve blood safety is to encourage donations from volunteers while discouraging donations from family members and friends of people treated with blood and blood products or from people who are paid to donate.[50,51] In both of these latter groups, HIV prevalence has been found to be higher than that of volunteer donors. HIV prevalence among

---

*Student associations from at least two universities in Canada have boycotted Red Cross blood collection efforts because they consider Red Cross donor self-exclusion criteria to discriminate unjustifiably against potential donors, such as men having sex with men, or people who have resided in the Caribbean region or in sub-Saharan Africa (*Gazette* [Montréal: November 24, 1993]:A5). In South Africa, a move to exclude black donors whose HIV prevalence was found to be 1:70, but not white donors with an HIV prevalence of 1:4,000, caused a public outcry (*Guardian* [Manchester: November 17, 1993]:8).

paid donors in Germany between 1985 and 1991 was almost eight times higher than among unpaid donors.[52] At a rural Kenyan district hospital in 1991, 13.6 percent of patient-recruited donors were HIV seropositive compared with only 4.6 percent of student volunteer donors under 21 years of age.[53] Similarly, 6.9 percent of patient-recruited donors in Kampala in 1992, 2.3 percent of student donors, and no volunteer donors, were found to be seropositive.[54] In Mexico HIV prevalence among paid and volunteer donors was 7 percent and 0.4 percent, respectively.[55] In New Delhi HIV seroprevalence was almost five times higher among paid donors than among donors who were family members or friends of transfusion recipients.[56] Finally, in Zanzibar volunteer donor HIV prevalence between 1987 and 1991 was only 3 percent of the prevalence among commercial donors and 10 percent of family member replacement donors. The complexity of this problem is illuminated by a report from Nigeria that patient-recruited replacement donors are sometimes paid donors.[57]

Reducing the demand for blood and blood product treatment

Decreasing the need for treatment with blood and blood products is another important strategy to improve blood safety.[58] Excessive demands for treatment with blood and blood products may exhaust resources or exceed the supply of screened blood donations and heat-treated blood products.[59] Demand for blood is increased by inadequate primary care, including a lack of prenatal care or failure to prevent infections such as malaria.[60] One consequence of this lack of primary care is that the majority of people receiving blood transfusions in developing countries are women and children.[61] In addition, many blood transfusions have been found to be unnecessary. In Kenya, 61 percent of blood transfusions in a rural district hospital were considered to be clinically inappropriate.[62] Studies in Tanzania, Zaire, and Canada have come to a similar conclusion.[63,64,65] Such studies have led to the development of relatively simple, inexpensive guidelines to reduce the unnecessary use of blood transfusions.[66-70]

Economic impact of strengthening blood safety

The cost of meeting the need for safer blood varies from country to country. In 1992 *AIDS in the World* estimated that U.S. $2.5 billion would be needed to ensure safe blood everywhere while only $50 million was available for this purpose in 1991.[71] HIV screening is a relatively minor part of the cost of collecting, processing, and distributing blood. The World Health Organization estimated that the cost of HIV screening reagents can be as low as U.S. $0.70 per donation.[72] In an effort to make screening feasible, a variety of cost-saving strategies such as pooling of specimens have been identified but not universally accepted.[73,74] Even when blood screening has been implemented, unmet needs persist in many countries. Immediate and long-term needs (and the proportion of countries with them) include better use of blood (85 percent); enhanced donor recruitment (84 percent) and education

(82 percent); increased financial support (83 percent); training of staff (75 percent); quality assurance (73 percent); increased technical staff (63 percent); and provision of testing supplies (63 percent) and equipment (55 percent).[75]

Implementing safer blood initiatives, in particular laboratory screening, can be cost-beneficial as an investment that avoids future health care costs.[76,77,78] Laboratory screening can also provide important and much needed epidemiological data, as has been shown in Tanzania.[79] These initiatives may be seen by some developing countries as beyond their resources, often necessitating foreign assistance to implement and sustain them.[80] This includes the efficient recruitment of uninfected donors, the screening, processing, storage, and distribution of donations, and a reduction in the need for blood and blood product treatment. Reducing demand for blood supply necessitates addressing problems that reflect and contribute to underdevelopment, that is, broader infrastructural initiatives such as road safety, improving maternal and infant nutrition and health, controlling parasitic diseases, and reducing military and political strife. This in turn emphasizes the importance of a national commitment to strengthen blood safety.[81,82,83]

Implementing and sustaining a safer blood supply may be perceived to be a smaller and less urgent need than dealing with other modes of transmission, especially when a country's HIV prevalence is low.[84] However, the resources required to successfully screen all blood donations are less than those needed for these other initiatives because of the intrinsic efficiency of screening and because the populations involved are smaller and more accessible. This means that strengthening blood safety by screening is less complicated and potentially more rapidly achievable. Further, "the control of transmission is so easy and effective that it's a starting point and a cornerstone for all other control campaigns."[85] Finally, there are also benefits from successfully addressing the infrastructural and organizational problems that can impede blood safety and that contribute to wider health and safety problems. These benefits include avoided infections, fewer transfusions, improved health, and safety in general, as well as future health care savings and economic opportunities. Like the eradication of smallpox, a safe blood supply has an important and universal symbolic impact.[86]

REFERENCES

1. R. W. Beal, M. Bontink, and L. Fransen, eds., *Safe Blood in Developing Countries. A Report of the EEC's Expert Meeting* (Brussels: EEC AIDS Task Force, 1992):11.

2. L. Dierick and M. Bontink, "Session B: Safe blood initiatives," Commission of the European Communities AIDS Task Force Newsletter, Report of the AIDS Task Force Pre-conference held in Berlin, Germany, June 6, 1993, *ATF News* (August 1993):6–14.

3. I. N'tita, K. Mulanga, C. Dulat, D. Lusamba, T. Rehle, R. Korte, and H. Jäger, "Risk of transfusion-associated HIV transmission in Kinshasa, Zaire," *AIDS* 5(1991):437–439.

4. P. Chiewslip, P. Isarangkuru, A. Poonkasem, W. Iamsilp, M. Khamenkhetkran, and S. Stabunswadigan, "Risk of transmission of HIV by seronegative blood," letter, *Lancet* 338(1991):1341.

5. J. M. Ward, S. D. Holmberg, J. R. Allen, et al., "Transmission of human immunodeficiency virus (HIV) by blood transfusions screened as negative for HIV antibody," *New England Journal of Medicine* 338(1991):1314.

6. P. M. Mannucci, "Clinical evaluation of viral safety of coagulation factor VIII and IX concentrates," *Vox Sanguinis* 64(1993):197–203.

7. W. Fricke, L. Augustyniak, D. Lawrence, A. Bornstein, A. Kramer, and B. Evatt, "Human immunodeficiency virus infection due to clotting factor concentrates: Results of the Seroconversion Surveillance Project," *Transfusion* 32(1992):707–715.

8. R. M. Selik, J. M. Ward, and J. W. Buehler, "Trends in transfusion associated acquired immune deficiency syndrome in the United States, 1982 through 1991," *Transfusion* 33(1993):890–893.

9. B. L. Kroner, P. S. Rosenberg, L. M. Aledort, G. Alvord, and J. J. Goedert for the Multicenter Hemophilia Cohort Study, "HIV-1 infection incidence among persons with hemophilia in the United States and Western Europe, 1978–1990," *Journal of Acquired Immune Deficiency Syndromes* 7(1993):279–286.

10. P. Chiewslip, P. Isarangkura, A. Poonkasem, W. Iamsilp, M. Khamenkhetkran, and S. Stabunswadigan, "Risk of transmission of HIV by seronegative blood," *Lancet* 338(1991):1341.

11. L. Petersen, M. Busch, G. Satten, R. Dodd, D. Henrad, et al., "Narrowing the window period with a third generation anti-HIV-1/2 enzyme immunoassay: Relevance to P24 antigen screening of blood donors in the United States," Abstract PO-C17-3001, presented at the IX International Conference on AIDS, Berlin, Germany, June 1993.

12. L. R. Petersen, G. Satten, R. Dodd, and HIV Lookback Study Group, "Time period from infectiousness as blood donor to development of detectable antibody and the risk of HIV transmission from transfusion of screened blood," Abstract S174, presented at the 45th Meeting of the American Association of Blood Banks, November 7–12, 1992, San Francisco, California, reprinted in *Transfusion* 32(suppl.)(1992):46S.

13. J. McCullough, "The nation's changing blood supply system," *Journal of the American Medical Association* 269(1993):2239–2245.

14. B. L. Kroner, P. S. Rosenberg, L. M. Aledort, G. Alvord, and J. J. Goedert, for the Multicenter Hemophilia Cohort Study, "HIV-1 infection incidence among persons with hemophilia in the United States and Western Europe, 1978–1990," *Journal of Acquired Immune Deficiency Syndromes* 7(1993):279–286.

15. L. Mangwiro, "Zimbabwe," in *Report of the Southern African Conference on AIDS*, (Harare, Zimbabwe: SANASO, May 14–16, 1990), reprinted in *ACT* (1990):40–42.

16. E. Marowa, "HIV/AIDS situation globally and locally, and the value of cooperation and collaboration between non government organizations and their respective National AIDS Control Programmes (NACP)," in *Report of the Southern African Conference on AIDS* (Harare, Zimbabwe: SANASO, May 14–16, 1990), reprinted in *ACT* (1990):19–22.

17. P. Mugabo and J. Nkurunziza, "Seroprevalence of HIV-1 in Rwanda blood banks from 1985 to 1990," Abstract PO-C21-3113, presented at the IX International Conference on AIDS, Berlin, Germany, June 1993.

18. R. W. Beal, M. Bontink, and L. Fransen, eds., *Safe Blood in Developing Countries, A Report of the EEC's Expert Meeting* (Brussels: EEC AIDS Task Force, 1992):28–29.

19. K. M. De Cock and F. Brun-Vézinet, "Epidemiology of HIV-2 infection," *AIDS* 3(suppl. 1)(1989):s89–s95.

20. C. Holden, ed., "New HIV group baffles French test" (News), *Science* 263(1994):1689.

21. L. G. Gürtler, P. H. Hauser, J. Eberle, A. von Brun, S. Knapp, L. Zenkeng, J. M. Tsague, and L. Kapute, "A new type of human immunodeficiency virus type 1 (MVP-5180) from Cameroon," *Journal of Virology* 68(1994):1581–1585.

22. M. Vanden Haesevelde, J.-L. Decourt, R. J. de Lys, B. Vanderbroght, G. van der Groen, H. van Hueverswijn, and E. Saman, "Genomic cloning and complete sequence analy-

sis of a highly divergent African human immunodeficiency virus isolate," *Journal of Virology* 68(1994):1586–1596.

23. N. T. Constantine, "Serologic tests for the retroviruses: Approaching a decade of evolution" (Editorial), *AIDS* 7(1993):1–13.

24. C. Almedal, N. Gilmore, R. Jurgens, T. Lemmens, P. Gill, D. Murphy, et al., "A worldwide survey of blood safety in relation to HIV/AIDS," Abstract PO-C21-3122, presented at the IX International Conference on AIDS, Berlin, Germany, June 1993.

25. P. C. K. Li and E. K. Yeoh, "Current epidemiological trends of HIV infection in Asia," in *AIDS Clinical Review 1992*, P. Volberding and M. A. Jacobson, eds. (New York: Marcel Dekker, 1992):1–23.

26. Panos Institute, "Making the world's blood safe," *World AIDS* 1(1989):4.

27. W. N. Gibbs, and P. Corcoran, "Blood safety in developing countries," *Vox Sanguinis*, 67(1994):377–381.

28. R. Beal, A. F. Britten, and I. Gust, "Blood safety and blood products," in *AIDS in the World*, J. Mann, D. Tarantola, and T. Netter, eds. (Cambridge, MA: Harvard University Press, 1992):432–433.

29. E. J. Watson Williams, J. J. Fournel, D. Sondag, and L. Fransen, "EEC's safe blood programme policies and strategies in view of controlling AIDS in developing countries," in *Safe Blood in Developing Countries, a Report of the EEC's Expert Meeting*, R. W. Beal, M. Bontink, and L. Fransen, eds. (Brussels: EEC AIDS Task Force, 1992):112–118.

30. S. Foster and A. Buvé, "Benefits of HIV screening of blood transfusions in Zaire," *Lancet* 346(1995):225–227.

31. N. Soderlund, J. Lavis, J. Broomberg, and A. Mills, The costs of HIV prevention strategies in developing countries, *Bulletin of the World Health Organization*, 71(1995): 595–604.

32. R. W. Beal, "Transfusion science and practice in developing countries: . . . a high frequency of empty shelves . . . ," editorial, *Transfusion* 33(1993):276–278.

33. A. O. Emerike, A. O. Ejele, E. E. Attai, and E. A. Usanga, "Blood donation and patterns of use in southeastern Nigeria," *Transfusion* 33(1993):330–332.

34. Z. Imam, "India's AIDS control programme is unsatisfactory," *British Medical Journal* 308(1994):877.

35. H. J. Heiniger, *Survey of Blood Transfusion Services of Central and Eastern European Countries and Their Concerns with Western Transfusion Services*, research report (Strasbourg, France: Council of Europe, March 1, 1993).

36. F. S. Boi-Doku, *Safe Blood and Blood Products and Their Efficient Use in Developing Countries. A Report* (London: Commonwealth Secretariat, 1987).

37. I. N'tita, K. Mulanga, C. Dulat, D. Lusamba, T. Rehle, R. Korte, and H. Jäger, "Risk of transfusion-associate HIV transmission in Kinshasa, Zaire," *AIDS* 5(1991):437–439.

38. D. Miller, A. Petitgirard, S. Anderson, J. Emmanuel, and S. Kalibala, "Blood donor counseling for HIV: A multi-country study to assess feasibility," Abstract PO-B42-2509, presented at the IX International Conference on AIDS, Berlin, Germany, June 1993.

39. D. L. Kirp and R. Bayer, "Second decade of AIDS: The end of exceptionalism," in *AIDS in Industrialized Democracies: Passions, Politics and Policies*, D. L. Kirp and R. Bayer, eds. (Montreal: McGill-Queen's University Press, 1992):361–384.

40. H. W. Reesink, "International Forum: How far shall we go in the predonation selection of blood donors to safeguard patients for blood transfusion-related infections?" *Vox Sanguinis* 65(1993):1–9.

41. R. M. Selik, J. M. Ward, and J. W. Buehler, "Trends in transfusion associated acquired immune deficiency syndrome in the United States, 1982 through 1991," *Transfusion* 33(1993):890–893.

42. R. Schutz, D. Savarit, J.-C. Kadio, V. Batter, N. Kone, G. LaRuche, A. Bondurand, and K. M. De Cock, "Excluding blood donors at high risk of HIV infection in a West African city," *British Medical Journal* 307(1993):1517–1519.

43. W. McFarland, J. G. Kahn, D. A. Katzenstein, D. Mvere, and R. Shamu, "Deferral of blood donors with risk factors for HIV infection saves lives and money in Zimbabwe," *Journal of Acquired Immune Deficiency Syndromes and Human Retrovirology* 9(1995):183–192.

44. C. Almedal, N. Gilmore, R. Jurgens, T. Lemmens, P. Gill, D. Murphy, et al., "Worldwide survey of blood safety in relation to HIV/AIDS," Abstract PO-C21-3122, presented at the IX International Conference on AIDS, Berlin, Germany, June 1993.

45. R. Beal, A. F. Britten, and I. Gust, "Blood safety and blood products," in *AIDS in the World*, J. Mann, D. J. Tarantola, and T. Netter, eds. (Cambridge, MA: Harvard University Press, 1992):432–433.

46. R. de Andres-Medina, L. Perez-Alvarez, and R. Najera-Morrondo, The HIV Blood Donations Study Group, "HIV seropositivity of blood donations in Spain, a 4 year surveillance (1988–1991)" (Letter), *AIDS* 7(1993):283–284.

47. P. Mugabo and J. Nkurunziza, "Seroprevalence of HIV-1 in Rwanda blood banks from 1985 to 1990," Abstract PO-C21-3113, presented at the IX International Conference on AIDS, Berlin, Germany, June 1993.

48. P. Kataaha, "Analysis of data for Nakasero bloodbank, 1992," Commission of the European Communities AIDS Task Force Newsletter Report of the AIDS Task Force Preconference held in Berlin, Germany, June 6, 1993, *ATF News* (August 1993):8–9.

49. R. Schutz, D. Savarit, J.-C. Kadio, V. Batter, N. Kone, G. L. Ruche, A. Bondurand, and K. M. De Cock, "Excluding blood donors at high risk of HIV infection in a West African city," *British Medical Journal* 307(1993):1517–1519.

50. A. E. Williams, S. Kleinman, R. O. Glicher, et al., "Prevalence of infectious disease markers in directed versus homologous blood donations," Abstract S172, presented at the 45th Annual Meeting of the American Association of Blood Banks, San Francisco, California, November 7–12, 1992, reprinted in *Transfusion* 32(suppl.)(1992):45S.

51. J. M. Starkey, J. L. MacPherson, D. C. Bolgiano, E. R. Simon, T. F. Zuck, and M. H. Sayers, "Markers for transfusion-transmitted disease in different groups of blood donors," *Journal of the American Medical Association* 262(1989):3452–3454.

52. H. Fiedler, "HIV seropositivity in paid donors," *Lancet* 339(1992):551.

53. E. M. Lakritz, T. K. Ruebush, J. R. Zucker, J. E. Adungosi, J. B. O. Were, and C. C. Campbell, "Blood transfusion practices and blood-banking services in a Kenyan hospital," *AIDS* 7(1993):995–999.

54. Uganda AIDS Commission, "Briefing note on the Uganda AIDS Commission and the multisectoral HIV/AIDS control strategy in Uganda" (Kampala, Uganda: AIDS Commission, May 1992):2–3.

55. C. Avila, H. C. Stetler, J. Sepùlveda, E. Dickinson, K. G. Castro, J. M. Ward, G. Romero, and J. L. Valdespino, "The epidemiology of HIV transmission among paid plasma donors, Mexico City, Mexico," *AIDS* 3(1989):631–633.

56. G. Singh, V. K. Sharma, and R. Natarajan, "Prevalence of HIV-1 infection and its correlation with HBs Ag carriage and VDRL reactivity among blood donors in Delhi," Abstract ESG.P16, presented at the World Congress on AIDS, Bombay, India, December 7–9, 1990.

57. A. O. Emerike, A. O. Ejele, E. E. Attai, and E. A. Usanga, "Blood donation and patterns of use in southeastern Nigeria," *Transfusion* 33(1993):330–332.

58. A. F. Fleming, "Prevention of transmission of HIV by blood transfusion in developing countries," in *Global Impact of AIDS*, A. F. Fleming, M. Carballo, D. W. FitzSimons, M. R. Bailey, and J. Mann, eds. (New York: Alan R. Liss, 1988):357–367.

59. R. Moodie and T. Abogaye-Kwarteng, "Confronting the HIV epidemic in Asia and the Pacific: Developing successful strategies to minimize the spread of HIV infection," editorial, *AIDS* 7(1993):1543–1551.

60. B. Gumodoka, J. Vos, F. C. Kigadye, H. van Asten, W. M. V. Dolmans, and M. W. Borgdorff, "Blood transfusion practices in Mwanza Region, Tanzania," *AIDS* 7(1993):387–392.

61. T. Klouda, "Discussion," in *Report of the Seminar on Issues of HIV Testing in Developing Countries, 5 November 1992, London*, S. Lucas, ed. (London: UK NGO AIDS Consortium, 1993):46–47.

62. E. M. Lakritz, T. K. Ruebush, J. R. Zucker, J. E. Adungosi, J. B. O. Were, and C. C. Campbell, "Blood transfusion practices and blood-banking services in a Kenyan hospital," *AIDS* 7(1993):995–999.

63. B. Gumodoka, J. Vos, F. C. Kigadye, H. van Asten, W. M. V. Dolmans, and M. W. Borgdorff, "Blood transfusion practices in Mwanza Region, Tanzania," *AIDS* 7(1993):387–392.

64. S. Foster and A. Buvé, "Benefits of HIV screening of blood transfusions in Zaire," *Lancet* 346(1995):225–227.

65. W. A. Ghali, A. Palepu, and W. G. Paterson, "Evaluation of red blood cell transfusion practices with the use of preset criteria," *Canadian Medical Association Journal* 150(1994):1449–1454.

66. WHO, *Global Blood Safety Initiative: Use of Plasma Substitutes and Plasma in Developing Countries*, WHO/GPA/INF 89.17 (Geneva: WHO, 1989).

67. WHO, WHO/LAB/89.91 (Geneva: WHO, 1989).

68. WHO, *Global Blood Safety Initiative: Guidelines for the Appropriate Use of Blood*, WHO/GPA/INF/89.18 (Geneva: WHO, 1989).

69. WHO, WHO/LAB/89.91 (Geneva: WHO, 1989).

70. American College of Physicians, "Practice strategies for elective red blood cell transfusion," *Annals of Internal Medicine* 116(1992):403–406.

71. A. P. Britten, "International blood transfusion: Size of the problem," in *AIDS in the World*, J. Mann, D. J. Tarantola, and T. Netter, eds. (Cambridge, MA: Harvard University Press, 1992):423.

72. H. Tamashiro, W. Maskill, J. Emmanuel, A. Fauquex, P. Sato, and D. Heymann, "Reducing the cost of HIV antibody testing," *Lancet* 342(1993):87–90.

73. *Ibid.*

74. F. Simon and F. Brun-Vézinet, "HIV testing: Reduce costs by all means, but not at all costs" (Letter), *Lancet* 342(1993):379–380.

75. C. Almedal, N. Gilmore, R. Jurgens, T. Lemmens, P. Gill, D. Murphy, et al., "Worldwide survey of blood safety in relation to HIV/AIDS," Abstract PO-C21-3122, presented at the IX International Conference on AIDS, Berlin, Germany, June 1993.

76. E. J. Watson Williams, J. J. Fournel, D. Sondag, and L. Fransen, "EEC's safe blood programme policies and strategies in view of controlling AIDS in developing countries," in *Safe Blood in Developing Countries, a Report of the EEC's Expert Meeting*, R. W. Beal, M. Bontink, and L. Fransen, eds. (Brussels: EEC AIDS Task Force, 1992):112–118.

77. S. Foster and A. Buvé, "Benefits of HIV screening of blood transfusions in Zaire," *Lancet* 346(1995):225–227.

78. WHO, Global Programme on AIDS, *The Costs of HIV/AIDS Prevention Strategies in Developing Countries*, GPA/DIR/93.2 (Geneva: WHO, 1993).

79. M. Borgdorff, L. Barongo, E. van Jaarsveld, et al., "Sentinel surveillance for HIV-1 infection: How representative are blood donors, outpatients with fever, anemia, or sexually transmitted diseases, and antenatal clinic attenders in Mwanza Region, Tanzania?," *AIDS* 7(1993):567–572.

80. R. W. Ryder, "Difficulties associated with providing an HIV-free blood supply in tropical Africa," *AIDS* 6(1992):1395–1397.

81. R. W. Beal, "Transfusion science and practice in developing countries: . . . a high frequency of empty shelves . . ." (Editorial), *Transfusion* 33(1993):276–278.

82. R. Moodie and T. Abogaye-Dwarteng, "Confronting the HIV epidemic in Asia and the Pacific: Developing successful strategies to minimize the spread of HIV infection," *AIDS* 7(1993):1543–1551.

83. R. W. Ryder, "Difficulties associated with providing an HIV-free blood supply in tropical Africa," *AIDS* 6(1992):1395–1397.

84. Transfusion Study Group, "Transmission of HIV-1 by transfusion," Abstract PO-C17-2928, presented at the IX International Conference on AIDS, Berlin, Germany, June 1993.

85. L. Dierick and M. Bontink, "Session B: Safe blood initiatives," Commission of the European Communities AIDS Task Force Newsletter Report of the AIDS Task Force Pre-conference held in Berlin, Germany, June 6, 1993, *ATF News* (August 1993):14.

86. M. A. Strassburg, "Global eradication of smallpox," in *Health and Disease. A Reader*, N. Black, D. Boswell, A. Gray, S. Murphy, and J. Popay, eds. (Philadelphia, PA: Open University Press, 1984):220–225.

29

Are We Learning from the Lessons of the Past?

JUNE OSBORN

Whereas biomedical science made bold strides toward understanding of the new and complex human pathogen called human immunodeficiency virus (HIV), the inability of society and its leadership to utilize new insights in the interest of prevention and care allowed a massive escalation of the epidemic. Overall, the lessons learned from the agony of that decade are instructive for the future and extend far beyond the boundaries of epidemic disarray.

America as a learning ground

The first decade of AIDS illuminated powerfully the distinctive features of America's complex human landscape, sharpening the contrast between erosive points of dissonance in daily interactions with abstract avowals of the value of each human life.

Hubris

At the outset of the AIDS epidemic in the United States there was a pervasive sense of pride and comfort in the modernity of its medical competence. Vaccine successes of recent decades, a profusion of new pharmaceuticals, and dramatic high-profile feats of diagnosis and surgical intervention attested to the power of the reductionist approach to biomedical science. In the years just preceding the recognition of AIDS, new "microbial invaders" such as the causative agents of legionnaires' disease, toxic shock syndrome, and Lyme disease seemed to yield readily to analysis and development of effective strategies for containment and control.

Even influenza, with its distinctive capacity to shift and re-erupt in fresh pandemics, added subliminally, if irrationally, to the American sense of comfort about the "contained" microbial ecosystem within which modern American society had evolved. Altogether these events and experiences generated a

This chapter is an adapted and expanded version of an article published by the author: "Lessons learned in the first decade of AIDS," *Current Issues in Public Health* 1(1995):60–63, courtesy of *Current Issues in Public Health*, Current Science Publishers.

sense of hubris that left the society especially vulnerable to the new, subtle pathogen that was on its way.

The false confidence assumed a number of forms once the AIDS epidemic was recognized. First, assurance (or assumption) that a vaccine would follow quickly blunted attention to urgent messages about prevention that could be quickly formulated after epidemiologic study revealed limited modes of transmission. As a corollary, the fact that elegant molecular virology and immunology had been successfully applied to discern the cause and pathogenesis of the new disease reinforced a tendency to downplay the worth of insights achieved by "lesser" technologies or sciences. Thus the clear evidence that human behavior was central to perpetuation or control of HIV/AIDS did not lead, as one might have expected, to expansion of social and behavioral research into ways to intervene more effectively in risky behaviors; quite the contrary: censorious constraints were placed on pertinent studies of human behavior.

Similarly, the centrality of injection drug use to the flashfire potential of HIV, which characterized the American East Coast epidemic almost from its outset, led not to efforts to expand and improve treatment for drug addiction, but rather to official outrage at such strategies of harm reduction as needle-exchange programs. The resultant refusal to grapple with the most efficient mode of HIV spread, coupled with passage of mandatory sentencing laws for drug-related offenses, led by the end of the decade to prisons crowded to two- or threefold capacity and prison populations that were enriched with immunosuppressed people and opportunities for an old familiar pathogen, *Mycobacterium tuberculosis*, to expand its range, which it did.

Communication and diversity

A second category of lesson learned concerned the changing nature of American urban society. Happily, the indolent process of redress and societal recovery from a history of slavery had been accelerated by strong voices coming from the Civil Rights movement. Yet a growing stream of access to the affluence of mainstream, middle-class America for increasing numbers of minority Americans converged with a tide of flight from "inner cities," and with policies of deinstitutionalization that set adrift large numbers of people whose personal ills left them fully vulnerable to the new storm as it came.

Counts of the numbers of homeless in the great cities varied widely, yet even minimal estimates were shocking, peopled as they were with increasing numbers of individuals whose illnesses left them defenseless. Perhaps, worst of all, the ranks of the homeless were swelling with women and children. As David Hilfiker commented in a 1989 editorial in the *Journal of the American Medical Association*, Americans had, tragically, adapted to homelessness as an acceptable price of affluence.[1] When people with AIDS began to add to those numbers, social response was commensurately blunted.

These ugly facts of American life were not simply a backdrop against which the AIDS epidemic was playing out: rather, they were the warp and

woof of its rapid expansion, for every factor that enhanced the marginalization and estrangement of components of society also enhanced the risk of
HIV and AIDS.

The heightening of risk involved a number of dynamics. The early description of "groups at risk" fingered "gays and addicts" with such singu-
larity that anyone who didn't identify with one of those epithets felt safe
and uninvolved (Box 38-1). Even after more than a decade, the tendency to
talk about "risk groups" persists, and the inferred walling-off of select
groups is a prime mechanism of denial.

As the exclusionary language illustrated, there was much that needed to
be learned about health communication. Each community in the uniquely
diverse American society shared the possibility of HIV risk, for sexuality is
universal and drug use was sadly pervasive. And yet community denial was
enormously powerful: when early efforts at posters and ads concerning
AIDS prevention showed only white (presumably gay) men, women were
lulled, and people in communities of color were able to look away. Through
indirect, unspoken communication, the message was brought home consistently that this disease was someone else's problem. Native American leaders
later commented, for instance, that during the early years the failure to depict
any Native American people in AIDS educational material from the government was reinforced disastrously as funds were diverted from the (already
strapped) Indian Health Service to pay for AIDS programs elsewhere.

In short, the wide-ranging diversity of culture, language, and ethnicity in
the United States posed an inherent challenge to effective communication;
but that complexity was compounded by false or misleading signals. Thus
even clear and unambiguous information about risk avoidance was put
through a censorious majority filter that rendered it almost useless.

In a way, the lesson that effective communication about health was difficult and culture-sensitive was timely—in fact, overdue—for AIDS appeared
at a time when essential insights into the behavioral components of many
illnesses were beginning to emerge. Yet comprehension of the important
role played by behavioral factors seemed to lead increasingly to a response
of blaming, which, it was becoming clear, could play a harmful role in either
prevention or care. And, as noted earlier, the blaming of others contributed
heavily to personal denial about involvement or risk.

As a final element in this brief discussion of communication and diversity,
is a theme that had barely surfaced before AIDS: that of distrust of the
minority for the majority. This was especially evident in African-American
communities, where anger and doubt had simmered, especially after the
revelation of the Tuskegee Syphilis study. This purportedly scientific study
is in fact a grotesque mark against biomedical "science." Information concerning the natural history of syphilis was developed by allowing African-
American men to go untreated for long, damaging years after effective therapy for syphilis was available and ethically mandated.[2]

The moral horror of the Tuskegee events was fairly widely appreciated,
but its pervasive undermining of minority confidence in majority good will
remained to be articulated. Resultant unease about majority intentions ex-

tended to AIDS when it came. In fact, it went far beyond AIDS; even the cruel epidemic of drug addiction was perceived by some as a purposeful attack on the integrity of the African-American and Hispanic/Latino communities. Federal funds were focused almost exclusively on patently ineffectual border interdiction while long waiting lists for drug treatment prevailed in the communities under siege from the drug epidemic.

In fact, a decade after the discovery of HIV and the powerful unleashing of scientifically sound interventions, continued anxious confusion pervades many minority communities. There is doubt about whom to believe; for it is variously held either that the scientists are wrong and intentionally misleading about AIDS causation or that HIV is a virus that escaped from a government laboratory, either by accident or intentionally. In 1989 *Dædalus* published a powerful article by Harlon Dalton entitled "AIDS in Blackface," in which he explored in depth the currents of estrangement between minority communities and the majority in power.[3] As he underscored in that essay, an awareness of the dynamic of mistrust in minority communities was sure to be a critical factor in arriving at successful interventions aimed at both prevention and care.

As Dalton pointed out, the persistence of unhealed schisms in our society has introduced a destructive and enervating dynamic into efforts to deal with the ravages of HIV. Communication is affected not only by the complexity stemming from diversity but also by a static of mistrust" that makes it difficult for people to hear the messages of prevention. That social dynamic must be understood and factored into strategies of epidemic containment and control if these strategies are to be successful.

Sex, sexuality, and gender issues

It came as a shock, as this new lethal, sexually transmitted disease with its 7- to 10-year silent start pervaded the land, to discover how little we knew (or seemed to want to know) about sexuality in America. Homophobia held quiet sway, despite gay activism that had begun with the Stonewall riots of 1969.[4] Even in those few urban areas where same-sex orientation was acknowledged, understanding of openly gay communities and lifestyles was limited. And in more than half the states, laws forbade even private, consensual same-sex relations between adults. So profound was the silence generated by homophobia that "hate crimes" against gay people seemed to be tolerated in contexts where similar racial intolerance would have inflamed a whole community.

At the same time, as presented by television, magazines, and other readily accessible media, American heterosexuality was depicted as flagrant and irresponsible. Blatant sex was used to sell virtually everything in advertisements, and heroes and heroines of the afternoon televised soap operas coupled frequently and without protection. In the real world, sexual activity among teens had clearly escalated: teen sexual behavior at the end of the first decade of AIDS had increased to levels where three-quarters of high school graduates (and almost certainly a higher proportion of out-of-school youth) were sexually active, and condom use was sporadic at best.

The wages of such sin were being paid in heavy currency: abortion, sexually transmitted diseases, and teenage pregnancy all occurred in disturbing numbers and offered concrete evidence that HIV could pose serious risk to the nation's teens. Yet in most school districts strong resistance prevailed against the provision of AIDS-relevant information, or even contraceptive guidance.

As to gender, the status of women in the society was revealed to be distinctly uneven. Despite the superficial inroads made by feminists and activists working for gender equality in many spheres, it became clear in early AIDS prevention efforts that naiveté about gender inequality could lead to real harm: that exhorting a woman to insist on condom use might well place her in harm's way with a sex partner who held abusive power.

Indeed, in many of the diverse communities throughout the United States, as well as in countries throughout the world, the inability of women to protect themselves against the risk of sexual transmission of HIV prompted the comment that, "by recognizing the societal and historical dimensions of gender and health, we are led to the conclusion that a male-dominated society is a danger to public health."[5]

Lessons learned

The lessons that can be learned from these dreadful years are central to society's ability to cope, and will be necessary as HIV continues to expand. Pronouncements that the epidemic had "peaked" in the United States offered false comfort as we passed a point sometime in 1995 when the number of young Americans diagnosed with AIDS exceeded the total number of deaths from all U.S. armed conflicts since the Civil War; and the "steady state" thus celebrated a predicted level of 40,000–80,000 new infections per year.

The latter prediction suggests that we have not, in fact, fully absorbed those essential precepts and that intense efforts must be made to overcome present inertia. We cannot simply declare victory and leave the field; for the virus of AIDS will never be gone and it is seeded throughout the world. Wise policies of diligence and sensitivity are needed, and our messages of prevention must be delivered in the language of our intended listeners.

Among those lessons, perhaps the most fundamental is that hubris is dangerous: there are more challenges like AIDS coming, and although biomedical bench science can be marvelously helpful, its successful deployment will depend on a wide range of disciplines, with social science and behavioral science insights central to the enterprise.

With respect to prevention and care, it is evident that human dignity is held in common by all members of society. As a corollary to that observation, it is clearly necessary to involve communities in their own programs of prevention and care. The most subversive enemies of epidemic control will be schisms within communities bred of mistrust and blame. The sense of powerlessness felt by marginalized people, and by women in unequal relationships, must be recognized and factored into planning. Finally, the pervasive harm of denial must be acknowledged: whether it comes from sobriquets concerning "groups" or from rejection of "blaming" language, denial of the facts of this epidemic seems to be the only adequate explanation for the persistent silence of leadership concerning such a massive tragedy.

In the final report of the U. S. National Commission on AIDS, in the text of which recommendations were reiterated from all the earlier reports extending over four years' work, two further recommendations were added: first, that we need leaders at all levels of government to help overcome the deadly inertia pervading epidemic response; and second, that we need a national plan. Both of those assertions remain true more than a year later, and their lack goes far to explain why the lessons of AIDS have not yet been learned.[6]

The world as a learning ground

The AIDS epidemic is "maturing" in many other parts of the world, even as it is appearing for the first time elsewhere. With that maturation has come much insight and knowledge that could be brought to bear effectively to lessen the impact of the epidemic globally. There have been many useful lessons learned in the first decade of AIDS on the world scale.

There is no longer any question that HIV and AIDS are global facts of life and are here to stay for generations to come. We also know that the upcoming years will dwarf the agonizing experiences of the epidemic to date, however difficult that may be to imagine.

We have learned that behavior change is difficult when it involves habitual (and pleasurable) activities; but under the pressure of epidemic need, encouraging progress in the crucial areas of health education and behavioral interventions has shown that remarkable change *can* be achieved and that additional concerted effort in this area is likely to pay off handsomely, especially when focused on adapting generally useful approaches to age-specific populations (such as adolescents) or ethnicities. It is also clear that cultural sensitivity and community participation are crucial ingredients for long-range prevention.

We have also learned much about the diversity of human sexuality, and it has become obvious that unequal power relationships characterize male–female sexual interactions almost universally. That recognition is critical for it means that everywhere women's health issues and educational status are fundamental to long-term success in bringing HIV and AIDS under control.

Finally, it is ever more clear that biomedical science and medicine—however brilliantly conceived and practiced—cannot stand alone. Treatments or early intervention strategies, vaccine development, and vaccine deployment all will necessitate involvement of politicians and community leaders, educators and communicators—in fact, all thoughtful citizens.

But we are forgetting those lessons! Country after country replays the sorry story of denial; each new society caught up in the need to deal with issues of sexuality finds that it is constrained by its own variety of repression or avoidance of discussion about sexuality. Women's inequality in sexual negotiations argues loudly for development of means of protection against HIV that can be under women's control—and yet work on vaginal virucides and so-called female condoms has been halting, always earning lower priority than antiviral and higher-tech research. And, of course, behavioral research is still disregarded or treated with contempt.

Why are we forgetting these fundamental lessons that were learned (or relearned) at such human cost? Globally as well as in the United States, *denial* is fundamental to any answer—no one really wants to acknowledge that the world underwent a permanent change with the advent of AIDS. For example, only through deep denial could there arise such a perniciously tempting distraction as the recent, irresponsible assertion carried by the media that there is no such thing as AIDS in Africa. For national leaders it is far easier to settle comfortably into such a wishful myth than to keep mustering the political energy to grapple with changed reality. The stigma and discrimination that cling to AIDS everywhere make such a pretense possible as people continue to hide their losses and their grief.

The "Duesberg" phenomenon in the United States has served a similarly draining disservice: reiteration by a few insistently iconoclastic scientists that the rest of the scientific community is totally wrong.[7] The wishful imagining arises that AIDS might, after all, not be real, or that some unrecognized microbe (presumably more readily treated than HIV) is the true cause of AIDS. That rejects all the scientific evidence of the past thirteen years and the consensus of the world's thoughtful scientists; but the denial is nonetheless persistent.

Mistrust of the voices of authority provides yet another vehicle for rejection of accumulated experience and wisdom, for there is anger and suspicion about this new scourge: anger at imputations of blame, and suspicion that unfriendly forces may have unleashed it with malicious purpose. When such mistrust is pervasive, it obscures the demanding but simple messages about behavior change—especially when they have an impact on procreation. Under such a cloud even advocacy of condom use can be misunderstood as having hostile or even genocidal intent.

And, of course, in every segment of society AIDS evokes deep responses to issues of sexuality, of unequal relationships between men and women, of homophobia or addictophobia, and of changes in social mores that are particularly severe at times of rapid urbanization and social instability. So the lessons learned are bound to be hard to hear, and inattention and forgetfulness are inviting ways to escape from their logical implications.

There are no easy paths around this: the clear, compassionate, and consistent voices of leadership at every level and in each dialect and idiom needed to communicate with all the varied peoples of the world would clearly help. So, too, would a sense of global solidarity, from which the sharing of lessons learned can flow readily and in all directions.

The agony of the first years of AIDS has been harrowing and enervating; but the situation will grow worse. In years to come, we will therefore need all our energy to refine and extend the lessons already learned.

REFERENCES

1. D. Hilfiker, "Are we comfortable with homelessness?" *Journal of the American Medical Association* 262 (1989):1375–1376.

2. G. E. Pence, *Classic Cases in Medical Ethics* (McGraw-Hill, Inc: New York, 1990):189–205.

3. H. Dalton, "AIDS in blackface," *Dœdalus* (Journal of the American Academy of Arts and Sciences: Cambridge, MA)118 (1989):205–227.

4. L. Garrett, *The Coming Plague* (Penguin Books USA, Inc: New York, 1994):260–261.

5. J. M. Mann, "AIDS: the second decade: a global perspective," *Journal of Infectious Diseases* 165 (1992):245–250.

6. Centers for Disease Control and Prevention: AIDS: An Expanding Tragedy. The Final Report of the National Commission on AIDS. Rockville, MD: Centers for Disease Control and Prevention National AIDS Clearinghouse; 1993.

7. J. Cohen, "The Duesberg Phenomenon," *Science* 266 (1994):1642–1644.

IV

THE INSTITUTIONAL RESPONSE

The institutional response to the HIV/AIDS pandemic also has a history. Almost immediately following the recognition of AIDS in the early 1980s, nongovernmental and community organizations arose to provide care and then prevention services to severely affected groups. At that time and for several years thereafter, virtually no national programs for prevention or care were developed. Then, generally in response to public pressure, national governments began to consider what they should do. During the same period in the early to mid-1980s, the World Health Organization became the first major organization and the first intergovernmental agency to begin mobilizing for HIV/AIDS prevention and care.

National governments and WHO tended to view their roles in relatively similar and complementary ways. True to the traditions of public health, governments initiated programs of information and education and related health services such as testing and counseling. From WHO's perspective, the need for a global mobilization implied catalyzing and supporting national AIDS programs in countries that were either already affected but were passive in their response, or were not yet affected. Together, WHO and national governments (or ministries of health) developed common policies and models for HIV prevention and care work. Donor nations rapidly responded to WHO's appeal for resources and by 1988 the Global Program on AIDS had become WHO's largest and most dynamic activity. Relatively soon thereafter, and partially in response to the UN General Assembly Resolution of late 1987[1], other members of the UN family, including notably United Nations Development Programme (UNDP), United Nations Children's Fund (UNICEF), United Nations Educational, Scientific and Cultural Organization (UNESCO), United Nations Population Fund (UNFPA), International Labour Organization (ILO), and the World Bank began to make their own contributions to HIV/AIDS prevention and care. The goal was to ensure that comprehensive national programs were in place worldwide. What is the status today of these collective efforts—at the nongovernmental, national governmental, and intergovernmental levels?

This part of *AIDS in the World II* explores the current work at each of these levels, with particular attention to the new challenges each is encountering. In summary, the major findings are as follows:

- National AIDS programs have experienced considerable difficulty fulfilling their central responsibilities for prevention and care (see Chapter 30).
- The challenge of ensuring that national AIDS programs are carried out (including policies, programs, and practices) in a manner which respects the human rights and dignity of HIV-infected people and people with AIDS has only been partially met (see Chapter 31).
- Nongovernmental organizations are undergoing a difficult transition period in their internal evolution, their relationship to official agencies, and their financial sustainability (see Chapter 32).
- The private sector is having difficulty fulfilling its potential role in promoting HIV prevention (see Chapter 33).
- The United Nations has created a new program, called UNAIDS, to better coordinate the work of the major UN agencies working on HIV/AIDS (see Chapter 34).
- International funding for HIV/AIDS prevention and care is relatively static, and this is failing to keep up with the rapid growth in prevention and care needs. Official development assistance for HIV/AIDS is becoming increasingly bilateral, so that in relative terms, support to multilateral efforts is diminishing (see Chapter 35).
- The cost of care for HIV-infected people and people with AIDS is increasing as the pandemic expands. The nature of HIV/AIDS care in the developing world is severely and increasingly disadvantaged compared with the industrialized world (see Chapter 36).
- Global spending on HIV/AIDS prevention, care, and research now exceeds U.S. $18.4 billion. Spending on care is five times greater than spending for prevention, and over 92 percent of prevention and care spending occurs in the industrialized world, while the developing world has over 90 percent of the global total of HIV-infected people and people with AIDS (see Chapter 37).

Of course, the collective response is really a complex mosaic, including some highly successful efforts in both prevention and care. Yet overall, the collective response seems enmeshed in trying to carry out the difficult tasks that it defined and that were defined for it nearly a decade ago. Meanwhile, the pandemic has intensified and expanded, organizational and institutional practices (even if less than effective) have tended to become fixed, and resources (especially since 1990) have not kept pace with the needs.

Thus the collective response seems to harken back to the mid-to-late 1980s, seeking to fulfill a mission which is necessary but now recognized to be insufficient to bring the pandemic under control. In the meanwhile, the pandemic is evolving (Part I), and as described in Parts II and III, a new approach is needed to address the social dimensions of vulnerability to HIV.

REFERENCES

1. United Nations General Assembly: *Resolution 42/8 of the Forty-second General Assembly of the United Nations: Prevention and Control of Acquired Immune Deficiency Syndrome (AIDS)* (New York: UN, 26 October 1987).

30

Governmental National AIDS Programs

This chapter focuses on the governmental response to AIDS and specifically on governmental national AIDS programs (GNAP). It is based on the most extensive survey of GNAP managers thus far conducted.

In *AIDS in the World* (1992), a framework to assess GNAP work was proposed using 11 criteria: (1) voicing commitment; (2) translating commitment into action; (3) coalition building; (4) planning and coordinating; (5) managing; (6) responding to prevention needs; (7) responding to care needs; (8) securing financial resources; (9) sustaining the effort; (10) evaluating progress; and (11) evaluating impact.[1] This framework was applied to the questionnaire of the survey conducted by AIW II (Box 30-1). Detailed responses by country are listed in Appendix D.

BOX 30-1

A survey of government national AIDS programs

The first edition of *AIDS in the World* presented a framework for the assessment of national programs.[1] This framework served as the template for the survey of government national AIDS programs (GNAP) presented in this volume. That survey, including both a mailing and follow-up telephone inquiries, was carried out between December 1993 and June 1994. The survey questionnaire was designed and tested with six GNAP managers, then revised and distributed in English, French, Spanish, and Japanese. Follow-up contacts with respondents were also made in Arabic, Chinese, French, Portuguese, and Spanish. While the first edition of *AIDS in the World* surveyed a panel of 38 countries, the present study sought responses from 187 countries/territories ("countries"), including the 184 member states of the United Nations as of June 1994, plus Hong Kong, Switzerland, and Taiwan. The effort involved the collaboration of WHO Regional Offices and multiple inquiries with embassies and ministries of health and resulted in the most complete directory of GNAP contacts available to date. Areas and Territories that are geographically distant from the mainland of the state of which they are part were also sent a questionnaire in order to collect information on differing epidemiological, cultural, or social features.* That information was used in commentaries included in various chapters of this book, but not included in the quantitative analysis.

*Responses were received from American Samoa, Cook Islands, Guam, New Caledonia, Niue, Tokelau, Tuvalu, Bermuda, Cayman Islands, Montserrat, and Netherlands Antilles.

Table 30-1.1 Governmental national AIDS programs (GNAP) response rate to *AIDS in the World II* survey

GAA	Total number of countries in GAA	Number of responding countries	Percentage of countries responding	Total population in GAA (millions)	Population of responding countries (millions)	Percentage GAA population in responding countries
1 North America	2	1	(50%)	286	258	(90%)
2 Western Europe	24	17	(71%)	383	301	(79%)
3 Oceania	9	9	(100%)	27	27	(100%)
4 Latin America	20	15	(75%)	427	405	(95%)
5 Sub-Saharan Africa	48	31	(65%)	560	337	(60%)
6 Caribbean	13	7	(54%)	30	12	(39%)
7 Eastern Europe	27	16	(59%)	418	287	(69%)
8 SE Mediterranean	21	9	(43%)	473	92	(19%)
9 Northeast Asia	11	6	(55%)	1,490	1,407	(94%)
10 Southeast Asia	12	7	(58%)	1,435	1,021	(71%)
Total world	187	118	(63%)	5,529	4,147	(75%)

Source: *AIDS in the World II* survey.

Responses were received from 118 of the 187 countries surveyed (63%) (Table 30-1.1). The total population of respondent countries was 75 percent of the world population. The highest response rate was achieved in Oceania (100 percent) and the lowest in the Southeast Mediterranean region (43 percent). The degree of completeness and specificity of the information provided in the returns varied from complete and detailed information (about one-quarter of respondents) to sparse and fairly general responses, of which about half were improved through active follow-up. The extensive collaboration of respondents was very much appreciated, especially given the enormous operational and administrative demands on their time and the growing number of GNAP surveys that followed from many sources in the wake of the first-ever survey carried out by *AIDS in the World* in 1992.

The summary information originates from GNAP managers, usually located within ministries of health. Although GNAP managers were invited to seek information on specific issues from the best-informed sources within other government sectors, they may not have done so. For example, questions on HIV/AIDS-related laws and practices assumed that GNAP managers would be fully aware of the legal context within which their program operates or that they would verify the legislation with ministries of justice (Chapter 31).

An important constraint involved the growing difficulty GNAP managers have in tracking financial resources allocated to and spent on HIV/AIDS prevention and care. In some countries, the integration of HIV/AIDS with broader health and social programs has been accompanied by a multiplication of funding sources, a dispersion of resource allocation, and a consequent decline in financial tracking capability. In all likelihood, the financial information provided in this volume is therefore only a partial representation of the resources allocated to and spent by government-controlled HIV/AIDS initiatives.

The questionnaire sought quantified, documented information obtained by GNAP managers from records and reports. When such information was unavailable, the questionnaire invited GNAP managers to provide an informed opinion on the degree to which a particular value or situation might have changed over time. Such entries are marked in the tabulation of results as an *opinion* sought from the GNAP manager, in order to differentiate such information.

Finally, in some cases, GNAP managers had been prevented by higher authorities from releasing information. When this censorship occurred, it had generally been provoked by the section of the questionnaire that sought information on human rights issues.

Detailed responses are displayed in Appendixes D and E, for each responding GNAP regrouped in

"Geographic Areas of Affinity." Tabulated results are presented and analyzed in various chapters throughout this volume.

The editors are grateful to GNAP managers who responded to this survey despite their heavy work-load.

References

1. J. M. Mann, D. Tarantola, T. W. Netter, and The Global AIDS Policy Coalition, eds., *AIDS in the World* (Cambridge, MA: Harvard University Press, 1992):282–283.

Voicing commitment

Are high governmental officials expressing publicly their commitment to prevent the spread of HIV and care for those infected? Since the beginning of the pandemic 60 percent had done so and 40 percent had not (Table 30-1). High governmental officials in those geographic areas of affinity (GAAs) that have experienced visible HIV epidemics (North America, Western Europe, Oceania, Caribbean, sub-Saharan Africa, Latin America, Southeast Asia) were nearly three times more likely to have addressed the issue publicly, compared to those in less affected GAAs (Eastern Europe, Southeast Mediterranean and Northeast Asia).

Translating commitment into action

The reporting of the first AIDS case in each country and the creation of GNAPs have followed two waves of similar shape (Figure 30-1). Most GNAPs were established between 1985 and 1990; by mid-1994, essentially all countries had a GNAP. The translation of commitment into the allocation of financial resources is reflected in the financial analysis carried out to estimate national spending on HIV/AIDS prevention, care, and research (Chapter 37).

Table 30-1   Public addresses on AIDS made by high governmental officials[a]

GAAs	Top governmental authority made a statement on AIDS	Top governmental authority did not make statement on AIDS	Total respondents
GAAs with visible or severe HIV epidemics[b]	59 (71%)	24 (29%)	83
Less affected GAAs[c]	8 (28%)	21 (72%)	29
All GAAs	67 (60%)	45 (40%)	112

Source: *AIDS in the World II* survey.

[a]"Top governmental authority" was defined by the respondent and may include heads of state, presidents, prime ministers, and ministers of health.

[b]North America, Western Europe, Oceania, Latin America, sub-Saharan Africa, Caribbean and Southeast Asia.

[c]Eastern Europe, Southeast Mediterranean, Northeast Asia.

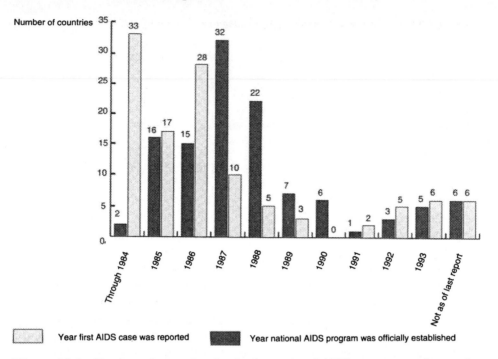

Number of countries

Figure 30-1   Number of countries developing national AIDS programs and reporting first AIDS case, by year, 1984–1993.

Coalition building

Coalition building by GNAPs requires expanded partnership between ministries of health and other government ministries, nongovernmental organizations (NGOs), and the private sector. An indication of attempts to build such coalitions can be obtained by noting the participation of groups outside the ministry of health in AIDS policy development. WHO has recommended that policy development be guided by national AIDS advisory committees (NACs) or the equivalent advisory bodies, in most cases appointed by the minister of health.

Overall, 85 percent of responding countries reported having an NAC. This proportion was lowest in Latin America and Eastern Europe (53 percent and 63 percent, respectively). NAC membership averaged 21 people, with a range of 7 to 74 participants. Gender representation for these committees varied widely; the proportion of women committee members averaged 30 percent (ranging from 0 to 67 percent). An average of 27 percent of NAC participants were from NGOs; 14 of 88 countries had no NGO representative on their NAC.

GNAP managers were also asked who had been consulted in AIDS policy development. Health professionals had been consulted in virtually all (96 percent) of the 94 countries; other government ministries in 82 countries (87 percent); other agencies in 77 (82 percent); state or regional authorities in 72 (77 percent); people with HIV/AIDS were involved in 41 countries (44 percent); and members of parliament in 29 countries (31 percent). In only 17 countries (18 percent) had all of the above groups been consulted.

Table 30-2 Contents of national AIDS policy and program documents

Key element	Does the document contain the key element listed? (Number and percentage of countries responding)			
	Yes	No	Did not respond to specific key element	Total
Statement of national policies on HIV/AIDS	79 (85%)	12 (13%)	2 (2%)	93 (100%)
Description of strategic approaches for the health sector	81 (87%)	11 (12%)	1 (1%)	93 (100%)
Description of strategic approaches for the health sector and other sectors such as ministries of development, education, and justice	61 (66%)	29 (31%)	3 (3%)	93 (100%)
Description of specific activities for the health and other sectors	77 (83%)	13 (14%)	3 (3%)	93 (100%)
Proposed budget for central/ federal expenditures on HIV/ AIDS	68 (73%)	24 (26%)	1 (1%)	93 (100%)
Evaluation plan for government activities	53 (57%)	37 (40%)	3 (3%)	93 (100%)

Source: *AIDS in The World II* survey.

Planning and coordination

By early 1994, 82 percent of 118 responding countries had developed an AIDS policy and program document. Further information was available from 93 countries on the content of these documents (Table 30-2). Document completeness varied widely; only 31 percent of GNAP policy and planning documents included all six of the key elements.

The responsibility for GNAP activities was vested primarily in the ministry of health for over half of the countries, but the dominant ministry of health role in major GNAP tasks diminished from 1991 to 1993 (Figure 30-2). In addition, the survey revealed that AIDS programs have occasionally been created in other ministries such as education (in 88 percent of the countries surveyed), defense (61 percent), and other ministries (between 11 and 39 percent), as shown in Figure 30-3. Nevertheless, GNAPs remain identified with ministries of health in most countries, raising important questions about the ability of governments to develop and disseminate a broader and expanded response to the HIV/AIDS pandemic.

Managing

The survey focused on two aspects of GNAP management: staff training and program decentralization (Figure 30-4). Strikingly, GNAP managers had been trained in only 40 percent of responding countries; levels of training for other important management staff were uniformly lower.

Decentralization of AIDS programs to regional or provincial levels was

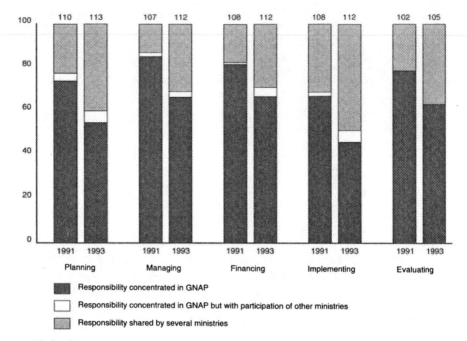

Figure 30-2 Division of responsibility for several tasks of GNAP, among ministries of health, 1991 and 1993.

Figure 30-3 Countries with AIDS programs in ministries other than the ministry of health. Eighty-three countries responded to this question.

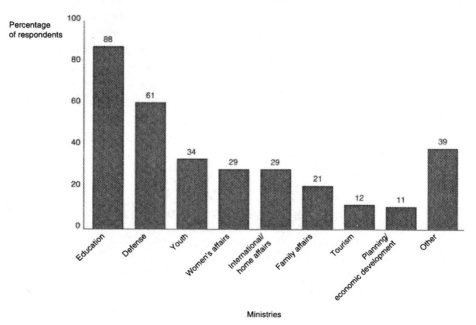

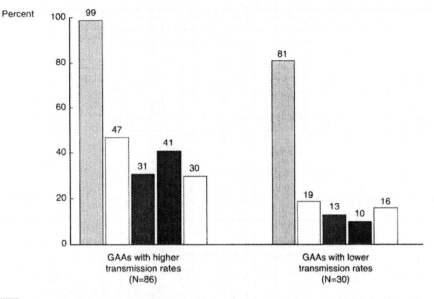

 Percentage of countries where government national AIDS program has been officially established

Percentage of countries where the GNAP has conducted targeted HIV/AIDS program management training for:

☐ GNAP managers

■ Managers of other governmental programs or departments

■ Region/province district managers

☐ Non-governmental organization managers

Figure 30-4 Percentage of countries with officially established national AIDS programs and where GNAP conducted targeted training on managing HIV/AIDS programs.

reported by about half (48 percent) of responding countries; 29 percent were partially decentralized and the remaining 23 percent were still completely centralized.

Responding to prevention and care needs

Assessments regarding prevention had been conducted in 70 percent of the countries surveyed and care needs in 54 percent (Table 30-3). To assess GNAP responsiveness to prevention and care needs, two measures were chosen: condom distribution and availability of voluntary testing with counseling.

Condom distribution

A large majority of countries reported that the distribution of condoms was allowed in certain sites (e.g., pharmacies and drug stores) (93 percent), and in sexually transmitted infection (STI) and other clinics (91 percent). However, substantially fewer reported that distribution was allowed in other settings such as hotels, bars, universities, and high schools. From 1990 to 1992 there was a very modest increase in the variety of sites where condoms were allowed to be distributed.

Table 30-3   Needs assessment conducted by government national AIDS programs

	Number and percentage of countries responding			
	Yes	No	No response	Total
Needs assessment for prevention	66 (70%)	24 (26%)	4 (4%)	94 (100%)
Needs assessment for care	51 (54%)	39 (41%)	4 (4%)	94 (100%)

Source: *AIDS in the World II* survey.

Voluntary HIV testing and counseling

Testing for HIV was available widely in only 58 percent of 113 countries and only in large cities in the remaining 42 percent (Table 30-4). Pre- and/or post-test counseling was said to be available in nearly all countries (106; 95 percent). However, only 45 percent of countries reported always providing pre-test counseling; 70 percent of countries always counseled persons who were found HIV seropositive; and 32 percent of countries always counseled persons found HIV seronegative (Figure 30-5). The lack of systematic pre- and post-test counseling was apparent in both industrialized and developing countries. For example, only 4 of 15 Western European countries (27 percent) reported systematic pre-test counseling; a similar proportion reported counseling of persons found HIV seronegative and 69 percent systematically counseled persons found HIV seropositive.

Seventy-seven countries also provided estimates of the number of HIV tests performed in 1993 (Table 30-4). Comparing 1990 and 1992, 22 percent of countries reported a considerable—greater than twofold—increase in the number of HIV tests performed and 42 percent reported a moderate increase (one- to twofold). Thirty percent of countries reported that the number of HIV tests had either stabilized or decreased.

It is evident that major gaps still exist in the availability of HIV testing facilities in several regions in the world and when available, testing is not accompanied with systematic pre- and post-test counseling in a significant number of developing and industrialized countries.

Securing financial resources and striving toward sustainability

Financial resources spent on HIV/AIDS prevention, care, and research are drawn from multiple sources: public, private, and, in the case of developing countries, international. Patterns of program spending are presented in Chapter 37. A comparison of the estimated overall spending on HIV/AIDS prevention, care, and research in low economies, inclusive of grants from official development agencies (ODAs) and of World Bank loans, show that developing countries are already bearing the brunt of AIDS program costs. It was estimated that in 1993 low economies spent $1.4 billion on national HIV/AIDS programs (Chapter 37). In that year, the external funding made available to them through ODAs totaled about $257 million, including the institutional costs and overhead levied by implementing agencies (UN Agencies, NGOs, private voluntary organizations, and other contractors) (Chapter 35). Thus the external financing from ODAs to NAPs in low economies

Table 30-4 Voluntary HIV testing—availability and number of tests performed, by GAA, 1993

| GAA | Availability (No. and percentage of countries responding) | | | No. of tests performed per 1,000 adults (aged 15–49) in country as reported by GNAP | | | Number responding |
	Everywhere in the country	Only in large cities	Total	Lowest	Mean	Highest	
1 North America	1 (100%)	0 (0%)	1 (100%)				
2 Western Europe	16 (94%)	1 (6%)	17 (100%)	8.7	115.9	322.5	11
3 Oceania	3 (33%)	6 (67%)	9 (100%)	17.6	68.8	215.9	6
4 Latin America	8 (57%)	6 (43%)	14 (100%)	1.8	24.6	42.0	7
5 Sub-Saharan Africa	7 (24%)	22 (76%)	29 (100%)	0.7	22.6	195.0	21
6 Caribbean	4 (67%)	2 (33%)	6 (100%)	27.4	48.2	93.1	6
7 Eastern Europe	12 (80%)	3 (20%)	15 (100%)	3.5	214.5	484.2	13
8 SE Mediterranean	4 (44%)	5 (56%)	9 (100%)	11.1	116.3	350.0	5
9 Northeast Asia	5 (83%)	1 (17%)	6 (100%)	1.3	43.4	148.2	5
10 Southeast Asia	5 (71%)	2 (29%)	7 (100%)	27.9	56.0	111.4	3
All GAAs	65 (58%)	48 (42%)	113 (100%)	0.7	94.1	708.1	77

Source: *AIDS in the World II* survey.

Figure 30-5 Frequency with which HIV counseling is provided in the country.

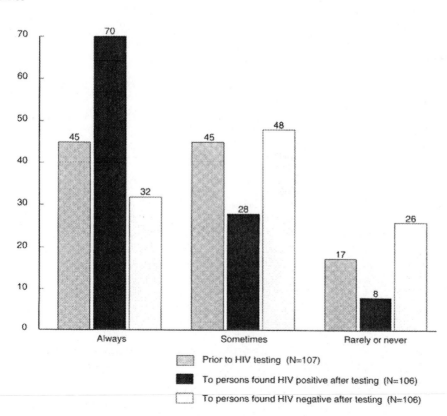

Number of countries

Prior to HIV testing (N=107)

To persons found HIV positive after testing (N=106)

To persons found HIV negative after testing (N=106)

323

Table 30-5 Outcome indicators used to evaluate government national AIDS programs*

Outcome indicator	Number and percentage of countries responding		
	Evaluated outcome	Outcome not evaluated	No response
Number of people provided with targeted HIV/AIDS prevention message/education	74 (82%)	11 (12%)	5 (6%)
Number of people HIV tested	70 (78%)	16 (18%)	4 (4%)
Number of condoms distributed	64 (71%)	19 (21%)	7 (8%)
Number of people reached by program	60 (67%)	24 (27%)	6 (7%)
Number of people who are HIV positive	59 (66%)	20 (22%)	11 (12%)
Noted behavior change	50 (56%)	29 (32%)	11 (12%)
Other	20 (22%)	0 (0%)	70 (78%)
Needles/syringes exchanged	18 (20%)	51 (57%)	21 (23%)

Source: *AIDS in the World II* survey.
*90 countries responded.

Table 30-6 Influence of evaluation on GNAP

	Number and percentage of countries reporting			
	Major change	Minor change	Population	No response*
Change in program strategies	35 (44%)	13 (16%)	27 (34%)	5 (6%)
Reformation of the national HIV/AIDS plan	31 (39%)	15 (19%)	26 (33%)	8 (10%)
Personnel changes	23 (29%)	21 (26%)	28 (35%)	8 (10%)
Redirection of a specific needed service	17 (21%)	13 (16%)	31 (39%)	19 (24%)
Change of a certain project focus	20 (25%)	20 (25%)	24 (30%)	16 (20%)
Ending a program component	7 (9%)	9 (11%)	45 (56%)	19 (24%)
Beginning a new program component	29 (36%)	14 (18%)	22 (28%)	15 (19%)

Source: *AIDS in the World II* survey.
*A country was counted as not responding to a segment of this question only if it had responded to another segment.

represented less than one-fifth of the estimated expenditures incurred in the developing world to cover the direct cost of HIV/AIDS prevention, care, and research. While this relatively modest external contribution has helped developing countries to better cope with the rising cost of HIV/AIDS, the mere fact that they mobilized more than 80 percent of the overall direct cost of AIDS from national sources increases the likelihood of long-term sustainability of their response to the pandemic at a time when international grants are harder to obtain.

Evaluating progress and impact

Of the 105 countries responding to this part of the survey, 85 (81 percent) reported that their GNAP had been evaluated at least once. This proportion was higher in developing (93 percent) than in industrialized countries (67 percent). These evaluations involved the participation of ministries of health in 93 percent of countries; other ministries in 73 percent; NGOs in 68 percent; representatives of international agencies in 85 percent (largely involving developing countries); and of all groups mentioned above, in 52 percent of countries. The variety of outcome indicators used to evaluate programs are listed in Table 30-5. The indicator most frequently used was the number or proportion of people provided with specific HIV/AIDS prevention education or messages (82 percent). Overall, the majority of countries still focus their evaluation on management processes and service coverage, with a lower proportion reporting attempts to evaluate epidemiological or behavioral impact.

Do evaluation findings influence program strategies and activities? Countries were asked to describe the influence of evaluation on program design and decisions in seven categories (Table 30-6). Over half of the countries reported having introduced major or minor changes in program strategies and/or having reformulated their national HIV/AIDS plan as a result of program evaluation. No programmatic changes occurred following the evaluation in 31–56 percent of countries, depending on the category of design or section; and 7 (9 percent) GNAPs reported no change in any of the categories listed. While program evaluation has become a more regular feature of GNAPs, the application of evaluation for reorienting programs or making structural or operational decisions is not yet widely apparent.

REFERENCES

1. J. Mann, D. Tarantola, and T. Netter, eds., *AIDS in the World* (Cambridge, MA: Harvard University Press, 1992):202–283, 605–683.

31

Human Rights and Responses to HIV/AIDS

SOFIA GRUSKIN, AART HENDRIKS,
AND KATARINA TOMASEVSKI

The relationship between human rights and HIV/AIDS prevention and control has proceeded through three relatively distinct phases. In the first phase, starting in 1981, the proposed application of public health measures such as isolation, mandatory testing, and quarantine to the new health problem led to a direct confrontation between health officials and human rights advocates. In the second phase, starting around 1987, international health officials explicitly recognized that discrimination against HIV-infected people and people with AIDS reduced the effectiveness of public health prevention efforts and was therefore counterproductive. This perspective was espoused by the World Health Organization (WHO), the UN agency primarily responsible for health issues. WHO's governing board, the World Health Assembly, adopted a resolution in 1988 which stated that preventing discrimination against HIV-infected people and people with AIDS was an essential element in a successful HIV prevention program; the principle of non-discrimination was consequently incorporated into WHO's Global AIDS Strategy.

The third phase developed in the late 1980s and early 1990s as independent analysis by groups such as the Global AIDS Policy Coalition led to a new perspective on the pandemic. This new perspective focused on vulnerability to HIV infection. When considering the personal, programmatic, and societal forces which contribute to vulnerability to HIV/AIDS, it became clear that a lack of respect for human rights and dignity was a major contributor to the HIV/AIDS problem. This awareness of a fundamental connection between HIV and human rights has slowly but increasingly led to new and deeper collaboration between public health officials and human rights advocates. Today, the basic, inextricable link between promoting and protecting human rights and health (HIV/AIDS or other major health problems of the modern world) is becoming more evident and serves as a new basis for action (see Part V).

This new collaboration between public health workers and human rights experts around HIV/AIDS issues is starting to influence the larger world of public health. One dimension of this work focuses on negotiation to ensure that public health policies, programs, and practices respect—to the maximum extent possible—human rights and dignity.

The following chapter focuses on this issue from the perspective of international law and human rights. To readers interested in the language of public health, the discussion may seem legalistic. Yet it is part of a fruitful dialogue between public health and human rights, based on an increasingly mutual ability to explore and consider differing underlying assumptions and terminology. This chapter focuses on the largest current area of human rights–HIV/AIDS interaction, involving efforts to prevent discrimination against people living with HIV or AIDS and certain people considered by societies to be at high risk of HIV infection (e.g., gay men, injecting drug users, sex workers). How the promotion and protection of human rights are linked with vulnerability to HIV/AIDS is discussed in detail in Part V.

Human rights and HIV/AIDS: key principles

The importance of bringing public health policies and programs in line with human rights law is, at least in theory, increasingly acknowledged by the international community. However, in the context of HIV/AIDS, a review of national laws, policies, and practices worldwide reveal a lack of consistent adherence to human rights standards.

A specific problem in this regard involves discrimination, which ensues when a distinction is made against a person that results in their being treated unfairly and unjustly. (This discussion is limited to negative discrimination. Laws and policies that treat people differently in an effort to ensure equal enjoyment and exercise of rights [positive or affirmative action] are not addressed in this chapter.) Discrimination commonly results from prejudice and misinformation, a denial of human variety, and feelings of superiority towards those considered "different." The principle of nondiscrimination is central to human rights thinking and practices. Each of the major human rights treaties specifically details the principle of nondiscrimination with respect to race, color, sex, language, religion, political or other opinion, national or social origin, property, birth, and, as it is called, "other status." The prohibition of discrimination does not mean that differences should not be acknowledged, only that different treatment must be based on objective and reasonable criteria.

Although international human rights law does not explicitly prohibit discrimination on the grounds of health status, the United Nations Commission on Human Rights has stated that "all are equal before the law and entitled to equal protection of the law from all discrimination and from all incitement to discrimination relating to their state of health."[1]

Rectifying inequalities—including health inequalities—and protecting people against discrimination are at the very core of human rights work. Human rights law generally concerns the relationship between the individual and the state, and includes civil, political, economic, social, and cultural rights which human beings everywhere are entitled to enjoy. Certain rights are absolute, which means that they can never be restricted—whether by governments or others. These rights include the right to life, the right to be free from torture, slavery, or servitude, and the right to a fair trial. However, interference with most human rights can, under narrowly defined circumstances, be justified if necessary for the achievement of an overriding public good. Public health is recognized as one of the legitimate grounds for restricting human rights. Nonetheless, such interferences with human rights are considered acceptable only if they are:

1. provided for and carried out *in accordance with the law;*
2. in the interest of a *legitimate objective* of general interest;
3. *strictly necessary* in a democratic society to achieve such a goal;
4. imposed *without a less intrusive means being available* to reach the same goal;
5. **not** imposed *arbitrarily,* i.e., in an unreasonable or otherwise discriminatory manner.[2]

Government health policies have not always taken this approach into account. Traditional public health measures have focused on curbing the spread of disease by imposing restrictions on those already infected or thought to be most vulnerable to infection. In fact, coercion, compulsion, and restriction have often been principal components of public health measures.[3] Interferences with the rights of individuals, justified as necessary to protect the public health, must be recognized as human rights violations if they do not satisfy the above-listed criteria.

Generally, the people most likely to experience discrimination are socially and/or economically disadvantaged and therefore have great difficulty preventing laws or actions that discriminate against them or seeking redress.

Data collected over the course of the AIDS epidemic has clearly shown that public health efforts to prevent and control the spread of HIV/AIDS are most likely to succeed (e.g., lower HIV incidence, increase the quality of life of those infected) if policies and programs respect, instead of violate, human rights.[4] Involuntary public health measures are hardly ever justified, let alone necessary.* In the context of AIDS, legitimate interferences with human rights can only occur in very exceptional circumstances.

International responses to AIDS and violations of human rights

Nongovernmental organizations

Information on human rights violations is usually made known to intergovernmental agencies through the work of individuals and national or international nongovernmental organizations (NGOs). Although the intergovernmental system has generated quite a bit of HIV/AIDS-related work, this pattern generally has not been followed with respect to AIDS-related human rights violations. In fact, the large international human rights NGOs

---

*The World Health Assembly adopted a number of resolutions stating that there is no public health rationale to restrict the rights of individuals in the context of HIV/AIDS. Cf. WHO/World Health Assembly, Resolution WHA45.35 (May 1992).

have only recently begun to consider HIV/AIDS-specific issues. The slow response of the established human rights NGOs to HIV/AIDS-related issues has resulted in intergovernmental organizations and agencies receiving the majority of their information from governments.

In most countries, human rights violations arising from HIV/AIDS have been identified and addressed by AIDS service organizations (ASOs). ASOs have mobilized to provide needed prevention and care services, and while often involved in advocacy efforts, they may not have had experience in working to redress human rights violations. Further, local or national human rights organizations have frequently not considered HIV/AIDS to be an important or relevant issue for their work. Nevertheless, an enormous amount of advocacy seeking to redress and prevent discrimination towards HIV-infected people, people with AIDS, and members of population groups considered at high risk of HIV infection has been generated and advanced by ASOs and other community organizations.

Stimulated by courageous efforts of many local and national groups, international human rights NGOs are gradually becoming active, for example:

- Amnesty International undertook a comprehensive study, including questionnaires addressed to ASOs worldwide, to determine in what circumstances AIDS-related issues are within Amnesty's mandate. Amnesty International has begun to note the impact of HIV/AIDS in their country reports and in their international advocacy efforts.
- The International Commission of Jurists (ICJ) has adopted items on its future agenda relevant to HIV/AIDS, including discrimination on the grounds of sexual orientation, drug use and addiction, and HIV/AIDS status.
- The International Human Rights Law Group submitted a petition in April 1993 to the UN Working Group on Arbitrary Detention. It was offered on behalf of the approximately 190 Haitian nationals seeking political asylum in the United States who were in detention because of their HIV status at the U.S. Naval Base in Guantanamo Bay. In addition, the International Human Rights Law Group has integrated HIV/AIDS concerns, including the application of human rights standards, into their international advocacy work.
- Asia Watch and the Women's Rights Project of Human Rights Watch highlighted AIDS-related issues in a report on the trafficking of Burmese women and girls into Thai brothels.
- The International Gay and Lesbian Human Rights Commission (IGLHRC), created in 1991, has acted as the action secretariat of the International Lesbian and Gay Association (ILGA), with a focus on the human rights of sexual minorities and people with HIV/AIDS. IGLHRC issues "action bulletins" to over 3,000 people and organizations around the world to catalyze campaigns in response to human rights violations.
- Other human rights NGOs have also studied related topics. For example, Article 19, the International Centre Against Censorship, has re-

cently completed a comprehensive report which includes AIDS-related issues in its analysis of how the denial of access to family planning information has an impact on the rights and health of women.

The intergovernmental system

Prior to HIV/AIDS, human rights principles only marginally influenced the design of international public health policies. While human rights norms are increasingly acknowledged by policy makers, the classic (non-human rights–associated) public health approach is still apparent in many public health laws and regulations.

Beginning in 1987, the WHO Global Programme on AIDS introduced a number of guidelines that increasingly reflected a commitment to human rights. Guidelines were adopted on such diverse issues as testing, travel and immigration policies, blood safety, prison health, mother-to-child transmission of HIV, and employment.[5]

Following the lead of the World Health Organization, between 1987 and 1990 virtually every agency of the United Nations issued resolutions or undertook some activity intended to limit the impact of HIV/AIDS on individuals and society. Several agencies adopted explicit nondiscrimination policies with respect to HIV/AIDS within their areas of work.* Since that time, the UN bodies responsible for human rights have continued to varying degrees to concern themselves with HIV/AIDS–related issues. For example, the UN Commission on the Status of Women declared the effect of HIV/AIDS on the advancement of women a priority theme for 1993–1997.[6] In March 1993 the UN Commission on Human Rights called on all states to ensure the full enjoyment of civil, political, economic, social, and cultural rights, not only for people with HIV/AIDS but also for their families and anyone associated with them or presumed to be at risk of infection, with particular attention to be given to vulnerable groups.[7] The treaty-monitoring body for the International Covenant on Economic, Social and Cultural Rights continues to include AIDS-related questions in its communications with governments.

Since the late 1980s, both the UN Commission on Human Rights (Commission) and the Sub-Commission on the Prevention of Discrimination and Protection of Minorities (Sub-Commission) have demonstrated a particular interest in AIDS-related human rights violations. Prompted by widespread reports of discrimination against people with HIV/AIDS, both bodies strongly urged governments to offer adequate legal protection to affected persons. In 1989 the Sub-Commission suggested the appointment of a Special Rapporteur to investigate discrimination in the context of HIV/AIDS, a proposal endorsed by the Commission at its next meeting.[8] This ensured that HIV/AIDS and human rights was on the agenda at each subsequent meeting of the Sub-Commission and the Commission, until the Special Rapporteur had submitted the final report. The 1990 preliminary report exten-

*For example, ILO, UNHCR, UNICEF, and UN Population fund.

sively discussed AIDS control measures that affect the enjoyment and exercise of human rights, including personal liberty and freedom of movement.[9] The 1991 progress report analyzed discrimination associated with the AIDS epidemic and raised some of the conceptual and legal issues that relate to discrimination.[10] The 1992 final report highlighted the need to tackle the underlying causes leading to discrimination in the context of AIDS.[11] The 1993 conclusions and recommendations urged states to take all necessary steps to eliminate AIDS-related discrimination, particularly against such groups as women and children.[12] These reports were all quite general and did not address specific HIV/AIDS–related human rights violations.

Although it is still not clear the degree to which work of the UN will focus on AIDS-related human rights issues, some action may result from the resolutions passed at the 1994 and 1995 sessions of the Commission on Human Rights.[13] The 1994 resolution asks that the UN Secretary General prepare a report on international and domestic measures taken to protect human rights and prevent discrimination in the context of AIDS, and it urges working groups, special rapporteurs, treaty-monitoring bodies, and others to consider AIDS-related human rights issues in their work. The 1995 resolution focuses on the need for the elaboration of guidelines concerning promoting and protecting respect for human rights in the context of HIV/AIDS. It further notes the need to consider appropriate methods by which to keep under continuous review the protection of human rights in the context of HIV/AIDS.

The importance of these resolutions will be determined by the degree to which they prompt reporting and monitoring by both intergovernmental bodies and NGOs of AIDS-specific human rights violations. Some initiatives have also been taken by regional intergovernmental organizations around the world. In 1989 the Parliamentary Assembly of the Council of Europe "instruct[ed] the Steering Committee for Human Rights to give priority to reinforcing the non-discrimination clause in Article 14 of the European Convention of Human Rights, either by adding health to the prohibited grounds of discrimination or by drawing up a general clause on equality of treatment before the law."[14] In seeking to implement this recommendation, the Steering Committee for Human Rights asked the Swiss Institute of Comparative Law to conduct a European study of AIDS-related discrimination. In May 1993, the Swiss Institute submitted a report outlining the main areas in which people with HIV/AIDS experience discrimination in various European countries. The report not only contains a wealth of information concerning discriminatory laws and practices, but also examines the scope and limitations of existing anti-discrimination legislation.[15] This report has been forwarded to the Steering Committee for Public Health for its opinion and for an indication of further steps to explore.

A selected chronology of international and regional documents on the human rights aspects of HIV/AIDS, 1990–1995, is provided in Box 31-1.

BOX 31·1

Updated chronology of selected international and regional documents on the human rights aspects of HIV/AIDS, 1990–1995*

1990: Preliminary Report on Discrimination Against HIV-Infected People and People with AIDS, from the Special Rapporteur of the Sub-Commission on the Prevention of Discrimination and Protection of Minorities, E/CN.4/Sub.2/1990/9.

1991: Progress Report on Discrimination Against HIV-Infected People and People with AIDS, from the Special Rapporteur of the Sub-Commission on the Prevention of Discrimination and Protection of Minorities, E/CN.4/Sub.2/1991/10.

1992: Rights and Humanity Declaration and Charter on HIV and AIDS, submitted by the Gambian government to the Commission on Human Rights at its 48th session, E/CN.4/1992/82.

1992: Declaration on the AIDS Epidemic in Africa, Organization of African Unity, Dakar, 1992.

1992: Final Report on Discrimination Against HIV-Infected People and People with AIDS, from the Special Rapporteur of the Sub-Commission on the Prevention of Discrimination and Protection of Minorities, E/CN.4/Sub.2/1992/10.

1993: Conclusions and Recommendations from the Special Rapporteur on Discrimination Against HIV-Infected People or People with AIDS, Sub-Commission on the Prevention of Discrimination and Protection of Minorities, E/CN.4/Sub.2/1993/9.

1993: Decision on The Protection of Human Rights in the Context of HIV or AIDS, United Nations Commission on Human Rights, E/CN.4/1993/L.74.

1993: Discrimination in the Context of HIV or AIDS, United Nations Sub-Commission on the Prevention of Discrimination and Protection of Minorities, E/CN.4/Sub.2/1993/L.11/Add.2.

1993: United Nations, World Conference on Human Rights, The Vienna Declaration and Programme of Action, Vienna, 1993, U.N. Doc. A/Conf.157/24 (1993).

1993: Swiss Institute of Comparative Law, Comparative Study on Discrimination Against Persons with HIV or AIDS, Council of Europe, Strasbourg, 1993, Doc. H (93) 3.

1994: The Protection of Human Rights in the Context of HIV and AIDS, United Nations Commission on Human Rights, E/CN.4/1994/L.60.

1994: Resolution passed at the Ninth Plenary Session of 10 June 1994, included in Annual Report of the Inter-American Commission on Human Rights and Special Report on the Human Rights Situation.

1994: Tunis Declaration on AIDS and the Child in Africa, Organization of African Unity, Tunis, Tunisia, 13–15 June 1994, AHG/Dec. 1.

1994: United Nations, Report of the International Conference on Population and Development and Various Recommendations of the World Health Organization, Cairo, 1994, U.N. Doc. A/Conf.171/13 (1994).

1994: Declaration of the Paris AIDS Summit of Heads of Government or Representatives, Paris, 1994.

1995: United Nations, Report of the World Summit for Social Development, Copenhagen, 1995, U.N. Doc. A/Conf.166/9 (1995).

1995: The Protection of Human Rights in the Context of HIV and AIDS, United Nations Commission on Human Rights, ECN.4/1995/44.

1995: Beijing Declaration and Platform for Action, Fourth World Conference on Women, Beijing, China, 15 October 1995, U.N. Doc. A/CONF. 177/20.

*For a chronology of international and regional documents on the human rights aspects of HIV/AIDS, see *AIDS in the World* (1992), Chapter 13.

Responses to human rights violations

In countries around the world, the number of individual and group complaints of human rights violations in the context of HIV/AIDS is steadily increasing. In some places, government-initiated investigations of the rights of people with HIV/AIDS has actually stimulated the complaints. Yet individual complaints and investigations of human rights violations concerning HIV/AIDS–related issues have seldom occurred at the international level. In this respect, it is important to recall that individual complaints only reach intergovernmental bodies as a last resort. In most cases, these bodies are authorized to consider complaints only after the exhaustion of all domestic remedies; that is, barring exceptional circumstances, the highest judicial body in the country must review a complaint before an international body will consider it.

However, HIV/AIDS issues have been relevant to several cases brought before international human rights bodies. In April 1994, for example, the UN Human Rights Committee, the treaty-monitoring body for the International Covenant on Civil and Political Rights (ICCPR), ruled on a related issue when it stated that the sodomy law of the Australian state of Tasmania violated the right to privacy under international human rights standards.[16] The Committee rejected the argument of the government of Tasmania that its laws were partly motivated by a concern to protect Tasmania from the spread of HIV/AIDS as well as being necessary to protect public health and morality. The Committee noted that the criminalization of homosexual practices can neither be considered a "reasonable means nor a proportionate measure" to achieve the aim of preventing the spread of HIV. It noted the observation of the Australian government that statutes which criminalize homosexual acts tend to impede public health programs "by driving underground many of the people at risk of infection" and stated that "criminalization of homosexual activity would thus appear to run counter to the implementation of effective education programmes in respect of HIV prevention."[17] The Committee went on to note the lack of any apparent link between the continued criminalization of homosexual acts and the effective control of HIV/AIDS.

Various cases brought before the European Commission and Court of Human Rights have also made reference (usually indirect) to HIV/AIDS. For example, in March 1992 the European Court of Human Rights ruled in a case concerning financial compensation to a person, meanwhile deceased, with hemophilia. The Court held that the person, who had been infected with HIV through blood transfusions in a French public hospital, was entitled to compensation on account of the excessive length of the proceeding, both before the administrative authorities and the Paris Administrative Court.[18]

When balancing conflicting interests, the European Court and Commission—in line with WHO guidelines—appear to attach great value to human rights. In the *Norris* case, for example, the Court dismissed a claim made by the Irish government that the laws criminalizing homosexual acts were necessary to protect, as the Irish Supreme Court had phrased it, "the spread of all forms of venereal disease." According to the European Court, this and other reasons were insufficient justification to interfere with a person's right to a private life, which includes the right to develop a sexual life.[19]

Actions within the intergovernmental system

In the context of HIV/AIDS, striking differences exist between the statements and the actual practices of various United Nations bodies and other intergovernmental agencies. While resolutions and declarations on non-discrimination and the promotion of human rights in the context of HIV/AIDS remain a constant of human rights bodies, UN recruitment, personnel, and organizational practices are frequently contradictory. The Director of the Joint UN Medical Services has drawn attention to the conflict between official UN policy which does not permit refusal of recruitment solely on the basis of HIV infection and other personnel rules and regulations.[20] For example, some UN agencies practice mandatory HIV testing for personnel, and current medical standards allow for the refusal of recruitment because of other medical conditions, some of which are comparable to HIV infection. In addition, as a general rule, military or police who are HIV infected are not deployed to peacekeeping mission areas, and those persons diagnosed as having AIDS while on mission are repatriated.[21] An internal UN study is under way to develop a uniform policy.

Similar problems have been reported in the European Union. Candidates for employment in Community institutions were systematically tested for HIV until 1988.[22] Under public and political pressure, the Community's medical service eventually stopped this practice.[23] However, candidate employees are currently *requested* to undergo an HIV test. Those who refuse will—without their knowledge and without their informed consent—be subjected to a T4/T8-cell count, a test to assess the impact of HIV infection on a person's immune system.[24] In 1989 a case was brought before the European Court of First Instance by a candidate employee, X, who was denied a job after the Community's medical officers had—in spite of the candidate's explicit refusal to undergo an HIV test—performed a T4/T8-cell count. In 1992 the Court decided that a T4/T8-cell count was fundamentally different from a test for HIV antibodies and disregarded the fact that X had not consented to the test.[25] X immediately appealed to the European Court of Justice.[26] On October 5, 1994, the Court of Justice annulled the judgment of the Court of First Instance. The Court held that it is illegal to subject candidate employees to a disguised HIV test without their knowledge and will, since obtaining a job applicant's informed consent is an absolute requirement for the lawful carrying-out of a preemployment medical examination.[27]

Current issues

Human rights questions continue to be a major part of the global HIV/AIDS debate. A number of controversies have emerged in the 1990s, each with an important human rights component. To illustrate the complexity of some of these issues, several are briefly reviewed.

HIV testing

The mandatory testing of individuals continues to raise human rights concerns. After numerous resolutions and analyses discouraged the implementation of mandatory testing programs, calls for obligatory testing are once again gaining support. For example, some claim that mandatory HIV testing of persons obligatorily tested for multidrug resistant tuberculosis (TB) is a legitimate measure to control the spread of disease, since undetected HIV infection may obscure the results of a TB test. Mandatory HIV and/or TB testing is being imposed particularly on confined populations, such as prisoners and persons in refugee camps. Persons in closed institutions are often thought to be at increased risk for both HIV and TB infection as a result of crowding and poor sanitary conditions. Testing, even without consent, is therefore proposed to be in the interest of the individual, as well as of the institutional population.

HIV/AIDS and the rights of migrants

Debate is also building over the rights of non-nationals in the context of HIV/AIDS. The health care systems in many countries are increasingly unable to care for the needs of people with HIV/AIDS. In these settings, the needs of foreigners with HIV/AIDS may be considered a low priority.[28] Xenophobic groups publicize reports of the few people with HIV/AIDS who have sought refuge in countries with more advanced health care systems and use these reports to demand stricter entrance and resident criteria for foreigners. This has led to catastrophic consequences for some migrants. A growing number of countries test refugees and asylum seekers for HIV/AIDS and then deny them status if they are HIV infected, even if they have entirely legitimate reasons for seeking refugee status or asylum. Also, some countries test various categories of foreigners (including workers and students), and if found to be HIV infected, require them to prove that they were unaware of their HIV status when entering the country. In addition, these foreigners may face denial of benefits, such as free or subsidized health care, and most commonly, deportation.

Human rights aspects of national responses to AIDS: national laws, policies, and practices

The magnitude of the HIV/AIDS epidemic requires governments to design comprehensive policies to minimize the impact of HIV/AIDS on individuals and society as a whole. Governments derive the authority to introduce policy measures by law ("the rule of law"). Whereas some laws relevant to the epidemic are quite old, the bulk of AIDS legislation has been enacted in response to the epidemic itself. Some AIDS laws specifically deal with HIV/AIDS–related issues, while others seek to complement existing, more general laws.

There are notable differences in the types of laws enacted and applied in the context of HIV/AIDS. Governments in many countries have outlawed certain forms of behavior and/or enforced compulsory control measures in efforts to prevent further spread of HIV infection. Examples of these practices include the mandatory testing of certain groups of people, including immigrants, foreign students, applicants for residence and/or work permits, and sex workers, as well as restrictions on certain rights, such as the right to marry. In other countries, legislation has been used primarily as a tool to emphasize individual responsibility.

An increasing number of laws, either explicitly or through judicial interpretation, prohibit HIV/AIDS–related discrimination. Provisions that prohibit discrimination against individuals on the basis of health, health status, or disability typically complement information and education programs carried out in these countries. Many of these laws, like the Americans with Disabilities Act of 1990, offer protection against discrimination in the context of employment, education, and housing. Under some of these laws, including the Australian Human Rights and Equal Opportunity Act of 1986 (revised), special mechanisms deal with allegations of human rights violations, including those that are HIV/AIDS-specific.

There has been—and sometimes continues to be—an intense debate about the measures most useful to responding to the AIDS epidemic. Tensions inevitably arise between those who emphasize protection of the public health in the traditional sense—and thus the restriction of rights of certain individuals considered dangerous—and those who advocate a minimum amount of interference with the lives of individuals. Policymakers often have to reconcile these conflicting concerns. Although the importance of full recognition of human rights as an integral part of HIV/AIDS policies and programs is increasingly acknowledged, numerous actions by governments reinforce existing patterns of discrimination and clearly violate human rights norms.

In practical terms, how can a policy be evaluated to determine if it complies with human rights standards? An initial assessment of a state's human rights obligations can be made by ascertaining which human rights treaties it has ratified. Treaties contain a number of provisions ("articles" or "sections") that define the rights that the ratifying states have committed to uphold. These rights are often phrased in general terms, leaving room for interpretation. In order to better understand the documents, a review of the genesis of various provisions, notably by studying the so-called *travaux preparatoires*, may help. In addition, learning the views of the official body established to monitor the particular international or regional human rights treaty under consideration may be useful.

Survey of national laws and practices

A review of legislation pertaining to HIV/AIDS conducted in 1992 by the Global AIDS Policy Coalition was summarized in the first volume of *AIDS in the World*. In 1993–94, managers of governmental national AIDS programs (GNAP) were requested to provide information on both laws and practices in the context of HIV/AIDS in their country. A survey questionnaire was sent to 187 GNAP managers; 116 responses were received, of which 115 had completed, either partially or fully, the section pertaining to laws and practice (Appendix E).

The survey found that involuntary testing remains part of many AIDS prevention and control programs. Governments continue to categorize individuals into "high-risk" groups in order to impose testing and to restrict their activities. The responses also dramatically highlight the differences that exist between law and practice in some countries. According to GNAP managers, policies that interfere with human rights are often being carried out without legal justification.

The survey of national legislation and practices as well as discussion with ASOs and human rights NGOs confirms two major conclusions. First, discrimination towards HIV-infected people, people with AIDS, and people considered within each society at high risk for HIV infection is an important and enduring problem. Second, bringing community, national, and even international organizations into conformity with the international consensus on nondiscriminatory approaches to HIV/AIDS prevention and control will require vigilance and enormous continuing effort. To achieve an optimal balance between public health objectives and human rights norms, public health policies and programs will benefit from the application of an analytical human rights framework (Box 31-2).

BOX 31-2

Assessing the human rights impact

SOFIA GRUSKIN

In order to assist policymakers, the Global AIDS Policy Coalition and the International Federation of Red Cross and Red Crescent Societies created an international working group to help assess the human rights impact of HIV/AIDS policies, programs, and practices.*

In mid-1995, the International Federation of Red Cross and Red Crescent Societies and the François-Xavier Bagnoud Center for Health and Human Rights (Harvard University) published a comprehensive manual on HIV/AIDS and human rights.[1] The manual, entitled "AIDS, Health, and Human Rights" includes a complete explanation of a methodology for balancing public health objectives and human rights norms, including illustrative examples involving both prevention and care.†

The intent of the public health/human rights impact assessment instrument is to ensure that conflicts are negotiated rationally, since—and this is the underlying assumption—public health and human rights are inextricably linked and largely share the same goal of promoting human well-being.

A schematic diagram in the form of a 2 × 2 table is presented in Figure 31-2.1. On one side of the diagram is "public health quality," on the other, "human rights quality." Each side represents a spectrum from "positive," meaning high quality public health or high respect for human rights and dignity, to "negative," meaning low public health quality and low respect for human rights and dignity. The goal is to ensure that any proposed policy or program reaches Box *A*, which means high quality public health plus high quality human rights. Briefly, the process involves four steps:

*The Working Group also included representatives from the Danish Centre for Human Rights, the McGill Centre for Medicine, Ethics and Law, the International Commission of Jurists, and the Society of Women Against AIDS in Africa.

†Copies of the manual may be ordered from the International Federation of Red Cross and Red Crescent Societies, Geneva, Switzerland, or from the François-Xavier Bagnoud Center for Health and Human Rights, Harvard School of Public Health, 8 Story Street, Cambridge, MA 02138, USA.

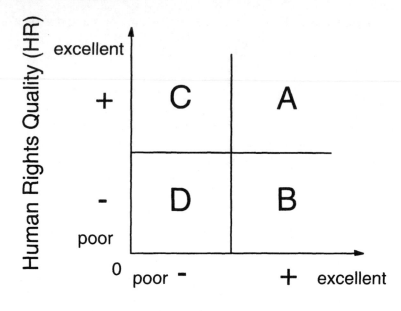

Public Health Quality (PH)

Figure 31-2.1   Assessment of interaction between public health and human rights quality. The four-setp approach is based on the Public Health/Human Rights Impact Assessment Instrument, developed at *AIDS, Health and Human Rights*, an explanatory manual, International Federation of Red Cross and Red Crescent Societies, and François-Xavier Bagnoud Center for Health and Human Rights, Harvard School of Public Health, 1994, Geneva, Switzerland and Boston, MA, 1994, p. 42.

1. Does the policy or program represent *good public health?* Locate the proposed policy or program along the horizontal axis from poor to excellent. The emphasis at this stage is entirely on the health benefits, risks, and harms, not on the human rights impact.
2. Is the proposed policy or program respectful and protective of human rights? In answering the question, the potential *benefits and burdens on human rights* which will occur as a result of the policy or program are described. The emphasis is entirely on the human rights component. Locate the proposed policy or program along the vertical axis from poor to excellent.
   Determine in which quadrant of Figure 31-2.1 the proposed policy or program is located (A, B, C, or D).
3. Next, how can the policy or program best move into quadrant *A*, thereby achieving the optimal *balance between protection of the public health and the protection and promotion of human rights and dignity.* The goal is to minimize to the greatest extent possible the burdens on human rights resulting from the policy as well as having the best policy.
   Specific steps are outlined to ensure a systematic approach to this complex negotiation process.
4. Review the basic approach. For completing this assessment, alternative approaches may have emerged that will be both more respectful of human rights and more effective in achieving public health goals.

References

1. François-Xavier Bagnoud Center for Health and Human Rights and the International Federation of the Red Cross, *AIDS, Health and Human Rights* (Cambridge, MA and Geneva: Harvard School of Public Health), 1995:42–43.

REFERENCES

1. UN Commission on Human Rights, *Non-Discrimination in the Field of Health*, preamble, Resolution 1989/11 (March 2, 1989).
2. Cf. P. Sieghart, *AIDS & Human Rights—A UK Perspective* (London: British Medical Association Foundation For AIDS, 1989):12.
3. K. Tomasevski, "AIDS pandemic and human rights," in *Collected Courses of the Academy of European Law*, Vol. II, Book 2, Academy of European Law, ed. (Boston: Kluwer Academic Publications, 1993):107.
4. Global AIDS Policy Coalition, *Towards A New Health Strategy for AIDS: A Report of the Global AIDS Policy Coalition* (Boston: GAPC, 1993).
5. J. Mann, D. Tarantola, and T. Netter, eds. *AIDS in the World* (Cambridge, MA: Harvard University Press, 1992):564–566 for overview.
6. UN Commission on the Status of Women, *Resolution of the Commission on the Status of Women*, adopted at the 34th Session of the Commission on the Status of Women (March 1990).
7. UN Commission on Human Rights, Resolution 1993/53 (March 9, 1993).
8. UN Commission on Human Rights, Resolution 1990/65 (March 7, 1990).
9. UN Commission on Human Rights, Sub-Commission on Prevention of Discrimination and Protection of Minorities, *Discrimination Against HIV-Infected People or People with AIDS*, UN Doc. E/CN.4/Sub.2/1990/9 (August 2, 1990).
10. UN Commission on Human Rights, Sub-Commission on Prevention of Discrimination and Protection of Minorities, *Discrimination Against HIV-Infected People or People with AIDS*, UN Doc. E/CN.4/Sub.2/1991/10 (July 24, 1991).
11. UN Commission on Human Rights, Sub-Commission on Prevention of Discrimination and Protection of Minorities, *Discrimination Against HIV-Infected People or People with AIDS*, UN Doc. E/CN.4/Sub.2/1992/10 (July 28, 1992).
12. UN Sub-Commission on Prevention of Discrimination and Protection of Minorities, *Discrimination Against HIV-Infected People or People with AIDS*, UN Doc. E/CN.4/Sub.2/1993/9 (August 23, 1993).
13. UN Commission on Human Rights, *Protection of Human Rights in the Context of HIV and AIDS*, UN Doc. E/CN.4/1994/L.60 (March 1, 1994).
14. Parliamentary Assembly of the Council of Europe, Recommendation 1116 on AIDS and human rights (September 29, 1989):para. 8A.
15. Swiss Institute of Comparative Law, *Comparative Study on Discrimination against Persons with HIV or AIDS* (Strasbourg, France: Steering Committee for Human Rights, Council of Europe, 1993).
16. Cf. UN Human Rights Committee, *Fiftieth Session Communication* No. 488/1992, CCPR/C/50/D/488/1992 (April 4, 1994).
17. *Ibid.*
18. Cf. European Court of Human Rights decision, *X v. France*, 81/1991/333/406 (March 31, 1992).
19. European Court of Human Rights decision, *Norris v. Ireland*, 6/1987/129/180 (October 28, 1988).
20. Inger-Agency Advisory Group on AIDS, *UN Personnel and Operational Policies Dealing with the Impact of HIV/AIDS* (October 28, 1993).
21. UN, *UN Medical Service Guidelines for Contributing States on Medical Preparation of Military and Police Personnel for Service with UN Peacekeeping Missions*, annex to UN Medical Standards.
22. H. Schröder, "Pratiques de dépistage du SIDA aux Communautés européennes," *Revue Belge de Droit International* 1(1990):171–189.

23. Cf. Cardoso e Cunha, response to written question 2322/90, *Official Journal of the European Communities* C90(1991):47–48.

24. A. Hendriks and S. Gevers, "(Pre-)employment medical examinations and the law, with particular reference to the European Union," *European Journal of Health Law* 1(1994):229–264.

25. Court of First Instance decision, *X v. Commission*, Case 94/92, *NJCM-Bulletin* 18(1993):36–45, annotated by A. Hendriks.

26. Court of First Instance decision, *X v. Commission*, Case 94/92, *Official Journal of the European Communities* C333(1992):17–18.

27. Court of Justice decision, *X v. Commission*, Case 404/92 (October 5, 1995); para. 20.

28. R. Rector, ed. *Migration, Health and AIDS, Phase I, Final Report to the Commission of the European Communities* (Copenhagen: HIV Denmark, 1994).

32

Nongovernmental Organizations

JEFFREY O'MALLEY, VINH KIM NGUYEN, AND SARAH LEE

To slow the spread of HIV, people need to change their most personal and private behaviors. Likewise, the most important aspect of care for people with HIV/AIDS is at an interpersonal level—ensuring self-respect, freedom from discrimination, and love and support. Thus, the heart of HIV/AIDS prevention and care is at the community level, where people help people, often through groups—typically known as CBOs (community-based organizations).

In addition to CBOs that are formed within (and are accountable to) particular communities, many other groups outside government are involved in responding to HIV/AIDS. Collectively, such groups are referred to as NGOs (nongovernmental organizations).

The first edition of *AIDS in the World* described the emergence of new community organizations in response to AIDS and outlined some of the issues faced by specialized AIDS groups as the epidemic spread and diversified.[1] How have the challenges changed in recent years? Are AIDS groups still serving the same functions as in the past? What is the role of other groups outside government in responding to AIDS? And how do NGOs decide on priorities as governmental commitments continue to decline and the epidemic expands and intensifies worldwide.

The range of NGOs responding to AIDS

In every nation, the impact of AIDS was first felt by a small number of people. At the beginning of the epidemic, first actions against AIDS were invariably organized locally by some of the people affected by the disease. While many governments ignored HIV/AIDS and health care systems reacted with fear and prejudice, people with AIDS, their loved ones, and their families often organized into groups that became known as "AIDS Service Organizations"—delivering care and support and offering prevention programs.

Groups formed by these early activists have become world famous, from TASO (The AIDS Support Organization) in Kampala, Uganda, to the Gay

Men's Health Crisis in New York City. Often AIDS service organizations (ASOs) evolved in response to growing demands and changing needs; for example, TASO has grown from a small group focused on service to families coping with HIV/AIDS in Kampala, to a national network with branches across Uganda. In Manila, "Reach Out" started by teaching about HIV prevention to mainly middle-class gay men, but it now operates a wide range of educational programs, including special services for women sex workers and for young people.

As the epidemic continued in initially affected communities, and spread to new cities and countries, established organizations working on different issues soon decided to do something about AIDS. For example, ENDA Tiers Monde, a large NGO working on community development and environmental issues in Senegal, started providing AIDS service activities in the late 1980s, as well as AIDS training to a range of small groups and community activists across the country. In 1987, the U.S. government launched what was to become the largest donor-driven AIDS program in the world, channeling a significant part of its foreign aid related to HIV/AIDS through nongovernmental subcontractors, which had more flexibility than national governments in starting new programs and in dealing with governmental and political restrictions. There are now examples of NGO involvement in AIDS in almost every sector and country (indeed, some have sought to secure their own funding base or legitimacy through AIDS activities), including "development" NGOs like Oxfam, human rights groups like the International Gay and Lesbian Human Rights Commission, and the Society for Women and AIDS in Africa (Box 32-1) women's groups such as Advocacy for Women's Health, and even trade union federations and farmers' networks.

BOX 32-1

Society for women and AIDS in Africa

EKA ESU-WILLIAMS

The Society for Women and AIDS in Africa (SWAA), a pan-African NGO led by women, works to empower women to address the causes and consequences of the HIV/AIDS epidemic on women in Africa. The birth of SWAA in 1988 resulted from the realizations that (a) women are critically affected by HIV/AIDS, (b) that they have limited access to information and education, (c) programs promoting their good health, social, and economic advancement are in short supply, and (d) because they face several constraints, a forum is needed both to enhance a large-scale mobilization of women for action against HIV/AIDS and to provide the voice to raise women's concerns about the epidemic and their lives in general.

From an initial nucleus of a handful of women in 1988, SWAA members now number several hundred in 30 African countries. Since 1990 it has grown from an NGO whose initial engagement was in providing education, information, and general awareness to one advocating for the development of policies to ensure that women and AIDS become an important program focus of national HIV/AIDS control programs. The rights of women at risk of or infected by HIV/AIDS and the advancement of strategies for the empowerment of women, especially young girls, toward reducing their vulnerability to HIV/AIDS have also been a major component of SWAA's advocacy work.

SWAA is working hard to extend its activities to areas it has not reached, such as northern Africa, and to consolidate activities in countries where new branches have only recently been established. Internationally, SWAA is extending its collaboration for the purpose of exchanging experiences with other women's groups, and influencing global and regional agendas in the area of women and AIDS. This networking allows for increased opportunities for SWAA branches and members to acquire new skills and information that will assist them in pursuing SWAA's objectives more effectively.

There have been many constraints. The voluntary nature of SWAA's operations has hampered timely and extensive input by members. Difficulties in communication within Africa have caused inadequate exchange among countries. As experienced by many other women's organizations, we face difficulties in accessing support, influencing policy-makers, and gaining acceptance for our mission from official structures. Because we have to discuss issues that are mainly within the domain and control of men, or that may invoke a feeling of threat among men, finding support from men is often difficult. Given these barriers, it is taking more time than we would like to break through to communities at the grassroots level, where the greatest impact needs to be made. To increase its outreach to the grassroots, SWAA is encouraging other women's groups to include HIV/AIDS concerns as a major activity focus. In this way, we hope to expand both our scope and our targets, preparing women and communities to deal with the escalating problems resulting from HIV/AIDS.

SWAA's approach to community participation also relates to its concern about the prevailing high degree of stigma and discrimination people with HIV/AIDS encounter. We hope that this community-based approach will support other initiatives in creating an atmosphere where women, men, and family members, whether infected or not, can be empowered to cope with or prevent HIV/AIDS. Such an approach can also assist the acceptance and support of children orphaned by AIDS, many of whom suffer abuse and neglect.

A key challenge facing SWAA and the AIDS prevention initiatives in Africa is that of enlisting the full participation of men and ensuring that they take on their responsibilities with respect to HIV/AIDS. Connected with this is the emerging picture of HIV/AIDS as a disease that affects the family, a social unit in which men play a dominant role. Responsibility for safe sex, sexual communication between partners, and ways of ensuring that the appropriate messages are communicated to children are areas in which men can play a significant role.

Overall, SWAA wishes to project its vision that, tragic as the consequences of the HIV/AIDS epidemic are for women in Africa, it has created the opportunity to address more appropriately the broader issues of women's subordination, gender inequity, and the neglect of the rights of women. HIV/AIDS programs that are more reflective of women's needs should be developed—providing long-term economic viability for women, mobilizing women for economic and social advancement, and supporting overall health concerns of women.

Typically, as NGOs spend a longer time involved in AIDS work, they diversify, grow, and become more professional in planning and evaluating their services. In their wake, new voluntary groups emerge with highly specialized or localized missions. Many countries thus benefit from a wide range of diverse and complementary organizations working on AIDS—from small groups catering to a very specific community, to comprehensive national service providers. Each voluntary organization working on AIDS has limitations as well as strengths, but the private sector as a whole is typically much more able than the government to reach and help vulnerable people avoid infection or cope with their illness.

The ubiquity and diversity of groups working on AIDS have led many authors to propose typologies of NGOs.[2-4] However, no single listing or typology can adequately illustrate the variety of organizational origins, members, goals, and functions.

Several relevant questions may help differentiate among organizations and the work they do: Does the group provide direct services or does it act as an intermediary between different institutions or organizations? Is the group essentially a self-help group or is it motivated by concern for others? Is the group functionally accountable primarily to its donors or funders, its members, or its intended beneficiaries? Is it primarily an HIV/AIDS group, or if not, are its HIV/AIDS activities distinct (and measurable), or are they included within activities aimed at broader health or development issues?

The term "HIV/AIDS services" is used here in the broadest sense, embracing all prevention and care activities from handing out condoms or providing "buddies" to the ill, to fighting for women's inheritance rights or challenging homophobia. The concept of "HIV/AIDS services" does not include activities intended to have an impact on the epidemic only through the mediation of another institution, such as training of trainers, provision of funds and technical support to other groups, policy analysis without advocacy for change, and similar intermediary functions carried out by many NGOs.

NGO roles and achievements

One of the greatest strengths of NGOs responding to HIV/AIDS is their roots within communities. Responses based on the assessed needs, priorities, and dynamics of local people are not only more likely to have an impact on a local epidemic, but will also help to ensure "ownership," unity, and sustainability in community efforts. Appropriate, sensitive approaches have proven to be effective and can have a multiplying effect. By carrying out effective and positive care programs, for example, NGOs play a key role in breaking down local barriers to fighting AIDS (whether based on fear, ignorance, or stigmatization) while at the same time promoting prevention strategies.

The most effective NGO responses are embedded in a local context, and thus reflect and are sensitive to the actual norms of a community, rather than what outsiders (individuals or organizations) perceive to be the norms. NGOs can help to make HIV/AIDS care and support part of everyday life, demonstrating that everyone has a role to play as both an individual and a member of the community.

Most of the NGOs now involved in AIDS work are not AIDS-specific organizations, but are oriented to broader health or development goals. Many religious organizations, women's groups, farmers' unions, or youth organizations have been working within their communities for years and know a great deal about mobilizing and supporting vulnerable people, especially the poor. Just as importantly, many such NGOs are likely to stay involved in their communities for a long time and will help provide a sustainable response to challenges such as HIV/AIDS. When these groups become capable of working on HIV/AIDS alongside their other activities, HIV/AIDS services reach a wider range of people for a longer period of time.

Cavite City, the Philippines provides a typical example of how community groups contribute to the fight against AIDS. KASAKA (Kalipunan Ng Mga Samahan sa Kabite), recently incorporated HIV/AIDS into their work among local farmers, after recognizing that many families in their community had tensions linked to post-harvest visits to brothels by men. KASAKA began with a participatory research project, which led to the development of HIV/AIDS information materials in the local language. They have now been asked to assist in the local health authority's HIV/AIDS training for health professionals. As the Chair of the KASAKA Health Committee, says: "We never thought that we who are just farmers would be asked to talk to doctors, nurses and other health experts about HIV/AIDS."

Most NGOs describe themselves as "community-based." In reality, however, many are based neither in geographic communities (like neighborhoods or villages) nor in identity communities (such as sex workers or migrant laborers). Many NGOs—even those dealing with specific communities on a daily basis—are both physically and philosophically "outsiders," much in the same way as governments tend to be. In reality, many NGOs carry on outreach work to community groups, and supposed beneficiaries may never have heard of an organization that claims to be working on their behalf. These NGOs may be medium-sized or even large-scale organizations with complex infrastructures, often with several branches or departments. Other NGOs are not directly involved in HIV/AIDS service, but have intermediary functions, such as passing on information, technical support, grants, or networking opportunities. NGOs not based in specific communities are more likely to be involved in programs that are larger scale and address broader sections or issues of society, to have paid professional staff, and to adopt approaches that are "for" rather than "with" and "by" communities. Despite rhetoric to the contrary, such larger NGOs are usually more accountable to their donors than to their beneficiaries. Their staff and governors are more likely motivated by concern for others than self-help.

Larger NGOs and intermediary groups tend to have different, often contrasting strengths and weaknesses. Such groups tend to be technically stronger, have more effective access to decision makers, and despite higher costs, can often be very cost-efficient because of the scale of their operations. Very few small community groups can distribute condoms as effectively and efficiently as a large social marketing NGO linked to an international network, but very few such large groups can actually convince a young man to use condoms if he has not tried them before.

Organizations that are based within (and known by) a specific community can typically boast of being flexible, working with volunteers, keeping potential beneficiaries in control, keeping costs down, being willing and able to work with the poor and marginal groups, innovating and advocating more effective approaches, building skills within vulnerable groups rather than relying always on outsiders, and being accountable to local people. In addition, such community-based NGOs are often the only institutions that are able to work closely with controversial groups in need of support, like sex workers, drug users, and illegal migrants—filling gaps left by governments due to political sensitivity or lack of contacts or expertise.

Nevertheless, public policy affecting NGOs, and public rhetoric, rarely differentiate between these different kinds of institutions. Few governments that fund NGOs really debate and decide whether they wish to fund community groups directly, and whether they are capable of doing so. Even fewer ask themselves the purpose of "NGO representation" on national AIDS committees and similar bodies; whether they are seeking the voices of affected or vulnerable communities, or the technical expertise of highly motivated philanthropists. The individual and joint strengths of NGOs combine to make them a dynamic, multidimensional, and potentially powerful force. HIV/AIDS has highlighted, almost more than any other issue, the benefits of drawing on the wealth of experiences and expertise available by investing in developing and strengthening NGOs as a sector. Throughout the world, NGOs have demonstrated that, with appropriate support, they can reinforce one anothers' work, complement the activities of other sectors, and put effective pressure on the state to meet their needs and those of communities.

Needs, capacities, and priorities of service delivery organizations

In 1994 and 1995, the International HIV/AIDS Alliance conducted a series of participatory assessments with local AIDS-service NGOs in twelve developing countries. These assessments were intended to identify their perception of needs, priorities, and capacities in HIV/AIDS prevention, care, and community support. The countries ranged from low to high HIV seroprevalence, and from strong to weak in terms of the organized NGO response to the epidemic. Assessments were conducted in Bangladesh, Burkina Faso, Côte d'Ivoire, Ecuador, Morocco, Mozambique, Pakistan, Peru, the Philippines, Senegal, Sri Lanka, and Tanzania.

Despite the many differences, a number of common priorities were identified: attention and technical support for the promotion of symptom recognition and treatment-seeking for sexually transmitted infections; support to self-organizing and self-help for people with HIV; support to community and neighborhood level groups and interventions; linkages of action research to program development; and availability of subsidized condoms to small NGOs, not just government and large social marketing agencies.

The NGOs surveyed in most of the countries also cited the need for more action on the contextual (societal) factors which increase vulnerability to HIV, such as gender inequality. However, this was frequently cited as an area which would require significant technical cooperation with others, as NGOs found it difficult to identify appropriate program development or intervention strategies.

The most striking difference among countries was the uneven development of the "AIDS specialist" sector, and consequent services to marginal populations. While certain countries, especially those with a legacy of external support from USAID-funded projects (AIDSCOM, AIDSTECH, and AIDSCAP) had well-developed specialist service organizations, relatively few broad-based health or development NGOs had added a specific HIV/AIDS component to their programs. A priority in these countries was reaching larger numbers of people, particularly the poor. For example, in Sri Lanka, Burkina Faso, and Bangladesh, health or development NGOs had taken the lead in responding to AIDS, and they identified a need for more specialist prevention and care services, and particularly, more effective work with marginal populations such as sex workers and men who have sex with men.

By the end of 1995, "linking organizations"—NGO support programs enabling the International HIV/AIDS Alliance to extend managerial and technical support to NGOs through local groups—had been created in six of these twelve countries.[5] An analysis of the priorities established for funding, requests for support received, and resources distributed, provides a unique insight into the strengths and weaknesses of NGOs in these countries, and the potential for a stronger response to HIV/AIDS from the NGO sector. The six NGO support programs were all autonomously responsible for deciding on funding priorities, reviewing applications, and allocating awards of funds and technical support. Of the 220 NGOs that were supported in these countries in 1995, sufficient data exist for 138. Only 8 of the 138 NGOs were AIDS-specific organizations, with the others coming from a wide range of sectors, particularly community development associations (46), youth groups (33), and women's groups (10). Most activities were intended to benefit either youth (50) or those in poverty (24), and almost three times as many focused activities on women in particular (17) then men in particular (6). Only 35 programs focused on broad contextual issues such as human rights or income generation, and only 42 of the prevention programs went beyond general information strategies to address behavior change. While, overall, funding decisions reflected the capacity of local NGOs, and as such resulted in good geographic coverage and access to vulnerable groups, only a minority of activities could be characterized as particularly innovative or likely to have a substantial impact.

Identity activism

In countries where HIV transmission was or is largely identified with "mainstream" sexual practices at the beginning of the epidemic, the development of "AIDS movements" and AIDS specialist NGOs has often been less widespread. In both high and low prevalence countries, from Burkina Faso to Bangladesh, there has rarely been a spontaneous social movement in response to AIDS where transmission had not disproportionately affected a marginal group that already had organizational or political cohesion. In contrast, in the United States, most western European countries, Australia, and Brazil, early AIDS organizing depended greatly upon gay politics and gay organizations and, in countries like the Philippines and Thailand, upon groups that were already working with sex workers.

In sub-Saharan Africa especially, and increasingly in parts of Asia, an NGO response to AIDS has often been built on a different sort of movement—the efforts of women and women's groups to address their own sexual health and sexual rights. The relationship between a response to AIDS and a response to other issues, whether gay rights or gender equality, has often been mutually beneficial. NGOs based in such identity movements or communities have been among the most successful at accessing vulnerable populations, providing education and social norm support to help change behavior, and pointing to the broader changes in social norms, human rights standards, and public policy that are required to sustain prevention and care efforts. In turn, many of these movements and organizations have been significantly strengthened by the attention to their issues catalyzed by AIDS.[6]

Increasingly, however, mutual support and cooperation between social movements and their respective NGOs is breaking down in competition for resources, the desire to "scale up" or replicate activities to the "general population," and genuine philosophical differences.

In many industrialized countries, debate surrounds the "heterosexualizing" or "gaying/re-gaying" of AIDS movements as the profile of local epidemics is purported to change (see Chapter 38). While gay groups fight to retain some resources in countries such as the United Kingdom, where gay men still represent the vast majority of AIDS cases and new HIV infections, debates also rage in developing countries. For instance, Latin American NGOs differ dramatically in their assessment of the relative importance of different HIV transmission routes. These debates are inevitably divisive because of their linkage to both perceptions of life and death as they relate to HIV infection, and to the movements themselves as they struggle for both legitimacy and funding.

As the struggle against HIV/AIDS enters its second decade, AIDS activism is connecting more and more to identity activism. The potential for variety of movements is already apparent—from sex work activism to a new generation of "queer" activism to, perhaps most strikingly, a strong and growing post-Beijing international women's movement. Activists concerned with areas such as human rights, gender and sexual health, base their work within their societal context—enabling them to challenge societal obstacles and discrimination. Although AIDS may be an important common thread among many participants, the central catalyst bringing people together is their social identity. A group of sex workers, for example, may form a movement because they share common concerns about stigmatization, safety on the streets, employment rights, and access to health care—as well as issues relating to HIV/AIDS. However, such groups may not seek common cause with other groups—also strongly affected by HIV/AIDS—yet based on other identities (e.g., gay men).

The greater involvement of people with HIV: principles and problems

One of the most striking social movements in response to AIDS involves the PWA or person with AIDS. In every language, the debate about which words (and acronyms) to use to describe people with either the HIV virus or associated illnesses has been controversial and catalytic. From *personnes at-*

teintes to the ironic "diseased pariah," from PWAs to P+ HIV/AIDS seems to have built on an earlier experience, such as with breast cancer, diabetes, lateral sclerosis, or coronary artery disease, to create identities, movements, and organizations based on a medical diagnosis.

Undoubtedly, some of the most effective specialized AIDS groups are self-help groups of people living with HIV/AIDS (see Box 32-2). These organizations ensure that HIV/AIDS work is not neglected and develop expertise specific to it. They are also usually the most convincing advocates and campaigners, encouraging governments and others to engage in AIDS work more effectively.

BOX 32-2

Women living with HIV/AIDS

WINNIE CHIKAFUMBWA

To be told that you are HIV positive by your doctor is just like receiving a death sentence on a judgment day. I was first told that I was HIV positive when I went to my postnatal clinic in January, 1989. The tests were taken without my consent at one of the Mission Hospitals in mid-1988 when I was attending an ante-natal clinic. At the time they were taking my blood, I did not suspect anything because I thought it was something to do with my pregnancy. They did not tell me the results until after I had the baby, and they tested my baby who was also found positive. There was no pre-counseling or post-counseling for me, the doctor just broke the news during my post-natal check-up. It was very shocking because he just told me that they took my blood and that of my child for an HIV test and the results were found positive, and that the child was not going to live past five years. Indeed my child did not live up to five years, she passed away when she was only four months old.

Although I was shocked, I instantly gathered courage and prayed to God to give me strength and stand by my side during the trying time. It really worked. I didn't break down until after I got home. Later in the evening when my husband came home, I broke the news to him and hell broke lose. I got the worst reaction from him. He walked out of my life that very same evening, calling me all sorts of names and blaming me that I had been unfaithful to him and that I was a prostitute. He left me with four children under my care and went to stay with another woman, and thus infected that other woman too, because I later learned that he had already been tested and found HIV positive but could not gather courage to tell me.

I spent most of my time crying, and the loss of my baby made my condition worse. But still I prayed to God to let me live for the sake of the remaining three children, and indeed God has given me strength because I have a will to live. Apart from my husband, I only told my elder sister about my status, and she advised me not to tell anyone else. People in Malawi, until now, think AIDS is a shameful disease, and anyone diagnosed with HIV is often taken as a promiscuous person. Therefore, I had to close my mouth and take it as my own problem. Up to now people in Malawi are still resisting to change their behavior, and the rate for HIV infection is increasing each day. According to the report from the National AIDS Control Program, the 1995 AIDS Analysis estimates that about 727 people are being infected every day. The cumulative figure will reach an estimated 1.3 million in a country of 10 million people. This is alarming.

In March, 1992, a lady from the Netherlands wrote her friend in Malawi, a woman who is working as a nurse with my sister, informing her that the Dutch HIV-positive women have organized a pre-conference of HIV-positive women from different parts of the world to be held in the Netherlands. When my sister heard about this, she asked me if I was interested in attending the conference. I accepted although I was afraid to talk about my status, and although I have never been involved in any AIDS activities, I accepted because I wanted to meet my "fellow dying people." I was wrong. I learned from these women that some had lived with the virus for 10 years. This gave me hope that I, too, could live longer. I can assure everyone that I am not dying any more.

The international pre-conference was attended by 54 HIV-positive women from different parts of the world. We shared experiences and exchanged information. It is at this conference in Amsterdam that the women decided to establish a recognized organization, which is now known as the International Community of Women Living with HIV/AIDS (ICW) to address the issues that affect women.

The conference gave me self-confidence and the courage to start getting involved in AIDS activities and talk about my status to friends and my whole family, including my own children. This approach also gave me a chance to come across some of the women who were experiencing the same trauma I was. It is this destitute nature of most HIV-positive women in Malawi that made me found The National Association of People with HIV/AIDS in Malawi (NAPHAM).

Because of the active part I have played in the fight against AIDS, my fellow African People living with HIV/AIDS elected me to be one of the key contacts for Africa in the International Community of Women Living with HIV/AIDS.

In Berlin, at the International AIDS Conference in 1993, I was also elected by the African PWAs to be one of their representatives on the Global Network of People with HIV/AIDS (GNP+). Although communication with other PHWAs in Africa is limited, due to lack of funds, I always pass any information through ICW London and the GNP+ London office to pass it over to PWHAs.

Being HIV positive has taught me to be forgiving, patient, loving, and caring. I am happy that my HIV status has taught me to prepare for my children and my own future. It has brought me closer to God. I feel God has kept me for a purpose, which I am now trying to fulfill; the purpose of supporting and empowering HIV/AIDS people in Malawi. It has also kept me on the run. I am no longer ashamed of my status, and my hope is to see that PWAs all over the world do not suffer as I did during my early days of living with HIV. The struggle continues.

Like NGOs in general, it is important to stress that there are many different types of PWA groups. Many start as groups of friends helping one another with peer support, income opportunities, or housing ("self-help groups"). Some self-help organizations evolve into offering AIDS services (prevention, care, policy, or advocacy work) to a wider public in return for grants, donations, or contracts. Other PWA groups bring together like-minded activists to engage in advocacy, monitoring, or providing treatments or treatment information, or human rights work. There are also local, national, and international PWA networks, some of which help smaller PWA organizations share information or collaborate on projects, others of which function as self-help groups where members provide direct support through e-mail and airplane tickets. Finally, many groups are closely identified with people with HIV or their loved ones, but do not actually restrict their membership or staff to people with HIV—TASO in Uganda and ACT-UP chapters around the world are somewhat imprecisely referred to as PWA groups by many commentators.

Supporting organizations of people living with HIV/AIDS seems to make eminent sense in the fight against the epidemic; indeed, a broad consensus has been reached on this issue among activists, health care providers, and funders. Large PWA organizations exist in many countries, and in most Western countries it is reasonable to refer to this as a movement, replete with various factions differing politically and its own panoply of styles of social intervention. The acceptance—perhaps even mainstreaming—of PWA groups is indicated by the representation of such groups on governmental advisory boards and even pharmacological monitoring agencies such as the U.S. FDA (Food and Drug Administration).

This consensus concerning PWAs arose from experiences with the epidemic in the 1980s in North America and Europe and, to a limited extent, in Africa. PWA organizations were in the vanguard, stimulating effective responses from government and other large institutions (such as hospitals and pharmaceuticals firms). While not all groups achieved the notoriety of ACT-UP New York, local groups in major western cities formed a constituency to which these large social actors were to be held accountable.

Over the years, recognition of the role of PWA groups has extended to the international arena. In December 1994, the Paris AIDS Summit, which brought together Heads of Governments and other officials from 42 countries, culminated in the signing of a declaration that included as one of its commitments a greater involvement of people with HIV/AIDS (GIPA), promising to:

> Support a greater involvement of people living with HIV/AIDS through an initiative to strengthen the capacity and coordination of networks of people living with HIV/AIDS and community based organizations. By ensuring their full involvement in our common response to the pandemic at all—national, regional and global—levels, this initiative will, in particular, stimulate the creation of supportive political, legal and social environments.[7]

This text represents a significant public policy victory for PWA activists as well as NGO activists, but its interpretation and implications remain controversial. An informal alliance had evolved for inclusion of the GIPA statement in the Paris summit, and to subsequently ask for alliance groups to receive financing to fulfill government pledges to "the GIPA initiative." While many NGOs, both PWA and others, felt excluded from this lobbying effort, there were also divisions amongst the key protagonists as to whether the initiative includes community-based organizations only as a route to supporting people with AIDS, or whether the initiative is intended to address both networks of people living with HIV/AIDS and, separately, networks of community based organizations. In any case, France was the only major government that pledged funds to the GIPA initiative (although, as of early 1996, France had reduced its 1995 commitment from 100 million FF to 15 million FF, or as characterized by French spokespersons, the government had decided to make pledged funds available over a longer period of time than had initially been anticipated).

Locally, PWA organizations have also had important achievements. As self-help groups, they provide the kind of supportive environments that motivate PWAs to "come out" and get involved in local prevention and care activities. This has contributed immensely not only to the visibility of AIDS but also to an awareness of its impact on people for whom, otherwise, the epidemic would have remained a distant reality until it struck closer to home. In this sense, PWA visibility has provided powerful experiential motivation for behavioral change on an individual level while at the same time advocating against discrimination at the social level.

However, despite support within their immediate environment, it is likely that people revealing their HIV status will continue to face sustained prejudice and discrimination from the broader society. The "coming out" of PWAs and the adoption of "positive" identities raises many issues both for individuals and for communities. It is not uncommon, for example, for "romantic myth-making" to surround the figures of PWAs—where they are seen as heroic characters.[8]

The success of PWA groups in carrying out this work has led to "mainstreaming" in another sense. The political pressure to include PWAs in policy making and service delivery, and the proximity of these groups to affected communities and their efficacy in outreach, has made them attractive to funders wishing to support service providers.

The attractiveness of PWA groups as service providers is also economic. As pressures to move services to less costly infrastructures are increasingly felt throughout the world, community groups provide tempting alternatives to funding hospitals, outreach workers, and traditional public health campaigns. The relationship between PWA groups and funders can also be contentious and divisive. PWA groups often start with minimal financial resources, usually contributed by the members themselves. The arrival of external funding—particularly on a large scale—to a PWA organization can have considerable impact on the group. The need to meet funding criteria can change, even distort, the rationale and priorities of the organization. In some cases, pressures—both positive and negative—can lead to the "professionalization" of PWAs, with considerable consequences, particularly in relation to the distribution of power within a group.

The potential and risks of "self-help" organizations in developing countries is illustrated by the experience of an association of PWAs created in a West African country in 1994. The founding of the group was linked to the presence and promotion of anonymous HIV testing as a prevention strategy, itself a controversial approach. With some instigation from the director of the testing program, the PWA group was founded by a small group of young people with HIV who felt impelled to "come out into the light," both in response to their own personal experience of isolation and because it was still too easy to deny the reality of the disease in many circles. The group's founding occurred when three young people declared their status at a meeting on AIDS involving government representatives as well as multi- and bilateral aid agencies. The interest of donors was sparked, and the minister of health promised that they would be welcomed at the headquarters.

Subsequently, the group became an official association, complete with bylaws and officers. Enthusiastic donors funded the organization to undertake prevention and care activities: members offered their testimonies through fora and education activities organized by the National AIDS Control Program and other NGOs, and "field" activities were undertaken. The articulate founding members gained notoriety and were quickly identified as national and international representatives of HIV-positive people, a responsibility involving frequent travel (paid for by donors and other NGOs) to conferences and meetings around the world.

Although they lack headquarters, the association has an office within the National AIDS Control Program (NACP). In weekly meetings—for which a stipend is received—members report on conferences and prevention activities, as well as specific cases. In reality, however, little can be done to address issues that arise, other than to offer supportive counseling—a situation that often ends in frustration and anger directed at those in power and perceived to be indifferent.

Although the overall mission of the group (to provide support to PWAs and to reduce their sense of isolation) is relatively clear, its exact goals and strategies remain vague. Some members emphasize the urgent need for individual material assistance—such as medicines and housing—and see membership as a way of ensuring privileged access to such resources. Others emphasize that it is the association that requires more facilities—including a headquarters, office equipment, and a drop-in center—ideas are already expressed in the organizational chart which contains an extensive tree of executives, committees, and subcommittees despite the lack of structure in the organization's current work.

Thus, in just over a year, divisions are apparent both within and outside the group. PWAs speak openly about how they must be "in" with the association's core group, articulate, young people who are often attending conferences where they seek additional support. Furthermore, the locally based donor community—who had pushed for funding for this PWA group—is increasingly disappointed. One representative, who had hoped that the group would break the complacent consensus that had settled around AIDS in the early 1990s, now expresses her deep concern that donor interest in the group has somehow destroyed solidarity and stifled initiative. Of particular concern was her impression that individually, the women in the association had strong ideas and initiative, but collectively, the women were silenced by the overall power dynamics.

Overall, although some evolutionary experiences of self-help groups are mirrored by those of service delivery organizations, others are unique to such bodies. Both types of organizations face the challenges of "professionalization," expansion and changing external climates. However, the sensitivities surrounding issues such as power structures, avoiding conflict of interests, and agreeing on systems for resource allocation, are heightened when members are both the governors and the beneficiaries. As self-help groups mature and evaluate their impact, they often face growing pressure (from both within and outside) to become service providers—a move that can fundamentally change the nature of their organization, its goals, and work (Box 32-3).

BOX 32-3

Empowerment and gay community in Australia

GEOFFREY WOOLCOCK AND DENNIS ALTMAN

The contrasting approaches of societies and governments in responding to the AIDS epidemic is intriguing. For example, Australia's response has been frequently touted as a model of effective community empowerment. The relationship among community agencies, health and medical institutions, and federal and state governments, popularly referred to as "The Partnership," continues to serve as the basis for the implementation of the Second National Strategy (1993–1996) and the proposed third national strategy.[1] This document consolidates the spirit of cooperation among different stakeholders in society as part of a collaborative effort to reduce the annual number of new HIV infections to fewer than 500 by 1996. The affected communities have been at the forefront of these efforts, arguably the pivotal factor in ensuring a swift and efficient response in Australia.

In Australia, as in other western countries, the great majority of early HIV infections were transmitted through homosexual intercourse. In Australia this remains true; in 1994 homosexual intercourse was involved in 82 percent of reported infections. The gay community throughout Australia was the primary activist group and source of initial information about AIDS. They were also the principal sources of support and creativity for the prevention and education-based community cooperation model, which fought successfully to establish a legitimate place alongside the traditional medical contain-and-control model championed by conservative forces. In this struggle, they were substantially assisted by the critical decision of the Federal Health Minister to fund gay community-based programs as the primary means of prevention. Prominent and politically active members of the gay community also became the leading figures in the work of AIDS Councils to complement the work of the broader, non-political gay community regarding care and support services.

Other affected communities created their own representative organizations, including the Australian IV League (injecting drug users), the Scarlet Alliance (sex workers), the National People Living with AIDS Coalition, and the Haemophilia Foundation. All played critical roles in framing and shaping policy and program responses and in ensuring that community groups remained the most effective and appropriate disseminators and education and preventive messages. The success of these proactive policies has in turn established a platform for the empowerment of various other sectors of the community facing the epidemic. As a result, some of the most innovative peer education and treatment and care programs in the industralized world have been developed and implemented in Australia.

The concept of community development has underpinned most of the effective strategies. This emphasizes health belief principles, empowering people to develop their own skills and to have the confidence to identify health concerns and then to develop appropriate programs. In adopting this model, however, most of the successful education programs in Australia have also recognized the need to enable individuals and communities to work toward changing the broader social and political context.

These developments have not emerged without some tensions. Official recognition of the community sector in government committees has been taken further in Australia than in most countries; accordingly, a number of gay men now have a legitimacy and access to government unimaginable before the epidemic. This has led to fears of co-option by the state, and the emergence of Australian chapters of ACT UP in the early 1990s was in part fueled by frustration at the perceived accommodationist stance of the AIDS Councils. Indeed, because the AIDS Councils have become large service delivery organizations—the largest, the AIDS Council of New South Wales, has about 75 full-time staff—their dependence on government for funding raises questions about how successfully they might resist government pressures.

Furthermore, there is a danger that the autonomy won by HIV/AIDS community-based organizations (CBOs) in Australia over the past decade will mask the problems that the community sector faces at present and for the future. The changing nature of the epidemic poses greater demands on both governments and community groups, but inevitably it is the latter that will continue to bear the brunt of the political shifts in priorities. Some of the problems that have emerged in Australia over the first few years of the current decade include:

- the growth of professionally staffed HIV/AIDS CBOs, which has reduced the impact of the role of volunteers and has raised problems in relation to meeting the wishes and needs of the affected communities
- the increasing bureaucratic nature of CBOs as they adopt organizational structures similar to those of their funding bodies, potentially reducing the capacity to respond rapidly to the changing needs
- the lack of ability to meaningfully involve HIV-positive people in the work of CBOs
- the tension between those who see CBOs as principal advocates for clientele and service delivery and those who view the CBOs primarily as political lobbyists
- the nature of identity in defining the constituency, and thus the commitment, of CBOs
- the escalation of efforts by other public health sources to channel scarce resources into other pressing health issues (e.g., breast cancer) and hence, the need to ensure ongoing funding
- the tend toward complacency, apparent in the assumption that the effective education work among homosexual men does not necessitate continual funding
- the concern about the sustainability of informed social research guiding prevention and care programs in CBOs

Many of these concerns have been addressed, if not resolved, in the debates currently taking place around a third national strategy. Australia's development of peer education and organization within the gay and PWHIV/AIDS communities has had some influence in Southeast Asia, where a number of AIDS/gay groups have developed close links with their Australian counterparts. The provision of some Australian government money for "partnership programs" with groups in India, Indonesia, Malaysia, the Philippines, and Thailand has made it possible for groups to exchange ideas, programs, and personnel, and has been a factor in the emerging assertiveness of gay groups in Asia over the past few years.

In Australia, the nature of empowerment as a driving force in the fight against HIV/AIDS has altered significantly. Emphasis has shifted from building self-esteem and community development processes to a position in which CBOs are increasingly adopting a more professional structure replicating those of the state. The focus on empowerment is increasingly shifting to communities of people living with HIV/AIDS. In fact, their organizational structure is largely based on a model of "coming out" and self-articulation, directly derived from gay politics. Their growing assertion and leadership role highlights the fact that the potential emplowerment of marginalized groups and their participation in all forms of decision-making is a great achievement whose potential remains undiminished.

References

1. Commonwealth of Australia, *National HIV/AIDS Strategy 1993–94 to 1995–96* (Canberra, Australia: Australian Government Publishing Service, 1993).

While some PWA groups in Australia, North America, and Western Europe have had unprecedented success in molding science and public health policy (and even the agendas behind research funding), this has been much less so where PWAs are severely marginalized (whether by the same structural conditions that underlie poverty or gender inequality or by more AIDS-specific discrimination). For example, PWA groups in West Africa have remained silent on a large multicenter clinical trial of AZT versus placebo in pregnant African women at the same time as their counterparts in Europe and America protested against the same trial; the African PWA groups simply do not have the expertise or access to the knowledge and resources necessary to affect local scientific research, especially when that research is driven by international research agendas.

Such experiences provide evidence that funding PWA organizations is not a panacea in the fight against AIDS. However, these complexities should not detract from the many positive examples and contributions of PWA groups that continue to emerge throughout the world.

The proliferation of NGO activities on AIDS and the dilemmas of funding

Why are NGOs now being supported? Is it due to prevention (and care?) success stories and to their proven efficacy and efficiency? Or is it due to the desire of ODA bodies to spend less for maximum political advantage?

Governments have not always been willing to fund generously NGOs for AIDS work. With few exceptions, NGOs, governments, and intergovernmental organizations responded to AIDS with remarkable independence from each other from the early 1980s until about 1987. If they did anything in response to HIV/AIDS at all, most governments largely restricted themselves to provision of care to the very ill, and to traditional public health responses of surveillance and infection control for blood. The intergovernmental response was largely restricted to WHO, which created a sectoral AIDS program focused on both international public health functions like epidemiology, and on technical advice and advocacy to mobilize national governments. As noted, NGOs typically pioneered home care, counseling, and prevention work, most notably inventing, adapting, and promulgating the notion of "safe sex."

In the latter half of the 1980s, these relationships began to change. NGO activists got to know each other at meetings and conferences, and they began to form networks and federations (including notably what has become the UK NGO Consortium on AIDS, a federation of international NGOs working on development from within the United Kingdom; and the first in a series of Brazilian NGO networks). This process was encouraged by WHO/GPA who, among other measures, organized the first meeting of AIDS NGOs in Vienna in 1988 which resulted in a declaration and the creation of the International Council of AIDS Service Organizations (ICASO). As these networks characteristically work to ensure three functions: sharing information on successes and failures in AIDS work; cooperating on advocacy work on such broad issues as human rights for people infected with HIV; and lobbying for funds and other support for NGOs from governments and intergovernmental organizations.

Over the same period, both governmental and intergovernmental organizations began to increase cooperation with NGOs in policy development and, crucially, by passing along grants or contracts of public funds to these private organizations. (It is important to note, however, that this cooperation proceeded much more slowly in the United States than in Europe.) The trend towards subcontracting activities and granting public funds outside the apparatus of the state accelerated quickly, probably in response to lobbying by NGOs, in recognition of the relative successes and advantages of NGOs, and in many countries as part of a broader ideological shift toward the privatization of state functions.

Rapid increases in public funding of private organizations had a considerable impact on the effect of NGO activity on AIDS. Some community organizations that had struggled to deliver services using volunteer resources rapidly expanded their scope. Thus, more and more communities around the world benefited from locally delivered AIDS services. Groups involved in AIDS services differentiated into the "haves" and "have nots," and countries with public funding for NGOs (either by local governments or international aid donors) quickly saw their NGO sectors eclipse those of countries where no such funding was available. New intermediary nongovernmental organizations and networks were created to capture, manage, and make more efficient these public funds (at a transnational level, early examples included the AIDS Communication Project (AIDSCOM) and the AIDS Technical Support Project (AIDSTECH), which administered some USAID funds for developing countries until the launching, in 1991, of the AIDS Control and Prevention Project (AIDSCAP), implemented by Family Health International. A more recent example is the International HIV/AIDS Alliance in London. Other existing NGOs, motivated by the growing importance of AIDS, as well as by their instinct to respond to new funding sources (both service deliverers and intermediary groups), also sought and received grants and contracts. Community AIDS groups founded and run for years by volunteers began to resent the arrival of "professional" NGOs like the international CARE federation or ENDA Tiers Monde, perceived as having arrived on the scene with generous government support.

Funding trends and their impact on NGOs

The first edition of *AIDS in the World* pointed to the importance of ASOs and other NGOs, and their pioneering role. Current data reflect a constant increase in NGO involvement in the epidemic, as well as in net increases in resources granted to NGOs. Developing country governments still receive far more grant assistance for AIDS work than NGOs, but such grants to governments are declining and are being offset by World Bank lending to governments for AIDS (see Chapter 35). In industrialized countries, the same governments that are increasing aid to developing world NGOs for AIDS work are cutting back on funding for domestic groups involved in prevention and care. Recent data on the transfer of resources to NGOs also hides other trends. According to a survey of overseas development agencies and government national AIDS programs (GNAP) $40.5 million of the $226 million support delivered by donors in a year circa 1993 went to NGOs in developing countries—in addition to indirect support allocated through NACPs (see Chapter 35).

Development assistance funds are increasingly controlled at the national level—limiting central funds available to international organizations, while not necessarily increasing access to resources for local NGOs. There is also a decline in the amount of funding available for AIDS-specific activities or organizations. Also, as the pursestrings tighten, ODA bodies are becoming notably more likely to fund "safe," tried-and-tested NGOs as opposed to new organizations. "The world inhabited by CBOs is no different than that of the private sector: those which already have visibility and resources are awarded more."[9] This scenario has undoubtedly increased the challenge faced by small-scale CBOs in terms of accessing even small allocations of resources and funds, as well as intensifying the tension between "upstart" AIDS-specific groups and more established development organizations as they compete for diminishing resources.

In response to the changing funding and political climates, different models and mechanisms have been developed to support NGO responses to HIV/AIDS. In 1989, the World Health Organization Global Programme on AIDS first established a grant program whereby local groups were to be supported through international NGOs (the Partnership Program), and then had considerable success in encouraging national AIDS programs to set aside 15 percent of their budgets to be made available in locally administered grant funds for local NGOs. More recently, in December 1993, the International HIV/AIDS Alliance was established as a means to provide CBOs with local access to resources and to ensure that donor money could reach communities in need. The alliance channels international resources to "linking organizations"—bodies coordinated by local leaders in areas such as health, NGOs, and development. A linking organization would make decisions about local priorities and function as an NGO support mechanism— allocating resources to CBOs as well as playing an active part in the NGO sector's response to HIV/AIDS.

It is difficult to discern a coherent logic to donor actions in supporting NGOs for AIDS work. Stated policies often differ from actual allocation of funds, and one of the few safe generalizations that can be made is that donors are consistently concerned about being identified institutionally with particular projects, and are thus hesitant about multilateral and cooperative efforts. Ironically, while many governments start supporting NGOs as a way to reduce state expenditure on HIV/AIDS, successful funding programs tend to result in articulate constituencies that demand expanded public services in health and health promotion.

While it is difficult to identify indicators of NGO success, assessing the impact of donor support is also quite complex. Donors are only too aware of NGO criticisms—of dictating local responses, flooding nascent groups with funds, insisting on inappropriate overly technical programs, and of lack of accountability to local people. Nevertheless, with some support from outside, community groups can be remarkably effective. This is especially true in countries that do not yet have widespread HIV/AIDS epidemics and where NGOs working intensively with small but vulnerable populations may curb the spread of disease. Providing NGOs with local access to appropriate resources can enable them to play their full role of providing care and support and saving lives.

Relations between NGOs and governments

A strong national response to HIV/AIDS in any country requires a dynamic alliance among community groups, government, and the private sector.

Governments are typically in the best position to monitor trends in HIV infection, to ensure consistent supplies of quality condoms at a national level, to strengthen health care practitioners' capacity to recognize and treat STIs, and to promote the respect of human rights, especially for vulnerable populations. Governments also have a unique opportunity to teach about HIV/AIDS, STIs, and sexuality to young people in schools.

Private sector companies are often responsible for providing health care and health information to their employees. Private sector leaders can also set an example for others by encouraging HIV/AIDS services in the workplace, by not discriminating against people living with HIV, by calling on governments to act responsibly, and by supporting community groups.

A cooperative relationship among NGOs, governments, and the private sector is required on an international level. NGOs not only share lessons learned across borders through their networks but also push institutions like the United Nations to pay more attention to the importance of human rights in HIV/AIDS work, and lobby international companies to be global leaders in offering prevention and care services, and ensuring non-discrimination in the workplace.

Responses to HIV/AIDS have demonstrated both the advantages and the disadvantages of cooperation between governments and NGOs. Close liaison has provided NGOs with access to both influence and resources, helping them to play a full and recognized role in shaping and building an integrated response. There is, however, a delicate balance to be achieved. Too close liaison has sometimes limited the independence and dynamism of NGOs—affecting their flexibility, as well as their access to support from nongovernmental sources.

NGO efforts in response to HIV/AIDS are not immune from existing national and regional issues and politics. In the UK, for example, the initial delay in the government response was partly attributable to the association of HIV/AIDS with controversial issues such as drug use and homosexuality. In Africa, addressing HIV/AIDS often involves sensitive cultural issues—such as polygamy and wife inheritance—which governments do not want to be seen to challenge. While effective NGO responses typically work within traditional structures of individual communities or tribes (or subcultures), some national governments are striving to promote "generic," national cultures. According to Alfred J. Fortin, "This state legitimisation strategy has the potential to undermine AIDS prevention efforts that stress involvement with the authority structures of tribal communities."[10] Officials in both Côte d'Ivoire and Kenya, for example, have hesitated to endorse or support tribally identified NGO activities on AIDS, with the Kenyan program being delivered mostly in the two official state languages, English and Swahili.

Other governments seem willing to allow NGO activity to flourish in many languages and discourses, from Uganda's twenty-two language AIDS posters to the Netherlands's tailored programs for sex workers of particular ethnic backgrounds.

Sustaining community action on AIDS

As the HIV/AIDS pandemic progresses, funders are increasingly supporting established organizations—such as women's groups—to become involved in AIDS, rather than asking AIDS service organizations to serve broader populations. There are valid arguments for this strategy; such organizations may have better, more specific community connections, and more sustainable approaches, than AIDS-specific groups. Nevertheless there is considerable concern that the wealth of experience gained by AIDS service organizations will be lost, and that groups will have to repeatedly learn basic lessons through trial and error. More insidiously, donors can use the rhetoric of empowerment and solidarity with affected communities, while publicly misrepresenting funding reductions as increases. One solution is to put pressure on donors to differentiate funding for AIDS activities that are integrated with other programs, but that can be tracked and evaluated, from funding for "AIDS-related activities," which often describes programs that contribute to reducing HIV vulnerability, but that were being funded long before the HIV/AIDS epidemic began.

The lessons learned from over a decade of experience of NGOs in the fight against AIDS must not be lost. When they develop policies, practices, and expectations about "NGOs" as a nondifferentiated group, governments and intergovernmental organizations risk undermining many of the unique contributions to be made by NGOs. The efforts of AIDS-specific and non-AIDS-specific organizations can be complementary—mutually reinforcing areas of expertise, experience, and access.

The HIV/AIDS pandemic, and its attendant trauma and loss for individuals, families, and communities, is with us for many years to come. Community action is an efficient way to deliver prevention, care, and support services. For an effective and sustained response to HIV/AIDS, people cannot rely too much on outside experts. Communities need to take control themselves, communicate messages among themselves which are understood and respected, follow their own leaders, and take actions that are appropriate and effective.

REFERENCES

1. J. O'Malley, "AIDS Service Organisations in Transition," in *AIDS in the World*, eds. J. Mann, D. Tarantola, and T. Netter (Cambridge, MA: Harvard University Press, 1992): 774–787.

2. D. Altman, *Power and Community* (New York: Taylor and Francis, 1994):27.

3. T. Brodhead and J. O'Malley, "NGOs and Third World Development," World Health Organization, Global Programme on AIDS, Geneva, 1989, GPA/GMC (2) / 89.5 Addendum 1.

4. P. Aggleton, J. Weeks, and A. Taylor-Laybourn, "Voluntary Sector Responses to HIV and AIDS: A Framework for Analysis," in *AIDS: Facing the Second Decade*, eds. P. Aggleton, P. Davis, and G. Hart (London: Falmer Press, 1993).

5. "The Alliance," "Community Action," "Alliance Programmes," "Programme Development," "Mission Vision and Values," sections of International HIV/AIDS Alliance information pack, November 1995.

6. M. Roberts, "Emergence of Gay Identity and Gay Social Movements in Developing Countries: The AIDS Crises as Catalyst," *Alternatives* 20 (1995):243–264.

7. Conference Declaration, Paris AIDS Summit, Paris, December 1994.

8. M. Benjamin, "A human condition," *New Statesman and Society* (August 20, 1993):34.

9. A. Klouda, "Shifting Patterns in International Financing for AIDS Programs," in *AIDS in the World*, J. Mann, D. Tarantola, and T. Netter, eds. (Cambridge, MA: Harvard University Press, 1992):795 (note 20).

10. A. J. Fortin, "AIDS, Development, and the Limitations of the African State," in *Action on AIDS: National Policies in Comparative Perspective*, B. A. Mesztal and D. Moss, eds. (Westport, CT: Greenwood, 1990).

33

The Private Sector: How Are Corporations Responding to HIV/AIDS?

BEA BEZMALINOVIC

An enlightened business community can provide critical leadership and help catalyze political will to deal with issues affecting the labor force, the economy, and the welfare of the nation as a whole. In the context of HIV/AIDS, the private sector can contribute effectively to prevention efforts for employees; to the provision of health care and social support to workers and their families; to advocacy for broader government actions on AIDS; and to philanthropic actions.

The workplace has been considered an appropriate and effective setting for HIV prevention programs. Fears and misconceptions about AIDS can be alleviated, discrimination against people with HIV can be prevented, managers can be helped to deal fairly with HIV-infected workers, and employees can be educated to reduce their risk for HIV transmission. These efforts may help corporations contain and even reduce other costs related to treatment and health insurance, decreased productivity, and "de-skilling" (the loss of workers with specific training or skills), or retraining of the workforce.[1] In many countries, workplaces also provide a unique opportunity to provide accurate information about HIV to sexually active adults who would be difficult to reach through other channels.

According to the World Health Organization, workplace HIV/AIDS policies should address a range of issues in order to create an environment conducive to promoting the health and human dignity of workers[2,3] (see Box 33-1).

BOX 33-1

Workplace guidelines on HIV/AIDS

A. Persons applying for employment: Pre-employment HIV/AIDS screening as part of the assessment of fitness to work is unnecessary and should not be required. Screening of this kind refers to direct methods (HIV testing) or indirect methods (assessment of risk behaviors) or to questions about HIV tests already taken. Pre-employment screening for insurance or other purposes raises serious concerns about discrimination and merits close and further study.

B. Persons in employment:

1. HIV/AIDS screening: HIV/AIDS screening, whether direct (HIV testing), indirect (assessment of risk behaviors), or asking questions regarding tests already taken, should not be required.

2. Confidentiality: Confidentiality regarding all medical information, including HIV/AIDS status, must be maintained.

3. Informing the employer: There should be no obligation of the employee to inform the employer regarding his or her HIV/AIDS status.

4. Protection of employee: Persons in the workplace affected by, or perceived to be affected by HIV/AIDS, must be protected from stigmatization and discrimination by co-workers, unions, employers, or clients. Information and education are essential to maintain the climate of mutual understanding necessary to ensure this protection.

5. Access to services for employees: Employees and their families should have access to information and educational programs on HIV/AIDS, as well as to relevant counseling and appropriate referral.

6. Benefits: HIV-infected employees should not be discriminated against including access to and receipt of benefits from statutory social security programs and occupationally related schemes.

7. Reasonable changes in working arrangements: HIV infection by itself is not associated with any limitation in fitness to work. If fitness to work is impaired by HIV-related illness, reasonable alternative working arrangements should be made.

8. Continuation of employment relationship: HIV infection is not a cause for termination of employment. As with many other illnesses, persons with HIV-related illnesses should be able to work as long as medically fit for available, appropriate work.

9. First aid: In any situation requiring first aid in the workplace, precautions need to be taken to reduce the risk of transmitting blood-borne infections including hepatitis B. These standard precautions will be equally effective against HIV transmission.

This box was excerpted from WHO/Global Programme on AIDS, *Statement on the Consultation on AIDS and the Workplace*, meeting on June 27–29, 1988 (Geneva: WHO, 1988).

However, relatively few corporations have addressed HIV/AIDS in their programs and policies. For example, a 1994 survey of 794 U.S.-based firms, including many large multinational corporations, found that only 32 percent had an AIDS awareness program, less than half (49 percent) offered AIDS-related services through their employee assistance program (EAP), and only 19 percent trained supervisors and managers to deal with HIV/AIDS.[4]

AIDS in the World II surveyed selected national and multinational corporations to determine *how* and *how well* corporations with HIV/AIDS programs were addressing issues related to HIV/AIDS in the workplace. The corporate respondents included: Anglo-American Corporation of South Africa, Avon Products, Banco de Brasil, Botswana Meat Commission, British American Tobacco Company, Ltd., Debswana Diamond Company, First Pacific Company, Ltd., Heineken NV, Gold Fields of South Africa, Ltd., International Business Machines (IBM), Kgalagadi Breweries, Matsushita Health Care Center, Metro Pacific, Nestlé, Polaroid Corporation, Saison Palette, Schlumberger, Shell International, Sony-U.S., Southwestern Bell, Sun Life, Syntex, 3M-Thailand, Tata Iron and Steel Company, Ltd., Volkswagen, and Zambia Consolidated Copper Mines.

Employee assistance programs and services

Traditionally, employee assistance programs (EAP) and services have been developed to deal with problems such as alcoholism, drug use, or mental disorders that affect workplace performance.[5] Survey respondents reported that in most cases (13), management leadership provided the impetus for developing HIV prevention programs and policies (other surveys have suggested that management may wait until they have an employee with AIDS to respond[6]).

Corporations generally have responded to HIV/AIDS by creating or modifying traditional EAPs. Nineteen respondents (70 percent) have trained staff in their EAP or the relevant department (personnel, health staff, etc.) about HIV/AIDS, and twenty-one corporations (78 percent) also have specially trained HIV/AIDS counselors. More than half the respondents (16) felt that individual counseling was well addressed in their company's current programs.

However, few corporations have extended their activities to include HIV-specific services beyond individual counseling and referral. For example, only six of the corporations with HIV education programs organize support groups for people with AIDS. In addition, fewer than one-third (8) of the firms distribute condoms at most work sites, only six (22 percent) make condoms available at some work sites, and nearly half (13; 48 percent) do not distribute condoms at any work sites. Corporations operating in developing countries were more likely to participate in community education activities and to distribute condoms in most work sites.

Corporate policies regarding HIV/AIDS

The responding corporations appear better prepared to provide support services for personal or health-related concerns of employees with HIV than to address the managerial or work-related policy issues that arise when an employee is HIV infected. Corporate policies should provide guidance to managers; respondents' reports on major policies on hiring and promotion and the accommodation of HIV-infected employees raise some concern about policy design and implementation.

Hiring and promotion
Virtually none of the corporate respondents have a policy requiring an HIV test (25) or CD4 count (26) as part of pre-employment procedures. However, only two corporations explicitly prohibit such tests as employment requirements. Twelve corporations (44 percent) also have written policies

regarding training and promotion opportunities for employees with HIV and AIDS.

Accommodation of HIV-infected employees

Are employees with HIV/AIDS allowed to continue to work and in what capacity? Most respondents reported that HIV-infected individuals are allowed to continue in their current job as long *as feasible* and can be transferred to more suitable workplaces *if necessary*. However, respondents did not have a stated policy regarding work-related travel (24; 88 percent) or long-term assignments abroad (22 or 81 percent) of HIV-infected individuals. The majority (13; 48 percent) of the corporations surveyed did not have a policy of conducting work performance assessments for employees who are ill or disabled. Presumably, such decisions are made on a case-by-case basis. Among the 11 corporations that did evaluate performance of HIV-infected workers, most did so as part of routine evaluations similar to those conducted for every employee.

Creating policies is only the first step. These policies must be clearly communicated to ensure clarity and compliance. Sixteen of the corporate respondents (52 percent) provide managers with specific training in HIV/AIDS, but only three corporations (13 percent) require managers to participate. Given the complexity of issues associated with HIV/AIDS, managers may need special training to ensure confidentiality, accommodation, and equity in regard to employees with HIV/AIDS.[7,8]

HIV/AIDS prevention programs

Nearly all (23; 88 percent) responding corporations had at least one type of HIV prevention program. Corporate prevention programs frequently use brochures and posters to distribute written information to employees. Interactive educational presentations and discussions are less commonly utilized. Most corporations (21; 88 percent) consider staff attendance at HIV/AIDS programs voluntary.

Few corporations have extended their efforts beyond reaching workers. Only seven corporations (30 percent) worked with community groups or others outside the workplace. Contact with governmental entities is also sporadic. Currently, more than half the corporate respondents (16; 60 percent) report that they coordinate policy and programs with the government of the country where the corporation is based, but only five corporations (19 percent) also work with governments where nondomestic operations are located. A minority of corporations, mostly in Africa, report that they work closely with the local government or NGOs.

Management information needs

Respondents reported that most managers have access to general information on HIV/AIDS; 16 (60 percent) receive information or statistics on HIV/AIDS from either the local ministry of health, the World Health Organization, or through other journals and newspapers. Nevertheless, managers lack information on critical workplace-related issues such as program efficacy, specific information on local conditions, and costs of HIV and HIV prevention programs.

Program efficacy

Few corporations (9; 38 percent) have performed a formal needs assessment prior to initiating an HIV prevention program. Corporate HIV prevention programs also tend to be informally designed, and fewer than half (13; 48 percent) have been formally evaluated. Among corporations that have evaluated their programs, surveys of knowledge, attitude, and practices were most frequently used. Although rapid and easy to administer, they have limited capacity to measure accurately behavioral changes.

Financial information

Managers do not generally collect information about the direct and indirect costs of HIV/AIDS or the potential cost-savings of HIV prevention programs.

Summary

With some important exceptions, the corporate sector is just beginning to respond to HIV/AIDS in the workplace. The corporate sector has also organized to address challenges presented by HIV/AIDS by creating business coalitions in countries including the United Kingdom, Thailand, Brazil, and South Africa.[9] Currently, business coalitions focus on coordinating efforts at a national level, sharing experiences, and disseminating information to members. These business coalitions have the potential to be powerful forces in organizing the corporate response to AIDS and influencing the nature of their response (Box 33-2).*

Given the number of employees and workers worldwide, it is clear that prevention programs in the workplace and policies on HIV infection and infected workers can contribute importantly to the global response to HIV/AIDS. However, many corporations and smaller businesses have not thus far developed or systematically applied guidelines and models for workplace HIV/AIDS policies and programs. In addition, the specific issues raised by HIV/AIDS may require a substantial rethinking of broad and traditional health and work policies and programs.

While the private sector can clearly do more within the workplace setting, including outreach to households of workers, their potential contribution extends far beyond the workplace. In many communities, business leaders are de facto leaders of public opinion.

*An incomplete list of coalitions would include: the AIDS Consortium in Brazil, the National AIDS Coordination Organization of India, the National AIDS Convention of South Africa, the Thai Business Coalition in Thailand, the AIDS Information Clearinghouse in Uganda, the Business Exchange on AIDS and Development (BEAD) Group in the United Kingdom, and the National Leadership Coalition and New England Consortium on AIDS in the United States. More information on international AIDS organizations and coalitions can be obtained from the Business Responds to AIDS Program at the Centers for Disease Control (CDC) by calling 1-800-458-5231 or writing BRTA Resource Service, P.O. Box 6003, Rockville, Maryland 20849.

BOX 33-2

Corporate response to AIDS in India

A. K. GANESH AND S. SUNDARARAMAN

The socialist era in India contributed to the formation and strengthening of labor unions and collectives. India has a large unemployed skilled labor force and a vast unskilled and semi-skilled labor force migrating from rural areas and the primary sectors of agriculture, in addition to labor displaced under the new economic agenda. Corporations believe that replacing labor lost to AIDS or infected with HIV will be fairly easy in India and therefore tend to dismiss HIV as another manageable issue while denying the crisis status of the explosion of HIV infection in India.

Thus, responses to HIV/AIDS in the corporate sector remain infrequent and limited. Well-developed business and trade forums, notably the Confederation of Indian Industries (CII) and other associations in which industrialists and industrial managers are members, such as the Rotary Club, the Lions Club, and the Round Table movement, have for decades nurtured social action. Recently, the CII indicated a collective corporate response to the AIDS pandemic, albeit on a small scale.

In 1990 the AIDS Research Foundation of India initiated a blue-collar HIV/AIDS education program based on a health education model developed with support from Family Health International Research, Triangle Park, North Carolina, U.S.A. The program employs small group dynamics and centers around behavior change. The program also assists management in developing systematic and noncoercive HIV workplace policies, including coping with HIV in the workplace, information on safe blood supply, staff (including family) orientation to HIV and AIDS, provision of condoms and other commodities that assist in the prevention of HIV within the workplace, and voluntary HIV testing.

Corporate support for the AIDS Research Foundation of India Program has varied; ANZ Grindlays Bank made meeting space available for NGO training; a travel service belonging to a large industrial group in South India offered subsidized rates; the first Asian display of the Names Memorial Quilt at Madras in 1991 would have been impossible but for generous contributions by local business houses. Industrialists, acting collectively through Rotary Clubs, have supported a rural outreach education mobile, a sexually transmitted disease (STI) clinic for truckers, and a mobile STI clinic, and have sponsored small events and provided office equipment. Finally, young entrepreneurs have offered to recruit people living with HIV who have been deprived of their employment on account of their infection.

To ensure the active involvement of the corporate sector in HIV/AIDS prevention and control, India urgently needs a catalyst, a multisectoral forum consisting of NGOs, corporations, and representatives from the government, to influence corporations to respond positively to the prevention and control of the HIV/AIDS pandemic and to impress upon the trade and business forums the need for including a response to AIDS as a social priority.

REFERENCES

1. J. K. Barr, J. M. Waring, and L. J. Warshaw, "Knowledge and attitudes about AIDS among corporate and public service employees," *American Journal of Public Health* 82(1992):225–228.

2. WHO, Global Programme on AIDS, *Guidelines on AIDS and First Aid in the Workplace*, WHO AIDS Series No. 7 (Geneva: WHO, 1990).

3. K. Brown and J. Turner, *AIDS: Policies and Programs for the Workplace* (New York: Van Nostrandt Reinhold, 1989).

4. American Management Association, "1994 AMA survey on HIV- and AIDS-related policies: Summary of key findings," *AMA News*, (1994):3.

5. D. A. Masi, *AIDS in the Workplace: A Response Model for Human Resource Management* (New York: Quorum Books, 1990):63–80.
6. American Management Association, "1994 AMA survey."
7. G. Banas, "Nothing prepared me to manage AIDS," *Harvard Business Review* (July/August 1992):26–33.
8. R. Stodghill, "Managing AIDS: How one boss struggled to cope," *BusinessWeek* (February 1, 1993):48–56.
9. J. K. Barr, J. M. Waring, and L. J. Warshaw, "Knowledge and attitudes about AIDS among corporate and public service employees," *American Journal of Public Health* 82(1992):225–228.

34

The UN Response

LISA GARBUS

The UN response to HIV/AIDS has been unique and remarkable in many respects. Under the leadership of the World Health Organization, a Global AIDS strategy was launched in the mid-1980s, which assisted countries in developing national AIDS programs and fostered extensive international collaboration. In October 1987, the UN General Assembly held an extraordinary session on AIDS, which led to a General Assembly Resolution acknowledging the multisectoral nature of the pandemic and calling for all parts of the UN system to become engaged in the global AIDS effort.

Even before 1987, several important UN agency initiatives were started. Historically, efforts to coordinate UN activities in any field have been difficult. Despite agreements on the leadership role of WHO and its relationship to other agencies (e.g., the WHO/UNDP Alliance), coordination on policies, strategies, and most critically, on support activities at the country level became increasingly problematic. In response to these difficulties, to the expanding pandemic, and to the growing awareness of the social and political complexity of HIV/AIDS, a new UN-level program was created. The new Joint United Nations Programme on HIV/AIDS (UNAIDS) brings together six agencies belonging to or affiliated with the UN system—WHO, UNDP, UNICEF, UNFPA, UNESCO, and the World Bank—under the aegis of a Program Secretariat. UNAIDS became operational on January 1, 1996.

To understand the challenges and opportunities facing UNAIDS, it is important to know the history of each UN partnership agency's involvement and perspective on HIV/AIDS (see Box 34-1). While new leadership and coordination will be applied by UNAIDS, each agency's past will undoubtedly influence UNAIDS, in obvious and less apparent ways.

BOX 34-1

Why UNAIDS?

PETER PIOT

Many lessons have been learned from the decade or more of struggle against HIV and AIDS. All point to the need for an expanded response—a response of greater quality, intensity, duration, and scope. Experience shows that in addition to focusing more and better quality action on the individual aspects of prevention and care, we need multisectoral action to address the societal causes and consequences of the epidemic, including its complex reciprocal links to human development.

To set an example and lead an expanded response of this kind, six organizations of the United Nations system have consolidated their efforts in a Joint United Nations Programme on HIV/AIDS. At the global level, UNAIDS serves as the global AIDS program of its six cosponsors: the United Nations Children's Fund (UNICEF), the United Nations Development Program (UNDP), the United Nations Population Fund (UNFPA), the United Nations Educational, Scientific and Cultural Organization (UNESCO), the World Health Organization (WHO), and the World Bank. At the country level, UNAIDS can be described as the joint action and collective resources of the cosponsoring organizations, with the backing of the UNAIDS central office in Geneva and UNAIDS country and intercountry staff.

The main focus of UNAIDS is on strengthening national capacity for an expanded response—that is, the capacity of a wide range of national partners from both government and civil society. Experience shows that efforts which are limited to one sector, or which exclude those most affected by the epidemic, are likely to fail. Thus, UNAIDS works with government departments and ministries of all kinds, people living with HIV, communities affected or threatened by the epidemic, nongovernmental and community-based organizations, academic institutions and the private sector, as well as bilateral and intergovernmental organizations. Technical soundness, inclusion, participation, gender sensitivity, ethics, and respect for human rights are among the values and principles that govern UNAIDS' staffing and operations and guide its work with national and international partners.

Mission and roles

As the main advocate for global action on HIV/AIDS, UNAIDS will lead, strengthen, and support an expanded response aimed at preventing HIV transmission, providing care and support, reducing the vulnerability of individuals and communities to HIV/AIDS, and alleviating the impact of the epidemic.

To this end it has four mutually reinforcing roles:

1. *Policy development and research*. UNAIDS identifies, develops, and serves as a major source of "international best practice." By this UNAIDS means the principles, policies, strategies, and activities that, according to collective experience from around the world, are recognized to be technically, ethically, and strategically sound. The Joint Program also promotes and supports biomedical, social science, and operations research on HIV/AIDS, especially research that fills critical gaps and that promises to be of benefit to developing countries.
2. *Technical support*. Technical support is the operational arm of international best practice. UNAIDS catalyzes and provides selected technical support in a way that builds on what countries have already put into place, and that takes advantage of the body of experience and expertise in the most-affected countries.
3. *Advocacy*. UNAIDS speaks out for and promotes a comprehensive, multisectoral response that is sound—technically, ethically, and strategically—and is provided with adequate resources.
4. *Coordination*. UNAIDS helps coordinate and rationalize action by the cosponsors and other UN bodies in support of the national response to HIV/AIDS.

Objectives

As this book went to press, UNAIDS had prepared a first draft of its strategic plan covering the period 1996–2000[1] and implementation and action plans, with specific outputs, were being developed. In support of the world's goals—preventing HIV transmission, providing care and support, reducing vulnerability and alleviating impact—UNAIDS has set itself four objectives:

- to foster an expanded national reponse to HIV/AIDS, particularly in developing countries
- to promote strong commitment by governments to an expanded response to HIV/AIDS
- to strengthen and coordinate UN action on HIV/AIDS at the global and national levels
- to identify, develop, and advocate international best practice

These are actions over which UNAIDS itself has some control. But in addition, through inclusion and participation, through a working culture of facilitation, UNAIDS hopes to leverage its own limited resources into far greater action, including by partners not yet involved in responding to HIV/AIDS. Because UNAIDS is built upon partnership, its own success needs to be seen in the light of the success of its partners.

References

1. Joint United Nations Programme on HIV/AIDS (UNAIDS): *Strategic Plan 1996–2000.* Background document for the second meeting of the Programme Coordinating Board, Geneva, 13–15 November 1995 (UNAIDS/PCB(2)/95.3, 31 October 1995).

Table 34-1 provides an overview of key elements for each of the six major UN agencies listed above. While a tabular form limits the amount of detail presented, it facilitates a comparison of AIDS program missions, primary clients or interlocutors at the national level, and funding and staffing levels.

Table 34-2 presents a cross-agency analysis which summarizes the information in Table 34-1. Together, this information provides insight into the kinds of coordination challenges and opportunities available to the new UNAIDS program. Melding the interests and capabilities of these six agencies will be difficult, but a truly synergistic, UN-wide approach to HIV/AIDS could make a major difference in the global AIDS effort and set a new precedent for global work through the UN system.

Table 34-1 UN response to HIV/AIDS: policies, programs, structures, and resources in 1994

	WHO/GPA	UNDP	World Bank	UNICEF	UNFPA	UNESCO
Mission	To mobilize an effective, equitable, and ethical response to the pandemic; to raise awareness and stimulate solidarity; to provide technical and policy guidance; to promote and support research	To strengthen the capacity of UNDP and of member states to respond to the development challenges of the HIV epidemic	To alleviate poverty (overarching institutional mission)	To support promotion of the health of youth and women, particularly their sexual and reproductive health	To provide support in line with national AIDS programs and within the scope of the Global AIDS Strategy	To foster development of efficient educational strategies to help young people avoid HIV infection
Primary clients	Ministries of health	Various ministries, especially planning	Various ministries, especially finance and planning	Various ministries, especially health, education, and information	Ministries of health, especially relating to maternal and child health	Ministries of education
Comparative advantage	Health expertise; technical and policy guidance; standard setting; sociobehavioral and vaccine-related research; intervention development; surveillance and forecasting; support to NGOs; discrimination-related activities	Central funding and coordinating mechanism for UN system operational activities in the field; extensive network of field offices; multisectoral experience; work with NGOs	Largest single source of long-term development finance for poor countries; ongoing policy dialogue with countries; research on socioeconomic impacts and on cost-effectiveness of interventions	Mobilize around children and youth; long-standing relationship with various ministries and with NGOs; experience with children in especially difficult circumstances and families affected by emergencies and disasters	Work centers on women's health and fertility. Key activity is support to training programs for maternal and child health/family planning providers, who in many countries are the only health service providers that women see	Policy and planning in education; curriculum development
HIV/AIDS strategy	Global AIDS Strategy: (1) to prevent HIV infection; (2) to reduce the personal and social impact of HIV infection; (3) to unify national and international efforts against AIDS	To increase awareness of the development implications of HIV; enhance community capacity to respond to HIV; promote and assist prevention, care, and support programs for women; assist governments in developing effective multisectoral HIV strategies	To create a better socioeconomic environment whereby personal vulnerability to HIV is decreased	To promote young people's health, placing HIV/AIDS in the broader context of young people's needs and problems	To support AIDS prevention within the larger framework of ongoing programs in the population sector	To provide technical assistance in developing and implementing AIDS educational prevention strategies that are culturally appropriate

Current program structure	AIDS program established in Communicable Disease Division in 1986; elevated to special program in 1987; renamed Global Programme on AIDS (GPA) in 1988	Interregional project on HIV and development established 1991; became a formal program within Division for Global and Interregional Programs in 1992	No AIDS program (though semiformal AIDS in Asia Unit exists); HIV/AIDS integrated into Population, Health, and Nutrition projects	Interregional Program on AIDS established 1990; current HIV/AIDS activities housed in Health Promotion Unit within Health Cluster	No formal HIV/AIDS activities or program; guidelines suggesting possible areas where AIDS-related activities could be incorporated issued to country offices	Program for Education for the Prevention of AIDS 1987–94; AIDS now integrated into new project on human development
Current program focus	Technical cooperation (rather than operational activities); increased emphasis on care, STIs, women's status, socioeconomic impact, and discrimination	Policy and program development; awareness creation and advocacy; program support; liaison with development community	Promotion of cost-effective interventions (e.g., STIs and TB treatment); training for high-level policymakers; research on socioeconomic impact of HIV/AIDS	Accelerate activities in 31 strategic programming countries by demonstrating successes that are or could be taken to scale	Activities suggested for country offices pertain to prevention of sexual and perinatal transmission	To strengthen education, training, and information activities to deal with population, environment, health, drugs, and AIDS, and their links with human development
Funding levels	Cumulative contributions for 1987–93 = $547.3 million; 1992–93 GPA budget = $140.4 million; revised 1994–95 budget = $140.1 million	1987–91 cycle = $41.85 million expended for regional and country activities; 1992–96 cycle = approximately $90 million allocated for interregional, regional, and country activities	Total lending for HIV/AIDS–related activities (1986–94) = approximately $560 million	Interregional AIDS program funding approvals: 1990–91: $3 million; 1992–93, $3.4 million; 1994–95, $6 million; supplementary funds approval ceilings: 1990–91, $3 million; 1992–93, $4.5 million; 1994–95, $25 million	Total funds for HIV/AIDS activities not disaggregated	N/A
Staffing levels	GPA has 167 professional staff; for 1994–95, an additional 25 staff are proposed.	HDP HQ = 5.75 staff; regional projects = 7 staff; funding for 22 country-level HIV-specific posts recently approved	13 staff (in full-time equivalents) throughout Bank	5 approved posts for interregional AIDS program in 1992–93; 7 posts proposed for 1994–95	No designated staff for HIV/AIDS; requests for technical inputs forwarded to head of MCH/FP	N/A

Note: UNESCO did not provide funding or staffing data for this study.   N/A, not available.

Table 34-2   UN response to HIV/AIDS: cross-agency analysis

	WHO/GPA	UNDP	World Bank	UNICEF	UNFPA	UNESCO
Agency-wide HIV/AIDS strategy document	√	√		√		√
Stated policies on and distinct activities in HIV & human rights	√	√		√		
Discrete AIDS program	√	√		√		√
Scope of activities:						
Prevention	√	√	√	√	√	√
Care	√	√	√		√	
Research	√	√	√	√	√	√
Socioeconomic impact	√	√	√		√	
External review conducted	√	√				
Channel funds directly through government	High	High	High	Low	High	Medium
Channel funds directly through NGOs	Low	Medium	Low	Medium	Medium	Medium
Funds its own activities in-country	Low	Low	Low	High	Low	Low
HIV/AIDS specifically assigned country-based staff	High	Medium		Low		
Systematic country-based planning and evaluation	√		√			
Marginal use of government				√		
Funding (as a percentage of overall agency resources)	9%[1]	2.10%[2]	0.38%[3]	0.43%[4]	N/A	N/A
	High	High	Medium	Medium		
Staffing (as a percent of overall agency staff)	6.90%[1]	0.43%[5]	0.22%[6]	0.07%[7]	0.00%	N/A
	High	Medium	Medium	Low		

*Note: Information on UNESCO refers to its program on preventive AIDS education, which ended in April 1994. Because of the limited data UNESCO made available for this study, this table may not accurately reflect all components of that program.

[1]From personal communication with WHO/GPA, April 6, 1994.

[2]Represents proposed 1992–96 planning cycle figures for global/interregional, regional, and country HIV/AIDS activities as a percentage of total UNDP 1992–96 anticipated resources.

[3]Represents cumulative lending for HIV/AIDS (1986–94) as a percentage of total Bank commitments for FY87–FY93.

[4]Represents 1993 approved interregional AIDS programs' general and supplemental funds as a percentage of estimated 1993 total UNICEF resources.

[5]Includes overall resources, regional, and recently approved country-level posts.

[6]Based on 13 full-time equivalents.

[7]Based on number of approved posts for interregional AIDS program in 1992–93.

35

International Funding of the Global AIDS Strategy: Official Development Assistance

MARGARET LAWS

The first edition of *AIDS in the World* chronicled the evolution of international development assistance funding for HIV/AIDS based on the World Health Organization's Global AIDS Strategy (1987) and the efforts to fund it.[1] This support came from and continues to involve predominantly official development assistance (ODA), which transfers funds from the industrialized donor countries to international agencies, governmental, and nongovernmental (NGO) AIDS programs in developing countries. Official development assistance is defined as aid administered with the promotion of economic development and welfare as the main objective; it is concessional in character and contains a grant of at least 25 percent.[2]

Official development assistance: donor countries

Twenty-four countries are members of the Organization for Economic Cooperation and Development (OECD). Twenty-one of these countries plus the European Union are members of the OECD's Development Assistance Committee (DAC) which issues an annual report on overall international financial assistance to the developing world.[3]

Development assistance from members of the OECD/DAC to low-income countries and multilateral institutions increased from an annual total of $7 billion in 1970 (the first year for which data were available) to $60.9 billion in 1992.* However, while ODA from members of DAC almost doubled in real terms between 1985 and 1990, disbursements rose only 0.5 percent between 1991 and 1992.[4] Then, in 1993, total ODA declined for the first time (by 10 percent) to $54.5 billion (Figure 35-1). In that same year, Japan made the largest single contribution on record ($11.26 billion), outranking the United States ($9.72 billion) for the first time. France was the third largest donor, with a total contribution of $7.91 billion.

The declining aid phenomenon is not unique to a particular donor country, region, or sector; with few exceptions, it has been a universal trend.

*Unless otherwise indicated, financial data in this chapter are expressed in U.S. dollars.

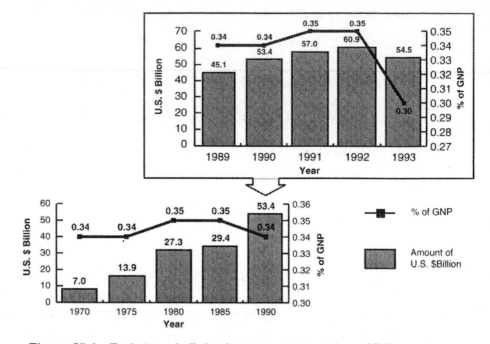

Figure 35-1 Evolution of all development assistance from OECD member countries, 1970–1993. Source: The World Bank, *World Development Report, 1995* (New York: Oxford University Press, 1995):216.

This decline in development assistance exacerbates an already serious funding shortfall: in 1970, the United Nations proposed that each country contribute 0.7 percent of its gross national product to development assistance.[5] Only four of the 21 DAC member countries achieved this target in each of the years 1990–1993: Denmark, the Netherlands, Norway, and Sweden. Overall in 1993, only a dismal 0.3 percent of OECD country GNP was provided as official development assistance.

Unfortunately, neither the OECD/DAC report nor any of the other published summary reports on development assistance (e.g., the *World Development Report*) provides detailed information on the allocation of funds to HIV/AIDS.

The *AIDS in the World II* 1994 financing survey: data sources

There is no single definitive source of information on international and national contributions to AIDS prevention and control in the developing world. In 1994 the Global Management Committee of the WHO Global Programme on AIDS undertook development of a database on international financing of HIV/AIDS programs, yet as of mid-1995, no financial data had been released.

Drawing primarily on the results of an international financing survey conducted for *AIDS in the World II*, this chapter attempts to address some of these information gaps.[6] The *AIDS in the World II* survey collected data on financing trends from ODA agencies and on their policies and practices for grant-making decisions. Survey participants were asked to provide data for the most recent 12-month period for which they had complete records. All respondents provided information from 1992, 1993, or a fiscal year circa 1993. The time period covered by the group of survey countries was therefore quite broad, a situation complicated by some agencies' provision of multiyear grant totals. In addition, the 1993 figures should be viewed with an important qualification: most large grants span several years, and many programs fail to disburse most or all of the funds allocated during the initial year of the grant. Therefore, 1993 data may significantly overestimate the amount of money actually *spent* in 1993, while data for previous years were generally adjusted to reflect the actual disbursement pattern of the grants.

Multilateral and multi-bilateral data were collected from WHO/GPA, and all bilateral data came directly from donor survey responses. Grants reported in a multiyear format were divided into equal increments according to the stated years of the project. The resulting figure was used as a 1-year average and then converted into U.S. dollars at the official International Monetary Fund (IMF) exchange rate for each year. Annual contributions were therefore expressed in current U.S. dollars, or the dollar equivalent of every contribution at the rate of exchange prevailing in each year for which data were collected.

Each ODA agency provided a funding profile, estimating the percentage of total resources devoted to all development assistance, health and social development assistance, and HIV/AIDS assistance. ODA agencies were also asked to break down their annual grants according to funding channels (multilateral, multi-bilateral, or bilateral) and recipients (international agencies, governments, NGOs, or others). They then provided information on projected trends in both overall funding amounts and channels through which AIDS funding will be distributed to developing countries in future years. The survey also inquired about funding policies, including criteria for funding of AIDS projects, organization of the agency budget, and tracking of development assistance funds.

Data collection was complicated by the fact that several countries have more than one government entity involved in ODA; for example, in France, both the Ministry of Foreign Affairs and the Ministry of Cooperation have ODA roles. Other countries may not have a distinct ODA agency but rather a department within their ministry of foreign affairs which handles development assistance disbursement (e.g., Switzerland and Luxembourg).

A portion of the funds committed to HIV/AIDS programs from European countries flows through the European Union (EU), which serves as a development assistance funding intermediary. The EU made available data on expenditures for HIV/AIDS-related programs for the period 1987 through 1993; these funds were classified as multilateral/bilateral. It is important to note that in some instances, these EU data may duplicate funds reported by European countries as bilateral grants. For example, if a European country designated funds for an African country but channeled the money through the EU, the funds might be reported by the donor country as a bilateral grant to the African country and also by the EU as a multilateral/bilateral grant.

Thus, the *AIDS in the World II* global financing survey pursued a variety of approaches in an attempt to accurately track funding and determine

Table 35-1   Twelve ODAs surveyed: contributions to the Global AIDS Strategy for a year circa 1993*

Country	Channel ($U.S. millions)			Total
	Bilateral	Multilateral	Multi- and bilateral	
Australia	$7.10	$0.53	$0.29	$7.92
Canada	$8.19	$3.07	$0.30	$11.56
Denmark	$2.09	$2.72	$4.07	$8.88
France	$18.50	$1.40	$0.10	$20.00
Germany	$7.81	$0.92	$4.07	$12.80
Japan	$1.00	$4.54	N/A	$5.54
Luxembourg	$0.99	$0.25	N/A	$1.24
The Netherlands	$2.70	$2.45	$0.93	$6.08
Norway	$4.58	$2.54	$2.25	$9.37
Sweden	$3.71	$5.05	$1.04	$9.80
United Kingdom	$7.76	$8.40	N/A	$16.16
United States	$82.00	$34.04	$1.00	$117.04
Total	$146.43	$65.91	$14.05	$226.39
Percent of total	64.68	29.11	6.21	100.00

*Total contribution to the Global AIDS Strategy, circa 1993 = $257.29 million. Percent of this total contributed by the 12 ODAs surveyed = 87.99%.   N/A, not available
Source: *AIDS in the World II* survey.

policy developments within each ODA agency. Despite all obstacles, data presented in this chapter are probably accurate within a 10 percent margin of error and therefore reflect the real trends in international aid to AIDS.

Survey responses

Responses from 12 countries provided data adequate for analysis: Australia, Canada, Denmark, France, Germany, Japan, Luxembourg, the Netherlands, Norway, Sweden, the U.K., and the U.S.. The Russian Federation, Spain, and New Zealand also returned survey questionnaires but did not report AIDS-related information in sufficient detail to be included. Together these 12 countries accounted for $226.39 million (87 percent) of the estimated $257.29 million* assigned to support the Global AIDS Strategy through all funding channels circa 1993 (Table 35-1). The 12 countries also provided approximately $49 billion (89 percent) of the $54.5 billion estimated total ODA from OECD/DAC countries to developing countries and multilateral organizations in that year.[7] Thus, although not entirely complete, the survey was sufficient to draw the profile of the international aid extended in support of the Global AIDS Strategy in 1992–1993.

Funding disbursement channels

Schematically, the survey examines funding distribution occurring in three broad channels: multilateral, multilateral/bilateral, and bilateral (Box 35-1).

*$16.66 million, or approximately 15 percent of the total multilateral and multilateral/bilateral funding in 1993 came from the European Union. These funds represent significant additional dollars contributed by the survey participants, most notably, France.

Of these, the multilateral/bilateral channel requires further examination. This channel allows ODA agencies to assign funds through WHO (or another UN agency) to a specific country, usually involving funds already designated by the donor for a recipient country under its overall ODA plan. In 1987, WHO created the multilateral/bilateral option to help increase support from ODA agencies for countries in desperate need of resources for AIDS work. For example, through a multilateral/bilateral arrangement, Sweden could support a national AIDS program in a country in which its ODA agency did not have an office.

BOX 35-1

BOX 35-1   Channels of official development assistance and sources of information on AIDS financing

Channel	Definition	Source of information
Multilateral	Transfer of funds from an ODA agency to the UN or any of its specialized agencies	Reports from WHO,[1] UNDP,[2] UNICEF,[3] and the World Bank[4]
Multilateral/Bilateral	Transfer of funds to a specific recipient country through WHO/GPA	WHO reports[5]
Bilateral	Transfer of funds from an ODA agency to a recipient country	*AIDS in the World* (1992)[6] *AIDS in the World II* survey (1994)[7]

References

1. WHO, Global Programme on AIDS, *Tenth Meeting of the Management Committee, Financial Implementation, Funds Available, and Obligations Incurred: 1992–1993*, WHO/GPA/GMC(10) 94.9, Rev 1 (May 19, 1994).
2. UN Development Program, Governing Council, *Annual Report of the Administrator for 1992 and Program Related Activities: HIV, AIDS and Development*, final draft, DP/1993/12 (New York: UNDP, May 1993).
3. UNICEF, *UNICEF 1993 Annual Report* (New York: UNICEF, 1993).
4. World Bank, *World Development Report 1993: Investing in Health* (New York: Oxford University Press, 1993).
5. WHO, Global Programme on AIDS, *Tenth Meeting.*
6 J. Mann, D. J. M. Tarantola, and T. W. Netter, eds., "The Global AIDS Policy Coalition," in *AIDS in the World* (Cambridge, MA: Harvard University Press, 1992): 511–535.
7. *AIDS in the World II* survey (1994).

Funding the Global AIDS Strategy

International funding for AIDS research, treatment, care, and program management grew steadily from 1986, when the Global AIDS Strategy was launched, through the end of the decade (Table 35-2). Total funding increased from less than $1 million in 1986, to about $59 million in 1987, to over $212 million in 1990—more than a threefold increase in the 4 years following the creation of the WHO Global Programme on AIDS. The total ODA funding assigned to AIDS increased rapidly through 1990; the annual rate of increase of 127 percent between 1987 and 1988 then declined to 4–11 percent during 1990–1993.

Taking inflation into account, a real decline in international AIDS financing occurred between 1991 and 1994. Two main factors may explain the flattening of the financing curve in the early 1990s. First, the ODA agencies responded to increasingly competing demands for resources, which were compounded by economic recession. Second, donors' commitment to subsi-

Table 35-2   Total contributions to the Global AIDS Strategy, 1986–1993*

Channel	1986	1987	1988	1989	1990	1991	1992	1993	Total
Bilateral	$0.11	$15.30	$39.40	$64.80	$98.90	$125.01	$129.80	$146.49ᵃ	$619.81ᵃ
Percent increase over prior year			158	64	53	26	4	13	
Multilateral/bilateral		$13.21	$30.69	$30.16	$31.58	$23.53	$26.69	$31.11ᵃ	$186.97ᵃ
Percent increase over prior year			132	−2	5	−25	13	17	
Multilateral		$30.26	$63.42	$65.58	$81.73	$75.00	$75.50	$79.69ᵃ	$471.18ᵃ
Percent increase over prior year			110	3	25	−8	1	6	
Total	$0.11	$58.77	$133.51	$160.54	$212.21	$223.54	$231.99	$257.29ᵃ	$1,277.96ᵃ
Percent increase over prior year			127	20	32	5	4	11	

*Amounts are in $U.S. millions.
ᵃProvisional figures as of August 1995; these amounts include multiple year grants extending beyond 1993.
Source: *AIDS in the World II* survey.

dizing HIV/AIDS programs—and more generally, international development—appears to be eroding, which perhaps reflects skepticism about the efficiency and impact of past efforts and/or complacency about the global HIV/AIDS pandemic. ODA funding figures are shown, by channel, in Tables 35-3, 35-4, and 35-5.

HIV/AIDS funding trends of major donors

In the early stages of the global mobilization, donors channeled most of their resources through WHO, the only multilateral agency that had embarked aggressively on a global program on AIDS. Thus in 1987, WHO/GPA received $43.47 million, representing 74 percent of the total ODA for AIDS of $58.77 million. Donors have become dissatisfied with this funding strategy, which relies largely on multilateral channels. Consequently, there has been a major shift towards bilateral funding since 1990: by 1993 less than one-third of ODA funding for HIV/AIDS ($79.69 million, or 31 percent of the $257.29 million total) was channeled through multilateral agencies and over half was provided bilaterally ($146.49 million; 57 percent; Figure 35-2).

Donor country projections for ODA funding for AIDS-related assistance over the next year are shown in Table 35-6. With the exception of Japan, all countries expected to sustain or reduce their 1993 levels of development assistance to all sectors. While most reported that grants to the health sector would remain constant, Australia and the Netherlands projected some increase. Of the 12 countries responding to the survey, only Japan, Luxembourg, and the Netherlands (which together accounted for less than 5 percent of ODA to AIDS in 1993) expected to increase multilateral funding for HIV/AIDS in 1994–1995; seven countries indicated that they intended to increase or maintain bilateral HIV/AIDS funding while decreasing multilateral funding in 1994–1995. Donors displayed a marked trend towards more focused bilateral and local project financing in their future support to HIV/AIDS programs.

Table 35-3 Multilateral contributions in support of the Global AIDS Strategy, 1987–1993, as reported in June 1992 and May 1994*

Contributions to WHO/ GPA by Country/ Organizaton	1987	1988	1989	1990	1991	1992	1993	Total
Australia	$0.00	$0.38	$0.38	$0.69	$0.22	$0.48	$0.53	$2.68
Austria	$0.05	$0.00	$0.03	$0.03	$0.04	$0.05	$0.15	$0.35
Belgium	$0.00	$0.00	$0.19	$0.52	$0.28	$0.00	$1.13	$2.12
Canada	$3.73	$4.01	$3.80	$7.77	$4.95	$4.80	$3.07	$32.13
Denmark	$2.18	$3.13	$2.96	$3.32	$2.89	$3.05	$2.72	$20.25
Finland	$0.07	$0.99	$0.70	$0.88	$0.88	$0.00	$0.00	$3.52
France	$0.17	$0.33	$1.56	$1.09	$1.20	$1.31	$1.40	$7.06
Germany	$0.08	$0.79	$0.32	$0.33	$2.59	$0.51	$0.92	$5.54
Italy	$0.00	$0.00	$1.27	$0.00	$0.48	$0.00	$0.29	$2.04
Japan	$0.00	$1.45	$1.75	$2.10	$2.20	$2.40	$4.54	$14.44
Kuwait	$0.00	$0.00	$0.05	$0.00	$0.00	$0.00	$0.00	$0.05
Luxembourg	$0.00	$0.00	$0.00	$0.00	$0.00	$0.00	$0.25	$0.25
The Netherlands	$3.75	$3.31	$3.05	$3.62	$4.13	$4.98	$2.45	$25.29
New Zealand	$0.00	$0.34	$0.00	$0.00	$0.00	$0.00	$0.00	$0.34
Norway	$1.83	$2.38	$2.30	$4.27	$5.78	$3.47	$2.54	$22.57
Russian Federation	$0.80	$0.82	$0.77	$0.82	$0.34	$0.00	$0.00	$3.55
Spain	$0.00	$0.00	$0.00	$0.00	$0.00	$0.24	$0.21	$0.45
Sweden	$5.06	$14.27	$8.60	$16.82	$7.99	$9.49	$5.05	$67.28
United Kingdom	$5.19	$8.22	$7.27	$8.47	$8.27	$7.83	$8.40	$53.65
United States	$6.64	$11.06	$25.65	$20.71	$23.00	$25.06	$34.04	$146.16
UN Development Program	$0.15	$2.91	$0.28	$0.51	$0.28	$0.14	$0.00	$4.27
IBRD[a]	$0.00	$0.00	$1.00	$1.00	$1.00	$1.00	$1.00	$5.00
Sasakawa Foundation	$0.00	$0.88	$0.00	$0.00	$0.75	$0.00	$0.00	$1.63
IBM	$0.00	$1.50	$0.00	$0.00	$0.00	$0.00	$0.00	$1.50
Swiss Red Cross	$0.00	$0.00	$0.00	$0.00	$0.03	$0.07	$0.00	$0.10
World AIDS Foundation	$0.00	$0.00	$0.00	$0.59	$0.25	$0.00	$0.00	$0.84
Miscellaneous/interest/ refund	$0.56	$2.77	$3.65	$4.54	$3.80	$3.47	$3.85	$22.64
Total WHO/GPA	$30.26	$59.54	$65.58	$78.08	$71.35	$68.35	$72.54	$445.70
To other multilateral agencies								
UNDP[b]	N/A	N/A	N/A	$0.65	$0.65	$3.25	$3.25	$7.80
UNICEF[c]	N/A	N/A	N/A	$3.00	$3.00	$3.90	$3.90	$13.80
UNFPA[d]	N/A	N/A	N/A	N/A	N/A	N/A	N/A	N/A
UNESCO[d]	N/A	N/A	N/A	N/A	N/A	N/A	N/A	N/A
Total to other multi- lateral agencies				$3.65	$3.65	$7.15	$7.15	$21.60
Total to all multilateral agencies	$30.26	$63.42	$65.58	$81.73	$75.00	$75.50	$79.69	$467.30

*Amounts are in $U.S. millions. N/A, not available.
[a]International Bank for Reconstruction and Development.
[b]UNDP financial information provided for a period of several years, which varied depending on the type of funding; funding totals were apportioned evenly across the grant period.
[c]Includes interregional AIDS program funding approvals and supplementary funds approval ceilings; biennial figures have been evenly divided between the two years.
[d]No financial information provided.
Source: *AIDS in the World* (1992); WHO/GPA, Tenth Meeting of the Management Committee, Financial Implementation, Funds Available, and Obligations Incurred: 1992–1993, WHO/GPA/GMC(10) 94.9, Rev 1 (May 19, 1994).

Table 35-4   Multilateral/bilateral contributions in support of the Global AIDS Strategy, 1987–1993*

Country	1987	1988	1989	1990	1991	1992	1993	Total
				($U.S. millions)				
Australia					0.06		0.29	0.35
Austria								0.00
Belgium				0.06				0.06
Canada	0.03		0.64	0.87	0.22	0.50	0.30	2.56
Denmark		0.43	1.55	0.16	0.38		4.07	6.59
Finland			0.02					0.02
France				0.25			0.10	0.35
Germany		2.18		0.25		0.04	4.07	6.54
Japan			0.60			2.10		2.70
Kuwait								0.00
Luxembourg								0.00
The Netherlands		0.60	0.15	0.12	0.16		0.93	1.96
Norway	2.67	3.38	2.20	2.12	1.99	2.01	2.25	16.62
Spain								0.00
Sweden		1.84	2.00	2.83	2.25	1.78	1.04	11.74
Switzerland							0.27	0.27
United Kingdom		2.50	1.50		3.13	3.42	0.00	10.55
United States		4.91	0.36	3.13		1.86	1.00	11.26
European Economic Community/ European Union[a]	10.51	14.30	15.29	14.05	8.08	10.33	16.66	89.22
Agency								
UNICEF					0.06			0.06
Swiss Red Cross					0.10			0.10
World AIDS Foundation								0.00
UNFPA			0.20	0.12	0.09	0.04	0.00	0.45
Miscellanous/interest/refund		0.45	2.36	2.41	1.41	0.38	0.13	7.14
Total	13.21	30.69	30.16	31.58	23.53	26.69	31.11	186.97

*Amounts are in $U.S. millions.
[a]Includes $11 million from France (1987–1993), the balance from other EU countries.
Source: *AIDS in the World* (1992); WHO/GPA, GMC (10), May 1994; *AIDS in the World II* survey, 1994.

Tracking funds from ODA agencies to developing countries

In order to track ODA funding from its sources to its beneficiaries, donor countries participating in the survey were asked to categorize their HIV/AIDS–related grants according to the funding channels described in Box 35.1, and to indicate the intended recipient as well as any intermediaries.

The 12 survey respondents providing data in channel format represented a total of $226.39 million, or approximately 88 percent of all ODA provided for HIV/AIDS in 1993 (Figure 35-3). Certain grants did not clearly fall into any of the categories (e.g., grants to research institutions or to multicountry initiatives), while in other instances, respondents were unable to provide the required information. These funds are listed as "other." The data in Figure 35-3 overestimates the resources actually available, in cash or in kind, to recipient governments and NGOs, for the survey could not identify

Table 35-5 Selected donors' bilateral contributions to the Global AIDS Strategy, 1986–1993, as reported to the Global AIDS Policy Coalition in June 1992 and May 1994*

Country	1986	1987	1988	1989	($U.S. millions) 1990	1991	1992	1993	Total
Australia	0.00	0.00	0.00	0.20	1.80	N/A	7.17	7.10[a]	16.27
Canada	0.01	1.70	4.00	3.50	20.00	7.51	9.75	8.19	54.66
Denmark	0.00	0.00	0.00	6.70	0.90	12.30	2.97	2.09[a]	24.96
France	0.00	2.20	1.70	8.30	9.40	12.80	12.50[a]	18.50[b]	65.40
Germany	0.00	0.00	7.00	7.00	7.30	7.00[a]	7.02[a]	7.81	43.13
Italy	0.00	0.00	0.40	1.40	N/A	N/A	N/A	N/A	1.80
Japan	0.00	0.00	0.00	0.00	0.00	0.00	0.00	1.00[a]	1.00
Luxembourg	0.00	0.00	0.00	0.00	N/A	N/A	N/A	0.99	0.99
The Netherlands	0.00	0.00	0.50	0.50	1.70	1.10	2.41[a]	2.70	8.91
Norway	0.10	0.00	0.00	0.20	12.20	N/A	4.58	4.58[a]	21.66
Spain	0.00	0.00	0.00	0.00	N/A	N/A	N/A	0.06	0.06
Sweden	0.00	0.00	0.10	8.50	11.40	15.20	4.80	3.71[a]	43.71
United Kingdom	0.00	0.00	0.00	4.20	3.40	3.90	1.90	7.76[a]	21.16
United States	0.00	11.40	25.70	24.30	30.80	65.20	76.70	82.00	316.10
Total	0.11	15.30	39.40	64.80	98.90	125.01	129.80	146.49	619.81

*Amounts are in $U.S. millions.   Figures for the year circa 1992 are estimates based upon available figures from 1991 and 1993.   N/A, not available.

Note: European Economic Community/European Union.

[a]Estimate based upon figures supplied for fiscal year reported on in survey.

[b]In addition to this sum, France contributed $12.1 million to the European Union. This contribution is reflected in Figure 32-4.

Source: *AIDS in the World II* survey; Global AIDS Policy Coalition, International Financing Coalition, International Financing Survey, 1994.

Figure 35-2 International contributions to the Global AIDS Strategy, by funding channels, 1986–1993.

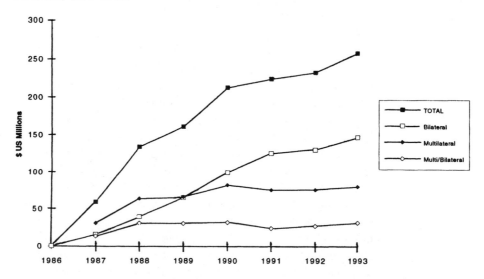

Table 35-6   Information provided by ODA agencies on foreseen trends in their HIV/ AIDS funding and evaluation practices*

| Country | $U.S. millions ODA HIV/AIDS circa 1993 | Projected funding trends, 1992–1995 | | | Project evaluations performed by agency or its ODA | |
		Multilateral ODA	Bilateral ODA	ODA through NGO	Multilateral ODA	Bilateral ODA
United States	117.04	↓	→	↑	+	±
France	20.00	N/A	N/A	N/A	N/A	N/A
Canada	11.56	N/A	N/A	N/A	−	±
Sweden	9.80	↓	↑	↓	+	±
United Kingdom	16.16	→	↑	↑	+	N/A
Norway	9.37	N/A	N/A	N/A	+	±
Germany	12.80	N/A	N/A	N/A	N/A	N/A
The Netherlands	6.08	↑	↑	↑	+	+
Australia	7.92	→	↑	→	+	N/A
Denmark	8.88	→	→	→	−	±
Japan	5.54	→	↑	→	N/A	N/A
Luxembourg	1.24	↑	↓	N/A	N/A	±
Total	226.39					

*→ = no change; ↑ = increase; ↓ = decrease; + = performed; − = not performed; ± = partially performed.

each ODA agency's overhead and administrative costs. Of the $226.39 million that could be tracked from ODA agencies to their recipients (governments, NGOs, and others), $79.96 million (35 percent) was channeled through UN agencies, including $65.91 million through the WHO/GPA multilaterally and $14.05 million in a multi- or bilateral form, generally through the ODA agency's regional or country office, then through WHO/ GPA, UN Development Program (UNDP), or United Nations Children's Fund (UNICEF).

The bulk of ODA for AIDS was disbursed through bilateral channels, $146.43 million (65 percent). These bilateral funds included: $85.46 million (38 percent of total funds) channeled to governments (channel 3); $2.95 million (1 percent) to local NGOs from funds disbursed from country-based ODA agency representatives (channel 4); $22.16 million (10 percent) from central funds to local NGOs through international NGOs (channel 5); $15.42 million (7 percent) from central funds provided directly to local NGOs (channel 6); and $20.44 million (9 percent) either allocated from central funds to "other" (channel 7), or for which the intended recipient was not indicated by the donor. Of these funds for HIV/AIDS in 1993, the largest proportion, $165.42 million (73 percent) was directed to government national AIDS programs (GNAPs) in developing countries, while $40.53 million (18 percent) was intended for NGOs. The amount of additional funds made available to local NGOs by GNAPs out of their own budget allocations could not be ascertained. Even without these data, it is apparent

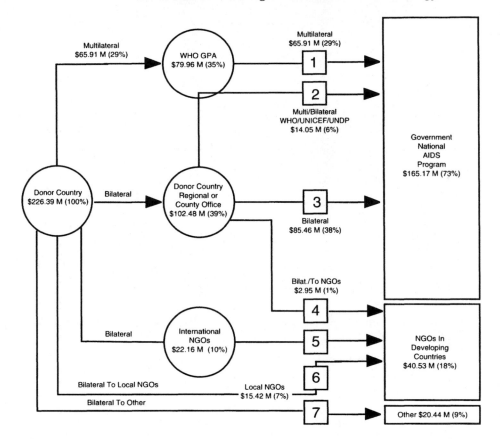

Figure 35-3   Global flow of official development assistance funds to HIV/AIDS programs, by funding channel, circa 1993.

that since the early 1990s, NGOs have received an increasing proportion of the resources allocated internationally to AIDS programs.

Concentrations of ODA funds: recipient countries

An attempt was made to discern patterns or concentrations of aid to specific countries during the period 1987–93. Nine of the ODA agencies surveyed reported bilateral and designated multilateral/bilateral donations to a total of 69 countries. The remaining three survey respondents contributed solely through undesignated multilateral or multilateral/bilateral grants. By 1993, United States Agency for International Development (USAID), the largest contributor to the Global AIDS Strategy, was implementing a centrally funded project—the AIDS Control and Prevention (AIDSCAP) Project of Family Health International—along with associate country projects as funds were assigned by local USAID missions. In 1993 France targeted its bilateral aid to 15 countries, the majority of which were in francophone Africa. Although it has funded a few projects in Southeast Asia, Germany also maintained a geographic focus on Africa. Finally, Scandinavian countries tended to concentrate their AIDS program funding in countries in which they were investing in overall socioeconomic development.

The grants that could be clearly attributed to specific recipient countries

**Donor Contributions
(Total $ US 88 Million)**

**Recipient
Countries**

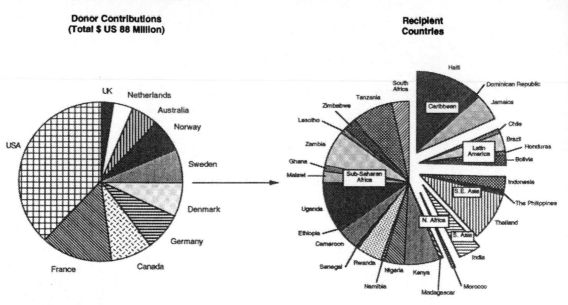

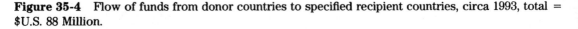

* These charts include <u>only</u> those grants reported by donors participating in the survey as being directed to specific, identified countries through bilateral and multilateral channels.

Figure 35-4   Flow of funds from donor countries to specified recipient countries, circa 1993, total = $U.S. 88 Million.

(circa 1993) amounted to approximately $88 million. Six countries (Uganda, Haiti, Tanzania, Thailand, Zambia, and Kenya) received about $24 million, representing 27 percent of this total. Twenty-eight of the 69 recipient countries received support from only one donor country; five (Tanzania, Thailand, Uganda, Zambia, and Zimbabwe) received support from five or more of the nine donors (Figure 35-4).

There was a significant discrepancy between the financing reported by donor countries in the funding survey and the data reported in the *AIDS in the World II* national AIDS program surveys by recipient countries (Chapter 30). Developing countries reported receiving substantially less than donor agencies had reported to have promised. Factors contributing to this discrepancy include ODA and multilateral agency underspending and carryover of a significant portion of an annual grant into the next funding cycle; ODA agency inclusion of funds for administrative, staff, and consultant costs in the reported allocations to grantees; differing fiscal years of donor and recipient countries; and finally, ODA agency grants for combined health programs which include HIV/AIDS funding but do not come under the control of or even come to the attention of the national AIDS program manager.

World Bank loans

From 1986 to 1994, the World Bank awarded an increasing number of loans to developing countries for HIV/AIDS prevention and care totaling approximately $565 million.[8] By mid-1995, 49 Bank-supported projects, devoted partly or wholly to HIV/AIDS, were in operation in 35 countries. Of these, 37 were located in 25 countries in Africa with total funding of $258.5 million.

Loans of $84 million and $160 million had also been awarded to India and Brazil, respectively, for HIV/AIDS work. An additional 19 projects involving $179 million in loans were to begin in 1995–1996, 16 of which were in Africa, including loans amounting to $120.5 million.[9] Although commonly defined as "soft" loans due to their low interest rates and long and flexible repayment periods, they will have to be repaid by recipient countries, many of which are already heavily indebted.

The apparent shift from government grant money to government and private loans for HIV/AIDS programs reflects two main factors. First, developing countries are turning to the World Bank as grant money is both becoming more difficult to obtain from other sources and is not increasing parallel to the growth of HIV/AIDS prevention and care needs in severely affected areas. Second, the World Bank has recognized the negative impact of HIV/AIDS on developing economies and is responding more favorably to loan requests for HIV/AIDS programs than in the late 1980s. World Bank loans have not been included as part of the international financial support of the Global AIDS Strategy but have been considered as part of the resources allocated by developing countries to their respective national AIDS programs.

Development assistance: supply, demand, and fatigue

In the period since 1989, the overall demand for development assistance has increased significantly. Countries traditionally receiving aid from the former Soviet Union have entered the OECD recipient pool, as have members of the former Soviet Union itself. The worldwide rise in ethnic conflicts and the need for peacekeeping and refugee assistance have added to the development assistance needs of already struggling countries. The proportion of all ODA spent on disaster relief has increased from approximately 2 percent in 1989 to 7 percent in 1993.[10] Aid to countries of Central and Eastern Europe and to the newly independent states has increased continuously in recent years: the total net disbursements from the 24 OECD countries to these nations rose from $18.6 billion in 1991 to $24.2 billion in 1992.[11]

The combination of a shrinking pool of donor countries, rising demands for aid, and the frustration within ODA agencies about their ability to demonstrate progress toward the goals of development have led to a complex state of donor fatigue (Box 35-2). Clear evidence of donor fatigue was revealed when the Summit of Heads of Governments on AIDS, held in Paris in December 1994 with the aim of mobilizing significant international funds in support of the Global AIDS Strategy, did not succeed in generating the expected resources.

BOX 35-2

"Donor fatigue syndrome"

Causes
- Increasing demand from national AIDS programs
- Increasing demands for allocations of ODA to new programs (e.g., Eastern Europe and newly independant states, humanitarian interventions, and ethnic conflict)

- Unfulfilled hope of demonstrating impact of funds assigned to AIDS programs
- Frustration arising from difficulties in coordination among UN agencies
- Frequent turnover of donor representatives on international ODA agency consultative and coordinating boards with loss of information about rationale underlying past decisions

Symptoms
- Pressure on UN agencies to develop evaluation and information systems that are in excess of ODA agencies' own practices
- Push toward the creation of new UN coordinating mechanisms
- Focus of ODA on a few countries in an attempt to "rationalize" funding efforts

Donor fatigue syndrome and the AIDS in the World II funding survey
- Complaints about multiple surveys from disparate sources requesting similar information
- Reluctance or inability to provide channel-specific funding information
- Average survey response time of over 6 months
- Surveys almost all incomplete and data often provided in donor's own format rather than in survey format

Conclusion

The second decade of the AIDS epidemic has been characterized by increasing demands for development assistance, growing fatigue among the major donors, and skepticism as to the effectiveness of the funding programs pursued by large, multilateral agencies. Donors are besieged by pleas for money and technical assistance.

The large ODAs have examined the experience of over 5 years of the Global AIDS Strategy and have attempted to devise and refine rational and effective funding policies. This effort, however, has not been coordinated effectively at a global level. Donors respond with frustration to efforts to standardize their reporting formats and clarify their policies and procedures, yet their inability to respond to such requests leaves the donors, their supporters, and their critics unable to engage in meaningful discussion of funding in support of AIDS work. The major lessons of the funding survey are that development assistance resources, including those for HIV/AIDS, are not increasing and should not be expected to increase significantly in the short term. Expenditures on HIV/AIDS–related projects are extremely difficult to track, and results of aid projects are very difficult to measure.

As the United Nations AIDS Programme (UNAIDS) undertakes to enhance the capacity of developing countries to coordinate their international aid allocations, it will be critical that both donor and recipient countries improve their financial accountability. If the financial resources assigned to HIV/AIDS programs remain difficult to track—and thus to critically evaluate—they will likely continue to decline, at least in proportion to needs, if not in absolute terms.

REFERENCES

1. J. Mann, D. Tarantola, and T. Netter, eds., "Funding the Global AIDS Strategy," in *AIDS in the World* (Cambridge, MA: Harvard University Press, 1992):511–535.

2. "Kindness of Strangers," editorial, *Economist* (May 7, 1994):19.

3. Organisation for Economic Cooperation and Development, *Efforts and Policies of the Members of the Development Assistance Committee 1993* (Paris: OECD, 1993):7.

4. "Kindness of Strangers," editorial, *Economist* (May 7, 1994):19.

5. *Ibid.*

6. Global AIDS Policy Coalition, "International Financing of AIDS Programs, A Survey of Official Development Agencies," conducted for *AIDS in the World* (Cambridge, MA, 1993).

7. *Ibid.*

8. World Bank, *World Development Report 1993: Investing in Health* (New York: Oxford University Press, 1994).

9. R. Feachem, P. Musgrove, and A. E. Elmondorf, "Comment from the World Bank," *AIDS*, 9 (1995):982–983.

10. "Kindness of Strangers," editorial, *Economist* (May 7, 1994):19.

11. Organisation for Economic Cooperation and Development, *Efforts and Policies of the Members of the Development Assistance Committee 1993* (Paris: OECD, 1993):131.

36

The Cost of HIV/AIDS Care

ANNE L. MARTIN

The HIV/AIDS pandemic has imposed a new burden on health and social service systems worldwide. As the pandemic proceeds, the global gap between needs for care and available resources steadily widens. Creating sustainable strategies for financing and delivering adequate health care for the growing number of people with HIV and people with AIDS (PWHIV/AIDS) is an increasing and unavoidable global challenge. This challenge of health care is driven by two main factors. First, the number of PWHIV/AIDS is continuing to increase (Chapter 1). Second, the period of time over which PWHIV/AIDS require care is lengthening. For example, in the U.S., life expectancy for a person with AIDS has nearly doubled since 1986, from 13 to 22 months.[1] HIV/AIDS is increasingly being viewed as a chronic rather than acute illness, requiring a broader scope of services during successive stages from HIV infection to AIDS and death. This is reflected in the increasing use of the term *HIV disease*.

To cope with this double challenge, health care planners are seeking both to improve the cost-effectiveness of health care delivery and to develop new models of care. Accordingly, attention is shifting from the hospital setting to lower-cost alternative health settings. Health care providers are expanding services from a hospital crisis intervention model to strategies for helping PWHIV/AIDS, as well as their families and loved ones, live with extended survival and improved quality of life. Hospital inpatient care is the most expensive mode of HIV/AIDS care delivery, constituting over 90 percent of total HIV/AIDS care costs,[2] yet a high proportion of PWHIV/AIDS in hospitals could receive effective care in an alternative setting. PWHIV/AIDS may actually require acute care for only 10 percent of the period of their illness.[3] In Barbados, over 40 percent of people hospitalized with HIV or AIDS had no valid medical reason to be in a hospital and could have been cared for in a lower-level facility.[4] In four Zambian hospitals, a review of all hospitalizations of HIV-infected patients determined that over 17 percent of these hospitalizations were not medically necessary.[5] Thus, the development of lower-cost health care facilities such as outpatient clinics, hospices, other long-term care facilities, or home-based care that can complement hospital services represents opportunities for improved efficiency and savings.[6]

Yet developing new models of care delivery for PWHIV/AIDS will not be easy. Reliance on hospitals for AIDS care persists for several reasons, ranging from insufficient confidence in local health facilities to a lack of alternative care providers and settings.[7] In many countries, hospitals may currently provide the only quality care—acute or otherwise—for PWAs.

Services must also become more responsive to the duration and diversity of needs of PWHIV/AIDS. Some countries have developed care models which expand HIV/AIDS services to reflect this range of needs. These care models assume many forms, and while they are often unique to their particular situation, all seek to reduce reliance on hospital inpatient care.

In this chapter, an estimate of the global cost of HIV/AIDS care is developed, involving direct medical care costs as related to per capita gross national product (GNP), care costs by stage of illness, and epidemiological data.[8,9]

Country information on the global cost of HIV/AIDS care

Direct medical care cost and per capita GNP

Data on the estimated direct annual medical care costs for a person with AIDS (PWA) are presented in Table 36-1.* Most available studies have included only direct costs or those directly involving payment for care. Neither the indirect costs of AIDS, such as lost income by the PWA or the person(s) caring for the PWA, nor the social opportunity costs have been included. These data are derived from studies using different methods, time periods, and definitions; nevertheless, there is reasonable consistency in results obtained from countries with similar levels of socioeconomic development.

Annual medical care costs ranged from $210 (Malawi) to $57,000 (Switzerland). These costs generally ranged from approximately 1.2–1.9 times the per capita GNP in industrialized countries and from about 1.1–2.8 times the per capita GNP in Africa (Fig. 36-1).

Available studies indicate that the total lifetime cost of medical care for PWHIV/AIDS in industrialized countries generally ranges from $20,000 to $40,000. A recent review of nine European studies concluded that the weighted average cost per year of care was $23,300 (at 1990 prices). In the industrialized countries, data are likely to approximate average AIDS treatment costs because most patients receive hospital care. Exceptions included small studies or those involving advanced rather than early stages of HIV/AIDS.[10,11]

The African studies likely overestimate the average direct cost of AIDS treatment because estimates are derived from studies which are: (a) based on small samples of patients receiving care in hospitals; (b) often limited to urban areas; (c) incomplete, as in the case of Tanzania and Zimbabwe, and

*Unless otherwise indicated, figures presented in this chapter are in current U.S. dollars for the year shown.

Table 36-1 Medical care cost of patients with AIDS in selected countries, 1990–1993

GAA	Country	Year published	Medical care cost per year ($U.S.)	GNP per capita ($U.S.)	Ratio cost/GNP per capita 1987–1991[a]	Study references
1	United States	1993	33,168	22,240	149%	Hellinger[1]
	Canada	1992	25,447	20,440	124%	Grover[2]
2	United Kingdom	1990	28,200	14,610	193%	Rees[3]
	Spain	1990	25,400–27,800	6,010	423%–463%	Ginestal[4]
	Switzerland	1990	57,000	29,880	191%	Cameron[5]
	Belgium	1990	21,900	14,490	151%	Lambert[6]
	Netherlands	1990	19,000	14,520	131%	Borleffs[7]
	France	1993	25,636	19,590	131%	Bez[8]
	Italy	1992	10,505–27,764	16,830	62%–165%	Tramarin[9]
3	New Zealand	1993	18,230	10,000	182%	Carlson[10]
4	Mexico	1991	1430–7350	2,490	57%–295%	Tapia-Conyer[11]
	Chile	1990	1,560	1,770	88%	Quinn[12]
	Honduras	1993	711	580	123%	Flores[13]
5	Kenya	1992	938[b]	340	276%	Forsythe[14]
	Malawi	1992	210	180	117%	Forsythe[15]
	Rwanda	1991	358	310	115%	Shepard[16]
	South Africa	1991	1,850–11,800	2,560	72%–460%	Broomberg[17]
	Tanzania	1992	290[b]	110	264%	World Bank[18]
	Zambia	1993	396	420	106%	Foster[19]
	Zimbabwe	1992	936[b]	650	144%	Hore[20]
6	Barbados	1992	4,550[b]	6,370	71%	Roach[21]
	Puerto Rico	1993	24,200	6,320	446%	Rodriguez[22]
10	Thailand	1992	658–1,015	1,570	42%–65%	Viravaidya[23]

[a]GNP ($U.S.) derived from World Bank, *World Development Report* (New York: Oxford University Press, 1989, 1990, 1991, 1992, and 1993).
[b]Mean lifetime costs.

References for Table 36-1

1. F. J. Hellinger, "Lifetime cost of treating a person with HIV," *Journal of the American Medical Association* 270(1993):474–478.
2. S. Grover, M. Swewitch, R. Fakhry, et al., *Natural History of Symptomatic HIV Infection and the Costs Associated with Medical Care* (Montreal: Center for Analysis of Cost-Effective Care, Montreal General Hospital, 1992).
3. M. Rees, "Methodological and practical issues in estimating the direct cost of AIDS/HIV; England and Wales," in *AIDS: The Challenge for Economic Analysis,* M. Drummond and L. Davies, eds. (Birmingham, U.K.: Health Services Management Center, University of Birmingham, 1990):69–74.
4. G. J. Ginetal, "Regional costs of AIDS in Spain," in *Economic Aspects of AIDS and HIV Infection,* D. Schwefel, et al., eds. (Berlin: Springer-Verlag, 1990):195–202.
5. C. Cameron and J. Shepard, *Resource Allocation Assessment of Swiss AIDS Programme: Final Report,* consultants' report (Geneva: WHO, Global Programme on AIDS, 1990).
6. J. Lambert and G. Carrin, "Direct and indirect costs of AIDS in Belgium: A preliminary analysis," in *Economic Aspects of AIDS and HIV Infection,* D. Schwefel, et al., eds. (Berlin: Springer-Verlag, 1990):151–159.
7. J. C. Borleffs, J. C. Jager, et al., "Hospital costs for patients with HIV infection in a university hospital in the Netherlands," *Health Policy* 16(1990):43–54.
8. G. Bez, *Soins et SIDA: Les Chiffres Clés* (Paris: Ministère des Affaires Sociales, de la Santè et de la Ville, March 1994).
9. A. Tramarin, F. Milocchi, et al., "Economic evaluation of home-care assistance for AIDS patients: A pilot study in a town in northern Italy," *AIDS* 6(1992):1377–1383.

10. R. Carlson, J. Dirkson, J. McDermott, et al., "Hospital associated costs of treating patients with AIDS," *New Zealand Medical Journal* 106(1993):76–78.

11. R. Tapia, A. Martin, et al., *Direct Cost of AIDS: Current and Projected Resource Requirements in Mexico* (Mexico City and Durham, NC: CONASIDA and Family Health International, 1990).

12. T. C. Quinn, J. P. Narain, and F. R. K. Zacarias, "AIDS in the Americas: A public health priority for the region," *AIDS* 4(1990):709–724.

13. M. Flores, S. Forsythe, C. Nunez, L. Hsu, et al., "Projecting the economic impact of HIV/AIDS in two largest cities of Honduras," Abstract PO-D28-4318, presented at the IX International Conference on AIDS, Berlin, Germany, 1993.

14. S. Forsythe, D. Sokal, L. Lux, and T. King, *Assessment of the Economic Impact of AIDS in Kenya* (Arlington, VA: AIDSCAP/ Family Health International, 1993).

15. S. Forsythe, *Economic Impact of HIV and AIDS in Malawi* (Durham, NC: AIDSTECH/Family Health International, 1992).

16. D. Shepard and R. Bail, *Cost of Care for Persons with AIDS in Rwanda,* consultant's report (Geneva: WHO, Global Programme on AIDS, 1991).

17. J. Broomberg, M. Steinberg, P. Masobe, and G. Behr, "Economic impact of the AIDS epidemic in South Africa," in *AIDS in South Africa: The Demographic and Economic Implications* (Johannesburg, South Africa: Center for Health Policy, University of Witwatersrand, 1991):29–74.

18. World Bank, *Tanzania AIDS Assessment and Planning Study,* 9825-TA (Washington, DC: Population and Human Resources Operations Division, Southern Africa Department, World Bank, 1992).

19. S. Foster, *Cost and Burden of AIDS on the Zambian Health Care System: Policies to Mitigate the Impact on Health Services* (London: Department of Public Health and Policy, London School of Hygiene and Tropical Medicine, 1993).

20. R. Hore, "Zimbabwe: Are the costs of AIDS medical care affordable?" *AIDS Analysis Africa* (March/April 1993):6–8.

21. T. Roach and A. Martin, *Report on Barbados Hostel/Hospice Feasibility Study* (Durham, NC: AIDSTECH/Family Health International, 1992).

22. M. Rodriguez, L. Torres, C. Diaz, W. Muirhead, and C. Rivera, "In-patient resource utilization by a pediatric AIDS patient population at a public teaching hospital," Abstract PO-D34-4310, presented at the IX International Conference on AIDS, Berlin, Germany, June 1993.

23. M. Viravaidya, S. A. Obremskey, et al., "Economic impact of AIDS on Thailand," Working Paper No. 4 (Cambridge, MA: Department of Population and International Health, Harvard School of Public Health, March 1992).

Figure 36-1 Comparison of cost of medical care for people with HIV/AIDS and GNP per capita for selected countries, 1990–1993.

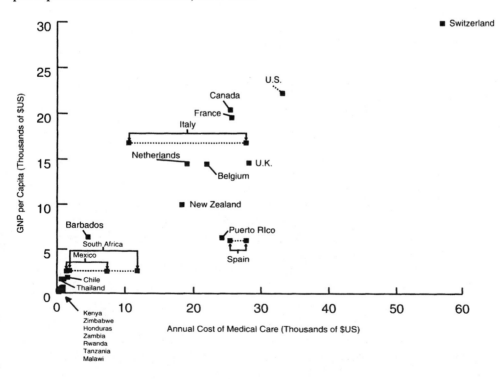

(d) involve costs of providing comprehensive medical protocols including full access to antibiotics. Unfortunately, many PWAs in Africa do not have access to this level of care; including all PWAs in the analysis would therefore decrease the average cost.

In addition, in sub-Saharan Africa sixfold differences in annual care costs were reported, ranging from $210 (124 percent of GNP) in Malawi to $936 (144 percent of GNP) in Zimbabwe. Per patient costs may also vary as much within countries as between geographic areas of affinity (GAAs). For example, in Rwanda the annual cost of medical care for PWAs varied from $149 to $620, and in Mexico, costs ranged from $1,430 to $7,350.

Cost issues for industrialized countries

The overall cost of caring for PWAs has increased steadily in most industrialized countries due to the increased number of AIDS cases, longer survival time, and increased use of expensive therapies.[12] In the U.S., for example, costs have increased by $4.9 billion from 1988 to 1992.[13] However, industrialized countries have been able to absorb escalating HIV/AIDS care costs, which will not overwhelm medical care resources.[14]

Yet cost savings have also occurred. They are attributed principally to improved case management of HIV/AIDS, leading to fewer hospital admissions; reduced use of intensive care units; decreased lengths of stay; an increased use of community-based support systems; and a general shift from inpatient to outpatient services.[15,16] Several studies suggest that outpatient care has started to supplant inpatient hospital care, since outpatient care accounts for up to half the total medical care costs of AIDS, and that this shift to outpatient care is leading to shorter hospital stays.[17,18,19] Instead of facing a shortage of resources, the industrialized world is challenged by issues of distribution, equity, access, and scope of care.

Resource shortfall in developing countries

The estimated cost of care for AIDS in developing countries is already weighing heavily on current government spending for health care, amounting to currently less than $10 per capita in many countries.[20] Estimates of the cost for providing current standards of care for people with AIDS illustrate the impact of AIDS on national health budgets in the developing world. For example, in Tanzania, treatment costs for HIV/AIDS consumed 50 percent ($26 million) of the country's 1991 operational health budget. By the year 2015 total costs for HIV/AIDS care in Tanzania could reach $155 million, more than three times the 1991 health budget. Drugs and nursing costs for HIV/AIDS care could require as much as two-thirds of the Tanzanian health budget by the year 2000.[21] Similarly, to meet the 1994 need for HIV/AIDS care in Rwanda, up to 65 percent of its health budget would be required, compared to the spending of about 5 percent of its health budget on HIV/AIDS in 1990.[22]

In South Africa the cost of health care for PWHIV/AIDS as a proportion of all annual health expenditures has risen three- to eightfold from an estimated 0.5–0.76 percent in 1991, to 2.33–4.13 percent in 1994. If AIDS cases increase as projected, the cost of care for PWHIV/AIDS in South Africa may require up to 40 percent of the total health care budget by the year 2000.[23] In

Malawi, AIDS currently consumes 20 percent of the medical care budget. To maintain current levels of treatment for patients with AIDS (costing an estimated $8.5–$9.6 million in 1993), 27–38 percent of Malawi's Ministry of Health expenditures will need to be allocated to AIDS care by the year 2000.[24] Similarly, in Kenya it was broadly estimated that public funds spent for the treatment of AIDS in 1991 totaled $8–29 million (roughly 20 percent of its medical care budget), and that the government will likely need to allocate $31–$162 million for this purpose by the year 2000.[25]

Experience from other GAAs indicates that the projected increases in HIV/AIDS incidence will require similar patterns of increases in health expenditure.

Cost of care for HIV/AIDS by stage of illness

Planning health care services requires an understanding of the spectrum of clinical and psychosocial conditions related to HIV and AIDS at each stage of the illness. Classification systems have been proposed to provide a framework for identifying the continuum of service needs for PWHIV/AIDS. These systems allow planners to define a spectrum of services and understand how the service needs change as HIV/AIDS progresses.

In the absence of a standardized global classification system, this chapter considers HIV/AIDS service requirements within three major disease stages:

• Stage 1: HIV-infected asymptomatic stage
• Stage 2: HIV-infected symptomatic stage prior to the onset of AIDS
• Stage 3: Clinical AIDS

While the cost of care for stages 1 and 2 is known to be important, only limited empirical data are available. Health care for stages 1 and 2 has been estimated to range from 10 percent of total lifetime HIV/AIDS costs in developing countries to over 50 percent of total lifetime HIV/AIDS costs in industrialized countries. In the U.S. and France, stage 1 medical care costs appear to represent between 16 and 25 percent of total lifetime costs for caring for PWHIV/AIDS while stage 2 costs total are between 26 and 29 percent of lifetime costs (Table 36-2).[26,27]

Global cost of care for people with HIV and people with AIDS

Methods

The estimated global cost of HIV/AIDS care in 1993 is presented in Table 36-3. The annual cost for treating AIDS (stage 3) in industrialized countries

Table 36-2 Lifetime cost in U.S. dollars per PWHIV/AIDS by stages: U.S. and France, 1993

	U.S.	(%)	France	(%)
Stage 1—asymptomatic	$19,083	(16)	$30,063	(25)
Stage 2—symptomatic	$31,196	(26)	$34,750	(29)
Stage 3—AIDS	$69,100	(58)	$54,298	(46)
Total	$119,379	(100)	$119,111	(100)

Table 36-3 Estimated global cost in U.S. dollars of HIV and AIDS medical care, by GAA, 1993*

GAA	Country	Persons with HIV,ᵃ January 1994		Persons with AIDS,ᵃ January 1994		1993 HIV care costs	1993 AIDS care costs	Total 1993 cost of HIV care		Total 1993 cost of AIDS care		Total 1993 cost of AIDS and HIV care
		Thousands	% total	Thousands	% total	Millions	Millions	Millions	% total	Millions	% total	Millions
1	North America	807	5.3	79	9.0	3,064	38,000	2,473	52.2	3,002	62.5	5,475
2	Western Europe	531	3.5	38	4.4	2,470	28,000	1,312	27.7	988	20.6	2,300
3	Oceania	21	0.1	2	0.2	2,000	20,000	42	0.9	40	0.8	82
4	Latin America	913	5.9	51	5.8	92	1,800	84	1.8	92	1.9	176
5	Sub-Saharan Africa	9,689	63.1	656	75.1	89	800	376	7.9	525	10.9	901
6	Caribbean	299	1.9	14	1.6	200	4,000	60	1.3	56	1.2	116
7	Eastern Europe	23	0.1	1	0.1	117	2,400	3	0.1	2	0.1	5
8	SE Mediterranean	50	0.3	4	0.5	262	5,200	13	0.3	21	0.4	34
9	Northeast Asia	90	0.6	2	0.2	302	6,000	27	0.6	12	0.3	39
10	Southeast asia	2,925	19.0	26	3.0	118	2,400	347	7.3	62	1.3	409
	Total	15,348	100	873	100			4,737	100	4,800	100	9,537

ᵃPersons with HIV calculated as cumulative persons with HIV on January 1, 1994, minus cumulative persons with AIDS.
Persons with AIDS calculated as cumulative persons with AIDS minus cumulative deaths.
Total HIV costs per person estimated as 40% of lifetime HIV and AIDS costs in industrial countries and now 40% (rather than 10%) in developing countries. Total HIV costs per person are then spread over 10 years in developing countries (10% per year) and 6 years in developing countries (15% per year).
Access factor in industrialized countries assumed to be 80–95% and in developing countries 100%.
*Persons aged 15 years and older. Thus, the figures presented in this table do not include the medical care costs of newborns and children under 15.

was calculated from studies presented in Table 36-1. For developing countries, per capita GNP was selected as a conservative estimate of annual AIDS care costs. (While costs in developing countries range from 106 percent to 276 percent of per capita GNP, this expenditure overstates the average cost as described above). To estimate the cost of stages 1 and 2 in 1993, data from the U.S. and France (Table 36-2) were applied to all industrialized countries. Since there have been few studies from developing countries, the proportion of costs for stages 1, 2, and 3 HIV/AIDS in developing countries was assumed to be the same as in industrialized countries (e.g., 40 percent of lifetime costs for stages 1 and 2).

Since the total cost of caring for PWHIV (stages 1 and 2) may be incurred over several years, total HIV care costs were divided by the estimated number of years during which HIV care would be required. In industrialized countries, where the mean interval between the acquisition of infection and the onset of AIDS is assumed to be 10 years, the annual expenditure was therefore estimated to be 10 percent of total HIV care costs. In developing countries, where the mean interval was assumed to be approximately 6.5 years, annual cost was estimated at 15 percent of total HIV care costs. Also, access to HIV care services was estimated at 80 percent in North America, 95 percent in Western Europe, and 100 percent in all other GAAs. This assumes that PWHIV/AIDS in industrialized countries with government-financed health systems have about 95 percent access to comprehensive public and private medical services while those with other financing have less access to these services (roughly 80 percent). In other countries it was assumed that, while access to formal medical services would be far less than in industrialized countries, alternate sources of care, including care obtained outside the formal medical system, are utilized at a very high rate.

Based on the above data and assumptions, the global cost of care for PWHIV/AIDS in 1993 was estimated to be $9.5 billion (Table 36-3). The total cost of care for stage 3 (AIDS) was estimated at $4.8 billion, an increase of 92 percent compared with estimates derived for 1990.[28] Including stage 1 and 2 costs ($ 4.7 billion) had the dramatic effect of almost doubling the global cost of HIV/AIDS care.

Trends affecting HIV/AIDS costs

Several trends related to the care of PWHIV/AIDS will profoundly affect future costs and financing of HIV/AIDS care, including:

- expanding care needs and evolving personal care strategies (Box 36-1)
- shifts in financing of HIV/AIDS care from formal and institutional financing to increased personal expenditure
- increased availability and utilization of antivirals and other expensive treatments
- improved case management efficiency
- heightened demand for services for groups such as women, infants, and children with HIV/AIDS

BOX 36-1

Personal care strategies of people living with HIV/AIDS

RUTH GUNN MOTA

How do people living with HIV decide what personal care strategies to choose? How do social influences and the availability of resources affect their decisions? Which decisions nonetheless appear to improve quality of life and/or survival time? To address these questions, International Health Programs (IHP) conducted a worldwide survey of people living with HIV. Respondents were identified among participants of seminars and workshops conducted by IHP or were known to IHP, by the International Council of Women (ICW),* or by the Appropriate Health Resources Technologies Group (AHRTAG). This convenience sample is not representative of people living with HIV worldwide but can illustrate the range of personal care strategies adopted in diverse geographic areas in the world. The survey included 100 HIV-infected people from 14 countries: Argentina, Brazil, Colombia, Denmark, Great Britain, Honduras, Italy, Kenya, Malawi, Mexico, Morocco, Rwanda, Uganda, and the United States. Seventy-two percent of respondents lived in developing nations; 28 percent were from industrialized countries. Sixty-five percent of respondents were men; 35 percent were women.

The survey asked respondents to rank, in order of importance, personal strategies they had chosen to cope with HIV disease. Participants were asked to describe factors that affected their emotions and willingness to seek help. They also related how they dealt with anger, how HIV had affected their sex life, and what they had learned and wanted to share with others about their experience of living with HIV.

Ranking of personal care strategies

From a list of 18 treatment options survey respondents ranked those they used in order of importance. Respondents also described other important strategies they had chosen but that were not on the list. For example, a number of Brazilian respondents mentioned the use of light, color, gems, and amulets to enhance mental and physical health.[1] Open-ended questions were asked about the specific application of treatment strategies.

Figures 36-1.1 36-1.2 show the distribution of responses. Overall, respondents from industrialized nations cited using many more strategies than respondents from developing nations. The most frequently mentioned strategies are discussed below and are accompanied by a brief review of related research.

Peer support groups and counseling

Among industrialized country respondents, participation in a peer support group was the most frequently cited personal care strategy. Respondents from developing nations also felt empowered by support groups, and those without such groups often mentioned isolation as a major source of stress in their lives. Peer groups are an excellent way to overcome the fear and isolation that may accompany an HIV-positive test result. Groups provide a forum for problem-solving about relationships, employment issues, treatment choices, and sexual concerns. They also let participants express their feelings about existential issues such as death and the meaning of life. Members of the group may give each other new perspectives on different ways to cope with HIV.[2] Although little specific research has been done on the impact of peer support on HIV disease progression, a study of U.S. women with

---

*The International Community of Women Living with HIV/AIDS (ICW) was founded in 1992 at the VIII International Conference in Amsterdam in response to the desperate lack of support and information available to HIV-positive women worldwide. Its major aim is to combat the isolation experienced by HIV-positive women through self-empowerment, international exchange, and mutual support. ICW headquarters are at POB 2338, London W84ZG, United Kingdom.

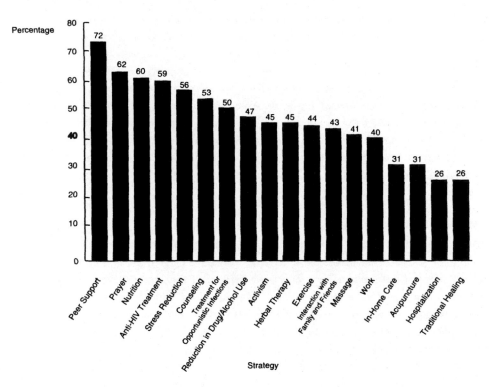

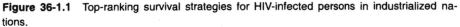

Figure 36-1.1 Top-ranking survival strategies for HIV-infected persons in industrialized nations.

Figure 36-1.2 Top-ranking survival strategies for HIV-infected persons in developing nations. Personal care strategies chosen by HIV respondents from developing nations to international health programs study.

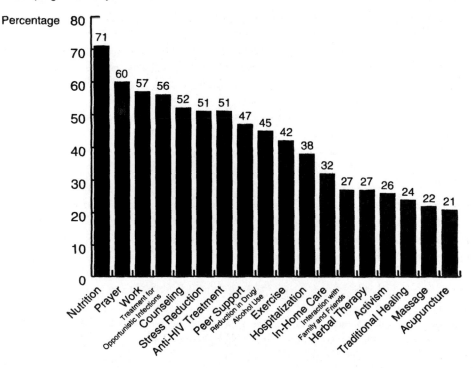

advanced breast cancer documented that those who attended peer support groups experienced less pain and fewer mood disturbances and lived nearly twice as long as women in control groups.[3]

Counseling was another frequently mentioned strategy, although the meaning of the term varies greatly among cultures. For non-English-speaking respondents, counseling tended to involve medical advice or health-education strategies more than emotional responses to illness. Respondents from Uganda who received services from The AIDS Support Organization (TASO) ranked counseling very highly and credited it with helping to have the courage to be tested for HIV, cope with the loss of loved ones, seek medical treatment, and look to the future and become involved in community education. As one respondent stated: "After receiving my positive results, I knew this was the end of my life. I felt I was going to die the next month. After counseling I was a different person ready to cope and live positively."

Nutrition

Among respondents from developing nations, many of whom mentioned fear of hunger as a major source of stress in their lives, nutrition was ranked as the most important personal care strategy. Respondents from industrialized countries also cited the importance of nutrition in the context of choosing nutritious food and taking vitamin supplements, often under the guidance of a dietitian.

A balanced diet was a cornerstone of HIV personal care strategies.[4,5] Obtaining sufficient nutrients was intended to help increase energy, bolster the immune system, fight infection, prevent weight loss, and mitigate the side effects of medications. Changes in diet were also sought to alleviate some symptoms of HIV: eating small, frequent meals helps control nausea and loss of appetite; drinking fluids and avoiding milk products may ameliorate the effects of diarrhea; and avoiding raw meat and fish may help prevent some opportunistic infections.

Spirituality

In both industrialized and developing nations, prayer was ranked as the second most important personal care strategy. However, prayer was not often utilized by respondents in Europe or Latin America. Some Latin American respondents expressed anger at the church for stigmatizing people with AIDS and obstructing prevention activities. Several respondents indicated that their diagnosis with HIV increased their religious belief. Spirituality was credited with decreasing fear of death, providing solace, support, and tranquillity, and lifting morale. A few respondents received support from organized religious groups. This took the form of offering prayers, free funeral services, food delivery, and other types of social support. The vast majority of respondents, however, received no support from any organized religious group, and said that their spiritual support came from a personal relationship with God or a higher power. In most cases respondents did not feel safe in sharing information about their HIV status with anyone in their religious community.

Antiviral drugs and other treatments

Respondents from Latin America had much better access to antiviral therapy than respondents from Africa. Many African respondents urged the medical community to make HIV treatments more accessible, and one mentioned a family member who died of AIDS without even an aspirin to relieve her pain. Respondents from Uganda, who received counseling on treatments for opportunistic infections, ranked these treatments as playing an extremely important role in alleviating pain and restoring health. Preventive treatment of opportunistic infections can also affect the length and quality of life of HIV infected people.

Acupuncture, herbal therapies, and traditional healing practices are sometimes used by people with HIV. Chinese herbs, including viola, epimedium, licorice, coptis, prunella, astragalus, and cassia seed have been used in North America.[6] Eleven Chinese herbs have been found to inhibit in vitro HIV replication.[7] However, evidence on the potential effectiveness of these drugs in humans remains anecdotal. Treatment choices among alternative therapies are complicated by the lack of clinical trials and good data. In the absence of this information, HIV-infected people are encouraged to distinguish between anecdotal evidence and data from clinical trials (it is also important to distinguish between data from in vitro [laboratory] trials and in vivo [human clinical] trials), and to develop their own philosophy of treatment.[8]

Work

Survey respondents from developing nations viewed work as a much more important personal care strategy than respondents from industrialized nations. Although some respondents said that work increased stress, many said it provided economic security, made them feel valuable and productive, and helped distract them from worries about HIV.

Activism

Many HIV-infected people who lost their jobs or had to quit work for health reasons found meaning in AIDS activism and volunteer work, which was perceived as a good way to channel feelings of anger and frustration. Those who participated in educational programs where they shared their experience of living with HIV were the most enthusiastic about the positive impact of this work on their health and well-being. A few African respondents who participated in international education through the ICW said that it changed their lives completely and gave them "the strength and will to live." One North American respondent said, "Speaking about my experience of living with HIV is a terrific opportunity to come to terms personally with the disease process, plus make a difference in my community regarding HIV prevention and the reality of HIV in everyone's life."

Stress reduction

Stress reduction was used frequently by respondents from all geographic areas. Stress reduction techniques include, but are not limited to, breathing exercises, relaxation techniques, laughter, visualization, chiropractic therapy, therapeutic touch, and aerobic exercise.

Societal impact on strategy options

Health care resources and a society's attitude towards illness both have an enormous impact on the range of personal care options from which an individual can choose. Often the initial strategy is not decided by the individual but by those who set health policy.

In some communities, HIV testing either is not available, or resources are so limited that testing is reserved for high-priority situations, for example, individuals presenting symptoms or donating blood. Regions where HIV testing is readily available present additional problems, such as people being tested without their knowledge or consent, and results being communicated in ways that cause great anxiety and despair.

A society's attitude towards HIV/AIDS can have a strong impact on an individual's choices. For example, if stigmatization, discrimination, and/or violence are commonplace, infected individuals will be unlikely to disclose their HIV status, which thus limits their access to support systems. In both developing and industrialized nations, fewer than half the survey respondents felt protected against discrimination. Sometimes stigmatization is internalized. Some respondents from the southeast Mediterranean, for example, referred to themselves as "the condemned ones."

Feelings of vulnerability were associated mainly with fear of losing one's job or housing and family rejection. Women were particularly concerned for the well-being of their children. Female respondents from developing nations told of being abandoned after they told their spouse of their HIV status. Married men, however, responded that they had either not informed their wives of their status or were receiving loving support from them. If this phenomenon is widespread, it raises many issues for women, including risk of transmission, access to early intervention, and care-giving needs.

Lack of public information about AIDS and the media's role in creating AIDS hysteria were repeatedly cited as factors that increased personal fragility and anxiety. Some respondents felt that judgmental religious groups added to a climate of discrimination. Health care providers created stress in several ways, such as testing without consent, refusal to treat, and breach of confidentiality, and this also often inhibited individuals from seeking out medical and social support.

On the other hand, respondents cited several major factors that helped them feel safe: support and love from family and friends, interaction with other HIV-positive people, and support from personal physicians and/or AIDS service organizations (ASOs). Elevated social status, economic stability through work, and good health also created a sense of safety. For some respondents from industrialized countries, knowing that ASOs might challenge cases of discrimination made them feel protected, and many also expressed an increased sense of security when ASOs were managed by HIV-positive individuals. Some respondents from the United States felt protected by AIDS legislation, specifically citing the importance of the Americans with Disabilities Act. No respondents from developing nations, however, cited legislation as a factor in reducing their fear of discrimination. Clearly, an individual's choice of personal health care strategies, as well as his or her initial willingness to get tested for HIV, is deeply influenced by such societal factors.

Conclusion: quality of life and long-term survival

One positive trend in the AIDS epidemic is that people are generally surviving longer. Results of a multicenter AIDS cohort study in Los Angeles found that average survival time with AIDS had doubled between 1984 and 1991.[9] In San Francisco, among 562 HIV-positive individuals followed for 14 years, 32 percent had not developed AIDS, and 9 percent were symptom free.[10]

If long-term survival is defined by the criterion of 7 years of HIV infection or 3 years with a diagnosis of AIDS, then 40 percent of the survey respondents (71 percent from industrialized nations and 28 percent from developing countries) are long-term survivors. Those who have survived the longest tended to express positive attitudes, take a more active role in their health care, and have experimented with a wide variety of survival strategies. Most are actively involved in AIDS activities or peer support and feel that they have the support of their family or loved ones. These respondents repeatedly asked that their health care providers listen to what they were saying and treat them with understanding, compassion, and patience. They asked to be seen as individuals, not as cases, and wanted more of a partnership with their provider, encouraging practitioners to offer choices rather than sermons. As one long-term survivor stated, "AIDS is not a death sentence. It's a call to do what you want with your life. Life is valued by its quality and not its quantity. Take each day as it comes and do the best you can. Get as much information as you can and be responsible for your own health. Love yourself, help others with HIV, and don't be ashamed."

References

1. L. A. Clark, *Ancient Art of Color Therapy: Updated, Including Gem Therapy, Auras, and Amulets* (Old Greenwich, CT: Devin Adair, 1975).

2. G. S. Getzel, "Survival Modes for People with AIDS in Groups," *Social Work* 36(1991):7–11.

3. D. Spiegel, "Effects of psychosocial support on patients with metastatic breast cancer," *Journal of Psychosocial Oncology* 10(1992):113–120.

4. J. D. Kaiser, *Immune Power: The Comprehensive Healing Program for HIV* (New York: St. Martin's Press, 1993).

5. L. O'Riordan and P. Paddock, "Whole Body Health," in *HIV: From A to Z: A Self Help Manual*, P. S. Blomberg, et al., eds. (Sacramento, CA: Sacramento AIDS Foundation, 1990).

6. H. Ziolkowski, "Oriental Medicine Takes on AIDS," *East West* (September 1990):59–63.

7. M. Katz, "General principles of HIV infection treatment," presented at the Positive Living for U (PLUS) Seminar, San Francisco, California, February 1994.

8. H. Ziolkowski, "Oriental Medicine Takes on AIDS," *East West* (September 1990):59–63.

9. J. Tighe and T. Simon, "Survival and HIV: Research Update," *HIV Counselor Perspectives* 3(1993):1.

10. *Ibid.*

Shifts in financing of HIV/AIDS care. Unless resources are reallocated to the health sector, complemented by resources made available internationally, developing countries will continue to be unable to finance adequate health services for PWHIV/AIDS. Increases in the need for services are likely to accelerate the shift in financing of care from formal mechanisms, such as public sector health programs and private insurance, to PWHIV/AIDS and their families.

Example 1   Employer health programs and medical aid societies in Africa

Employment-based health and medical programs, such as medical aid societies (MAS), are facing increasing pressure in countries most affected by AIDS. In Zimbabwe the MAS identified 536 AIDS cases in 1993, along with an estimated 19,000 HIV-infected beneficiaries. Claims expenditure for the provisionally identified cases totaled $9.9 million. This level of claims may soon necessitate increases in contribution rates which will make care unaffordable to all but a few or even threaten the viability of the MAS. At the same time, since MAS are only for the employed, the death of an MAS member, unless the spouse is similarly employed, may leave a family entirely without medical coverage.[29]

Example 2   Publicly owned industrial enterprises in Africa

Publicly owned industrial enterprises in Africa are coming under increasing pressure to meet AIDS-related medical costs in their labor force. For example, the Uganda Railway Corporation lost an estimated 10 percent of its 5,600 employees to AIDS over the last several years, and an average of three HIV-infected workers per month seek early retirement with benefits. Annual individual employee medical expenditures for the company have increased from $69 in 1988 to $300 in 1992.[30] It remains uncertain whether state-owned enterprises will address these growing demands by creating special funds to cover future AIDS care costs or by reducing medical coverage to employees, or whether AIDS-related expenses will force severely affected enterprises into bankruptcy.

Example 3   Increase in informal sector employment

Increasing unemployment coupled with increased informal sector employment will result in diminishing employment insurance coverage and increased personal payment for health services. Largely due to the structural adjustment program, unemployment rates in sub-Saharan African urban areas increased from about 10 percent in the 1970s to about 30 percent in the mid-1980s while informal sector employment rose by 6.7 percent for the same period.[31] If this decline in formal sector employment continues, medical care paid directly by individuals will increase in proportion to the net loss of employment-based medical care.

Example 4   Increase in cost recovery programs and user fees

Over the last several years, a number of developing countries have introduced or increased user fees for health services in an attempt to recoup a portion of recurrent costs, expand access to services, or improve their quality. In African countries where user fee policies have been implemented, they have generated an average of about five percent of recurrent annual health care budgets. These charges, while small in absolute amount, may constitute a significant financial burden if considered along with other direct costs borne by PWHIV/AIDS and their families. For example, in Zambia, cost recovery schemes have imposed a nominal weekly fee for hospital patients. This cost, in addition to other expenses such as food and transport for the patient and family, amounted to approximately 31 percent of the total cost of an average hospital admission. One survey found that 64 percent of the patients had difficulty paying the relatively small weekly hospital fee; the cost recovery effort may be placing an undue burden on HIV/AIDS patients and their families who are already coping with the loss of regular employment income.[32]

User fees at urban health centers in Zambia led to an 80 percent decline in patient utilization. In this instance, fees may have been set higher than the local population's ability or willingness to pay, increasing the possibility that users would either bypass health centers altogether in favor of similarly priced care at referral hospitals or forego care entirely.[33]

Increased availability and utilization of antivirals and other medications. In industrialized countries, the cost of HIV/AIDS care will be affected by the growing availability and utilization of antivirals and prophylaxis and treatment for HIV-related illnesses and infections. The net effect of these trends is unclear, as increased expenditure on drugs may be offset by a lower number of hospital admissions or shorter hospitalizations.

Expenditures for HIV/AIDS medications have increased. In the U.S., medications now account for an estimated 14 percent of lifetime HIV/AIDS treatment costs.[34] In France, from 1990 to 1993, the number of PWHIV/AIDS using antivirals increased by more than 180 percent. Total expenditures for antivirals in France increased by almost 90 percent during this period, and 21 percent of France's total AIDS budget in 1993 was allocated for these drugs.[35] This trend is likely to increase as more drugs are developed and approved for use in industrialized countries.

The impact of antivirals and other medications on the cost of HIV/AIDS care in the developing world is not well understood. These costs are expected to be quite limited because of high cost and a lack of the medical infrastructure needed to manage widespread use of these therapies. The need for medications for opportunistic infections will also increase dramatically. Clearly, however, in developing countries their utilization will remain contingent on funding. In Tanzania, for example, average lifetime medication costs per case range from $46 to $102, depending on the level of drug availability.[36]

Improved case management efficiency. A decline in HIV/AIDS–related hospital admissions and lengths of stay (LOS) can result from more efficient case management. In the U.S., care costs per person from AIDS diagnosis to death are declining as a result of decreasing average LOS for PWAIDS and PWHIV—a decline between 1988 and 1991 of over 36 percent and 50 percent, respectively. These decreases are largely attributed to the shift from inpatient hospital care to outpatient care and the increased use of coordinated community-based services for post-discharge support.[37] The decline in the average LOS and hospitalization rates may also reflect increasing confidence of providers as they treat more PWHIV/AIDS. In general, hospitals that treat more PWHIV/AIDS tend to have lower adjusted mortality rates and to use fewer resources, while those with less experience tend to have longer LOS and higher costs (Box 36-2).

BOX 36-2

Caring for persons with AIDS (PWA) in Botswana: Is home-based care the answer?

CHARLES CAMERON, DONALD SHEPARD, AND JOHN MULWA

Botswana has the highest per capita income in sub-Saharan Africa ($2,790 gross domestic product [GDP] per person).[1] Although Botswana was affected by HIV infection later than much of Africa, since 1991, HIV transmission rates have risen rapidly. By June 1994, sentinel surveillance in prenatal clinics found HIV prevalence rates of up to 29 percent. It has been estimated that one in six sexually active people is seropositive nationwide, with higher rates of one in four in Francistown, in the north, and one in three in Gaborone, the capital.

Care provision

The Government of Botswana is trying to answer a difficult policy question: how can the health system address the needs of both the rapidly growing numbers of persons with AIDS (PWAs) and the other health problems of a country just entering the health transition induced by economic development and, concurrently, changing health needs and demands? The public health sector is well developed with an impressive primary health care (PHC) system based on family welfare educators—about 600 minimally trained health workers who are the entry point to the formal health system. The system includes an integrated referral network from the clinic to the district and national reference levels. The well-stocked medical stores provide clinicians with access to a wide array of treatment options. Outpatient departments charge approximately $0.75 for each visit, including drugs. However, many patients receive services free of charge.

Left unchanged, this referral system is expected to flood hospitals with PWAs, a concern validated by experience in Uganda, Zambia and Tanzania. The Government of Botswana wants both to provide a high quality of care for PWAs and to limit hospital-based treatment to those who can most benefit from it. In response, it is actively developing home-based care options which are integrated into the PHC system. The government has developed a prototype home-based model and plans to pilot-test it in two of 14 districts during 1994 and 1995.

The home-based care model

The focus of home-based care (HBC) is at the community level. Family members and friends of PWAs form the foundation of the system. Family welfare educators, in conjunction with clinic-based nurses, provide oversight, clinical support, counseling, and referral to higher levels in the care system. It is essential that PWAs and their care providers be convinced that community-based care provides high quality of care, good access to drugs, and the possibility for referral to hospitals when needed. Otherwise, it is likely that PWAs or their care providers will bypass the HBC program and present themselves at hospitals. Realizing that drugs and other supplies provide a measured level of comfort, nurses in the pilot test will carry a medical kit containing essential drugs (e.g., analgesics, antibiotics, and Nistatin), and supplies of selected items (e.g., a bottle of disinfectant, box of gloves). Drugs for treating tuberculosis (TB) were not included in the kit as the country's existing TB treatment program functions well and alterations might undermine its effectiveness.

Assessing costs and effects

A spreadsheet has been developed to assist the Ministry of Health to identify inputs for care, assess direct costs, and assist in comparing home-based care to conventional, hospital-based alternatives. Based on preliminary data from the major referral hospital, it is estimated that 46 percent of hospital days could be averted. Using data provided by the Ministry of Finance and Development Planning and Ministry of Health for 1991–1992, the spreadsheet was used to project the cost of inpatient care without HBC and a home-based care scenario in 1995. Without HBC, the analysis assumed that 35 percent of PWAs would be hospitalized at least once, and those hospitalized would average one additional hospital admission. Each admission was assumed to last 8.2 days at a cost of $42 per day. This totaled U.S. $628 for one PWA for one year.

Initial results

In the baseline home-based care scenario, it is assumed that a PWA receives care at the community level with biweekly visits during the last year of life (24 total visits, considering staff vacations). The baseline home care program would cost the equivalent of $3.0 million (7.9 million Pula) per year. The savings in hospitalization cost would be $0.6 million. Thus, 21 percent of the cost of home-based care would be averted by fewer hospitalizations, reducing the net cost of the home-based care program to $2.4 million. This is $362 per PWA, or $1.70 per capita—an affordable amount in this growing, upper middle-income country.

The cost analysis is sensitive to a number of assumptions, including the length of inpatient stay, the cost of an inpatient day, the hospitalization rate, and the ability of HBC to avert hospital stays. Alternative scenarios identified the circumstances required for costs of home care to be totally offset by savings in hospital costs, or break-even points. For example, the average interval between visits would have to be increased to 9 weeks, or the program would have to be limited to patients who would have been hospitalized at least once with certainty and would have 2.3 subsequent hospitalizations on average. These results make it unlikely that a home-based care program could be financed entirely from savings in hospital care, but the pilot study will generate actual results.

Qualitative factors

Home-based care program costs can be as high, if not higher, than a strictly hospital-based care program. Nevertheless, development of HBC makes sense for several reasons. It allows PWAs to remain with loved ones for as long as possible, extends the integrated primary health care system, and provides the government with a mechanism to explore and test different treatment options before the number of PWAs grows even larger.

The relative newness of HIV and AIDS has had predictable results: denial, fear, and prejudice in some parts of the population. Potential care providers must be ready, willing, and able to deal with all aspects of care provision. Communities must be prepared to have PWAs live among them. An essential part of Botswana's program will be information, education, and communication efforts for the general population, supplemented with efforts aimed at community-level care providers. At the hospital level, the desire to reduce unnecessary inpatient stays will likely require changes in admitting protocols to use available beds most efficiently. In addition, clinical management guidelines for PWAs will need adjustment to shift treatment to the community level, when possible.

Implementation and evaluation

During the second half of 1994, the Government of Botswana plans to finalize the form of its HBC model. This will be pilot-tested in two districts for up to 1 year and evaluated based on factors such as feasibility, quality of care, acceptability, and sustainability. If warranted by the evaluation, a model (or several models) will be expanded to additional districts. The projections show that while home-based care promises to be useful and affordable, it will not be a panacea. The Ministry of Health is examining additional options to reduce demands on tertiary hospitals, including patient education and transfer systems, and paid community workers to help support patients whose condition would allow home care, but who lack family at home to care for them.

References

1. World Bank, *World Development Report Infrastructure for Development 1994*, Table 1. (New York: Oxford University Press, 1994): Table 1, page 162.

The increased application of clinical guidelines for treatment of HIV/AIDS will also affect patient care costs. Since the late 1980s, guidelines have been developed by WHO and by individual countries to promote cost-effective utilization of health care resources.

Finally, the use of formalized case management systems have contributed significantly to increasing patient management efficiency. Case management involves multidisciplinary teams which coordinate community providers as well as manage patient care to assure appropriate utilization of services (Box 36-3, Box 36-4).

BOX 36-3

The San Francisco care model

INGE B. CORLESS AND MARY PITTMAN

The San Francisco Model provides coordinated care across settings which addresses the physical, psychosocial, financial, and daily living needs of the person with HIV disease. It transcends the boundaries of the traditional health care system, incorporating both traditional and various ancillary and alternative providers of care. The San Francisco Model emerged out of the crisis created by HIV disease. It developed in response to the needs of those affected at a time when little was available to treat the multiple infections and problems confronting the afflicted.

The San Francisco Model is composed of an amalgam of formal institutions and community-based organization, extant services and those developed to meet the emerging needs of the individual, public and private agencies, and professionals and volunteers. Hospitals such as San Francisco General Hospital developed a medical and dedicated AIDS unit. The San Francisco AIDS Foundation and countless other institutions were created as a response to the epidemic. Groups such as Shanti, whose focus was on individuals with terminal illness, primarily cancer, redirected their efforts to meet the needs of persons living with HIV disease.

Boundaries between patient and provider and various institutions were erased and redefined. Indeed, this is what is distinctive about the model. That this was possible may be attributed to several factors. One of the most important was that many of the individuals affected and some of the professional providers of care were from the same community and shared the lifestyle of the infected. In San Francisco, many of the infected were young, well-educated, productive and affluent members of society. Both of these factors fostered concern and a push for action. Lastly, a political infrastructure was in place and functioning to advocate for the interests of gays and lesbians. The infrastructure, like that of numerous service organizations, redirected its focus to encompass the needs posed by the epidemic.

As quickly became apparent, these needs included protection from and response to discrimination, whether on the job, in housing, or in insurance. The development of the role of benefits counselor helped to access financial resources available to individuals with AIDS. Providing money management and home health aides helped keep people with minimal dementia in their homes. Alternative living situations offered a gradation of assistive living to meet the varied dependency needs from acute to chronic to terminal illness. The delivery of meals to the home attended to this vital need. Other activities included the care of pets, particularly during stints of illness or hospitalization, grocery shopping, laundry, and assistance with transportation, particularly to medical appointments. The development of the "Buddy Program" provided volunteers to assist with these activities of daily living. What emerged was a delivery system to meet the needs of the whole person in his or her own setting and on his or her own terms.

Another enhanced role was that of the case manager, extant in hospice programs, who took the lead in coordinating the care of the various professionals and caregivers involved over time and across settings. Together with the activities of volunteers, this enabled individuals to remain in the community. The development of inhalation and infusion therapy services redefined the care that could take place at home and also served to lower the costs of care by adapting to the home.

The motivation of those living with HIV to assume self-responsibility for good nutrition, exercise, and safer sex, and the education which developed around health promotion and maintenance contributed to the well-being and longevity of the infected person and decreased further transmission of infection. Finally, attention was given both to the mental health of the client and that of the provider in order to maintain well-being and prevent burnout.

Does the San Francisco Model still hold in San Francisco and is it applicable to other settings? The answer is yes, if certain conditions met: a safe environment; the presence of a lay caregiver, whether family member, partner, friend, or volunteer; and accessibility to a range of health care and social services. These conditions, particularly the support provided by volunteers, are at risk even in San Francisco, where the ranks of the volunteers have been diminished by illness and death.

The public–private partnership is an aspect of the model which is likely to transcend settings in an era of diminishing resources. This partnership, which brings the community into the tertiary care setting as well as health care into the community, while precipitated by the epidemic, had a strong economic substrate.

As individuals with fewer educational or economic resources are increasingly the affected population, the test of the San Francisco Model will be the willingness of citizens to volunteer to provide services across divisions by economics, ethnicity, race and sexuality. Unless the ethos of volunteerism and the health care provider and consumer coalition are maintained, the San Francisco Model will become a curious artifact in the history of health care innovation.

BOX 36-4

An African model of home-based care (HBC): Zambia

ANNE L. MARTIN, ERIC VAN PRAAG, AND ROLAND MSISKA

In the mid-1980s, the nongovernmental sector in Zambia began to respond to the AIDS health crisis by developing HBC programs. Today, in an effort to bridge the gap between hospital and home, over 40 programs serve over 5,000 PWHIV/AIDS and their families. Recently, six of these programs were studied to measure their direct cost and the impact of HBC.[1]

The need for complementary care or even alternatives to hospital care in Zambia is clear. Projections suggest that although bed capacity will remain constant, there will be at least a 15 percent annual increase in demand for hospital beds for PWHIV/AIDS and a 20 percent annual increase in demand for hospital treatment of HIV-related tuberculosis (TB) and Kaposi's sarcoma over the next decade. Already, in major hospitals, over 50 percent of hospital patients and 70 percent of patients on TB wards are HIV infected, and overall hospital occupancy rates are usually over 90 percent.

Two types of HBC programs were examined in a study by the Swedish International Development Agency (SIDA) and WHO in 1993: hospital-instituted, or "vertical," programs, and community-based, or "horizonatal," programs. Four hospital-initiated outreach programs, or programs which have evolved from hospital-based infrastructures, are being slowly integrated into community activities. These were initially started by hospital staff concerned about the quality of care provided to hospitalized PWHIV/AIDS and the needs expressed by PWHIV/AIDS. Two community-based programs which rely on volunteers with support from community organizations, churches, and health facilities were started by Catholic nuns with donations or small budgets from the Church.

On average, the total annual direct cost (including capital and recurrent costs) to operate an HBC program was U.S. $37,600,* with a more than twofold difference in program cost. The proportion expended on specific services was: home visits (45 percent); health education (23 percent); conferences/meetings (12 percent); counseling in hospital (9 percent); condom distribution (5 percent); partner notification (3 percent); and training (3 percent).

HBC was found to provide a cost-effective complement to hospital care. On average, each home visit costs $2.00 compared with an average cost of a day in hospital of $4.08. More importantly, HBC offers an opportunity to relieve overcrowded hospitals by discharging patients who no longer require acute care. There was a 40 percent reduction in unnecessary hospital care for eligible patients referred to HBC compared to those who were not referred, resulting in a cost savings to the hospital of $840 over 1 year. If all eligible patients in the survey had been referred to HBC, the total days of unnecessary care could have been reduced by 87 percent, at a cost savings to the hospital of $4,450.

A qualitative impact analysis found patient satisfaction to be high. Nearly 90 percent of PWHIV/AIDS and their families preferred HBC to hospital care. A key perceived advantage of HBC was the provision of basic amenities to the patient, and emotional support to both the patient and the family. Over 90 percent of home caregivers reported more understanding of HIV/AIDS, less stigmatization of PWHIV/AIDS, and more knowledge of how to care for a PWHIV/AIDS as a result of HBC. Not surprisingly, 100 percent said they would like to receive HBC if infected with HIV/AIDS.

Four vital lessons have been learned in Zambia:

*All monetary amounts are in U.S. dollars, unless indicated otherwise.

1. There is opportunity for efficiency savings in the design of HBC programs. There are opportunities for efficiency savings and more rational allocation of resources for HBC programs, as suggested by the threefold difference in unit costs among the six HBC programs. Integrating HBC with community resources can lower costs by increasing involvement of existing health providers and community lay persons. Hospital-initiated programs cost on average three times more per patient visit than community-based programs ($3.00 compared with $1.00). This difference is largely due to the cost of transporting mobile teams from hospitals to visit homes of patients. Community-based programs, where care providers usually travel short distances on foot have significantly lower transport costs. This may also influence the quality of care delivered since the community-based home care teams were able to spend three times more time with clients per visit (1.3 hours compared to 30 minutes) than the hospital-based staff, who spent over 75 percent of total home visit time traveling to clients' homes. Emotional support and practical household assistance could especially be achieved through community-based home care. The availability of volunteer and community lay persons also lowered salary costs of community-based programs by over 80 percent.

Lastly, there is an opportunity for cost saving through improved coordination with hospitals. There would be significant cost savings to hospitals if all eligible hospital patients were referred to HBC.

2. There is a vital role for NGO's in the development of HBC and an interdependent relationship between NGO's and government. Nongovernmental organizations, including church medical services, play a critical role in developing HBC services for PWHIV/AIDS. In Zambia, these groups have been responsible for recognizing a critical gap in services and were in an advantageous position to mobilize community as well as government support. The government, which subsidizes to a certain extent many mission hospitals, continues to share many of the less visible recurrent costs of HBC with donor groups and has now developed explicit strategies to promote long-term sustainability of HBC.

3. The challenge of sustaining HBC programs must be faced early on. All the HBC programs currently face critical resource shortfalls either to sustain or to expand their services to meet increasing need. A major challenge will be to improve and sustain home-based care in the context of declining health resources, maintain donor support, and increase government contributions, as well as community commitment, in particular where volunteers are concerned.

The Zambian government has acknowledged the importance of HBC programs and the challenge of their sustainability. The current concern among health officials is how to improve and sustain existing programs which depend on outside donor funding. Efforts are currently underway to implement the decentralization of the health care system towards the districts, which allows planning and support in direct response to local needs with a greater flexibility to coordinate between the governmental and nongovernmental organizations operating at community level, as well as allowing for developing local financing or cost recovery schemes.

Many of the hospital-initiated programs developed with little or no coordination with existing local providers. Thus, local capacity and feeling of ownership for addressing HIV/AIDS care needs has not been strengthened. Other programs have been developing local capabilities through the training of health center staff and community and family members. These programs, which should be promoted, have maximized resources through the integration of HIV/AIDS care services with primary health care, maternal and child health, and tuberculosis programs.

4. Lessons learned for others planning home care. The Zambian study and experience confirmed that the highest priority service need for HBC from the perspective of clients is for domestic support, such as providing food, bedding, and medicines, as well as family emotional support. Can HBC programs provide this assistance? This study concluded that for all models of HBC it would not be possible to sustain this level of support without substantial improvement in logistical support and resource availability. Moreover, the more integrated community-based approaches of HBC, the more likely the sustainability of activities intended to meet the various needs PWAIDS and their families.

References

1. C. M. Chela, R. Msiska, A. Martin, et al., "Costing and evaluating home-based care in Zambia," unpublished report (Geneva: GPA/WHO, 1993).

Health care requirements for groups such as women, infants and children with HIV/AIDS. The increase of HIV/AIDS among women, infants, and children will have a significant impact on the direct cost of health care, as well as on indirect costs to families and communities. Beyond the total cost of care, changes in health service utilization patterns will also occur, placing new demands on health care systems and providers.

To date, there has been little research on the special medical, psychosocial, or welfare needs of infants, children, and women with HIV/AIDS. It is now widely accepted that the HIV/AIDS clinical course and subsequent clinical needs for women with HIV/AIDS differ from those of the adult male population. Also, the complex medical and psychosocial care needs of pregnant women with HIV infection require a range of services that are only beginning to be made available.[38] Women generally have less access to health care than men. For example, in the U.S., women with AIDS utilize $2,295 less inpatient care per year than men with AIDS, they are 5 percent less likely to be hospitalized than men with AIDS, and women injecting drug users (IDUs) with AIDS are 20 percent less likely to be hospitalized than male IDUs with AIDS.[39] Among the reasons cited for this imbalance are a lack of transportation and the absence of child care.[40,41] In the U.S., women with HIV/AIDS are also less likely to be diagnosed rapidly and are more likely to have a health care provider with little HIV knowledge.[42]

Even when women gain access to health services, the care they require may not be available. In the U.S., asymptomatic women are 20 percent less likely to receive AZT than asymptomatic men.[43] Pregnant women with CD4 counts < 200 are less likely to receive *Pneumocystis carinii* pneumonia (PCP) prophylaxis than AZT, even though PCP prophylaxis is considered relatively safe and cost-effective, while the safety of AZT treatment during pregnancy is still unclear.[44]

HIV-infected newborns also have special care needs which may influence survival. HIV-infected newborns typically have lower birth weights (up to 30 percent lower), higher perinatal morbidity and mortality rates, and have higher rates of malnutrition.[45] These conditions, while primarily due to HIV infection, may also reflect environmental factors such as poor prenatal care or poor nutrition. Services directed at these factors may influence infant and child survival.

Conclusion

Medical care cost is only one, albeit important, measure of the impact of HIV/AIDS. The preceding analysis must also be considered in light of the expanding epidemic (Chapter 1). Overall, in the coming decade, the global cost of caring for PWHIV/AIDS will increase at an annual rate exceeding 20 percent.

References

1. F. Hellinger, "Lifetime cost of treating a person with HIV," *Journal of the American Medical Association* 270(1993):474–478.
2. A. Tramarin, et al., "Economic evaluation of home-care assistance for AIDS patients: A pilot study in a town in northern Italy," *AIDS* 6(1992):1377–1383.
3. L. Beresford, "Alternative, outpatient settings of care for people with AIDS," *Quality Review Bulletin* 15(1989):194–199.
4. T. Roach and A. Martin, *Report on Barbados Hostel/Hospice Feasibility Study* (Durham, NC: AIDSTECH/Family Health International, 1992).
5. C. M. Chela, R. Msiska, A. Martin, et al., "Costing and evaluating home-based care in Zambia," unpublished report (Geneva: GPA/WHO, 1993).
6. S. McDonnell, M. Brennan, G. Burnham, D. Tarantola, "Assessing and planning home-based care for persons with AIDS," *Health Policy and Planning* 9(1995):429–437.
7. A. Jorge and R. Cabral, "AIDS in Africa: Can the hospitals cope?" *Health Policy and Planning* 8(1993):157–160.
8. C. Cameron, "The Cost of AIDS Care and Prevention," in: *AIDS in the World*, J. Mann, D. Tarantola, T. Netter, eds., (Cambridge, MA: Harvard University Press, 1992): 477–509.
9. D. Tarantola, M. Mann, C. Mantel, et al., "Projecting the Course of the HIV/AIDS Pandemic and the Cost of Adult AIDS Care in the World", in *Modeling the AIDS Epidemic*, E. Kaplan, M. Brandeau, eds. (New York: Raven Press, 1993):3–27.
10. M. Drummond and L. Davies, eds., "AIDS: The challenge for economic analysis," report of a WHO meeting (Birmingham, U.K.: University of Birmingham, 1989).
11. C. Cameron and J. Shepard, *Resource Allocation Assessment of Swiss AIDS Programme: Final Report*, consultants' report (Geneva: WHO, Global Programme on AIDS, 1990).
12. D. C. Lambert, *Le Coût Mondial du SIDA 1980–2000* (Paris: CNRS Editions, 1992).
13. F. J. Hellinger, "National forecasts of the medical care costs of AIDS: 1988–1992," *Inquiry* 25(1988):469–484.
14. Hellinger, "Lifetime cost."
15. Hellinger, "National forecasts."
16. R. L. Sowell, S. H. Gueldner, et al., "Impact of case management on hospital charges of PWAs in Georgia," *Journal of the Association of Nurses in AIDS Care* 3(April–June 1992).
17. C. A. Rietmeijer, A. J. Davidson, et al., "Cost of care for patients with Human Immunodeficiency Virus Infection," *Archives of Internal Medicine* 153(1993):219–233.
18. Hellinger, "Lifetime cost."
19. L. G. Kaplowitz, I. J. Turshen, P. S. Myers, L. A. Staloch, A. J. Berry, and J. T. Settle, "Medical care cost of patients with acquired immunodeficiency syndrome in Richmond, Va. A quantitative analysis," *Archives of Internal Medicine* 148(1988):1793–1797.
20. T. Kahane, "Hidden cost of AIDS," *World AIDS* 25(1993):7–10.
21. World Bank, *Tanzania AIDS Assessment and Planning Study*, 9825–TA, (Washington, DC: Population and Human Resources Operations Division, Southern Africa Department, World Bank, 1992, hereafter cited as World Bank, *Tanzania AIDS Assessment*).
22. T. Kahane, "Hidden Cost of AIDS," *World AIDS* 25(1993):7–10.

23. J. Broomberg, M. Steinberg, P. Masobe, and G. Behr, "Economic impact of the AIDS epidemic in South Africa," in *AIDS in South Africa: The Demographic and Economic Implications* (Johannesburg, South Africa: Centre for Health Policy, University of Witwatersrand, 1991).

24. S. Forsythe, *Economic Impact of HIV and AIDS in Malawi* (Durham, NC: AIDSTECH/Family Health International, 1992).

25. S. Forsythe, D. Sokal, L. Lux, and T. King, *Assessment of the Economic Impact of AIDS in Kenya* (Arlington, VA: AIDSCAP/Family Health International, 1993).

26. G. Bez, *Soins et SIDA: Les Chiffres Clés* (Paris: Ministère des Affaires Sociales, de la Santé et de la Ville, March 1994).

27. F. Hellinger, "Lifetime cost of treating a person with HIV," *Journal of the American Medical Association* 270(1993):474–478.

28. J. Mann, D. Tarantola, and T. Netter, eds. *AIDS in the World* (Cambridge, MA: Harvard University Press, 1992).

29. R. Hore, "Zimbabwe: Are the costs of AIDS medical care affordable?" *AIDS Analysis Africa* (March/April 1993):6–8.

30. C. Sebunya, "Cost to companies in Uganda," *World AIDS* 25(1993):9.

31. D. Sanders and A. Sambo, "AIDS in Africa: The implications of economic recession and structural adjustment," *Health Policy and Planning* 6(1991):157–165.

32. A. Buve and S. Foster, "What do relatives pay when a patient is admitted to hospital? A study of admissions to a district hospital in Zambia," unpublished (1993).

33. S. Foster, *Cost and Burden of AIDS on the Zambian Health Care System*, (Arlington, VA: John Snow, 1993).

34. Hellinger, "Lifetime cost."

35. G. Bez, *Soins et SIDA: Les Chiffres Clés* (Paris: Ministère des Affaires Sociales, de la Santé et de la Ville, March 1994).

36. World Bank, *Tanzania AIDS Assessment*.

37. National Association of Public Hospitals, *Preserving Access in the Era of Reform: America's Urban Health Safety Net* (Washington, DC: NAPH, 1994).

38. R. Brotman, D. Hutson, F. Suffet, et al., "Childbearing women at risk for HIV infection in New York City: The need for family-oriented comprehensive care," *AIDS and Public Policy Journal* 8(1993):186–193.

39. F. Hellinger, "Use of health services by women with HIV infection," *Health Services Research* 28(1993):543–561.

40. S. Enders, "Issues and implications facing women with HIV," Abstract PO-D03–3523, presented at the IX International Conference on AIDS, Berlin, Germany, June 1993.

41. J. Klapholz, T. Sugden, C. Coleman, et al., "Service needs of HIV symptomatic women," Abstract PO-D03–3532, presented at the IX International Conference on AIDS, Berlin, Germany, June 1993.

42. F. Hellinger, "Health services use by women with HIV," *Journal of the American Medical Association* 270(1993):474–478.

43. *Ibid.*

44. P. Wortley, S. Chu, and K. Farizo, "Use of zidovudine (AZT) and primary prophylaxis for *Pneumocystis carinii* pneumonia (PCP) among pregnant HIV-infected women," Abstract WS-B06-6, presented at the IX International Conference on AIDS, Berlin, Germany, June 1993.

45. C. Canosa, "HIV infection in children," *AIDS Care* 3(1991):303–308.

37

Global Spending on HIV/AIDS Prevention, Care, and Research

Estimating how much is spent on HIV/AIDS prevention and care in any country and at the global level poses an enormous challenge. Studies of public spending on AIDS often focus on the cost of medical care and rarely consider prevention spending except for central government expenditures. In the absence of clear information on funding of prevention and care, some researchers suggest that spending on prevention and care represents only a small fraction of overall health expenditures; others claim that this spending adds a tremendous burden onto already strained national budgets; and still others propose that a significant impact on the pandemic could be achieved with global investment of a relatively modest amount of resources (see Box 37-1).

BOX 37-1

The cost of HIV prevention

J. BROOMBERG AND D. SCHOPPER

Despite widespread implementation of a broad range of HIV prevention strategies and programs in the last decade, economic evaluation of these activities remains limited. While cost-effectiveness data would be most useful for efficient resource allocation, cost data alone provide vital information for planning and program management. A study recently commissioned by WHO's Global Programme on AIDS and conducted by the Health Economics and Financing Programme of the London School of Hygiene and Tropical Medicine, used a case study approach to examine the costs of current intervention programs representing six broad HIV prevention strategies in developing countries.[1] The strategies chosen for study were: promotion of safer sexual behaviors through mass media and through person-to-person education; provision of condoms through social marketing; provision of sexually transmitted infection (STI) treatment and prevention services; prevention of unsafe drug use practices among injecting drug users; and provision of safe blood for transfusion. Case studies were selected on the basis of availability of cost and output data and potential generalizability. Cost data were obtained from published studies or directly frorn program personnel. Only costs incurred by the providing agency were considered; other costs such as donated goods and services and costs borne by users were omitted. All costs were converted to U.S. dollars in the year incurred and converted to 1990 U.S. dollars.

As would be expected, the results show wide variability (both in unit costs and in the relationship between capital and recurrent costs) between case studies of the same intervention strategy and between strategies. Nevertheless, important patterns can be detected. The per capita costs of the mass media programs studied range from $0.06 to $0.32, which may be attributable to a combination of economies of scale as well as to significant variations in local cost structures. Unit costs of person-to-person strategies are predictably higher than those for mass media, and show similar variability, with costs per contact ranging from $0.47 to $1.89 and costs per condom distributed ranging from $0.10 to $0.70. In this case, factors influencing costs include the total numbers of individuals targeted by the strategy, as well as the accessibility of target groups. The costs per condom sold in a wide range of condom social marketing programs indicate a progressive decrease in unit costs over time which begins to level off about 3–5 years after the start of the program and is primarily due to increasing numbers of condoms sold as programs mature. There was also a variability in costs between programs of a similar age, which may be due to market size, as well as to the sources and costs of condom procurement. The unit costs of STI services depend on whether these are integrated into existing primary health care infrastructures or are targeted at specific risk groups. In the former case, costs per visit in two case studies (in South Africa and Mozambique) were both approximately $10, while the cost for a targeted intervention in Kenya was $50, reflecting the much smaller target population and hence, lower usage of services. Costs per client contact in programs aimed at intravenous drug users ranged from $2.25 to $12.59, with the variation attributable mainly to the length of operation of the project and hence, the number of clients recruited. The costs of ensuring a safe blood supply vary between $34.50 to $51.60 per blood unit. These estimates depend upon and include both the costs of ensuring general blood safety and the specific, additional costs of ensuring HIV safety, which would include counseling, HIV testing materials, additional laboratory overheads, and the costs of replacing blood discarded because of a positive test.

Based on these data, the global resources required to implement a mix of all six strategies in all developing countries were estimated to be between $1.5 billion and $2.9 billion per year. Low and high cost assumptions are based on different levels of STI incidence and condom needs. Only about 15 percent of the global resources would be required in Africa, whereas more than half would be spent in Asia. This difference is due to the larger population size in Asia and the higher income level as compared to Africa.

As shown in Figure 37-1.1, condom social marketing and STI treatment are the major contributors to total cost. This is due to the fact that these two interventions provide services to the general population. In contrast, blood safety programs and needle exchange or bleach provision programs, for example, are targeted at a much smaller subset of the total population and thus contribute little to total costs.

These results should be interpreted with caution, since they were derived from a small sample of case studies from which generalizations may be limited and because the reported cost data were difficult to validate in some cases. In addition, using official exchange rates to translate local costs into U.S. dollars may have under- or overestimated the real value of inputs, especially labor, in developing countries. Nevertheless, this analysis provides a preliminary insight into the financial costs and outputs of a sample of HIV prevention strategies, indicating relevant relationships between costs and various factors that should be of use to all parties involved in the planning and budgeting of HIV prevention activities. This analysis is also important in that it shows the need for an expanded database of program costs that would overcome several of the limitations of these data.

A review of national expenditures on HIV prevention in a sample of countries from Asia, Africa, and Latin America suggests that approximately $120 million were spent on HIV prevention in developing countries in 1992, or 10–20 times less than the estimated global resource requirements. This resource gap should be viewed in the context of very little having been spent to date in Asia, where most of the

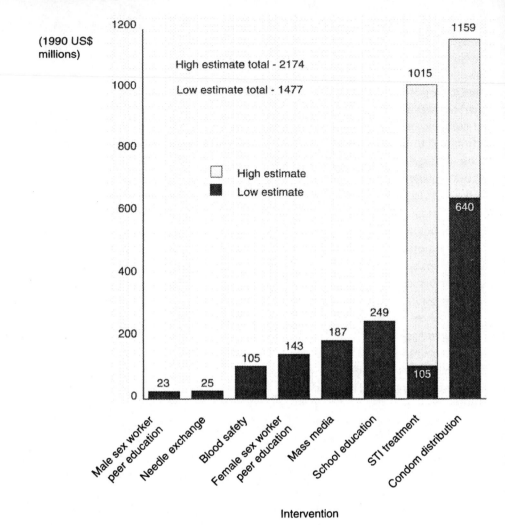

(1990 US$ millions)

High estimate total - 2174

Low estimate total - 1477

☐ High estimate
■ Low estimate

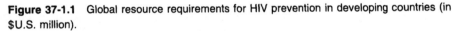

Intervention

Figure 37-1.1   Global resource requirements for HIV prevention in developing countries (in $U.S. million).

world's population lives. The gap will only be closed if the costs are shared among a multitude of partners. International donors must strengthen their contribution to the worldwide control of the spread of AIDS. National governments need to assume greater leadership and financial responsibility for HIV prevention. The corporate sector has at least a threefold interest in investing to reduce the spread of HIV among its workers, namely, to retain a maximally productive work force, to reduce health care costs, and to ensure a strong market for its products. And finally, individuals worldwide who are able to pay must also be willing to pay for certain commodities such as condoms and STI drugs. Ultimately, the absence of common output or effectiveness measures renders rigorous comparisons between different strategies, and hence efficient resource allocation, impossible. Cost-effectiveness analysis must therefore be regarded as an urgent research priority.

References

1. WHO, Global Programme on AIDS, *Costs of HIV Prevention Strategies in Developing Countries*, WHO/GPA/DIR/93.2 (Geneva: WHO, 1993).

In an attempt to provide reference points for this discussion, *AIDS in the World II* has developed crude estimates of global spending on HIV/AIDS prevention, care, and research. These estimates were derived from a survey of government national AIDS programs (GNAP) which collected data on resources *spent* by GNAPs in a fiscal year, circa 1993. No country can account for all AIDS expenditures incurred within the country (which would include expenditures from central, regional, and local government sources as well as NGO, private, and personal out-of-pocket spending). Therefore, the GNAPs were asked to provide information on GNAP expenditures and to estimate the proportion that this represented of overall prevention, care, and research expenditures in their country. Information of sufficient completeness was obtained from 73 countries (see Appendix C). The analysis proceeded as follows:

1. GNAP expenditures were divided into three elements: prevention (including program management), care (including laboratory costs), and research. Responses from GNAPs from sub-Saharan Africa and for Southeast Asia and Oceania were particularly complete and useful (see Tables 37-1 and 37-2).
2. For each element, respondents indicated the proportion of total spending which they believed was accounted for by GNAP expenditures. These proportions were expressed in quartiles (i.e., 1–25 percent; 26–50 percent, 51–75 percent, and 76–100 percent). The extrapolation from GNAP's own spending to overall national spending therefore provided a low figure (the lower end of the quartile selected) and a high figure (the upper end of the quartile).
3. Low and high estimates in each country were divided by the adult population (ages 15–49) to obtain low and high per-capita spending in prevention, care, and research.
4. Information available from responding countries was extrapolated to the whole GAA to which they belong. However, for the purpose of this study, countries were categorized within their GAA, based on the level of their economy as defined in the 1994 *World Bank Atlas.*[1]
5. Low and high per-capita figures were then applied to each country population by category of economy and by GAA (see Table 37-3).
6. As no data were available for two countries with large populations— China and India—very conservative figures were applied to prevention expenditures and even lower figures for care, given the recency of HIV spread in these countries.
7. The average of low estimates and high estimates were then considered as the "best estimates" for each grouping of countries and each program element.
8. Finally, totals for prevention, care, and research were assembled for countries and divided into high economies, low economies, and for the world.

The results of the above analysis are summarized in Table 37-4.

Table 37-1 Expenditures on AIDS by governmental national AIDS programs (GNAP) in selected sub-Saharan African countries, one fiscal year, circa 1993, as reported by government AIDS programs

Countries by economy[a]	Total $/yr	Per capita	GNAP management	GNAP prevention	GNAP laboratory and care	GNAP support to other organizations	GNAP research
				GNAP spending ($U.S.)[b]			
Upper middle–income economies							
Botswana	1,822,210	1.34	247,821 (14%)	1,415,857 (78%)	63,777 (4%)	0 (0%)	94,755 (5%)
Gabon	3,559,220	2.96	954,939 (27%)	8,542 (0%)	2,595,739 (73%)	0 (0%)	0 (0%)
Mauritius	255,780	0.23	179,046 (70%)	51,156 (20%)	22,509 (9%)	2,558 (1%)	512 (0%)
Seychelles	84,790	1.23	21,198 (25%)	42,395 (50%)	21,198 (25%)	0 (0%)	0 (0%)
Lower middle–income economies							
Angola	577,720	0.06	109,536 (19%)	132,587 (23%)	318,324 (55%)	0 (0%)	17,274 (3%)
Cameroon	3,632,430	0.30	726,486 (20%)	1,997,837 (55%)	181,622 (5%)	363,243 (10%)	363,243 (10%)
Senegal	1,593,330	0.20	366,466 (23%)	764,798 (48%)	159,333 (10%)	239,000 (15%)	63,733 (4%)
Low–income economies							
Benin	647,070	0.13	258,828 (40%)	194,121 (30%)	97,061 (15%)	64,707 (10%)	32,354 (5%)
Burkino Faso	1,383,780	0.15	553,235 (40%)	775,470 (56%)	0 (0%)	2,768 (0%)	52,307 (4%)

Chad	676,210	0.11	236,674 (35%)	371,916 (55%)	67,621 (10%)	0 (0%)	0 (0%)
Comoros	154,000	0.30	30,800 (20%)	69,300 (45%)	53,900 (35%)	0 (0%)	0 (0%)
Côte d'Ivoire	2,725,630	0.21	545,126 (20%)	1,635,378 (60%)	163,538 (6%)	272,563 (10%)	109,025 (4%)
Ghana	1,406,710	0.09	211,007 (15%)	773,691 (55%)	351,678 (25%)	42,201 (3%)	28,134 (2%)
Guinea	240,000	0.04	72,000 (30%)	72,000 (30%)	24,000 (10%)	72,000 (30%)	0 (0%)
Guinea-Bissau	60,000	0.06	—	—	—	—	—
Lesotho	480,800	0.26	134,624 (28%)	192,320 (40%)	57,696 (12%)	96,160 (20%)	0 (0%)
Madagascar	541,370	0.04	92,033 (17%)	124,515 (23%)	297,754 (55%)	0 (0%)	27,069 (5%)
Mali	2,409,000	0.27	240,900 (10%)	1,445,400 (60%)	481,800 (20%)	192,720 (8%)	48,180 (2%)
Mauritania	356,840	0.17	214,104 (60%)	17,842 (5%)	124,894 (35%)	0 (0%)	0 (0%)
Rwanda	44,340	0.01	—	—	—	—	—
Tanzania	2,055,830	0.08	863,449 (42%)	616,749 (30%)	431,724 (21%)	102,792 (5%)	41,117 (2%)
Togo	876,880	0.22	175,376 (20%)	350,752 (40%)	175,376 (20%)	175,376 (20%)	0 (0%)
Uganda	893,930	0.05	178,786 (20%)	402,269 (45%)	250,300 (28%)	17,879 (2%)	44,697 (5%)
Zaire	606,680	0.02	254,806 (42%)	91,002 (15%)	97,069 (16%)	155,310 (26%)	8,494 (1%)
Zambia	2,350,000	0.27	470,000 (20%)	822,500 (35%)	1,057,500 (45%)	0 (0%)	0 (0%)

ᵃCountries have been divided into economies following the structure used by the International Bank for Reconstruction and Development as published in The World Bank Atlas, 1994.

ᵇFigures may not add up in every row because of rounding to nearest thousand above 1,000.

Source: AIDS in the World II survey.

Table 37-2 Expenditures on AIDS by governmental national AIDS programs (GNAP) in selected Asian and Pacific countries, one fiscal year, circa 1993, as reported by government AIDS programs

Large/medium-sized countries[a]	Total $	Per capita	GNAP spending ($U.S.)[b]				
			GNAP management	GNAP prevention	GNAP laboratory and care	GNAP support for other organizations	GNAP research
ASIAN COUNTRIES							
High-income economies							
Japan	98,398,000	0.79	0 (0%)	32,471,000 (33%)	19,680,000 (20%)	0 (0%)	46,247,000 (47%)
Australia	62,658,000	3.52	3,759,000 (6%)	8,772,000 (14%)	38,848,000 (62%)	3,759,000 (6%)	7,519,000 (12%)
New Zealand	2,492,000	0.72	—	—	—	—	—
Middle-income economies (upper-middle and lower-middle)							
Malaysia	8,889,000	0.47	711,000 (8%)	1,778,000 (20%)	5,867,000 (66%)	89,000 (1%)	444,000 (5%)
Thailand	56,000,000	0.97	1,120,000 (2%)	8,400,000 (15%)	43,120,000 (77%)	2,240,000 (4%)	1,120,000 (2%)
Low-income economies							
India	20,266,000	0.02	—	—	—	—	—
Nepal	354,000	0.02	46,000 (13%)	142,000 (40%)	106,000 (30%)	53,000 (15%)	7,000 (2%)
Bhutan	246,000	0.16	41,000 (17%)	145,000 (59%)	53,000 (22%)	7,000 (3%)	0 (0%)

PACIFIC ISLAND COUNTRIES

Upper-middle-income economies						
Guam	170,000	1.10	136,000 (80%)	8,500 (5%)	25,500 (15%)	0 (0%)	0 (0%)
Lower-middle-income economies						
Fiji	54,000	0.07	7,000 (13%)	31,000 (57%)	13,000 (24%)	3,000 (6%)	0 (0%)
Western Samoa	375,000	2.30	94,000 (25%)	131,000 (35%)	113,000 (30%)	19,000 (5%)	19,000 (5%)
Vanuatu	71,000	0.45	11,000 (15%)	57,000 (80%)	4,000 (5%)	0 (0%)	0 (0%)
Micronesia, Fed. State of	58,000	0.52	9,000 (15%)	29,000 (50%)	12,000 (20%)	9,000 (15%)	0 (0%)
Kiribati	12,000	0.15	2,000 (17%)	3,000 (28%)	3,000 (28%)	3,000 (22%)	< 1,000 (6%)
Cook Islands	30,000	1.74	6,000 (20%)	12,000 (40%)	9,000 (30%)	3,000 (10%)	0 (0%)
Tuvalu	2,000	0.20	< 1,000 (20%)	1,000 (60%)	< 1,000 (10%)	0 (0%)	< 1,000 (10%)
Niue	3,000	1.50	3,000 (85%)	< 1,000 (10%)	< 1,000 (5%)	0 (0%)	0 (0%)

[a]Countries have been divided into economies following the structure used by the International Bank for Reconstruction and Development as published in *The World Bank Atlas*, 1994.

[b]Figures may not add up in every row because of rounding to nearest thousand above 1,000.

Source: *AIDS in the World II* survey.

Table 37-3 Estimated annual per capita spending ($U.S.) on HIV/AIDS prevention, care, and research, by level of economy and by GAA, circa 1993*

Economy[a]	N	GAA	Country	Per capita GNAP spending	1992 pop. (× 1000) per economy	Low per capita: prevention	High per capita: prevention	Low per capita: care	High per capita: care	Low per capita: research	High per capita: research
High	1	1	North America	20.75	283,258	$1.87	$2.46	$13.90	$18.29	$4.98	$6.55
High	11	2	Western Europe	0.47	360,939	0.25	$0.38	$0.19	$4.39	$0.12	$0.50
Upper-middle	2	2	Western Europe	0.19	20,460	$0.13	$0.26	$0.01	$1.15	$0.09	$0.18
Low-middle	1	2	Western Europe	0.12	360	$0.10	$0.13	($0.01)	($1.15)	($0.09)	($0.18)
High	2	3	Oceania	3.11	21,162	$2.86	$71.45	$4.43	$8.52	$1.71	$42.87
Upper-middle	1	3	Oceania	(0.48)	364	($0.29)	($0.42)	($0.48)	($11.97)	($0.46)	($11.57)
Low-middle	4	3	Oceania	0.48	5,897	$0.29	$0.42	$0.48	$11.97	$0.46	$11.57
Upper-middle	7	4	Latin America	0.06	309,519	$0.02	$0.03	$0.03	$0.42	$0.03	$0.72
Low-middle	6	4	Latin America	0.06	99,831	$0.05	$0.08	$0.05	$1.35	$0.02	$0.52
Low	4	4	Latin America	(0.06)	10,140	($0.05)	($0.08)	($0.05)	($1.35)	($0.02)	($0.52)
Upper-middle	4	5	Sub-Saharan Africa	1.53	4,419	$0.58	$2.20	$2.88	$71.93	$0.05	$0.10
Low-middle	3	5	Sub-Saharan Africa	0.19	75,256	$0.21	$0.79	$0.04	$0.64	$0.05	$1.28
Low	17	5	Sub-Saharan Africa	0.09	464,239	$0.07	$0.44	$0.05	$0.70	$0.01	$0.05
High	1	6	Caribbean	(0.46)	454	($1.04)	($1.90)	($1.43)	($35.71)	($0.30)	($7.55)
Upper-middle	4	6	Caribbean	0.46	6,411	$1.04	$1.90	$1.43	$35.71	$0.30	$7.55
Low-middle	3	6	Caribbean	0.28	20,840	$0.10	$0.51	$0.15	$3.75	$0.01	$0.04

				GNAP	Pop. (×1000)	Low per capita	High per capita				
Low		6	Caribbean	(0.28)	6,715	($0.10)	($0.51)	($0.15)	($3.75)	($0.01)	($0.04)
Upper-middle	2	7	Eastern Europe	0.14	24,119	$0.05	$0.26	$0.07	$0.13	$0.01	$0.37
Lower-middle	6	7	Eastern Europe	0.04	381,259	$0.01	$0.17	$0.04	$0.25	$0.00	$0.03
Low		7	Eastern Europe	(0.04)	10,017	($0.01)	($0.17)	($0.04)	($0.25)	($0.00)	($0.03)
High	2	8	SE Mediterranean	0.52	9,237	$0.09	$0.12	$0.99	$20.70	$0.12	$0.16
Upper-middle	1	8	SE Mediterranean	0.19	22,429	$0.13	$0.25	$0.30	$7.48	($0.12)	($0.16)
Lower-middle	4	8	SE Mediterranean	0.05	219,165	$0.02	$0.02	$0.04	$0.53	$0.01	$0.16
Low		8	SE Mediterranean	(0.05)	208,838	($0.02)	($0.02)	($0.04)	($0.53)	($0.01)	($0.16)
High	1	9	Northeast Asia	0.79	150,123	$0.26[a]	$0.34[a]	$0.16[b]	$0.21[b]	$0.37[b]	$0.49[b]
Upper-middle		9	Northeast Asia	(0.79)	44,150	($0.26)	($0.34)	($0.16)	($0.21)	($0.37)	($0.49)
Lower-middle		9	Northeast Asia	(0.16)	24,925	($0.10)	($0.13)	($0.04)	($0.05)		
Low	1	9	Northeast Asia	0.16	1,250,260	$0.10	$0.13	$0.04	$0.05		
High		10	Southeast Asia	(0.48)	3,087	($0.40)	($10.03)	($0.63)	($1.21)	($0.10)	($2.39)
Upper-middle	1	10	Southeast Asia	0.48	18,610	$0.40	$10.03	$0.63	$1.21	$0.10	$2.39
Lower-middle		10	Southeast Asia	(0.02)	122,179	($0.01)	($0.01)	($0.03)	($0.69)		
Low	2	10	Southeast Asia	0.02	1,261,813	$0.01[c]	$0.01[c]	$0.03[c]	$0.69[c]		

*Per capita GNAP: per capita overall spending on HIV/AIDS prevention, care, and research; 1992 pop. (× 1000) per economy: 1992 population in aggregates of countries according to their level of economy; low per capita/high per capita: lowest and highest value of the range of per-capita spending; parentheses indicate value assigned from neighboring GAA economic index category.

[a]Levels of economy follow structure as used in *World Bank Development Report*, 1994.
[b]Japan's government was assumed to fund 75%–100% of AIDS activities to derive these estimates.
[c]India's financial data come from both the survey and from the publication *National AIDS Control Programme*, Government of India, New Delhi, India, April 1993.

Table 37–4 Cost of HIV/AIDS prevention, care, and research, circa 1993 in high economy and low economy countries*

	People (thousands)			Costs (thousands $U.S.)				
	Total 1992 population	Cumulative HIV as of January 1, 1994	Cumulative AIDS as of January 1, 1994	Prevention	Care	Prevention and care	Research	Prevention, care, and research
High economies	1,278,741	1,826	457	2,206,922	10,875,615	13,082,537	3,886,239	16,968,777
(% of world total)	(24%)	(8%)	(7%)	(86%)	(94%)	(92%)	(93%)	(92%)
Low economies	4,161,734	20,374	6,385	353,107	738,099	1,091,206	303,483	1,394,689
(% of world total)	(76%)	(92%)	(93%)	(14%)	(6%)	(8%)	(7%)	(8%)
World total	5,440,475	22,200	6,842	2,560,029	11,613,715	14,173,744	4,189,722	18,363,466

*Countries have been divided into economies following the structure used by the International Bank for Reconstruction and Development: high- and upper-middle (GNP per capita over $2,695) income economies are combined into the category "high economies," and low- and lower-middle-income economies into the category "low economies."
Sources: Global AIDS Policy Coalition; *AIDS in the World II* survey.

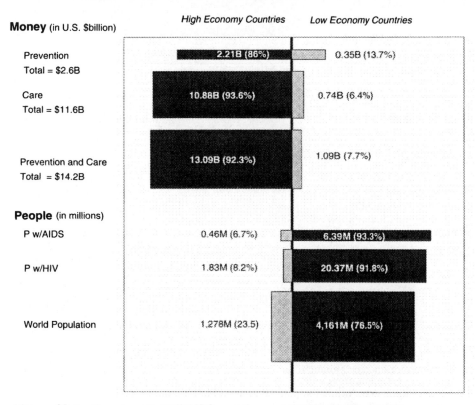

Figure 37-1   People with HIV/AIDS and the cost of HIV/AIDS prevention and care in high- and low-economy countries: the world disparity, circa 1993.

Estimated spending on HIV prevention

The annual per capita expenditure for HIV *prevention* varied from $ 0.02 to 0.09 per person and per year in Latin America, to $ 0.25 to 2.46 in high economy countries of North America and Western Europe. Worldwide, as shown in Table 37-4, $2.6 billion was estimated to have been spent on HIV prevention; 86 percent of these funds were spent in high economy countries.

Estimated spending on HIV/AIDS care

The global expenditure on HIV/AIDS *care*, circa 1993, was estimated at $11.6 billion; 94 percent of this expenditure occurred in high economy countries (Table 37-4). This estimate was consistent with the data in Chapter 36, which estimated the annual global cost of care for HIV/AIDS in adults at $9.5 billion, circa 1993.

Total expenditures for HIV/AIDS *prevention and care* were therefore estimated at $14.2 billion, of which less than 8 percent was spent in low economy countries, which contain more than three-quarters of the world's population and, in 1993, approximately 92 percent of the world's people with HIV and about 93 percent of the world's people with AIDS (Figure 37-1).

Spending on HIV/AIDS research

The study estimated that in the year circa 1993, $4.2 billion had been spent worldwide on HIV/AIDS–related *research* (Table 37-4). High economy coun-

Table 37-5   Estimated spending on HIV/AIDS care, prevention, and research in comparison with gross development product (GDP), health expenditures, and military expenditures in high and low economies, circa 1993 (in $U.S. billions)

	High economies	Low economies[a]	World
GDP, 1993[b]	18,247.5	4,865.0	23,112.6
Spending on HIV/AIDS care and prevention	13.1	1.1	14.2
Total expenditure on health (as percentage of GDP, 1991)[c]	9.40	4.20	8.60
Estimated total spent on health (1991)	1,715.2	204.3	1,919.5
Spending on HIV/AIDS care, prevention, and research	17.0	1.4	18.4
Spending on HIV/AIDS prevention, care, and research[c] (as percentage of total health expenditures)	0.99	0.69	0.96
Spending on military expenditures (as percentage of GDP, 1991)[d]	3.40	3.50	3.40
Estimated total spent on military expenditures (1991)	620	170	790
Spending on HIV/AIDS prevention, care, and research (as percentage of total military expenditures)	2.70	0.82	2.32
Spending on HIV/AIDS prevention, care, and research (as percentage of GDP)	0.09	0.03	0.08

[a]Includes medium-high and medium-low economies.
[b]*World Bank Development Report*, Table 3, p. 186. The World Bank.
[c]*Human Development Report*, United Nations Development Programs, 1994, p. 191. In this report, countries are not categorized as economies but as industrial and developing countries.
[d]*Human Development Report*, United Nations Development Programs, 1994, p. 171.

tries accounted for $3.9 billion (93 percent) of this global expenditure and Low Economy countries for $300 million (7 percent).

Summary

Global spending on HIV/AIDS prevention, care, and research totaled $18.4 billion in 1993, of which $17 billion (92 percent) was spent in high economy countries and $1.4 billion (8 percent) was spent in low economy countries, respectively. On average, worldwide, nearly $5 was spent for HIV/AIDS care for every $1 spent for HIV prevention. Globally, for every $1,000 of gross development product, less than $1 had been spent on HIV/AIDS in 1993. Total estimated expenditures on HIV/AIDS prevention, care and, research represented less than 1 percent of overall health expenditures, both in high and low economies (Table 37-5). They represented 2.7% of military expenditures in high economy countries and less than 1 percent of military expenditures in low economy countries.

REFERENCES

1. World Bank, *World Bank Atlas 1994* (Washington, DC: World Bank, December 1993):17–24.

PART V

FROM EPIDEMIOLOGY
TO VULNERABILITY
TO HUMAN RIGHTS

Since 1981, in the effort to prevent and control the pandemic of HIV/AIDS, we have all been learning. Who among us has not seen personal preconceptions challenged? Who has not changed views, who has not also been changed in the process? In the first four parts of this book, we have summarized the current status of the dynamic epidemic, the frontiers of scientific progress, the experience of different population groups, and the responses of organizations—national, nongovernmental, private sector, and intergovernmental—as they face the pandemic and its growing impact.

A central theme emerges within each of these areas: that HIV prevention will require efforts at individual, community, and societal levels. Only a combination of all three will be sufficiently powerful to combat the pandemic. For individual capacity, whether involving people trying to change risky behaviors or scientists seeking research support, is strongly influenced and sometimes dominated by the community and societal context. Further, whether designing a community prevention and care program or directing a national AIDS effort, the societal ecology determines, to a substantial extent, the range of the feasible.

Yet while public health can draw on its traditions to suggest how to work at the individual level, or even the community level, there is little public health experience sufficiently relevant and powerful to guide us as we seek to translate awareness of the societal dimensions into concrete action. Therefore, in this final part of the book, the tone of *AIDS in the World II* changes. For in Part V we present a proposal, which is conceptually coherent, practical, and pragmatic, for making progress on the central issue for the future of HIV prevention and care: how do we address—directly, concretely, coherently—the societal dimension? To construct this proposal, we proceed through four steps.

- First, we review the pathway leading to recognition of the need to work at a societal level (Chapter 38).
- Second, we review the concept of vulnerability and how its personal and programmatic dimensions have been applied (Chapter 39).

- Third, we explore how the societal level of vulnerability has thus far been understood and acted upon (Chapter 40).
- Fourth, we present and develop a new approach to societal vulnerability, based on a human rights framework for societal analysis and pragmatic response (Chapter 41).

38

The History of Discovery and Response

The understanding of, and response to, HIV/AIDS has proceeded along two independent yet related tracks.[1] One track is biomedical, through which modern science has identified HIV, delved ever deeper into the mechanisms of its action and the human immune response, and led toward therapeutic and preventive technologies.[2] The second track centers on individual and collective human behavior to develop and improve the capacity to prevent HIV transmission.

Just as biomedical progress has involved a sometimes gradual, sometimes exhilirating, yet continuous, process of discovery, the public health perspective on human behavior, which is central to designing HIV prevention and care efforts, has evolved through successive and recognizable stages. Each step, building upon earlier efforts and using new knowledge and experience, has resulted in substantial changes in HIV prevention strategies.

Three periods can be identified in this history of response to the challenge of HIV. They are briefly outlined and then explored in more detail.

The period of discovery

The period of discovery (1981–84) started with the recognition of the new clinical entity. Epidemiological studies then provided descriptive information, discovered routes of spread, and identified behaviors associated with increased risk of HIV infection. Public health efforts focused on providing information about risk behaviors to stimulate individual behavior change (e.g., messages to reduce the number of sexual partners or to use condoms) (Fig. 38-1).

The period of early response

During the period of early response (1985–88), individual risk reduction became codified as the central goal, which was supported by certain health and, to a lesser extent, social services. These services constituted the essential purpose of national AIDS programs, whose creation was fostered by the

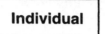

Figure 38-1 Early 1980s: risk reduction strategy, focus on the individual.

World Health Organization's Global Program on AIDS (WHO/GPA). In addition, as part of its Global AIDS Strategy, WHO/GPA articulated a three-part program for risk reduction.[3,4] The three basic elements were information and education, health and social services (e.g., testing and counseling, condoms, needle exchange), and nondiscrimination towards HIV-infected people and people with AIDS. Prevention messages during this period were primarily targeted at people (presumed) uninfected, and many institutions, large and small, acted as if prevention and care were distinct, programatically separate, activities.

The current period

The current period (1989 to the present) is beginning to extend and deepen its approach by adding a societal dimension to the risk reduction approach. The concept of vulnerability has been central to this effort. As described in *AIDS in the World* (1992), vulnerability focuses on constraints and barriers to individual control over health.[5] In addition, there is an increasing understanding of the connection between care and support for people with HIV, and efforts to decrease the spread of the epidemic. Vulnerability analysis requires consideration of the political, social, cultural, and economic influences on decision-making, behavior, and health. Therefore, this period witnessed the beginning of a shift from a nearly exclusive focus on individual risk reduction towards an increasing concern with societal issues. This expanded combination of risk and vulnerability reduction has become the strategic basis for the new UNAIDS program (Box 34-1).[6]

This sequence of discovery, from the message dissemination of basic information, to individual risk reduction, and more recently, to vulnerability reduction, represents real progress in analysis of and the capacity for response. For each level of analysis is useful and each builds upon and goes beyond the previous approach.

The period of discovery (1981–84)

Epidemiology has been an extremely powerful tool for understanding the dynamics of HIV transmission. Epidemiological studies rapidly identified the modes of HIV transmission (even before the virus was discovered!) and the specific behaviors associated with increased risk of HIV spread. In this context, risk involves the statistical probability of becoming HIV infected through specific behaviors (e.g., intercourse without a condom) and patterns of behavior (e.g., multiple sexual partners), or in specific situations (e.g., one sexual partner has multiple partners, but does not tell this to his or her regular partner).[7] It is important to emphasize that because epidemiological analysis involves collecting information from individuals and seeking associations between behaviors and the likelihood of HIV infection, its ability to identify or examine broader, contextual issues (i.e., social attitudes towards sexuality, or gender relations) is limited (Chapter 9).

Epidemiological analysis can also identify those populations among whom HIV is more, or less, concentrated at any point in time. For example, HIV infection among sex workers or injection drug users may be relatively high; or, among men and women donating blood, it may be noted that HIV prevalence peaks at 15–24 years of age for women and 25–34 years of age for men (Chapter 3). The usefulness and practical applications of these kinds of data are obvious: epidemiology provides the fundamental basis for rational interventions that are designed to break the chains of transmission. Yet we must not lose sight of the fact that the methods of epidemiology have predetermined that our understanding of "risk" will be focused on individual behavior (Box 38-1).

BOX 38-1

"Risk groups" or "risk behaviors?"

SIMON WATNEY

Epidemiologists use the term *risk groups* to refer to defined groups at demonstrably increased risk from particular medical conditions, compared to the rest of the population. Thus, smokers may be described as a "risk group" in relation to lung cancer. Risk groups may be defined in relation to many different types of *risk factors,* such as environmental or occupational factors associated with specific patterns of illness. Further, those at highest statistical risk are sometimes referred to as *high-risk groups.*

While epidemiology has often been sensitive to certain social factors such as class, gender, and race in relation to differing patterns of health and illness, it has generally lacked a strong awareness of homosexuality as a ground for social identity and organization. In the early stages of the AIDS epidemic, it was apparent to epidemiologists that gay and bisexual men were greatly disproportionately affected. Accordingly, they were described as a "risk group" for AIDS, together with other disproportionately affected people, including hemophiliacs and injecting drug users. The aim of defining such risk groups is to contribute to prevention, including to marshall adequate and appropriate resources for those in greatest need. In an epidemic, such resources will include preventive measures, care, and service provision, which need to be targeted to those at greatest predictable risk.

Two factors initially influenced the use of the term *risk groups* in the early years of the epidemic. First, the mass media sadly used the phrase in such a way that named risk groups were seen to pose a risk to the rest of the population, which therefore contributed to prejudice and misunderstanding. It also became apparent that an exclusive focus on risk groups might imply that HIV was *not* a risk for those who were not defined as members of risk groups.

These two concerns led to a widespread reaction against the notion of risk groups, and new emphasis placed on *risk factors* and particularly on behaviors potentially facilitating the transmission of HIV. Thus the concept of *risk behaviors* became increasingly used in public health and in HIV/AIDS education and prevention policies. By 1988 it had become an axiom that risk for HIV comes not from who you are, but from what you do. This attitude subsequently became incorporated in most public health campaigns around the world.

Unfortunately, however, this shift of terminology introduced at least as many problems as it seemingly resolved. While it is true that unprotected sexual intercourse is a risk behavior which may increase the likelihood of contracting HIV infection, it is also clear that not everyone engaging in this risk behavior is at equal risk. The discursive shift from "risk groups" to "risk behaviors" thus suggested that everyone is at equal risk from HIV. The global epidemiology of HIV, however, clearly demonstrates that this is not the case—HIV is not an "equal opportunity" disease. Moreover, exclusive attention to "risk behaviors" increased the difficulty of prevention, since those at greatest risk could no longer be named, and therefore their entitlement to services and support could hardly be identified, let alone met.

The discourse of "risk behaviors" has thus contributed to a widespread international "de-gaying" of the HIV epidemic, especially in countries where gay and bisexual men continue to make up the great majority of cases cumulatively, and of newly diagnosed HIV and AIDS.[1] It is therefore understandable that there has been a widespread revival of the use of the term *risk group* since 1990, in order to help direct scarce resources to those in demonstrably greatest need.[2] While it is also clear that not all members of named risk groups are at identical risk from HIV, the term is necessary and helpful in drawing attention to certain realities, and may serve to counter exaggerated notions of risk, which are latent within the concept of risk behaviors.[3] As a British report noted in 1991:

> "Failure to recognise that, in some instances, the use of the term 'risk group' may be valuable is a major barrier to assigning appropriate priorities in health promotion actions. . . . The bottom line is that avoiding the notion of risk groups has failed to prevent stigmatisation and prevented effective targeting of different groups. . . . There has been insufficient work with gay men and other men who have sex with men. If this omission is not addressed immediately many more gay men will become infected with a virus which will cost [them] their health and probably their lives."[4]

References

1. E. King, *Safety in Numbers: Safer Sex and Gay Men* (London: Cassell, 1993).
2. S. Watney, "Emergent Sexual Identities and HIV/AIDS," in *AIDS: Facing the Second Decade,* P. Aggleton, P. Davies, and G. Hart, eds. (London: Falmer Press, 1993):13–29.
3. A wider context for this entire debate is provided by R. Castel, "From dangerousness to risk," in *Foucault Effect: Studies in Governmentality,* G. Burchell, C. Gordon, and P. Miller, eds. (London: Harvester Wheatsheaf, 1991):281–298.
4. M. Rooney and P. Scott, "Working where the risks are," in *Working Where the Risks Are,* B. Evans, S. Sandberg, and S. Watson, eds. (London: Health Education Authority, 1992):13–66.

The next logical question is how risk-taking behaviors can be modified, or risk situations minimized, so as to reduce risk to individuals, and by limiting individual spread, control the epidemic. In this first period of response to HIV/AIDS, this new, epidemiologically derived information about risk formed the basis of informational campaigns, including some of the most aggressive and large-scale public information efforts ever undertaken in public health. The emphasis was on information, information, information, as the basis of protection against HIV.

The period of early response (1985–88)

During this period, an enormous, unprecedented effort was undertaken to promote and support individual risk reduction through individual behavior change. The ensuing global mobilization involved an effort to implement

HIV prevention programs in countries around the world, most of which focused heavily on prevention.[8] For in traditional public health terms, support for individual risk reduction would be delivered through specific services and activities. The overall shape of this approach was guided by the three-part prevention program model developed as part of the WHO Global AIDS Strategy.[9,10]

Of the three parts of HIV prevention programs, two involved traditional public health ideas and one was highly innovative. Based on prior public health efforts to change various personal behaviors (involving, for example, cigarette smoking, diet, and sexual behavior), HIV prevention programs were designed to provide information and education, along with health and social services needed to promote and support the recommended behavioral changes.[11,12] These services included condom distribution, HIV testing and counseling, treatment for other sexually transmitted infections, needle exchange, treatment for injecting drug users, and the provision of safe blood and blood products.

The innovative element in HIV prevention programs was the requirement that discrimination against HIV-infected people and people with AIDS be prevented.[13,14] For field experience had demonstrated that the fear of profound personal and social consequences (such as dismissal from work or school, denial of health care, or even physical abuse or imprisonment) led those most likely to be infected to avoid participating in HIV prevention programs. Accordingly, discrimination was identified as a tragic and counter-productive effect of the pandemic which endangered public health. Thus, for the first time in history, preventing discrimination against infected people became an integral part of a strategy to control an epidemic of infectious disease (Fig. 38-2).

Developing and sustaining comprehensive policies and programs to deliver these services to assist individual risk reduction was an enormous task.[15] There is clear evidence that when implemented with care, sensitivity, and community involvement, the three-part approach can substantially reduce HIV spread. Yet, as reviewed in earlier chapters, neither the scope nor comprehensiveness of program delivery has been optimal; many people still

Figure 38-2   Mid-1980s: expanded risk reduction. Focus on the individual, access to services, and protection against discrimination.

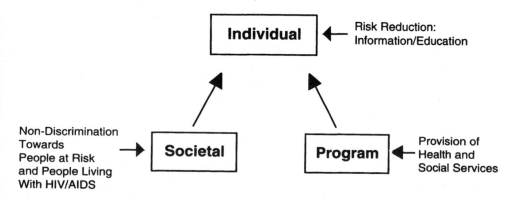

do not have access to these programs, and many programs still do not provide the necessary services, nor do they provide these services in a useful and appropriate manner.

In summary, during the period of early response, the initial emphasis on information was widened and expanded to that of a comprehensive programmatic approach seeking to provide individuals with information, education, and specific services that would help promote and support the process of individual behavioral change. The focus remained individual, but the need for external (programmatic) support was acknowledged and acted upon.[16]

The current period (1989 to the present)

Worldwide experience has demonstrated that while the HIV risk reduction approach is necessary and useful, it is not sufficient to control the pandemic; it has worked for some, but not for many others (Box 38-2).[17-20]

BOX 38-2

The spread of HIV/AIDS in the world's indigenous populations

RONALD M. ROWELL

Indigenous peoples, the term used by the United Nations, are those who were the first inhabitants of lands that were later colonized by foreigners. There are an estimated 250 million indigenous people in the world who live on every continent. In almost every instance, indigenous people occupy the lowest social and economic status in the societies that have developed around and hold power over them.

Not surprisingly, the health status of indigenous peoples is generally lower than for others in the same country. Infectious disease epidemics have played a major historical role in the destruction of indigenous communities, especially in the Western hemisphere in the 500 years since initial contact with Europe and Africa. AIDS has the potential to play a similar role.

Epidemiology of AIDS among indigenous people

Poor health status, high rates of sexually transmitted infections (STIs), significant alcohol and drug abuse, child prostitution, and sexual abuse, all suggest the potential for a catastrophic spread of HIV among indigenous people.

Sexually transmitted infection

In the Amazon region of Brazil, STI rates among Amerindian tribes, such as the Yanomami, Suruí, and Kayapo, are at alarmingly high levels. In Guatemala, STI rates are very high among Amerindian military conscripts; little is known about rates in the civilian Indian population. In Papua New Guinea, STI rates are extraordinarily high among tribal peoples. In Canada, STI rates among first nations people are three times the national average.[1] In the United States, citizens of the first nations suffer rates of STIs which average twice that of the non-indigenous population; in some states, these rates are from seven to ten times higher.[2]

Substance abuse

Alcohol and drug abuse rates are also exceedingly high in many indigenous communities in the world. In Thailand, for example, opium addiction is such a problem among many hill tribespeople that it has led to the selling of young girls into prostitution in cities to support parents' drug habits. Among the San people of southern Africa, alcoholism is widespread. Among Aboriginals of Australia, alcoholism and drug abuse are major health problems. Similarly, in North America, alcoholism and drug abuse, including intravenous drug abuse, are the most significant factors in the overall poor health of the indigenous inhabitants. In India, intravenous heroin use is reported to be growing among young Naga tribesmen.

Sexual abuse and prostitution

The poverty that has arisen from the destruction of traditional economic pursuits and social, legal, and political persecution has led to prostitution, rape, and sexual abuse among indigenous children as well as adults. Among the Guatemalan Indians, prostitution is common; it has also been increasing among Amerindian women in Brazil's Amazon region. The gold prospectors who have invaded the area have committed rape and other crimes of violence against the local indigenous women and communities. In Papua New Guinea rates of prostitution are also very high and increasing. A study conducted by the Papua New Guinea Institute of Medicine indicated that 26 percent of women in villages were providing sex in return for cash and that 40 percent of the men had paid for sex. In Thailand, many young tribal women are forced by their families into prostitution in Bangkok, including some as young as 11 years old. An anthropologist working with the Akha hill people states that few girls over 12 are left in the villages.[3] In Africa, sexual abuse of San women by employers is reportedly common. In Australia, prostitution among homeless Aboriginal youth and adults on the streets of the nation's cities places them at risk for HIV. It is a sadly similar story for many American Indians and Inuit peoples in the larger cities of the United States and Canada.

HIV infection and AIDS

HIV-infected and AIDS-diagnosed individuals have been reported in the indigenous communities of Brazil, Thailand, India, the United States, Canada, Australia, and New Zealand.[4] Unfortunately, existing information is extremely limited and not surprisingly, the best information comes from the industrialized countries. The Centers for Disease Control and Prevention (CDC) has reported diagnosed AIDS cases among American Indians and Alaska Natives since before 1984. As of June 30, 1993, the CDC had reported 1,202 cumulative cases. The figures illustrate the growth in AIDS cases, transmission categories, and cases by sex (Figures 38-2.1–38-2.4).

Figure 38-2.1   AIDS cases in Native Americans, USA, 1984–1995.

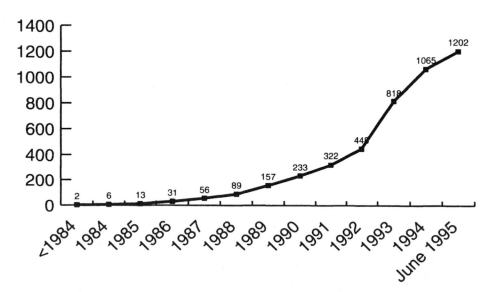

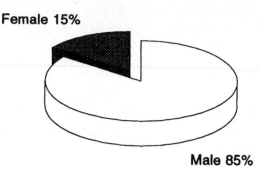

Female 15%

Male 85%

Figure 38-2.2 Gender distribution of AIDS cases in Native Americans, USA, 1984–1995.

Figure 38-2.3 Male Native American AIDS cases by transmission category.

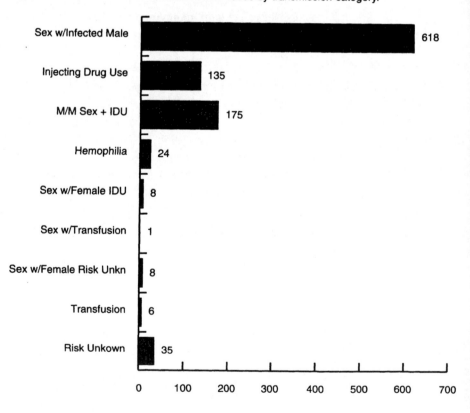

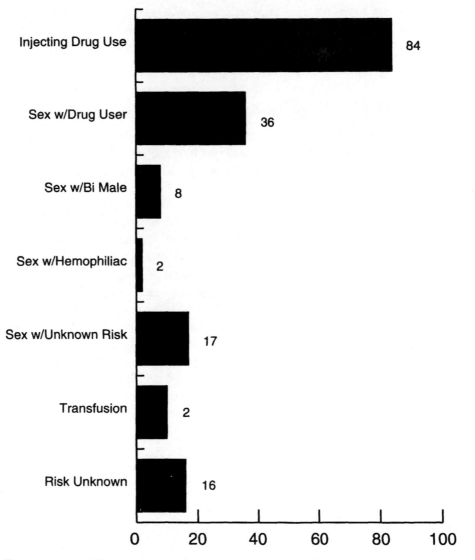

Figure 38-2.4 AIDS cases in female Native Americans, 1984–1995.

In the United States, the CDC and the Indian Health Service have been conducting a nationwide seroprevalence survey for which preliminary data have been made available. The investigators found that HIV prevalence among American Indian/Alaska Native women in the third trimester of pregnancy was from 2.4 to 8.4 times higher than for other rural women in similar studies. Prevalence was similar for women in both urban and rural sites. Based on these findings, it was projected that between 1,210 and 4,250 American Indian/Alaska Natives were infected with HIV as of June, 1991.[5] Another study found a 75–100 percent rate of misreporting of American Indian/Alaska Native ethnicity in HIV/AIDS surveillance in Los Angeles and Seattle.[6,7,8]

A study conducted in Vancouver, British Columbia, Canada, in 1990 of that city's homeless population estimated an HIV prevalence rate of 50 percent among homeless Aboriginal drug users. As of January of 1994, 93 of the 9,083 AIDS cases reported in Canada were among Aboriginal people. Although the AIDS incidence rate (9.2/100,000) in this population was less than one-third the rate for all Canadians (33.6/100,000), many AIDS cases are reported without ethnic or racial origin specified.[9]

AIDS cases have also been reported among the indigenous populations of Australia, New Zealand, Brazil, Thailand, and India. In Thailand, the New Life Center in Chiang Mai reports that 60 percent of the young hill tribes girls returning from Bangkok brothels are HIV-infected. One-third of the injecting drug users in Nagaland, India, are estimated to be infected. Seropositive San have also been reported in Namibia.[10]

Barriers and successes in prevention and care

There are numerous barriers to effective HIV/AIDS prevention and care in indigenous communities. The international aid system is structurally unfriendly to indigenous groups. The marginal political and legal status of indigenous populations remains the single largest barrier to effective HIV prevention or providing care. In many places in the world, national governments work to destroy first nations people either through outright genocide or gradual and total assimilation. Recent events in the Mexican state of Chiapas among the Mayans illustrate the desperation felt by many indigenous peoples in the face of ongoing violations of basic human rights and dignity. Existing international multilateral and bilateral structures ill-serve the needs of indigenous communities since they require the participation and agreement of those same national governments most responsible for their oppression. Thus, very little is known concerning the spread of HIV in indigenous communities, few resources are dedicated to HIV prevention, and even less are available to care for those already infected.

Language and illiteracy are barriers. Most indigenous languages are not written and many indigenous people do not read. The prevalence of oral tradition and communication necessitates approaches that are personnel intensive. Obviously, the person providing education and information must be fluent in the indigenous language, knowledgeable about AIDS, and able to translate information and concepts accurately and appropriately within the culture and world view of the target population. The sheer multiplicity of languages also poses a challenge in many places. For example, in Papua New Guinea there are 860 languages spoken in a population of 3 million indigenous people.

Distrust of outsiders based upon historical experience and communal tradition can block educational efforts initiated by those who do not belong to the community, share its values or speak its language. Such barriers are difficult, but not impossible to overcome.

Determinants of successes and failures

One of the most important lessons learned by those working on HIV prevention and care in indigenous communities is the need to provide training, technical assistance, and ongoing support to members of those communities who can take on themselves the responsibility for education and community organizing to influence the behaviors involved in the spread of HIV. There is no substitute for self-determination. It is perhaps self-evident that taking responsibility for one's own health and that of one's community makes it much more likely that the effort will take on meaning and lead to success.

Traditional culture can and should play a central role in both the expression of the problem and the strategies for proposed solutions. Thus, the best role that nongovernmental, governmental, and private voluntary organizations can play is to provide support to local, community-based efforts where indigenous resources are not available to do so. Conversely, failure is most likely in situations where indigenous communities have no voice in the definition of the threat of HIV/AIDS and in the proposed solutions.

References

1. N. McKenna, "Disaster waiting to happen," *World AIDS* (May 1993):5–9.
2. K. E. Toomey, A. G. Oberschelp, and J. R. Greenspan, "Sexually transmitted diseases in Native Americans: Trends in reported gonorrhea and syphilis morbidity 1984–88," *Public Health Reports* 104(1989):566–572.

3. McKenna, "Disaster."

4. *Ibid.*

5. G. A. Conway, T. J. Ambrose, E. Chase, et al., "HIV infection in American Indians and Alaska Natives: Surveys in the Indian Health Service," *Journal of Acquired Immune Deficiency Syndromes* 5(1992):803–809.

6. L. Lieb, P. Kerndt, M. Hedderman, E. Chase, J. Yao, and G. Conway, "Evaluating racial classification among Native American Indians with AIDS in Los Angeles County, California," poster presented at the V International Conference on AIDS, Montreal, Canada, June 1989.

7. M. G. Hurlich, S. G. Hopkins, J. Sakuma, and G. A. Conway, "Racial ascertainment of AI/AN persons with AIDS Seattle/King County, WA 1980–1989," *IHS Primary Care Provider* 17(May 1992):73–74.

8. M. Smyser, S. D. Helgerson, and M. Hess, "Racial misclassification among AI/AN reported with class IV HIV infection in Washington state," *IHS Primary Care Provider* 17(May 1992):74–75.

9. L. M. Calzavara, 1993; P. Yan, update, March 1994; "Second Annual HIV/AIDS Epidemic Research and Surveillance Meeting," *Quarterly Surveillance Update AIDS in Canada* (Division of HIV/AIDS Epidemiology, Health Canada) (April 1994):26–33.

10. McKenna, "Disaster."

It has become evident that the rather exclusive focus on individual risk reduction was too narrow, for this focus was unable to deal concretely with the lived, social realities of women, men, and children around the world (Chapters 9 and 21).

The history of this period is dominated by two related, although separate, efforts. The principal effort worldwide has been directed at implementing, more fully and with increasing attention to care, the program-based approach described above (Part IV). The second activity, which is more innovative, has sought to develop and expand the strategic approach to HIV/AIDS by considering the social influences on personal behavior and program methods and content. This effort has taken many forms, from incorporating social context into sexual behavior research (Chapter 9), to proposals that pay greater attention to the influence of social norms and human development on individual behavior.[21,22,23] Since vulnerability has been central to this effort, the next chapter (Chapter 39) reviews the concept of vulnerability and describes how its personal and programmatic dimensions were understood and applied. Chapter 40 then explores how the societal level of vulnerability has thus far been understood and acted upon.

REFERENCES

1. J. Mann and K. Kay, "Confronting the pandemic: The World Health Organization's Global Programme on AIDS, 1986–1989," *AIDS* 5 (suppl. 2) (1991):s221–s229.

2. M. Grmek, *Histoire du SIDA, Début et Origine d'une Pandemie Actuelle*, (Paris: Petite Bibliothèque Payot), 1989.

3. WHO, *Special Programme on AIDS. Strategies and Structure: Projected Needs*, WHO, SPA/GEN/87.1 (Geneva: WHO, March 1987).

4. J. Mann, *Address to Special Session of the Fortieth World Health Assembly on AIDS: The Global Strategy for AIDS Prevention and Control*, WHO/SPA/INF/87.2 (Geneva: WHO, May 5, 1987).

5. J. Mann, D. Tarantola, and T. Netter, eds., *AIDS in the World* (Cambridge, MA: Harvard University Press, 1992):577–602.

6. Economic and Social Council of the United Nations, Document E/1995/L.24/Rev.1, Geneva, 1995.

7. D. Tarantola, "Structural and environmental influences on HIV risk behavior and vulnerability," presented at the USAID 3rd HIV/AIDS Prevention Conference, Washington DC, August 8, 1995.

8. Mann, "Confronting the pandemic."

9. WHO, *Special Programme on AIDS. Strategies and Structure: Projected Needs*, WHO, SPA/GEN/87.1 (Geneva: WHO, March 1987).

10. Mann, *AIDS in the World*.

11. J. Sepulveda, H. Fineberg, and J. Mann, eds., *AIDS Prevention through Education: A World View* (Oxford, U.K.: Oxford University Press, 1992).

12. *AIDS Prevention and Control*, World Summit of Ministers of Health on AIDS Prevention Programmes, jointly organized by the World Health Organization and the Government of the United Kingdom, London, January 26–28, 1988. (Oxford, U.K.: Pergamon Press, 1988).

13. 41st World Health Assembly, *Avoidance of Discrimination Against HIV-infected People and Persons with AIDS*, resolution 41.24 (Geneva: World Health Organization, May 13, 1988).

14. M. Kirby, "HIL revisited," in *AIDS in the World*, J. Mann, D. Tarantola, and T. Netter, eds., (Cambridge, MA: Harvard University Press, 1992):346–347.

15. D. L. Kirp and R. Bayer, eds., AIDS in the Industrialized Democracies, (New Brunswick, New Jersey: Rutgers University Press, 1992).

16. World Health Organization, *Guidelines for the Development of National AIDS Prevention and Control Programmes*, (Technical Series Document no. 1, (Geneva: Global Programme on AIDS, 1988).

17. Mann, *AIDS in the World*.

18. J. Stryker, T. Coates, P. DeCarlo, et al., "HIV prevention: looking back, looking ahead," *Journal of the American Medical Aassociation* 273 (1995):1143–1146.

19. J. C. Caldwell, P. Caldwell, and P. Quiggin, "The social context of AIDS in sub-Saharan Africa," *Population and Development Review* 15(1989):185–234.

20. J. Cleland, and P. Way, eds., "AIDS Impact and Prevention in the Developing World: Demographic and Social Science Perspectives," *Health Transition Review* 4(suppl.) (1994).

21. J. M. Mann and M. Carballo, "Social, cultural, and political aspects—overview," *AIDS* 3 (suppl. 1)(1989):s221–s223.

22. Panos Dossier, *The Hidden Cost of AIDS: The Challenge of HIV to Development* (London: The Panos Institute, 1992).

23. E. Reid, "The HIV epidemic as a development issue," in R. Glick, ed., *Law, Ethics and HIV: Proceedings of the UNDP Intercountry Consultation* (Cebu, Phillippines: United Nations Development Programme 1993):3–6.

——— *The HIV Epidemic and Development: The Unfolding of the Epidemic*, (New York: United Nations Development Programme undated).

——— "Sharing the challenge of the HIV epidemic: Building partnerships," plenary presentation to the 2nd International Congress on AIDS in Asia and the Pacific, New Delhi, India, 8–12 November 1992.

39

Vulnerability: Personal and Programmatic

Vulnerability is the converse of empowerment.[1] By vulnerability we mean the extent to which individuals are capable of making and effecting free and informed decisions about their life. A person who is genuinely able to make free and informed decisions is least vulnerable (empowered); the person who is ill-informed, or whose ability to make informed decisions freely and carry them out is most vulnerable.[2]

To facilitate analysis, *AIDS in the World* (1992) proposed that vulnerability could be considered on three interdependent levels: personal, programmatic, and societal.

Personal vulnerability to HIV/AIDS (or in general) involves both cognitive and behavioral dimensions. Cognitive factors involve informational needs—about HIV/AIDS, sexuality, and services—for reducing vulnerability to HIV infection. Behavioral factors can be considered in two overlapping categories: personal characteristics, which include emotional development, perception of risk and attitudes towards risk-taking, personal attitudes towards sex and sexuality, and history of sexual and substance abuse (including alcohol); and, personal skills, such as the ability to negotiate sexual practices, including safer sex, and the skills needed to use condoms.

Several approaches have been used to reduce personal vulnerability. These focus on the individual by providing information and education; counseling and peer support (Chapter 21); skills training for sexual negotiation and condom use; treatment for substance abuse; and research about knowledge, attitudes, beliefs, and practices regarding sexual and drug-injection behaviors (Chapters 21–25).

Programmatic vulnerability focuses on the contributions of HIV/AIDS programs toward reducing or increasing personal vulnerability. Programmatic vulnerability has been defined broadly in terms of the three major prevention elements identified by WHO: information and education, health and social services, and nondiscrimination towards HIV-infected people and people with AIDS. Efforts to reduce programmatic vulnerability have principally involved ensuring and strengthening the availability and accessibility of key program elements, the quality and content of each element, and the process through which the elements are designed, implemented, and evaluated. For example, considerable effort has been made to improve and refine informational and educational services. In this regard, a major emphasis has been placed on participation of the intended audience ("targets") in the design of the messages and in the choice of channels for their dissemination.

To strengthen the health and social services element, enormous efforts have been made to define the constituent parts of each service, to improve delivery of the service, to evaluate service quality, and to broaden participation in their design and implementation. For example, to help ensure condom-related services, WHO and others have worked hard to develop uniform condom quality standards, have provided guidance on condom program elements, organized training to improve management and logistics, and promoted the application of various methods (such as social marketing) for expanding condom acceptability and use.[3] In addition, a substantial research effort continues to seek improved understanding of determinants of condom use, nonuse, and misuse.

Finally, nondiscrimination toward HIV-infected people and people with AIDS has been pursued, with varying degrees of success. The major emphasis has been on responding to discrimination (and other violations of rights) which occur—either through official policies, programs and practices, or despite rights-affirming and anti-discriminatory efforts by governments. Chapter 31 describes some of the work being carried out to help bring international law and human rights to bear on discrimination and rights violations experienced by people living with HIV, people with AIDS, and people considered by the government and/or the public as "high risk" for HIV/AIDS.

The common denominator in these various, and in many ways, necessary and impressive, efforts to reduce programmatic vulnerability is their focus on services and service delivery. However, they have not generally incorporated a social dimension into their work. Thus far, the concept of personal vulnerability has just begun to be applied in identifying and responding to the societal factors that underlie and strongly influence the nature of personal vulnerability.[4] Clearly, the concept of programmatic vulnerability has not yet been incorporated into an active understanding and meaningful response to the many ways in which social factors influence, constrain, and restrict program design, accessibility, content, quality, process, and implementation.

Nongovernmental organizations have often been aware of the critical importance of the social context for HIV prevention and care. Many official national and international agencies have also struggled with these issues, and some researchers have sought to provide a conceptual and empirical foundation for including social issues along with behavioral issues. However, the major, dominant effort has thus far been focused on a limited appreciation of the nature of vulnerability to HIV/AIDS.[5] The next chapter explores how the social level of vulnerability has been understood and acted upon.

REFERENCES

1. J. M. Mann, D. J. M. Tarantola, and T. W. Netter, eds., *AIDS in the World* (Cambridge, MA: Harvard University Press, 1992):325–420.

2. *Towards a New Health Strategy for AIDS: A Report of the Global AIDS Policy Coalition* (Boston, MA: François-Xavier Bagnoud Center for Health and Human Rights, Harvard School of Public Health, 1993).

3. *AIDS, Images of the Epidemic* (Geneva: World Health Organization, 1994).

4. M. Sweat and J. Denison, "Reducing HIV incidence in developing countries with structural and environmental interventions," *AIDS* 9 (suppl.) (1995):s251–s257.

5. Committee on Substance Abuse and Mental Health Issues in AIDS Research, "Understanding the determinants of HIV risk behavior," in *AIDS and Behavior: An Integrated Approach*, Institute of Medicine, (Washington, DC: National Academy Press, 1994):78–123.

40

Societal Vulnerability: Contextual Analysis

Research and empirical observation over the past 15 years have demonstrated that personal behavior is so profoundly influenced and conditioned by broader, societal factors that a focus on change in personal behavior without influencing the relevant societal factors could never be sufficiently effective.[1-6] For example, inferior economic and social status limits the ability of many women to refuse unwanted or unprotected sexual intercourse, regardless of how much they know about AIDS or wish to adopt recommended individual risk-reduction practices[7] (Chapters 19 and 20). Similarly, it has become evident that HIV/AIDS programs are created within, and therefore constrained by, the larger society. Thus, for example, governmental refusal to inform the public about condom use for HIV prevention or allow harm reduction strategies for injecting drug users severely handicaps and influences the national AIDS program; in contrast, the program would benefit from overall public and official support for anti-AIDS efforts.[8]

The concept of societal vulnerability builds upon the insight that collective, societal factors strongly influence both personal vulnerability and programmatic vulnerability. Societal vulnerability focuses directly on the contextual factors which define and constrain personal and programmatic vulnerability. Vulnerability analysis recognizes that broader, contextual issues such as governmental structure, gender relationships, attitudes towards sexuality, religious beliefs, and poverty, influence the capacity to reduce personal vulnerability to HIV, both directly and as mediated through programs (Fig. 40-1) (Boxes 40-1 and 40-2).

BOX 40-1

Cultural influence on society vulnerability

TONY BARNETT AND RACHEL GRELLIER

Societal vulnerability includes both vulnerability to disease and vulnerability to social and economic impacts of disease. To see how culture and vulnerability relate requires an examination of the notion of culture, its relation to economic and social conditions of life, and the links between these and vulnerability.

Cultures and codes: risk, danger, and culture

Culture is adaptive. It is not something which is fragile and cracks under stress. Human life is characterized by risk, and culture is that assemblage of material, or conceptual, institutional, and organizational arrangements which enable individuals and groups to code and cope with risk in their natural and social environments.[1] Danger to health may be encoded in various ways: as individual or communally, as witchcraft, as malign intent, as statistical incidence, or as the result of transgression of dominant views of purity and impurity, as, for example, in relation to sexual behaviors.[2] Evaluations of dangers and responses to them are encoded in institutions and practices through stigmatization and/or isolation of the sick, hospitalization, and community care. Institutions, practices, and social structures are coping responses to perceived dangers.

Culture, power, and entitlement

A brief definition of these three concepts elides issues that are important in the context of major epidemic diseases. It is crucial to recognize that cultural ideas, practices, and forms of organization are closely related to power. Power, the ability of individuals and groups to gain their ends, despite contrary volitions by other individuals and groups, is unequally distributed in human societies. Natural resources, ideas, artifacts, human resources, and institutions can be manipulated by, and are accessible to, different social groups. The term *entitlement* has increasingly been introduced to describe aspects of this differential access.[3] Entitlement apportions individuals and groups differing abilities to command resources via access to systems of various kinds, often through markets, but also via legal or ritual rules. These access systems implicitly or explicitly evaluate the relative claims of individuals or groups by using criteria which commonly include ethnicity, class, gender, and sexual predisposition. A common result of differential entitlement is that the more powerful or privileged groups frequently scapegoat those less powerful or otherwise marginalized, for dangers or risks from which the latter may actually suffer the major casualties.

Vulnerability to infection and its consequences

Current thinking on issues of societal vulnerability presents a dichotomy. Those working within the *culture-as-belief* perspective define culture narrowly, as what people do and believe, and assume that this is a useful starting point for understanding factors which make particular individuals and groups more vulnerable to infection and less able to cope with the consequences. Although those adopting this perspective are usually aware of the link between this approach and the development of victim-blaming responses, they consider the policy benefits of such an approach to outweigh the social costs, so that these costs can be mitigated, usually through public education programs. This perspective tends to see cultures as crumbling under the impact of trauma. In contrast, people working from the other position, or *culture as action,* point to the virtual impossibility of disengaging the cultural from economic and environmental factors that are conducive to vulnerability in both senses described above. In particular, poor people's livelihood strategies often shorten their horizon of decision. In such circumstances, it is not only, or most importantly, beliefs which influence behavior, but also, and most powerfully, people's material circumstances and their resultant entitlements. This perspective emphasizes the adaptability and changeability of culture.

It is safe to assume that in practice, vulnerability to infection and to the impacts of the epidemic are at once related to what people believe and do and to the arenas of power and entitlement in which they do them. It is vital to bear in mind that culture is not a constant, but continually changes in relation to material, political, and environmental circumstances. It may be most useful to view culture-as-belief as an entry point to understanding observed behaviors and as an indicator of the need for more substantial and sophisticated analysis of material influences on vulnerability, as indicated by culture as action.

Societies, cultures, and networks

Societies differ in degree of homogeneity. Use of terms such as *subculture* or *group* to describe these differences has limitations because they obscure the processes and practices that make up real people's lives. Currently, the best practice is probably to use the analytical idea of networks through which people negotiate their livelihoods and their identities, thus employing the concept of culture as action. This is where the most important research issues on social vulnerability may be identified, as the concept of network permits a deconstruction of the abstract notion of a social group into observable processes of human life and recognizes the adaptability of human beings under conditions of stress.

The main parameters of societal vulnerability

The main parameters that are generally held to affect both vulnerability to infection and to its social consequences are ethnic relations and social evaluation of ethnicity; attitudes toward fate and destiny; religious differentiation and social evaluations of religious communities; levels of inter- and intracommunal conflict, including civil and international warfare; gender relations; intergenerational attitudes and relations; patterns of voluntary and force migration; resources and beliefs about rights and obligations of existing support networks; degrees of income and wealth differentiation; and levels of environmental marginality experienced by social subgroups and the effect of this on livelihood strategies. While it is difficult to generalize as to the precise manner in which these factors affect vulnerability in any specific case, it can be suggested that for policy purposes it is useful to understand the way that their interrelations affect the distribution of social and economic entitlements. In particular, when any social relation defined along one or more of these parameters is conflictual or a focus of stress, then this social area is likely to be a locus both of infection and of manifestations of socially traumatic responses to an epidemic. In most cases, this will lead to both infection and to its impact being concentrated on economically, culturally, politically, or environmentally disadvantaged or marginalized groups or networks. This marginalization may often be in relation to the state itself.

Research issues

From the preceding observations, it follows that (a) the concept of culture has to be used with great care; (b) "culture" should never be used loosely to imply integrated and unchanging sets of beliefs, practices, and values; and (c) culture exists in a complex relation to economic and environmental circumstances within which people make their livings and negotiate their identities. Research on cultural influences on social vulnerability has to focus on (a) situations where livelihoods and identities are disputed or under stress; (b) networks of relationships (as opposed to broad groups) through and within which livelihoods and identities are pursued and negotiated; (c) relations between social networks and groups and the state; and (d) the degree to which vulnerable networks are able to command the various kinds of entitlement available in any given society.

References

1. M. Douglas, *Risk Acceptability According to the Social Sciences*, ed. P. Kegan (London: Routledge, 1986).
2. R. Davenport-Hines, *Sex, Death and Punishment: Attitudes to Sex and Sexuality in Britain since the Renaissance* (London: Collins, 1990).
3. A. Sen, *Poverty and Famines: An Essay on Entitlement and Deprivation* (Oxford, U.K.: Oxford University Press, 1981).

BOX 40-2

AIDS as a challenge to religion

DANIEL DEFERT

The primary mode of transmission of HIV in the world is sexual, and sexual practices are the object of prescriptions, ritualization, and spiritual and moral elaboration in all the world's religions. The repertory of sexual practices, whether admitted or excluded, is given normative value by religion. This not only affects believers, but constitutes a measurable element in the cultural differentiation of sexual habits.

Religious people not only express themselves in the day-to-day morality and the imparting of meaning to the essential moments of life—birth, marriage, suffering, and death—they also actively impact educational and medical establishments as well. Through them, religion is involved in educational programs and in the construction of attitudes towards diseases.

Most religions underline the importance of charity towards the weak, the poor, the infirm, the sick, which they justify philosophically in different ways. Religious communities also have the responsibility to enforce obedience of their rules and commandments, and they can be intolerant when faced with their violation. This reaction to errors, infractions, or sins normalizes various forms of exclusion. The severity with which moral or religious taboos are regarded reflects the perceived threats to various boundaries, and defenders of religious values greatly fear breaches of such rules. Thus, religion frequently intervenes, not only in regard to secular efforts to prevent HIV transmission but also to the social definition of the dignity of those infected by the virus. Generally, the leaders of religious communities try, to the extent that social forces will permit, to impose their values upon political decision makers to maintain the identity and boundaries of their institutions, their values, or their groups.

If religion is prescriptive and normative, the epidemiology of HIV is descriptive. It describes the reality and the diversity of sexual practices, which contrasts with most religious prescriptions. This reveals the limits of religious commands and illuminates other social determinants of sexual practices. With the current transformation of societies, the following social determinants tend to be predominant: a person's social, economic, and legal status; the number of years of schooling; the diversity of behavior models; and the dominant influence of media such as television, the press, and radio, which are independent of religious authorities.

AIDS therefore reveals the challenging circumstances that face religions in their moral substance and their social influence. This testing of religious morals is probably even more crucial for the monotheistic religions, and particularly—for reasons of doctrine and social organization—for Islam and for the Catholic church. The HIV epidemic makes manifest the extension of a conflict of values surrounding human sexuality. This conflict may be more crucial and also discussed more within religious communities than we can infer from their official statements. On the other hand, health officials have made efforts to involve the greatest number of exposed individuals and to respect contemporary moral pluralism. Accordingly, they have reached a consensus that they need not judge the sexual practices of individuals but should merely provide them with the most neutral, technical means of preventing the sexual transmission of HIV. The method which is least destabilizing both to the acquired habits and to the psychology of the individual, and which is the most easily achieved, is unquestionably the condom. But this technical approach to sexual relationships involves a profound secularization of sexuality, that is to say, a neutral approach, independent of any religious ideology. Never before have states and legislatures addressed sexuality in such a factual and objective manner.

But just as religions have been prescriptive regarding questions of sexuality, so too have political powers and lawmakers. Examples include the penalization of adultery, abortion, homosexuality, transvestism, prostitution, soliciting, pornography, and more recently, of sexual harassment. Indeed, the political authorities have penalized the visibility of sexuality.

Governments also intervene in demographic aspects of sexuality, that is, whether to encourage population growth in developed countries or to limit it in developing ones. The current governmental promotion of condoms is an event in the history of sexual morals because it explicitly thematizes sexuality as a pleasurable activity without the goal of procreation or the construction of a family-oriented society. Undoubtedly, the debates regarding legalization of abortion are also an important step in this process of secularization of sexual relationships. The various faiths may see in this process a form of proselytism against their own values. They may stress that historically they have supported other sexual strategies that can also prevent the spread of HIV: abstinence and fidelity, for example. Should these religions subordinate their commandments and value judgments regarding sexuality to the single goal of slowing the spread of HIV?

Thus, we are witnessing a kind of confrontation of two proselytisms. One is sanitary, which tends to condemn certain behaviors such as the use of tobacco, alcohol, and some dietary habits. It proposes a new sexual technique—the use of condoms, which officializes a secularization of the meanings attached to sexuality. The other proselytism, which is religious, recalls traditional prohibitions surrounding sexuality to give it a spiritual meaning that involves two elements: the relation of an individual to him- or herself through abstinence or asceticism, and also to the partner through fidelity.

The intensity and forms of expression of this conflict of values surrounding sexual activity are an important part of what can be called the social construction of the epidemic, with paramount impact on public policies. In the context of AIDS, should health officials fear religious intervention as a hindrance to the prevention of the epidemic and at times to the social integration of infected persons, or should they consider religious leaders and the morality they espouse to be allies who may be enlisted in their prevention strategies? There is no simple answer, and the question merits close examination through two perspectives: first, in regard to the ethical content given to sexuality by each faith; second, through the real influence exercised by religious rules upon contemporary sexual practices. Thus, we must be attentive to debates going on within each of the major faiths regarding the meanings to be given to new modalities of sexual behavior, as well as to new medical technologies, notably medically assisted procreation and extension of the procreative limits of women. Contemporary ethical debates surrounding human sexuality cannot be reduced to a conflict between a secularized hygenic ethos and traditional spiritual values. The conflict of values seems to be much deeper, and this conflict is the object of ongoing inquiry at the heart of each spiritual family in regard to the dynamics of the AIDS pandemic, as well as to reproductive issues for women.

The major monotheistic religions have most closely regulated sexual practice, within both their doctrinal foundations and their social organization. Ancient Judaism, according to historians, instituted a profound rupture with the orgiastic cults that surrounded it geographically through its forceful interdictions of alcohol, nudity, illicit sexual union, and the regulation of all spheres of sexuality, as controlled by the priesthood and reactivated periodically by prophecy. The monotheistic religions are marked by a naturalism or a vitalism which principally inscribes sexuality within the field of the transmission of life. All practices which thwart this end are condemned: onanism, sodomy, adultery, bucogenital practices. Despite their naturalism, none of the main monotheistic religions considers sexual instinct as an energy which must necessarily receive satisfaction or expression; it undergoes ritual or ethical control, a modeling of the self, or asceticism. Islam (the Qur'an) recognizes the need for sexual satisfaction of both partners, but within marriage.

Christian sexual morality, originally elaborated within the framework of monastic life, controls not only sexual activity but also concupiscence by inventing the fundamental Christian distinction between the body, which can be used correctly, and the flesh, which is doomed to sin: are not wet dreams and erections manifestations in my body of something which escapes my will? Are they not manifestations of the flesh where Freedom and Evil come into conflict?

Islamic law, on the other hand, in its four Sunni schools, as in Shiism, focuses on the sexual act itself, and ignores "flesh": this because there are sexual acts which are either legal or illegal. The problem is one of obedience or disobedience. In order to prove that a sexual act was illegal, classical Islam required at least three witnesses, a condition which would have been difficult to meet, and which shows that between the letter of the law and actual practices, a large space was available for the reduction of penalties. Islam experienced periods where the law could not be applied, and the question of the law's application was crucial in the history of Shiism from the moment of the eclipsing of the Twelfth Imam in the tenth century. It is only recently (the period of Khomeini was decisive in this process) that a theory was elaborated of the collective representative of the absent Imam, which permits the reestablishment of the law, or *chariat*, which to that point had been suspended. This important shift allows Shiite fundamentalism to communicate as never before with Sunnite fundamentalism. The subject of classic erotic Arabic poetry was in fact an illegal act: alcohol, relations between men and women out of wedlock, the submission of the lover to the beloved object, or whether a woman or a young man (*ephebe*) committed acts not regulated by the *hadith*, which is the tradition of the words of the prophet.

But there is one point upon which the four major Sunni schools and the Shiites do agree: they did not accord the woman the same theologico-juridical status as for a man; she has neither the moral purity, nor the *virtu*, in the Latin sense of virility of the Soul. Consequently, she has both fewer rights and fewer duties. Her testimony is less consequential than that of a man, but the sanctions against her will also be less. In any case, it is true that the Qur'an offsets this juridical inferiority, which is probably pre-Islamic, with new rights which protect a woman economically, allowing in her favor a form of divorce. In countries where civil and Islamic laws are still very close today, this asymmetry between the genders is incontestably experienced by women as a handicap in the mastery of their sexual relations and in their own protection when faced with AIDS. In Islamic thought, a woman has no reason to protect herself because she cannot be exposed to any risk; she must enter marriage as a virgin and know only her husband. Marriage thus conceived can only pose a risk of infection for the woman by a less restrained husband.

But the Qur'an is not the only aspect governing gender relations in Islamic societies, and today many Islamic countries adhere to a legal system of British or French origin. On the other hand, specialists of the Qur'an claim to find no explicit condemnation of contraceptive methods. The objective of marriage is to make licit the relation between man and woman; procreation marks the successful outcome of this union. As mentioned above, however, the question of contraception and of any form of sexual activity which is intended to avoid procreation is much more crucial in Catholicism, where ritual control over the body, notably in matters of eating restrictions and fasting, is considerably weaker in comparison with Judaism and Islam.

Yet the promotion of condoms is more than a problem of contraception. It incorporates the acknowledgment that sexuality is neither uniquely nor essentially inscribed within the perspective of the transmission of life but is pleasure. Second, it acknowledges sexuality as a physical exercise, a learning process, and as a play, and not essentially as a spiritual openness toward the Other (which every religion emphasizes) or as a relation to the Self, that is to say, asceticism, continence, and chastity. Third, the promotion of condoms recognizes a certain equivalence of heterosexuality and homosexuality. Hostility towards homosexuality is a strong feature of the modern Christian world, but it is also something which none of the monotheistic religions accepts.

As a result, the three monotheistic religions feel challenged in a field which is precisely their own: the advocacy of life. It is interesting to follow the contemporary reemergence at the heart of Judaism of the concept of the saving of the Soul, according to which, the traditional imperatives concerning, for example, the observing of the *shabbat* can be hierarchized and made secondary relative to the dominant imperative of saving a life. (Of course, one difficulty of a casuistic nature is to appreciate the moment when there is no other alternative but to lift the generic imperatives in order to confront a particular situation.) Despite this liberal progress, the recent declarations of the State of Israel, according to which HIV screening is a precondition to immigration, pose a considerable juridico-theological problematic regarding the definition of Jewish identity.

If, as they pretend and aspire to do, religions really exercised spiritual authority over the daily lives of individuals, it is quite likely that the HIV epidemic would not have reached its current proportions. (It would be interesting to correlate the epidemiology of HIV with religious practices around the world.) Health officials must act wherever there is an epidemic that is primarily transmitted through sexual activity which religious morals are unable to contain. Yet, health officials must seek to slow the progression of this epidemic and not to promote religious values when people have ceased to ascribe significance to those values in their daily lives. This fact is difficult to admit in societies where the religious and the legal, the spiritual and the temporal, have not become distinct from one another, a distinction which is characteristic of modern societies. In these societies, the sexual morality of religions faces competition from other value systems; this moral pluralism has been manifested strongly in the progression and the legalization of contraception and abortion, the decreasing frequency of marriage, and the increasing number of people who choose not to marry. Lastly, in these societies, the methods of modern mass communication, television, radio, and the press, dominate whatever influence the religious press might have. The progress of medicine and genetics is pushing back the limits of Nature as defined by the major religions at the moment of such limits' codification. In many countries, there is a crisis in religious vocations, a graying of the clergy, and the closing down of places of worship in working class suburbs and rural areas. Of course, religion continues to inspire the life of communities with as much fervor as ever, since it perceives its mission to include a sort of reconquest in an environment rife with pluralistic moral values; hence, the rise of fundamentalism in many creeds. The growing visibility of the Vatican in world media should not mislead us; more is demanded of the leader of the Catholic church to the extent that its local representatives have lost influence over individual behavior. Moreover, it is not surprising to see the reaffirmation of doctrinal positions in opposition to the procedures endorsed by the medical community for the prevention of HIV. What is more difficult to accept in a democratic society is that religious representatives may influence legislators despite their incapacity to alter their followers' morals, and that they attempt to impose legislation tied to a particular set of dogma upon all citizens of a country while excluding non-believers from the means of prevention. When they act in such a manner, religious leaders encroach upon freedom of conscience—a fundamental aspect of the Universal Declaration of Human Rights, which most states have ratified through international conventions—as well as upon the respect for democracy.

Generally, the reaffirmation of traditional religious values occurs in the context of the defense of a given social order that is being threatened by a new set of values, by foreign contacts, by a transformation of the forms of economic property, of knowledge, and technology. For centuries, sexual relations were articulated through marriage and the maintenance of a family-oriented society. Marriage and the family are fundamental modalities in the exchange of economic goods. The stabilization of the social order was accomplished through these legal, religious, and economic modes of exchange between the genders. The emergence of women's rights and individualism are experienced by certain sectors of various societies as the eruption of licentiousness and as a destabilization of all social order. This applies for those defending a traditional, secular order as well as for those defending religious values. Yet here we must consider an ongoing transformation of the composition of property and capital. Modern societies are witnessing the development of new categories of social agents whose "capital" is made up of years of study, technical competence, and complex knowledge and skills. This human and cultural capital is more and more inseparable from individuals. This is just as true for men as for women, the latter increasingly being holders of a "cultural dowry," in other words, a profession which assures their autonomy. These modern forms of capital and property, which are indivisible from individuals, are less visible than traditional forms of property like land, cattle, houses, stocks, and shares; these modern forms of capital also escape the control of extended families. Current sociological research supports the idea that as a result of these transformations, sexual relations continue to be developed in a stable social homology, proving that what is essential in sexual behavior is tied to social determinants: the economy, the social division of work, and recognition of gender equality.

At the end of the eighteenth century, Europe underwent a similar transformation with the "sentimental tidal wave," as the historian Edward Shorter terms it, which shattered the social rules of marriage by making a place for love. By the end of the nineteenth century, there were hardly any marriages not based on love. The contemporary emergence of sexuality, which is linked to the development of individual cultural capital and is manifested by the growth of divorce and the decision to remain single or to live together without marrying, and by the increasing visibility of homosexuality, shatters social codes which continued to govern love until quite recently. But the successive disappearances of traditional family functions have always been followed by the appearance of other institutions which incorporate those functions, e.g., the health and welfare institutions.

Today, most religious communities have noted these profound transformations of society which go far beyond the moral polemics surrounding the prevention of AIDS. Within each religious tradition there is already a theological pluralism which is not often appreciated. While official statements do not change, religious everyday life practices do change. The press gives greater visibility to the former. We who are involved in the fight against AIDS have to bring these moral debates to the attention of the public.

For instance, in France, a group of Christians (both lay people and theologians) and medical doctors recently acknowledged the importance of new technologies that medically assist procreation, in offering a redefinition of the possibilities of life and proposing, after 3 years of work, a sort of "popular encyclical" in opposition to the Roman encyclical *Donum Vitae,* which spells out church doctrine concerning procreation. Returning to Max Weber's famous distinction, a Catholic theologian in this group acknowledged that believers "must make room beside the ethic of conviction for an ethic of responsibility."

The history of religions is one of constant interpretation of meaning and reinterpretation of events. Today, no religion is in a position to offer a unique moral pronouncement regarding the world event which is the sudden appearance of AIDS. Each religion is tormented by this event, as are the believers of whatever faith who suffer through their flesh, their sexuality, or their loved ones; the believer who cares daily for the sick or gives the young an education in life, and the senior official of a particular faith do not have the same experience of this crisis, nor do they give it the same interpretation. Indeed, they are not engaged in the same work or spiritual development. These are pluralistic voices that contribute to an elaboration of meaning.

To save a life makes sense in all religions. A Ugandan Catholic official recently said, "We as a church cannot offer condoms, except, of course, in the case of a couple in which one partner is seropositive." "And how would you know that he or she is?", a doctor inquired. "Here it's better to proceed as if all couples were discordant regarding HIV-serology," replied the Father. An ethic of responsibility, in other words, which tempers the ethic of conviction. Too often, those who make decisions in the fight against AIDS feel they must obtain the agreement of the most eminent religious leaders of their hierarchy, forgetting that it is precisely the duty and function of the latter to reaffirm the traditional positions of their faith. Nevertheless, at the heart of each denomination, real spiritual work is underway and there are multiple voices. It would be erroneous both from a moral point of view as well as from a sociological one—two approaches which we have tried to bring together—to pretend that the most highly placed voices in the religious hierarchies are the only ones worth consulting; there is a pluralism of voices attentive to the issues.

Given the dedication of lay people and of clergy at the side of the sick—priests have even revealed themselves to be homosexual in order to help reinforce self-esteem among people living with HIV—it is essential to maintain a multiplicity of dialogues, to inform lay people and clergy of the extent of current epidemiological information, of the various strategies of prevention, and of all available medical knowledge. It is important that there be an exchange between health practitioners and members of religious groups, and that health practitioners be aware of the numerous debates that occur within each religion. It is not a matter of soliciting the opinion of religious hierarchies concerning their doctrine but to facilitate in this, as in all other sectors of our societies, the awareness of the multiple dimensions of this epidemic, of all the obstacles that continue to exist, and of all the resources available, in order to stop the pandemic's progression.

To analyze and respond to the social dimension of vulnerability, three broad categories of contextual factors can be identified: political and governmental, sociocultural, and economic. A partial listing of such factors, readily recognized by those working in HIV/AIDS prevention programs, include the following:

Political and governmental factors
1. lack of attention or concern about HIV/AIDS
2. laws that criminalize certain behaviors
3. interference with the free flow of complete information pertinent to HIV/AIDS
4. a lack of HIV-related services. This includes either insufficient, inadequate, or poorly integrated services, or a lack of availability of quality of services tailored to specific groups.
5. official (or sanctioned) discrimination against HIV-infected people and people with AIDS in employment, insurance, health care, marriage, travel, or residence.

Figure 40-1 Late 1980s: risk reductions strategy and initial efforts toward vulnerability reduction.

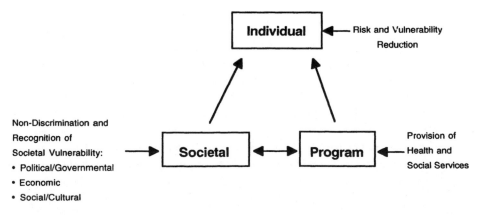

6. official (or sanctioned) discrimination against certain groups for example, on the basis of organization, gender, race, religion, national origin, sexual orientation, age, or substance abuse.

Sociocultural factors
7. gender roles
8. attitudes towards sexuality
9. stigmatization and marginalization of different groups
10. illiteracy and lack of educational opportunity

Economic factors
11. poverty and income disparity
12. lack of resources for prevention programs
13. lack of work or job opportunities

Implementing vulnerability reduction

A vulnerability reduction strategy is the basis of the new, expanded approach to HIV prevention that is now moving from the status of proposal by the Global AIDS Policy Coalition toward implementation through the new UNAIDS program.[9,10,11]

Initially, it may be difficult for many HIV/AIDS programs to expand beyond the earlier and narrower risk-reduction strategy and work described in earlier chapters. The first step involves a thorough analysis of available information, leading to preliminary identification of those who are most vulnerable to HIV infection. This process is illustrated in Box 40-3, which describes a project to develop field experience with the use of contextual analysis of social vulnerability.

Using the example of young people's vulnerability to HIV/AIDS, Box 40-4 outlines the range of information required to identify and bring together the personal, programmatic, and social dimensions of analysis.

BOX 40-3

Country assessment and strategic planning

Steps to be considered in expanding the response to HIV/AIDS through concerted action on contextual factors

- review of available information on epidemiological, behavioral, and HIV/AIDS care patterns
- identification of population subsets exposed to higher risk of HIV infection
- review of ongoing and planned actions aimed at reducing risk in these population subsets
- review of contextual factors influencing the vulnerability of these population subsets to HIV infection
- identification of other population subsets who share vulnerability characteristics of the population currently most affected
- identification of needs and approaches to lowering risk and vulnerability in both the population subsets recognized as being at higher risk and others recognized as being similarly vulnerable
- inventory of existing or planned human development programs (including health, social, and

economic development programs) aimed at reducing risk and vulnerability; inclusion of an HIV/AIDS element in their design, monitoring, and evaluation systems

* inventory of human development programs that may have adverse effects on HIV/AIDS risk and vulnerability and identification of approaches likely to minimize these effects
* identification of additional programs needed to further reduce HIV/AIDS risk and vulnerability
* mapping of human, institutional, and financial resources—both currently available and anticipated—from national or international sources (including UN programs) that can be mobilized in order to expand the national response to HIV/AIDS
* formulation of a national strategy for an expanded national response to HIV/AIDS

The above process is to be applied by a core group of national and international personnel with a mix of expertise in HIV/AIDS prevention and care and in other aspects of human development.

BOX 40-4

Vulnerability of young people to HIV/AIDS: a proposed analytical framework

Young people are affected disproportionately by the HIV/AIDS pandemic worldwide

Every year, more than 150 million young people become sexually active at an age and in situations that are influenced by a broad range of individual and contextual (social) factors. The prevention of HIV, other sexually transmitted infections (STIs), and unwanted pregnancy requires a more complete understanding of these factors and advocacy for the design of programs that are specifically targeted at young people.

Young people do not form a homogeneous population in any country or community. Personal histories, access to quality information and services, the availability of material and emotional support, present role in society, and representations of the future, are many elements that may influence the ability of each individual young man and woman to associate with others on the basis of affinity and to determine freely the course of their lives. Furthermore, the sensitivity of young people to societal (cultural, social, economic) changes affecting them, their claim for better and faster responses to their evolving needs and aspirations, and the creativity and cultural specificity with which they voice these claims, instill much diversity and dynamism in the already complex mosaic of issues and opportunities concerning them.

The quest for a deeper understanding of young people's vulnerability to HIV/AIDS and other STIs creates a convenient point of entry to analyze the tensions that prevail between their personal evolution and the societal context in which one develops, from birth to maturity. The ability of HIV/AIDS prevention programs to negotiate these tensions depends on their intrinsic sensitivity to differences among young people's needs and, concurrently, on the commitment and capacity of such programs to respond to these needs at an individual level while generating the contextual changes needed for young people to develop and express their sexuality safely.

Factors largely drawn from empirical knowledge that may determine the vulnerability of young people to HIV/AIDS are also likely to affect their vulnerability to several other health and social issues confronting this population, including physical illness, mental disorders, unwanted pregnancy, and violence. It is expected that, rather than acting independently, certain factors may act in synergy with or in opposition to young people's vulnerability to HIV/AIDS. Vulnerability analysis should therefore attempt to determine how and in what direction certain factors interact and, consequently, what action could be applied to them in order to reduce vulnerability to its lowest possible level.

The vulnerability analysis framework provided below is built on a list of factors that are deemed influential in young people's vulnerability to HIV/AIDS from three perspectives: (1) on the individual; (2) as it relates to the availability and quality of prevention programs; and (3) from a societal perspective.* This framework is intended to focus on the need for combining primary (proximal) preventive action with contextual (societal) intervention. Each of the factors listed evokes a wide spectrum of research issues including the nature, strength, and interaction of determinants of vulnerability, and possible approaches to vulnerability reduction. The use of the analytical framework could proceed as follows:

- Define the population subset and the setting (social, cultural, economic environment) to which the study applies.
- Define any particular vulnerability factor retained for analysis, to be chosen in any of the three categories (personal, program-related, societal).
- Suggest way(s) the chosen vulnerability factors may influence the risk of acquiring HIV infection.
- Explain how the chosen factor is influenced by, or influences other, factors listed within the same or other categories.
- Suggest possible vulnerability reduction actions, both for the short term and the medium and long term.

I. Individual vulnerability
  A. Factors related to physical and mental development
    - biological and physiological vulnerability to HIV and other STIs: hormonal and physical (genital) changes associated with pubertal development, particularly in young women
    - existence of a physical or mental disability or chronic illness
    - history of physical, mental, or sexual abuse
    - intellectual evolution from concrete to abstract
    - emotional development from immortality to pragmatism
  B. Cognitive factors
    - awareness of sexuality, reproductive health, and sexual health
    - awareness of sources of condom supply
    - awareness of available health and social services serving young people
    - awareness of right to services and confidentiality
    - awareness of same-sex attractions
    - educational attainment
  C. Behavioral and personal characteristics
    - history of having been subjected to discrimination
    - self-esteem
    - development of sense of self as a sexual person
    - ability to decide on one's sexuality and control other events in the course of development
    - development of independence
    - perception of risk and social norms
    - history of risk-taking behavior, substance use and/or addiction, and sexual behavior
  D. Skills
    - skills to use condoms
    - negotiating skills to persuade partner to practice safer sex, particularly in situations of age and gender imbalance
    - ability to modulate risk-taking behavior, including sexuality and substance use

*This framework, initially developed by the editors of *AIDS in the World II*, was revised on the basis of most helpful comments received from Bruce Dick and Mark Connolly, Health Promotion Unit, UNICEF, New York; Peter Aggleton, World Health Organization, Global Program on AIDS, Geneva; John Chittick, Harvard School of Public Health; Dona Futterman and Neil Hoffman, Adolescent AIDS Program, Montefiore Medical Center, New York; and Sofia Gruskin, François-Xavier Bagnoud Center for Health and Human Rights, Harvard School of Public Health, Boston.

E. Social roles
  • quality of relations to parents, other family members, and friends (peers)
  • availability of role models and age-appropriate socialization opportunities
  • perception of personal safety within social environment and social network

II. Program-dependent vulnerability
  A. Program focus
  • availability of school health-based initiatives and outreach programs for young people out of school and others in especially difficult circumstances
  • availability of programs for orphans and for physically or mentally disadvantaged young people
  • availability of health and social programs targeted at runaway and homeless young people
  • availability of health and social services for the prevention, detection, referral, and care of child abuse
  B. Program content
  • information and education on sexuality, sexual health, and reproductive health built into curriculae of formal and nonformal education programs
  • availability of STI diagnosis and treatment and of HIV testing and counseling programs linked to other clinical services
  • availability of condoms and other contraceptive methods
  • providers' training in health and mental health issues relevant to young people
  • providers' specific knowledge and skills in addressing diverse sexual practices and concerns of young people
  • availability of programs that expose the risks of any needle use (for addictive drugs, hormones, or tattoos and rituals) and of mind-altering substances, including drugs and alcohol
  • availability of harm reduction and drug treatment programs for injecting drug users, on demand
  C. Program approaches
  • recognition of young people's specific aspirations, needs, and sexual orientation
  • collection, analysis, and use of information collected, specifically on young people
  • availability of health systems for young people that are accessible, friendly, visible, confidential, affordable, flexible, and coordinated
  • partnership between young people, health systems, and educational services
  • creation of venues for young people to share information without censorship by adults

III. Societal vulnerability
  A. Sexuality
  • recognition of the diversity of sexual behaviors and practices among young people
  • patterns of sexual initiation
  • recognition of, and non-discrimination toward, different emerging sexual orientations (as heterosexual, bisexual, lesbian, or gay)
  • social, cultural, and religious beliefs that militate against safer sex
  B. Gender
  • gender inequalities in patterns of ownership, access to education, employment opportunities, and fair wages, and in gender roles
  C. Education and information
  • level of educational achievement for both genders
  • media involvement in sex education, including promotion of safer sex targeted at young people

- media involvement in raising societal issues pertaining to young people
- ability of parents and educators to dialogue with young people on issues relevant to them, particularly on sexuality

D. Supportive environment
- material and emotional support from family, kinship, and friends
- expansion of the concept of family to include friends and community
- social norms pertaining to the role of youth in the family and in society
- collective, positive vision of the future (hope)
- prevalence of domestic and public violence and population displacement
- marginalization of particular groups
- recognition of patterns and frequency of child abuse
- social, physical, and spiritual support extended to young people during illnesses, including those related to HIV infection and AIDS
- enactment of policies and laws conducive to the reduction of young people's vulnerability

E. Livelihood
- education, training, and employment opportunities for young people
- poverty
- patterns of distribution of wealth; economic gaps within society
- quality of working environment
- demand for and attitude toward exchange of sex for payment
- prevalence and nature of child labor

Then, once this information is collected, it becomes possible to identify systematically the contextual issues relevant to reducing vulnerability (Box 40-5).

BOX 40-5

Societal context and response

JEFFREY O'MALLEY

Although many activists have criticized governmental and other AIDS programs as being too *medically* oriented, it would be more accurate to characterize many institutional responses as derivations of narrow, traditional *public health* strategies, with a related focus on individual behavior change. Indeed, most official AIDS programs are organized within institutions with a public health mandate, and even nongovernmental efforts heavily emphasize information and education, which are expected to change individual behavior. Thus, the early response to HIV/AIDS has been characterized as "program based"; the major institutional objective was the creation of programs to provide the benefits of the "prevention triad" to as many people as possible, in as many countries as possible.

Despite various assertions that AIDS is a development issue, and gradually increasing attempts to address the social consequences of AIDS, such as discrimination against people with HIV, there has been remarkably little attempt to analytically or programmatically link the *causes* of HIV/AIDS to issues of income growth and distribution. There have been even fewer attempts to broaden the analysis of the social context of the epidemic to such issues as culture, the social construction of sexuality, patterns and structures of health service delivery, and gender identity and gender relations.

In order to move beyond simple assertions of linkages between social context and HIV/AIDS, it is useful to consider how social factors are both narrowly and broadly relevant. For example, the first obvious link between poverty and the epidemic is that AIDS costs money, both to affected individuals and their communities. The money is spent on prevention, care, and the consequences of death. However, the costs of preventing HIV infection, for example, to finance community prevention programs and individual condom purchases, remain lower than the costs of care or the consequences of death. Therefore, prevention efforts can be justified with an economic analysis.

There are also links between economics and the efficacy of prevention and care interventions. When HIV-infected individuals spend their savings on care and lose their incomes due to illness, they suffer from reduced access to proper nutrition and support. They also become less able to control their environment and responsibly avoid infecting others. A similar phenomenon can affect their families. For instance, an economically dependent wife may find that she has to have an increased number of sexual partners when widowed due to disinheritance and impoverishment. Thus, economic support activities for people with HIV and their loved ones are an important component of any response to AIDS.

Yet there is also a broader set of linkages between poverty and HIV. Both absolute poverty and relative differences between rich and poor shape both sexual behavior and care-seeking behavior (for example, the poor are less likely to be diagnosed and treated for STIs). Thus HIV/AIDS prevention and care efforts must also occur within a broader context of equitable economic development.

The actions needed to help reduce social vulnerability by working directly on the contextual factors inevitably extends beyond the traditional bounds of public health, or at least beyond the normal scope of influence and authority of ministries of health.[12] Indeed, to address the social context, work with at least three additional groups and organizations is required:

- other governmental departments (e.g., ministries of information, social welfare, defense, employment, justice, finance, education) and official agencies (e.g., governmental organizations involved with employment, public safety, medical care)
- nongovernmental organizations, including both AIDS-specific and other organizations
- the private sector (including business, religious groups, and the media, etc.)

Box 40-6 briefly outlines the principal steps involved in an effort to reduce social vulnerability.

BOX 40-6

Generating government commitment

To illustrate how vulnerability reduction work proceeds, consider an example in which an important contextual factor is governmental inattention and lack of concern about HIV/AIDS. The following questions should be raised:

1. *What needs to be done?* Governmental commitment to HIV/AIDS needs to be ensured and the priority of HIV/AIDS among governmental concerns raised. This could be measured in several

ways, including budgetary and personnel commitments to HIV/AIDS, and leaders speaking out on HIV/AIDS.

2. *How can this be done?* Decision makers need to receive accurate information and reasonable projections about the HIV epidemic in the country. The general public and/or sectors with influence on government need to become more aware of the current status of HIV/AIDS and its future potential. Governmental agencies must feel pressure to pay attention to HIV/AIDS.

3. *With whom would the work be done?* Important governmental departments include those dealing with the economy, defense, information and communication, and planning. Important nongovernmental organizations (NGOs) include AIDS service organizations and other AIDS-related NGOs, and large, already established NGOs. Important private sector collaboration may come from the media, popular figures (film, television, sports, music, dance, theater, fashion), religious organizations, and private businesses.

Considerable experience and empirical data suggest that poverty—both in absolute and relative terms—is an important contextual issue in HIV/AIDS prevention, as poverty increases social vulnerability to HIV. The absolute level of poverty clearly burdens the poor in many ways that adversely affect their vulnerability to HIV/AIDS. These range from a lack of disposable income for purchasing condoms, to lack of access to health services and HIV prevention programs.[13] In addition, large gaps between the highest and lowest socioeconomic strata (relative poverty) generate the conditions in which people adopt survival strategies which in turn, amplify their vulnerability to becoming HIV infected.[14] Such survival strategies may involve providing unprotected sexual intercourse in return for money, lodging, food, or other necessities. Of course, the analysis of HIV/AIDS and poverty is a particular case of the well-known and well-studied, consistent global relationship between socioceconomic status and health status.[15] Yet the identification of poverty as an important contextual factor for understanding social vulnerability to HIV/AIDS also suggests the limits of contextual analysis as a guide to effective public health action. For while the question, what needs to be done?, can be answered simply: reduce or eliminate poverty, reduce the gap between the rich and the poor, the methods for accomplishing this goal are unclear. This difficulty is compounded by the consideration of related questions: how can this be done?, and with whom would the work be done?

To put the case bluntly: what should public health workers be advised to do in order to address the problem of poverty directly? The usual public health response is to create clinics and provide needed services, which, although useful and important, cannot by themselves compensate for the social disadvantage created by poverty. To the extent that poverty is understood as a societal problem which expresses itself as income and economic disparity, it is clear that fundamental questions about society are raised in this analysis. The challenge is to discover how to understand, define, and then address poverty directly and to spell out the specific roles and responsibilities of public health workers in this effort.

Viewing the HIV/AIDS pandemic from a perspective of vulnerability has several institutional and organizational advantages and creates major challenges for public health:

- Vulnerability analysis requires a mix of short- and longer-term approaches.[16] While most national and international responses to the pandemic are still driven by short-term risk reduction approaches, an expanded and long-term response is required to address the complex societal issues revealed to be important determinants of behavior.[17] In addition, it is important to recognize that the extent of personal vulnerability may vary over time. Thus, a person not highly vulnerable to HIV infection may become so as a consequence of loss of employment, which affects self-esteem, forces displacement and a loss of social support networks, or causes severe intrafamilial stress. Therefore, vulnerability must be viewed in a short-, medium-, and longer-term perspective in order to transform a seemingly daunting challenge into a manageable set of tasks that takes into account personal capacity, contextual factors, and the temporal dimension.
- Implementing vulnerability reduction requires a shift from isolated HIV/AIDS programs to a fuller integration of HIV/AIDS programs within health systems and the restructuring of these systems to ensure that they strengthen development efforts. Once contextual factors are highlighted, the need to ensure that HIV/AIDS work is truly part of the entire health system becomes evident.
- Vulnerability analysis also requires a shift away from a traditional, multisectoral approach to HIV/AIDS prevention to a recognition of and response to deeper commonality among different sectors. In the past, many national AIDS programs have sought to involve ministries other than health (education, communication, defense, etc.) in HIV/AIDS work. Too often, however, this has involved only superficial and token measures, such as including a few words about HIV/AIDS in an existing brochure published by another ministry. In contrast, the contextual approach required by vulnerability analysis demonstrates the human development dimensions of HIV/AIDS and creates the potential for synergy by focusing efforts of different sectoral groups onto the contextual issues of common concern. HIV/AIDS is no longer an addition to the development agenda; it signals where development efforts should focus and who should be their prime beneficiaries.
- The interventions needed to address contextual factors are in many ways markedly different from interventions to reduce personal or program-related vulnerability and raise complex analytic, communication, and implementation challenges (Box 40-7). In addition, given the nature of contextual issues (political, economic, cultural, and social), some advocates are discouraged by the realization that the societal changes needed to address contextual issues will require sustained work over a long period.

BOX 40-7

Constraints to contextual changes

Contextual level action can be very useful in an effort to reduce or eliminate barriers to effective implementation of HIV prevention programs. Yet such efforts are also constrained and difficult for several reasons, including:

1. leadership: who will organize and lead the effort?
2. a lack of clarity or common purpose about the goals and the types of intervention needed
3. a sense of powerlessness on the part of health workers about their ability to influence the national or international economy or politics
4. problems with cross-departmental government collaboration
5. difficulties and mistrust between the government and nongovernmental organizations
6. the usually narrow focus on AIDS resulting in relief for HIV/AIDS prevention programs but usually without a broader impact on health in the community. This may compound an attitude among the public and/or decision makers that too much attention is already being paid to HIV/AIDS in comparison with other problems.

In summary, the more recent approach to HIV/AIDS, which is substantially enriched by experience demonstrating how the lived realities of women, men, and children around the world strongly influence their vulnerability to HIV, includes a combination of risk-reduction and vulnerability-reduction actions. The ultimate aim of vulnerability reduction is to expand people's capacity to exert control over their own health. By identifying the larger social issues that constrain or promote this ability, contextual analysis stresses the need for positive and synergistic interaction between the individual, services, programs and other collective initiatives, and the social environment.

Yet, even as efforts to implement contextual analysis and related approaches to reducing societal vulnerability are being developed, it has become clear that a deeper understanding of the nature and fundamental cause of vulnerability has been brought to the forefront. It is clear that HIV prevention, in its full, modern form, challenges personal as well as organizational status quos. Further progress in HIV prevention requires that we learn to apply fully the knowledge and experience borne out of our confrontation with the pandemic. The next chapter will present the new approach to societal vulnerability, based on a human rights framework for societal analysis and program response.

REFERENCES

1. J. Fraser Mustard and J. Frank, *The Determinants of Health*, CIAR publication no. 5 (Toronto: Canadian Institute for Advanced Research, 1991).
2. M. Fishbein and S. E. Middlestadt, "Using the theory of reasoned action as a framework for understanding and changing AIDS-related behaviors," in *Primary Prevention of AIDS: Psychological Approaches*, J. N. Wasserheit, ed. (1989).

3. A. Bandura, "Social cognitive theory and exercise of control over HIV infection," in *Preventing AIDS: Theories and Methods of Behavioral Interventions*, R. J. DiClemente, ed. (New York: Plenum Press, 1994).

4. J. A. Catania, S. M. Kegeles, and T. J. Coates, "Toward an understanding of risk behavior: An AIDS risk reduction model," *Health Education Quarterly* 17 (1990):53–72.

5. R. G. Evans, M. L. Barer, and T. R. Marmor, eds., *Why Are Some People Healthy and Others Not? The Determinants of Health of Populations*, (New York: Aldine de Gruyter, 1994).

6. J. W. Frank, "The determinants of health: A new synthesis," *Current Issues in Public Health* 1 (1995):42–65.

7. M. Berger and S. Ray, *Women and HIV/AIDS: An International Resource Book* (London: Pandora Books, 1993).

8. D. A. Feldman, ed., *Global AIDS Policy* (Westport: Bergin & Garvey, 1995).

9. *Towards a New Health Strategy for AIDS: A Report of the Global AIDS Policy Coalition* (Boston, MA: François-Xavier Bagnoud Center for Health and Human Rights, Harvard School of Public Health, 1993).

10. Joint United Nations Programme on HIV/AIDS (UNAIDS): *Strategic Plan 1996–2000*. Background document for the second meeting of the Programme Coordinating Board, Geneva, 13–15 November 1995 (UNAIDS/PCB(2)/95.3, 31 October, 1995).

11. "Declaration," Paris AIDS Summit of Heads of Government, Paris, France, December 1, 1994.

12. J. Mann, D. Tarantola, J. O'Malley, and The Global AIDS Policy Coalition, "Towards a new health strategy to control the HIV/AIDS pandemic," *Journal of American Society of Law, Medicine, and Ethics*, 22(1994):41–52.

13. T. O'Shaughnessy, "Beyond the fragments: HIV/AIDS and poverty," in *Issues in Global Development* 1 (World Vision, Melbourne Australia Research and Policy Unit, November 1994).

14. Panos Institute, "Triple jeopardy: Women and AIDS," in *Panos Dossier*, (London: The Panos Institute, 1990).

15. World Development Report, *Investing in Health* (Washington, DC: The World Bank, 1993).

16. J. M. Mann and D. Tarantola, "Making history: Revitalization of the global AIDS effort" working paper submitted for the preparation of the Paris Summit of Heads of Governments on AIDS, Paris, January, 1994.

17. I. O. Orubuloye, J. C. Caldwell, P. Cadwell, and G. Santow, eds., *Sexual Networking and AIDS in Sub-Saharan Africa: Behavioral Research and the Social Context* (Canberra: Health Transition Centre, The Australian National University, 1994).

41

From Vulnerability to Human Rights

The future of HIV/AIDS prevention and control will depend on our ability to understand, at the deepest possible level, the nature of individual and collective vulnerability to HIV. Modern human rights analysis provides a conceptual framework, consensus about the direction of necessary change, and a consistent vocabulary needed to analyze and address the underlying societal conditions that strongly influence vulnerability to HIV. Since contextual factors have an impact on personal, programmatic and societal vulnerability to HIV, a human rights analysis strengthens the ability to identify and to address the root causes, or the underlying conditions of society which create and sustain vulnerability to HIV, as well as more broadly, to preventable disease, disability and premature death (Fig. 41-1). The insight that vulnerability to HIV/AIDS depends upon the extent to which human rights are realized and human dignity is respected within each society (and among societies) creates an opportunity to intervene at the deepest societal level, and thereby combat the pandemic.

Background

In working on health problems directly linked with human behavior, public health has always recognized that forces beyond the immediate control of individuals—political, economic, cultural, or social—have a major and sometimes overwhelming influence on individual behavior and the capacity for health-promoting behavioral change. Precisely because the social environment that allows people to make and effectuate real and informed choices is so important, it ought to be a dominant concern for public health.

Yet public health has experienced great difficulty engaging in efforts to change the economic, political, cultural, and social environment (the contextual factors) in a health-promoting and -protective direction. Unfortunately, public health approaches have often stopped at the point of noting the impact of larger, societal forces on health, citing the epidemiological evidence, and deploring the lack of social or political will to effect change.

While many explanations for this paralysis can be advanced, four reasons

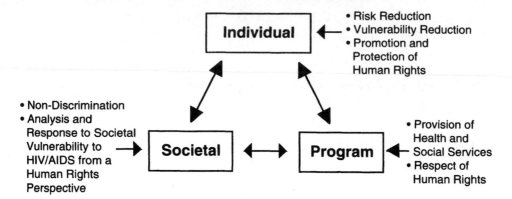

Figure 41-1　1990s: human rights approach for reducing individual program-related and societal vulnerability to HIV/AIDS.

for confusion and inaction in public health in regard to influencing the societal determinants of health include:

- lack of a coherent conceptual framework to describe and analyze the nature of the societal factors
- lack of consensus about the ways in which the societal factors should change to better promote and protect health
- lack of a consistent and accessible vocabulary to speak of these societal factors
- lack of a practical approach, adaptable to different settings and circumstances, that could be recommended

Discovery of the human rights basis of vulnerability to HIV

Two lines of evidence have provided insight into the human rights foundation of HIV vulnerability and of health in general.[1] First, a meta-analysis of the evolving HIV epidemics in countries around the world has revealed a feature of the pandemic which was previously unknown. The history of AIDS has shown that HIV can enter a community or country in many different ways. In each country, where and among whom HIV enters obviously defines the early history of the epidemic. Thus, in the United States and France, white gay men were first noted to be affected; in Brazil, first cases occurred among members of the "jet set" in Rio and São Paulo; in Ethiopia, AIDS was initially noted among the social elite. However, with time, as the epidemic matures, it evolves and moves along a clear and consistent pathway, which, although different in its details within each society, nevertheless has a single, vital, and common feature. For in each society, those people who were marginalized, stigmatized and discriminated against—before HIV/AIDS arrived—have become over time those at highest risk of HIV infection. Regardless of where and among whom it may start within a community or country, the brunt of the epidemic gradually and inexorably turns towards those who bear this societal burden. Thus in the United States, the epidemic has turned increasingly toward "minority" populations in inner cities, injecting drug users, and women. In Brazil, the HIV epidemic now rages through heterosexual transmission in the *favelas* of Rio de Janeiro and São Paulo. In Ethiopia, HIV is concentrated among the poor and dispossessed. The French have a simple term which says it all: HIV is now becoming a problem mainly for *les exclus*—the "excluded ones" living at the margins of society.

The second source of insight about human rights and HIV prevention is the detailed analysis of limits and failures in prevention programs. For example, married and monogamous women who receive the normal benefits of HIV prevention programs—information, education, access to testing and counseling, and condom availability—may nevertheless be at risk of HIV infection. Indeed, in some countries, being married and monogamous is considered a risk factor for HIV infection. To understand this apparent paradox, the real-life situations facing women must be appreciated.

Consider, for example, the recommendation given to women (and men) to reduce the number of sexual partners as part of a risk reduction approach. This recommendation fails in the real world for several reasons (Chapters 16, 19, 20). First, women's risk is related to their male sexual partner's behavior. In the city of Kigali, Rwanda, for instance, 20 percent of HIV-infected women had only a single lifetime sexual partner, and in Morocco 45 percent of infected women have been infected by their husbands. Second, multiple sexual partnerships may be the only route of access to resources—for school, financial credit, or jobs. Third, women often lack control over their sexual relationships. In marriage, without legal recourse or legal rights to property, the pervasive threat of physical violence or divorce may totally disempower a woman, even if she knows about AIDS, condoms are available, and she knows her husband is HIV infected.

Therefore, the central problem for HIV infection among women cannot be solved with risk reduction approaches such as posters, information campaigns, or condom distribution systems. Since the central issue is the inferior role and subordinate status of women, the disadvantage created by society cannot be redressed through information and education or HIV-specific health and social services.[2] For to the extent that women's human rights and dignity are not respected, society creates and enhances their vulnerability to HIV and, more generally, to ill-health.[3] This is one among many groups suffering greater vulnerability to HIV infection due to discrimination, including gay and lesbian people worldwide, commercial sex workers, or adolescents, whose competence and voice are rarely acknowledged in any meaningful way.

This relationship between how people are treated within a society, and risk for HIV infection and inadequate HIV/AIDS care, is something that has been known for a long time, but it has been hard to speak about for at least three reasons. First, as mentioned above, a common conceptual approach and vocabulary have been lacking, which are needed to identify commonalities between the HIV prevention status of, say, gay men in Eastern Europe and married women in East Africa, or between adolescents in Latin America and drug users in Asia. Because a broad conceptual framework was lacking, only the particular and unique features of each group and place could be seen. Second, members of vulnerable communities and AIDS workers feared that these observations about society and AIDS would be misused by others to reinforce the false yet persistent notion that AIDS is only a problem for the marginalized and thus no longer a threat to the "general public." Third, many AIDS workers and organizations were reluctant to broaden the debate around AIDS out of concern that limited resources would become too thinly spread.

However, a conceptual framework, consistent vocabulary, consensus about the necessary direction of change, and practical measures to advance health have all been available. The concepts and language of modern human rights can be used to describe vulnerability and the societal meaning and impact of the epidemic's evolution. Human rights offers an extremely powerful approach to discuss marginalization, stigmatization, and discrimination and what must be done about these societal problems.[4] Indeed, human rights thinking and public health have been evolving rapidly in the context of HIV/AIDS (Chapter 31, Box 41-1).

BOX 41-1

Tolerance and discrimination

JEFFREY O'MALLEY

Historically, AIDS discrimination first manifested as dramatic and debilitating abuses of the rights of people with HIV/AIDS, or those perceived to be at risk for HIV/AIDS. As a result of the widespread incidence of hatred and intolerance, people with HIV/AIDS were victimized by the burning of their homes, exclusion from schools, withdrawal of health coverage, social ostracization, job loss, and even violence and murder. Individuals from communities initially associated with HIV/AIDS, such as people originating from Africa, sex workers and self-identified gay men, were also prone to victimization, regardless of their HIV status. The response to this severe discrimination was both humanitarian and pragmatic. These human rights abuses were denounced as early as 1987, followed by statements and resolutions such as the World Health Assembly Resolution on avoidance of discrimination in relation to HIV-infected people and people with AIDS.[1] The resolution's analysis focused on the immediately evident human rights *consequences* of the HIV/AIDS pandemic, and pointed to the need for a response which encourages understanding and support of people with HIV or AIDS.

Discrimination against people with HIV or AIDS has more than morally and ethically unacceptable direct consequences. Systematic discrimination against people with HIV/AIDS jeopardizes prevention and care efforts. This argument, the public health rationale for preventing discrimination, was developed at the international level by WHO. The argument gained a high profile in 1989, when people with HIV were excluded from traveling to the United States and certain other countries. Activists around the world joined virtually all major HIV/AIDS and public health institutions in decrying these restrictions not only as a violation of human rights, but as a barrier to the improvement of programs through the free exchange of information at forums such as international AIDS conferences.

This second level of analysis is also reflected in the increasing arguments that the fear of human rights violations undermine HIV/AIDS efforts by driving people at risk and people from affected communities "underground," and away from prevention and care services. This analysis influenced the first ever United Nations human rights decision (in April, 1994) decrying discrimination against consensual homosexual acts among adults. In its decision, the UN Human Rights Committee considered that criminalizing homosexuality would impede an effective education program regarding HIV/AIDS prevention.[2]

Such an argument appearing in the UN Human Rights Committee's findings is strong evidence of the argument's increasing international acceptance, which is paralleled in rising numbers of AIDS programs and health ministries around the world. This analysis was outlined in detail in the first volume of *AIDS in the World* in "AIDS and Human Rights" (Chapter 13), which also noted the extent to which different countries protected or violated the rights of people with HIV, and the extent to which rights were respected in the broader implementation of AIDS programs.[3]

The Committee's findings go beyond a rejection of discrimination as a legitimate public health strategy and actually argue that discrimination against homosexual men undermines public health. This points towards a third analysis of the linkage between AIDS and discrimination, one that views intolerance not only as a misguided *consequence* of HIV/AIDS, but as an actual *cause* of the epidemic. This is a qualitatively different approach to AIDS and discrimination. This approach was earlier developed by the Global AIDS Policy Coalition in 1993 in its statement that "[A]nalysis of the epidemic at all levels—community, national and global—shows that the spread of HIV in populations is strongly influenced by an identifiable societal risk factor: the scope, intensity, and nature of discrimination practiced within the society."[4] Identifying discrimination *in general* as a causative factor in the HIV/AIDS epidemic suggests a need to promote respect of human rights more broadly.

References

1. WHO, World Health Assembly, *Avoidance of Discrimination against HIV-Infected Persons and Persons with AIDS*, preamble, resolution WHA41.24 (May 13, 1988).
2. UN Human Rights Committee, *Fiftieth Session Communication No. 488/1992*, CCPR/C/50/D/488/1992 (April 4, 1994):11.
3. K. Tomasevski, S. Gruskin, Z. Lazzarini, and A. Hendriks, "AIDS and human rights," in *AIDS in the World*, J. Mann, D. Tarantola, and T. Netter, eds. (Cambridge, MA: Harvard University Press, 1992):537–573.
4. Global AIDS Policy Coalition, *Towards A New Health Strategy for AIDS: A Report of the Global AIDS Policy Coalition* (Boston: GAPC, 1993).

An important reason why human rights analysis has rarely been used in public health and why vulnerability to HIV/AIDS has not been sufficiently linked to issues of human rights and dignity is that experts in public health are unfamiliar with modern human rights thinking and practice. Even today, although several schools of public health around the world (i.e., in Australia, the United States, and Mexico) are teaching about human rights, there has been little formal teaching about human rights in health-oriented academic institutions and professional schools. For this reason, Box 41-2 provides some basic information which is useful for discussing the human rights foundation of vulnerability to HIV.

BOX 41-2

Human rights primer

The human rights movement has a long, early history, including philosophic efforts to define the natural rights of all people, international campaigns such as abolition (anti-slavery), and the publication of key documents, such as the late 18th century *Declarations of the Rights of Man and the Citizen* in

France and the U.S. Bill of Rights. However, the modern period of human rights started after the Second World War, in response to the atrocities of the Holocaust in Europe. The same determination to prevent recurrent human tragedy, which led to the creation of the United Nations in 1945, also resulted in a dramatic change in the definition and meaning of human rights.

The promotion of human rights was identified as one of the four principal purposes of the United Nations. In 1948 the Universal Declaration of Human Rights (UDHR) was proposed and adopted by the UN General Assembly as a global bill of rights—"a common standard of achievement for all peoples and all nations." For the first time in history, a set of norms was defined at the international level, providing a universal, secular description of the preconditions for human well-being, and international and national institutions and organizations were created to promote and protect human rights.

The rights contained in the UDHR derive from the central idea that "all human beings are born free and equal in dignity and rights." The UDHR is a list of rights which form the core of the modern human rights movement. Some of these rights involve protecting the individual against the power of the state. Examples of these rights include the right to liberty and security of persons and the right not to be tortured or subjected to cruel, inhuman, or degrading treatment or punishment. Other rights call for societies to create conditions necessary for their realization. These rights include the rights to education, social security, work, and to health care; care in the event of sickness is a human right! A remarkable feature of the UDHR is its accessible vocabulary: in the words of Eleanor Roosevelt, the Universal Declaration of Human Rights is intended for ordinary people, not just for jurists or philosophers. Subsequently, these basic rights have been further elaborated in two major international covenants and then further refined in a large number of treaties and declarations on specific issues such as discrimination against women, genocide, torture, and the promotion and protection of the rights of children.

Yet the modern view of human rights goes beyond a list; a number of core principles applies to all these internationally protected rights:

- Rights inhere in people simply because they are human.
- Rights are inalienable; they cannot be granted nor taken away by a government.
- Rights are universal, applying equally to all people in all places at all times (this also means that violations of rights in any country are of relevance to us all).
- Rights are individual and focus on the relationship between individuals and their governments.
- Governments must strive to realize and protect rights.
- Rights are generally inviolable; they predominate over other social goods. However, the protection of public health is one of the recognized acceptable reasons for restricting some rights under limited circumstances, insofar as this is absolutely necessary for as short a time as possible and is done in the least restrictive manner.
- Rights are inseparable and indivisible.

From this description, it should be clear that human rights emerge from a set of beliefs about people and what is required to promote and protect their well-being. Rights are a set of statements which cannot be proved or disproved empirically.

Yet human rights is not just an idea that we or others can simply decide that we like or dislike. Human rights exist and derive their special nature and legitimacy by having been agreed upon (and voted upon) by the nations of the world. Thus this list of rights is human-made and not a result of revelation or a product of religious authority; thus also, it can change and evolve.

Human rights analysis of vulnerability to HIV

Three-step approach

First, the societal/contextual factors that are important for understanding vulnerability to HIV within a specific community or society need to be recognized.

Second, violations of the specific human rights underlying each of the contextual factors need to be identified. The Universal Declaration of Human Rights (UDHR) is a readily available and practical guide for this process (Appendix F). For example, low priority or lack of attention to HIV/AIDS resulting from governmental denial and neglect of the issue may be identified as an important contextual factor which intensifies vulnerability to HIV. A list of rights that are immediately germane to this problem include the rights to participate in the government of one's own country (UDHR, article 21) and to free flow of information (UDHR, article 19). Indeed, lack of realization of these two rights may be understood as the underlying, fundamental basis of the contextual problem.

Another example is the contextual problem of women's inferior societal role reflecting profound and pervasive discrimination against women in a particular society. Therefore, the right of nondiscrimination (UDHR, article 2) is one of the preconditions for progress against this contextual factor.

Box 41-3 lists the previously cited contextual factors relevant to HIV prevention and identifies rights listed in the UDHR which underlie each contextual factor.

BOX 41-3

Human rights underlie contextual factors

The following section uses the UDHR to identify some of the rights that underlie a list of contextual factors relevant to HIV prevention. The numbers in parentheses refer to the particular article in the Universal Declaration of Human Rights (Appendix F).

I. Political and governmental factors
  A. Rights pertaining to inattention to or lack of concern about HIV/AIDS
   • right to take part in and influence (through elections) the country's government (21)
   • right to health (22,25)
   • right to medical care (25)
   • right to security in the event of sickness or disability (25)
   • freedom of assembly (20)
   • freedom of association (20)
  B. Rights pertaining to laws that criminalize certain behaviors
   • right to nondiscrimination (2)
   • right to liberty and security of persons (3)
   • freedom from degrading treatment or punishment (5)
   • right to equal recognition as a person before the law (6)

- right to equal protection (7)
- freedom from arbitrary arrest, detention, exile (9)
- freedom from arbitrary interference with privacy, family, home (12)
- freedom from attacks on honor/reputation (12)
- freedom of thought, conscience, religion (18)
- freedom of opinion or expression (19)
- right to realization of economic, social, and cultural rights indispensable for dignity (22)

C. Rights involved in interference with information
- freedom from arbitrary interference with correspondence (12)
- freedom of thought, conscience (18)
- freedom of opinion and expression (19)
- freedom to seek, receive, and impart information and ideas (19)
- right to health (25)

D. Rights involved in lack of HIV-related services, as in either insufficient, inadequate, or poorly integrated services, or lack of availability of quality of services to specific groups
- right to nondiscrimination (2)
- right to security of persons (3)
- right to take part in government (21)
- right to medical care (25)
- right to necessary social services (25)
- right to security if sick or disabled (25)
- right to share in scientific advancement and its benefits (27)

E. Rights violated in official (or sanctioned) discrimination against HIV-infected people and people with AIDS, such as in areas of employment, insurance, health care, marriage, travel, or residence
- right to nondiscrimination (2)
- right to freedom of movement and residence (13)
- right to marry and found a family (16)
- right to just and favorable condition of work (23)
- right to medical care and necessary social services (25)
- right to security if ill or disabled (25)

F. Rights violated in official (or sanctioned) discrimination against certain groups based on the following affiliations: organization, gender, race, religion, national origin, age, sexual orientation (partial list)
- rights listed in E, above
- right of assembly and association (20)

II. Sociocultural factors

A. Rights involved in gender roles
- right to nondiscrimination (2)
- UDHR articles 3,5,6,7,9,12,13,16,18,19,20–27. Examples: the right to equal rights to marry, in marriage, and in the dissolution of marriage (16); the right to equal pay for equal work (23); the right to freedom of movement (13); the right to participate in the cultural life of the community (27)

B. Rights involved in attitudes towards sexuality
- right to nondiscrimination (2)
- right to information (19)
- rights listed in A, above

C. Rights violated in stigmatization and marginalization of different groups
  - right to nondiscrimination (2)
  - right to education (26)
  - rights listed in A, above
D. Rights involved in illiteracy and lack of educational opportunity
  - right to nondiscrimination (2)
  - right to seek, receive, and impart information and ideas (19)
  - right to education (26)
III. Economic factors
A. Rights pertaining to poverty and income disparity
  - right to an adequate standard of living, including food, clothing, and housing (25)
  - right to security if unemployed, ill, disabled, widowed, or elderly (25)
  - right to realization of economic, social, and cultural rights indispensable for dignity (22)
  - freedom from degrading treatment (5)
  - right to equal protection of the law (7)
  - right to take part in government of country (21)
  - right to work, including protection against unemployment (23)
  - right to rest and leisure (24)
  - right to education (26)
B. Rights involved in lack of resources for prevention programs
  - right to take part in government of country (21)
  - rights listed in I. A., above
C. Rights pertaining to lack of work/job opportunities
  - right to nondiscrimination (2)
  - right to work, including protection against unemployment and the right to form trade unions (23)
  - rights listed in A, above

Third, one must determine the concrete actions needed to improve respect for the human rights identified as underlying important contextual factors. To determine the next steps, the following three questions need to be considered:

1. What needs to be done? The goal is to increase the realization of specific human rights and dignity in the community and/or country.
2. How can it be done? Methods for advancing human rights include education, seeking changes in law and in practice, catalyzing awareness, and monitoring, identifying, and drawing attention to human rights problems.
3. With whom would this work be carried out? This work requires collaboration with public health workers and those individuals and groups from the official, nongovernmental, and private sector, who are working to promote respect for human rights and dignity within the society.

Box 41-4 outlines the types and range of concrete activity that can be done to promote and protect human rights.

BOX 41-4

The human right to information: pathway to action

The following is a list of specific activities designed to increase respect for the right to information, developed and carried out in concert with both health and human rights colleagues:

- Identify the problem of information censorship in the society. This may involve meetings with government officials, efforts to educate the public, and efforts within the educational system.
- Define the goal clearly, to reduce government censorship and other arbitrary interferences with the free flow of information.
- Describe concretely how respect for this right is essential for protecting and promoting public health, using specific, locally relevant examples.
- Bring together individuals and groups who are concerned about, or adversely affected by, the current obstacles to the free flow of information. If no existing asociation is engaged in this work, create a new association.
- Point out to the government that it has obligations to respect human rights, to which it agreed by signing human rights treaties and declarations.
- Establish links with organizations in other countries and with international organizations to network and help discover new avenues for achieving progress.
- Other activities may include letter-writing campaigns, demonstrations, and publicity to inform people outside the country.

A specific example

Consider the situation in which the government is interfering with dissemination of accurate information about the routes of HIV spread or the methods that people can use to protect themselves, such as condoms. This increases people's personal vulnerability, because an uninformed or misinformed persons cannot act rationally to protect themselves. In terms of the program, the lack of information means that the prevention triad has not been applied. In societal terms, vulnerability is enhanced by governmental failure to allow dissemination of information needed to protect public health. This in turn, reflects several contextual issues, including political and governmental inattention or lack of concern about HIV/AIDS, socio-cultural factors (e.g., attitudes towards sexuality), and economic factors (lack of resources for prevention).

In human rights terms, vulnerability to HIV results from violation of several rights, including:

- the right to seek, receive and impart information
- the right to security of person
- the right to freedom from arbitrary interference with privacy, family, and home
- freedom of opinion and expression
- the right to share in scientific advancement and its benefits
- the right to take part in and influence the government

The problem is clearly posed. Personal vulnerability will be difficult to reduce until the critical information is made available. Similarly, program-related vulnerability cannot be reduced precisely because the government will not allow the needed information/education program to be carried out. The contextual analysis of societal vulnerability may identify the problem as excessive influence of certain political, economic, or other groups on governmental policy.

If limited to a contextual analysis, the likely actions will focus on trying to convince the decision-makers that HIV/AIDS is such a serious problem that information about its modes of spread and methods to prevent spread must be disseminated widely. One hopes that these efforts to change decision-makers' attitudes will succeed. However, even if successful, the results will be limited to the immediate HIV/AIDS issue of information about condoms. And what can be done if the effort to get decision-makers to change their assessment of the HIV/AIDS problem does not succeed, or succeeds only in superficial ways (e.g., a government statement not followed by changing policy or resource allocation)?

A human rights–based analysis identifies a cluster of rights, from which the right to seek, receive, and impart information and ideas can be selected as most critical, which underlie the specific problem of governmental objection to the provision of information essential for preventing HIV transmission. Action to promote respect for the right to information will contribute both to reducing the spread of HIV and will have larger positive effects on public health.

A second example of this approach, involving young married women and vulnerability to HIV, is outlined in Box 41-5.

BOX 41-5

Example of the human rights analysis

Consider the specific situation of young married women and their vulnerability to sexual transmission of HIV/AIDS.

1. The epidemiology will show that increasing numbers of married women are becoming HIV infected. Individual risk factors will generally involve the partner's sexual behavior, including unwillingness to use condoms.
2. Personal vulnerability can be described in cognitive terms (what knowledge is needed), or in terms of skills for negotiation of condom use.
3. Program-related vulnerability considers whether programs to provide services, including testing and counseling and condom distribution, are available to these women.
4. Societal vulnerability analysis will identify the contextual factors that are important to enhancing married women's vulnerability to being exposed to HIV through sexual intercourse with their partner. Examples include women's lack of influence in government, their economic subordination, and sociocultural factors.
5. A human rights analysis will identify the violation of a cluster of rights—including rights to non-discrimination, education, and equal rights in marriage—as deep, underlying factors that place married women in a "risk ecology" of increased vulnerability to HIV.

The health and human rights–based response links HIV vulnerability of married women to one or several of the rights issues cited, for example, the right to education. Working to promote educational opportunity (by improving access and ensuring equal opportunity for women within existing educational systems) will then help advance the public health goal of reducing vulnerability of married women to HIV (as well as to other health issues, such as reproductive health and injuries, including domestic violence and rape).

Advantages and barriers to the human rights approach

Adding a human rights dimension to HIV prevention work will have major advantages as well as creating some difficulties. Major advantages include:

1. acting at the deeper level of societal causes, so as to help uproot the pandemic
2. linking health issues with the mobilizing power of human rights discourse
3. expanding the ability of people throughout society to see the connection between a rights issue and their health
4. creating an increased capacity for cross-disciplinary and institutional work which occurs when people can identify a larger commonality of interest
5. revitalizing the concept of globalism within the collective response to HIV/AIDS

In addition, major potential difficulties include:

1. the inevitable accusation that public health is "meddling" in societal issues that go far beyond its scope or competence
2. the unfamiliarity of public health workers with rights concepts and language
3. skepticism among human rights workers about the interest of public health professionals in working on common issues
4. public health workers' desire to "own" the problem of HIV/AIDS; for by keeping the discourse at a medical and public health level, the preeminent role of health workers is assured
5. human rights issues are inherently and inevitably contentious and may put the person evoking rights potentially at odds with governmental and other sources of power in the society

Conclusion: bringing it all together

As the capacity for understanding and preventing the pandemic deepens, the challenges become ever more difficult. For example, it is clearly easier for public health agencies and organizations to provide only information about HIV/AIDS (as in the period of discovery) than to ensure comprehensive services to support risk reduction (as proposed in the period of early response). Similarly, it is easier for those concerned about HIV/AIDS to de-have been developing gradually during the current period) than to undertake a human rights–based analysis and response to the pandemic.

Yet real progress towards uncovering and addressing the roots of the pandemic will depend upon further development and application of all the approaches described in this part of *AIDS in the World II*, including the human rights–based approach. The central challenge today is to bring together the optimal mixture, including risk reduction, vulnerability reduction, and human rights realization, to create a strategy best suited to each specific setting.

The creation of a synthesis cannot be used to justify ignoring or failing to implement at least some actions based on each of the approaches listed above. For while each level is complementary, drawing upon special analytic skills and methods, only when joined together can they fully equip public health efforts against HIV/AIDS. Therefore, the response to HIV/AIDS must ensure that efforts are *simultaneously* underway for risk reduction, vulnerability reduction, and human rights realization. From the previous analysis it is clear that HIV prevention, in its full, modern form, challenges personal, organizational, and societal status quos. The challenge of HIV prevention and care is truly daunting.

The history of response to HIV has clearly evolved in the direction of bringing both the best of traditional public health together with new insights and understanding of the societal influences on personal behavior. However, some people and organizations working in public health (whether on HIV/AIDS or in other areas) still hold tenaciously to the traditional risk-reduction approach, despite its inherently limited ability to prevent HIV transmission. Most often, however, people working on HIV/AIDS recognize the importance of the societal dimension but are unclear about how to proceed or think that this work on social factors should be done by someone else.

This brings us to the threshold of empowerment, which is a critical concept not only for others, but also for ourselves. Empowerment occurs when people realize that some important aspect of their lives *can be different*. For example, when women who are physically abused by their partners realize that this treatment is not an inherent, inescapable part of life, the first step towards empowerment has occurred. Other examples are easy to identify in the context of HIV/AIDS: when gay men in a closed community realize that gay men in other places can live openly, or when sex workers discover that in other places, associations of sex workers have been able to improve working conditions and make sex work safer.

A second element in empowerment is a sense of self-efficacy, the idea that *change is possible*. This belief, while it may be inspired by historical examples, or fostered by peers and participation in community organization and social movements, is ultimately quite personal. It is not clear exactly how people who have considered themselves powerless may begin to believe in the possibility of change, but this step is at the heart of personal, and ultimately, societal transformation.

Once these two elements come together—realizing that the status quo is not immutable and that change is possible—the stage is set for empowerment to occur. Yet empowerment can only develop from within each individual, organization or society; it cannot be forced upon any person or group from outside. At the same time, empowerment can be facilitated by providing information, by linking people with others, and by supporting active initiatives developed from within.

Empowerment applies not only to those vulnerable to HIV infection because they cannot make and effectuate real and informed choices about their health; these same principles apply to those working to prevent HIV infection. For *we* must recognize that the limited ability of the risk reduction approach to HIV prevention can change; that the status quo of inherently limited impact of the programmatic approach (information/education and health and social services) can change. Next, we must have confidence that we *can* influence positively those societal factors that determine to a large extent, who will become HIV infected and who will not and who receives quality care and who does not. This confidence is derived from the analytic work revealing the societal dimensions of the pandemic. These are contextual—political, social, cultural, and economic—and they must be understood and acted upon at a deeper level as consequences of a lack of respect for human rights and dignity.

Thus we are equipped to advance—in new and meaningful ways—the community, national, and global effort to control the HIV pandemic. The next step requires a leap of confidence based on analysis, reflection, and hard work. Only we can empower ourselves. The future history of HIV/AIDS in the world is in the balance.

REFERENCES

1. J. M. Mann, "Public health and human rights," *Current Issues in Public Health* 1 (1995):97–101.
2. K. Tomasevski, *Women and Human Rights* (London: Zed Books, 1995).
3. R. J. Cook, "Gender, health and human rights," *Health and Human Rights* 4(1995):350–364.
4. J. Mann, L. Gostin, S. Gruskin et al., "Health and human rights," *Health and Human Rights* Volume 1, No. 1(1994):6–22.

APPENDIXES

Appendix A. AIDS Reporting

AIDS cases reported to the World Health Organization, by geographic area of affinity (GAA), and year, 1979–1996
(Figures shown are Jan 1 to Dec 31 of each year)

GAA	Country	1979–1984	1985	1986	1987	1988	1989	1990	1991	1992	1993	1994	1995 to date	Cumulative to date	Date of last report
1	Canada	259	357	579	876	1,007	1,133	867	714	1,229	2,059	1,747	1,292	12,119	9/30/95
1	United States	10,546	11,315	18,423	27,464	33,297	37,556	36,658	31,512	44,300	160,836	13,767	75,636	501,310	10/31/95
	Totals for GAA1	10,805	11,672	19,002	28,340	34,304	38,689	37,525	32,226	45,529	162,895	15,514	76,928	513,429	
2	Austria	16	23	21	87	104	139	152	148	188	225	204	135	1,442	9/30/95
2	Belgium	109	67	74	121	138	159	184	195	196	302	246	139	1,930	9/30/95
2	Cyprus	0	0	5	3	2	3	7	3	1	1	14	8	47	10/29/95
2	Denmark	36	37	69	100	126	172	196	202	188	217	264	174	1,781	9/30/95
2	Finland	6	4	7	8	17	17	18	23	14	36	38	28	216	9/30/95
2	France	367	564	1,218	2,188	1,976	3,631	3,857	4,045	4,010	6,647	5,643	4,226	38,372	9/30/95
2	Germany	203	319	586	1,075	1,357	1,633	1,263	1,032	1,533	1,816	1,493	1,355	13,665	9/30/95
2	Greece	6	7	22	53	82	107	135	147	139	183	174	181	1,236	9/30/95
2	Iceland	0	1	3	1	5	3	3	6	1	8	4	2	37	9/30/95
2	Ireland	6	5	6	20	37	50	55	62	58	78	59	55	491	9/30/95
2	Italy	44	196	452	1,036	1,741	2,413	2,977	2,759	3,445	5,254	5,690	4,440	30,447	9/30/95
2	Luxembourg	0	3	3	3	4	11	9	12	11	19	13	12	100	9/30/95
2	Malta	1	1	3	2	7	0	1	7	3	4	3	3	35	9/30/95
2	Monaco	0	0	0	0	1	2	2	2	4	13	7	6	37	9/30/95
2	Netherlands	55	66	137	242	322	385	405	356	395	557	450	364	3,734	9/30/95
2	Norway	6	15	21	35	25	43	54	49	39	69	66	60	482	9/30/95
2	Portugal	4	29	32	70	114	167	205	188	224	602	612	479	2,726	9/30/95
2	San Marino	0	0	0	0	0	1	0	0	0	0	0	0	1	9/30/95
2	Spain	65	158	437	974	1,992	2,618	2,811	2,510	3,878	7,277	6,637	5,261	34,618	9/30/95
2	Sweden	18	32	55	79	86	131	119	125	108	200	183	140	1,276	9/30/95
2	Switzerland	51	75	163	257	423	511	459	290	507	804	737	518	4,795	9/30/95
2	United Kingdom	258	234	461	663	863	1,007	1,111	857	1,168	1,953	1,701	1,218	11,494	9/30/95
	Totals for GAA2	1,251	1,836	3,775	7,017	9,422	13,203	14,023	13,018	16,110	26,265	24,238	18,804	148,962	

(continued)

Appendix A AIDS cases reported to the World Health Organization, by geographic area of affinity (GAA), and year, 1979–1996—continued
(Figures shown are Jan 1 to Dec 31 of each year)

GAA	Country	1979–1984	1985	1986	1987	1988	1989	1990	1991	1992	1993	1994	1995 to date	Cumulative to date	Date of last report
3	American Samoa	0	0	0	0	0	0	0	0	0	0	0	0	0	3/30/95
3	Australia	53	122	226	371	522	568	591	544	644	1,086	674	482	5,883	3/31/95
3	Cook Islands	0	0	0	0	0	0	0	0	0	0	0	0	0	12/31/94
3	Fiji	0	0	0	0	0	3	0	1	1	1	1	0	7	3/20/95
3	French Polynesia	0	0	0	1	0	7	8	11	3	6	9	0	45	12/31/94
3	Guam								11	2	6	6	6	31	8/31/95
3	Kiribati	0	0	0	0	0	0	0	0	0	1	0	0	1	9/27/95
3	Marshall Islands	0	0	0	0	0	0	0	2	0	0	0	0	2	9/30/95
3	Micronesia	0	0	0	0	0	0	0	2	0	0	0	0	2	10/11/95
3	Nauru	0	0	0	0	0	0	0	0	0	0	0	0	0	6/8/95
3	New Caledonia	0	0	0	0	2	0	12	6	5	6	8	4	43	6/8/95
3	New Zealand	8	12	18	33	45	69	61	58	48	79	44	36	511	9/30/95
3	Niue	0	0	0	0	0	0	0	0	0	0	0	0	0	4/26/95
3	Northern Mariana Islands	0	0	0	0	0	0	0	1	3	0	2	0	6	10/1/95
3	Palau	0	0	0	0	0	0	0	0	0	1	0	0	1	10/20/95
3	Papua New Guinea	0	0	0	2	9	5	13	11	6	12	35	48	141	9/28/95
3	Solomon Islands	0	0	0	0	0	0	0	0	0	0	0	0	0	9/29/95
3	Tokelau	0	0	0	0	0	0	0	0	0	0	0	0	0	9/19/95
3	Tonga	0	0	0	1	0	0	1	0	1	3	0		6	12/31/93
3	Tuvalu	0	0	0	0	0	0	0	0	0	0	0		0	12/31/94
3	Vanuatu	0	0	0	0	0	0	0	0	0	0	0	0	0	4/10/95
3	Wallis & Futuna	0	0	0	0	0	0	0	0	0	0	1	0	1	9/28/95
3	Western Samoa	0	0	0	0	0	0	0	0	1	0	0	1	2	7/31/95
	Totals for GAA3	61	134	244	408	578	652	686	647	714	1,201	780	577	6,682	
4	Argentina	14	28	31	72	169	229	377	378	642	1,591	1,910	1,394	6,835	9/30/95
4	Belize	0	0	0	4	5	2	0	28	20	23	18	8	100	6/30/94
4	Bolivia	0	1	2	3	10	2	7	14	12	29	17	8	105	6/30/95
4	Brazil	158	481	945	2,162	3,580	4,516	4,421	6,868	9,100	14,762	13,876	10,242	71,111	9/2/95
4	Chile	5	6	18	40	53	65	68	245	101	230	295	164	1,290	9/30/95
4	Colombia	0	0	61	181	263	330	450	904	998	1,043	1,049	484	5,763	6/30/95
4	Costa Rica	6	3	11	23	52	56	81	80	117	127	153	142	851	9/30/95

4	Ecuador	0	0	15	19	25	15	53	52	50	114	113	35	491	3/31/95
4	El Salvador	0	1	6	16	48	94	118	56	60	193	326	330	1,248	9/30/95
4	French Guiana	0	0	31	62	20	37	82	0	0	232	218	39	721	9/30/95
4	Guatemala	0	0	16	12	18	18	78	94	67	206	85		594	12/31/94
4	Guyana	0	0	0	10	34	40	61	86	159	49	188	71	698	6/30/95
4	Honduras	0	5	12	102	184	231	513	548	482	1,196	817	334	4,424	6/30/95
4	Mexico	121	220	452	1,027	1,411	900	1,776	3,154	2,394	5,779	4,502	4,924	26,660	9/30/95
4	Nicaragua	0	0	0	0	2	2	7	11	11	26	30	28	117	9/30/95
4	Panama	0	0	26	30	61	75	57	69	84	211	203	131	947	9/30/95
4	Paraguay	0	0	2	5	4	3	12	10	16	16	43	65	176	6/30/95
4	Peru	5	4	3	60	68	117	141	164	214	231	642	1,060	2,709	6/30/95
4	Suriname	1	1	2	5	4	35	35	15	30	39	29	13	209	6/30/95
4	Uruguay	0	0	7	7	20	32	82	91	80	124	118	97	658	9/30/95
4	Venezuela	16	20	55	132	268	326	244	512	769	990	863	765	4,960	9/30/95
	Totals for GAA4	326	770	1,695	3,972	6,299	7,125	8,663	13,379	15,406	27,211	25,495	20,326	130,667	
5	Angola	0	3	6	32	63	0	0	317	131	151	149	43	895	3/31/95
5	Benin	0	1	2	6	18	57	50	82	254	121	330	145	1,066	7/10/95
5	Botswana	0	1	10	25	22	29	91	82	205	950	1,187	508	3,110	6/5/95
5	Burkina Faso	0	0	10	21	394	481	72	250	1,658	1,307			4,193	12/31/93
5	Burundi	0	0	269	652	1,054	809	521	2,359	1,209	689			7,562	12/31/93
5	Cameroon	0	0	21	20	33	60	61	691	1,288	1,006	2,195		5,375	12/31/94
5	Cape Verde	0	1	1	16	0	10	4	19	14	78			143	12/10/93
5	Central Afr. Rep.	0	0	0	108	622	432	702	1,866	270	249	214		4,463	11/10/95
5	Chad	0	0	2	2	7	10	38	165	675	682	1,089	787	3,457	5/31/95
5	Comoros	0	0	0	1	0	1	1	1	0	1	2		7	11/15/95
5	Congo	0	0	250	1,000	330	360	465	1,077	1,785	919	1,196	391	7,773	4/22/95
5	Côte d'Ivoire	0	2	118	404	1,193	1,930	3,189	3,956	3,306	3,628	5,359	2,151	25,236	5/31/95
5	Djibouti	0	0	0	0	6	51	46	168	170	171	155		768	10/30/95
5	Equatorial Guinea	0	0	0	1	2	2	4	15	20	45	68		157	11/9/95
5	Eritrea	0	0	0	0	0	0	0	0	0	0	0	1,664	1,664	7/31/95
5	Ethiopia	0	0	2	17	62	238	796	558	3,188	5,229	6,237	3,106	19,433	7/30/95
5	Gabon	0	0	13	4	10	24	66	98	138	135	275	227	990	10/27/95
5	Gambia, The	0	0	11	16	30	21	46	46	49	58	53	39	369	9/30/95

(continued)

481

Appendix A AIDS cases reported to the World Health Organization, by geographic area of affinity (GAA), and year, 1979–1996—continued
(Figures shown are Jan 1 to Dec 31 of each year)

GAA	Country	1979–1984	1985	1986	1987	1988	1989	1990	1991	1992	1993	1994	1995 to date	Cumulative to date	Date of last report
5	Ghana	0	0	26	35	266	899	1,011	903	4,022	4,349	3,190	1,189	15,890	6/30/95
5	Guinea	0	0	0	4	29	49	138	118	192	446	566	139	1,681	3/31/95
5	Guinea-Bissau	0	0	0	0	0	123	34	19	118	203	210		707	12/31/94
5	Kenya	0	10	264	1,223	2,817	4,825		14,947	9,377		17,111	6,336	56,910	4/25/95
5	Lesotho	0	0	1	1	3	6	0	33	137	300	34		515	12/31/94
5	Liberia	0	0	2	0	0	3	0	19	38	129			191	3/31/94
5	Madagascar	0	0	0	0	0	0	0	2	1	5	7	7	22	11/14/95
5	Malawi	0	72	72	858	3,034	3,812	4,226	5,709	5,267	8,180	4,357	4,402	39,989	11/6/95
5	Mali	0	1	5	23	99	106	104	567	445	569	649	26	2,594	1/10/95
5	Mauritania	0	0	0	0	5	6	5	14	10	11	28	51	130	8/22/95
5	Mauritius	0	0	0	1	1	2	1	5	6	2	9		27	12/31/94
5	Mozambique	0	0	1	3	23	37	98	186	271	207	700	289	1,815	5/31/95
5	Namibia	0	0	4	15	43	127	122	0	3,515	1,275			5,101	12/31/93
5	Niger	0	0	0	18	24	38	213	204	298	315	347	272	1,729	10/13/95
5	Nigeria	0	0	0	10	3	35	36	82	386	465	415	159	1,591	5/31/95
5	Reunion	0	0	0	3	10	34	2	14	2				65	3/20/92
5	Rwanda	83	161	501	236	299	1,005	2,204	2,089	2,908	1,220			10,706	6/30/93
5	Sao Tomé and Pr.	0	0	0	0	1	1	0	3	7	12			24	12/10/93
5	Senegal	0	0	6	60	115	126	118	195	202	315	310	126	1,573	6/27/95
5	Seychelles	0	0	0	0	0	0	0	0	1				2	9/12/94
5	Sierra Leone	0	0	0	2	13	12	7	6	36	33	29	24	162	10/31/95
5	Somalia	0	0	0	1	4	3	5	0	0	0	0	0	13	7/6/95
5	South Africa	15	9	34	48	94	176	304	393	658	1,267	2,774	2,633	8,405	8/3/95
5	Sudan	0	0	1	1	64	122	130	174	164	203	195	204	1,258	10/30/95
5	Swaziland	0	0	0	1	2	7	18	84	131	146	114	87	590	10/26/95
5	Tanzania	109	295	1,121	2,931	4,824	4,822	7,073	9,837	7,577	6,171	6,158	2,329	53,247	5/18/95
5	Togo	0	0	0	2	15	39	44	1,178	551	857	2,137	786	5,609	6/30/95
5	Uganda	0	21	126	3,477	3,625	6,029	8,441	8,471	5,729	7,956	2,245		46,120	12/31/94
5	Zaire	0	0	440	1,988	3,501	6,408	2,425	2,500	2,587	2,268	4,014		26,131	7/6/94
5	Zambia	0	1	240	468	985	1,115	1,393	1,601	1,015	23,252	1,706	715	32,491	6/2/95

(continued)

Rgn	Country	1	2	3	4	5	6	7	8	9	10	11	12	Total	Date
5	Zimbabwe	0	0	0	119	202	1,281	4,362	4,861	7,751	9,329	5,971	7,422	41,298	10/19/95
	Totals for GAA5	207	578	3,559	13,851	23,942	35,717	38,669	63,965	69,351	84,900	71,813	36,695	443,247	
6	Anguilla	0	0	0	0	1	2	1	0	1	0	0	0	5	3/31/95
6	Antigua and Barbuda	0	0	0	0	3	0	0	3	22	6	4	3	41	3/31/95
6	Bahamas, The								834	143	412	326	161	1,876	6/30/95
6	Barbados	2	9	21	24	15	40	81	64	66	96	100	68	586	6/30/95
6	Bermuda	0	0	42	33	17	30	25	45	10	38	34	17	291	6/30/95
6	Br. Virgin Islands	0	0	0	0	0	1	1	2	0	2	3	1	10	6/30/95
6	Cayman Islands	0	0	0	2	2	0	2	5	4	0	2	1	18	6/30/95
6	Cuba	0	0	0	27	24	12	10	30	65	77	91	43	379	7/8/95
6	Dominica	0	0	0	5	1	2	4	0	10	4	5		31	6/30/94
6	Dominican Republic	9	40	67	294	292	499	284	122	232	428	342	339	2,948	9/30/95
6	Grenada	0	0	2	5	9	0	3	11	5	20	8		63	12/31/94
6	Guadeloupe	14	6	27	41	47	54	6		145	94	113	76	623	9/30/95
6	Haiti	443	110	242	477	731	453	630	0	0	0	0	0	3,086	12/31/92
6	Jamaica	2	4	5	32	30	66	62	133	99	236	341	304	1,314	9/30/95
6	Martinique	3	6	16	23	30	5	38	78	30	47	39	29	344	9/30/95
6	Montserrat								1	0	3	3	0	7	6/30/95
6	Nthrlnds Antilles								90	44	29	9	5	177	9/30/95
6	St. Kitts & Nevis								33	4	3	4	3	47	6/30/95
6	St. Lucia	0	0	0	6	5	5	2	24	7	8	6	10	73	9/30/95
6	St. Vincent	0	0	3	4	6	6	7	14	3	12	7	5	67	6/30/95
6	Trinidad & Tob.	27	45	79	85	160	167	173	229	263	247	280	137	1,892	6/30/95
6	Turks & Caicos I	0	0	0	4	1	2	1	13	4	14			39	9/30/93
	Totals for GAA6	473	175	422	969	1,207	1,169	1,149	1,475	887	1,503	1,430	1,060	11,919	
7	Albania	0	0	0	0	0	0	0	0	0	1	2	2	5	9/30/95
7	Bulgaria	0	0	0	1	1	5	2	4	3	8	9	2	35	9/30/95
7	Croatia										62	14	13	89	9/30/95
7	Czechoslovakia	0	1	6	2	3	7	5	2	8				34	12/17/92
7	Czech Republic										47	12	10	69	9/30/95
7	Slovak Republic										7	3	2	12	9/30/95
7	Hungary	0	0	1	7	9	15	17	30	28	37	26	25	195	9/30/95
7	Poland	0	0	1	2	2	24	21	39	31	48	101	77	346	9/30/95
7	Romania	0	5	2	5	13	277	1,042	360	407	531	440	519	3,601	9/30/95

Appendix A AIDS cases reported to the World Health Organization, by geographic area of affinity (GAA), and year, 1979–1996—continued
(Figures shown are Jan 1 to Dec 31 of each year)

GAA	Country	1979–1984	1985	1986	1987	1988	1989	1990	1991	1992	1993	1994	1995 to date	Cumulative to date	Date of last report
7	Slovenia										31	9	7	47	9/30/95
7	USSR	0	0	1	3	3	23	23						53	4/30/93
7	Armenia									2				2	4/30/93
7	Azerbaijan										0	1	1	2	9/30/95
7	Belarus										10	2	2	14	9/30/95
7	Estonia										3	1	2	6	9/30/95
7	Georgia									2				2	4/30/93
7	Kazakhstan										2	3	0	5	9/30/95
7	Kyrgyz Republic													0	4/30/93
7	Latvia										7	1	1	9	9/30/95
7	Lithuania										5	0	1	6	9/30/95
7	Moldova										4	1	1	6	9/30/95
7	Russian Federation								19	39	21	30	29	138	9/30/95
7	Tajikistan										0	0	0	0	9/30/95
7	Turkmenistan									1				1	4/30/93
7	Ukraine										25	10	13	48	9/30/95
7	Uzbekistan									1	1	0	0	2	9/30/95
7	Yugoslavia, Fed. Rep.	0	2	6	18	39	44	70	70	41	31	88	100	509	9/30/95
	Totals for GAA7	0	6	11	20	31	351	1,110	435	479	772	616	657	4,488	
8	Afghanistan	0	0	0	0	0	0	0	0	0			0	0	2/15/92
8	Algeria	0	0	3	5	5	32	0	57	29	33	53	0	217	12/31/94
8	Bahrain	0	0	0	0	0	0	0	0	8	5	7	8	28	11/21/95
8	Egypt, Arab Rep.	0	0	2	3	6	9	7	7	24	32	23	7	120	8/1/95
8	Iran, Islamic Rep.	0	0	0	1	3	5	10	25	12	29	25	8	118	11/29/95
8	Iraq	0	0	0	0	0	0	0	7	0	14	14	7	42	11/2/95
8	Israel	16	10	19	17	22	30	32	23	29	68	42	32	340	9/30/95
8	Jordan	0	0	1	3	1	5	1	4	9	6	3	6	39	10/28/95
8	Kuwait	0	0	1	0	0	0	0	6	0	3	4	4	18	11/5/95
8	Lebanon	0	0	8	0	4	4	8	5	7	27	14	14	91	11/2/95
8	Libya	0	0	0	0	0	0	1	6	0	4	3	1	15	4/10/95

Grp	Country													Total	Date
8	Morocco	0	0	1	9	13	20	27	24	29	55	53	49	280	8/27/95
8	Oman	0	0	1	5	6	4	7	1	3	5	11	12	55	11/13/95
8	Pakistan	0	0	0	3	3	7	1	3	8	13	9	5	52	11/5/95
8	Qatar	1	7	0	8	5	2	0	8	0	9	20	20	80	11/11/95
8	Saudi Arabia	0	0	7	14	4	7	7	5	9	12	40	39	137	11/15/95
8	Syrian Arab Rep.	0	0	0	4	1	4	0	8	2	6	4	1	30	7/8/95
8	Tunisia	1	4	0	14	17	14	27	28	11	48	54	37	255	8/11/95
8	Turkey	2	1	9	4	9	12	11	18	28	33	24	25	172	9/30/95
8	United Arab Emir.	0	0	0	0	0	0	0	0	0	8	0	0	8	2/12/93
8	Yemen, Rep.	0	0	0	0	0	0	0	0	0	8	3	9	20	10/18/95
	Totals for GAA8	18	13	56	95	102	162	146	217	208	410	406	284	2,117	
9	Bhutan	0	0	0	0	0	0	0	0	0	0	0	0	0	11/22/95
9	Cambodia	0	0	0	0	0	0	0	0	0	0	22	64	86	10/15/95
9	China	0	1	0	2	0	2	2	5	24	0	27	14	77	6/30/95
9	Hong Kong	0	3	6	16	7	12	13	6	12	0	33	20	148	6/30/95
9	Japan	0	11	14	34	31	92	189	68	82	131	218	192	1,062	10/31/95
9	Korea, Dem. Rep.	0	0	0	0	0	0	0	0	0	0	0	0	0	11/22/95
9	Korea, Rep.	0	0	1	3	2	2	0	2	6	0	11	4	32	5/31/95
9	Lao PDR	0	0	0	0	0	0	0	0	0	7	5	0	13	8/30/95
9	Macao	0	0	0	0	0	0	0	0	2	2	2	0	8	6/30/95
9	Mongolia	0	0	0	0	0	0	0	0	0	0	0	0	0	10/1/95
9	Taiwan	0	0	0	0	0	0	0	24	24	0	0	0	48	12/31/93
9	Viet Nam	0	0	0	0	0	0	0	0	0	66	133	93	292	9/20/95
	Totals for GAA9	0	15	14	43	41	109	205	111	129	261	451	387	1,766	
10	Bangladesh	0	0	0	0	0	0	1	0	0	0	1	5	7	11/22/95
10	Brunei	0	0	0	0	0	0	1	0	1	1	2	1	6	4/30/95
10	India	0	0	5	4	19	12	17	45	152	275	491	1,075	2,095	11/22/95
10	Indonesia	0	0	1	2	3	6	9	4	18	0	19	20	82	11/22/95
10	Malaysia	0	0	1	1	4	6	12	16	32	28	59	100	259	7/31/95
10	Maldives	0	0	0	0	0	0	0	0	0	0	1	1	2	11/22/95
10	Myanmar	0	0	0	0	0	0	0	9	12	132	143	274	570	11/22/95
10	Nepal	0	0	0	2	0	2	3	6	11	0	10	14	48	11/22/95
10	Philippines	1	2	6	9	10	7	11	16	23	32	62	41	220	8/31/95

(continued)

Appendix A AIDS cases reported to the World Health Organization, by geographic area of affinity (GAA), and year, 1979–1996—continued
(Figures shown are Jan 1 to Dec 31 of each year)

GAA	Country	1979–1984	1985	1986	1987	1988	1989	1990	1991	1992	1993	1994	1995 to date	Cumulative to date	Date of last report
10	Singapore	0	0	1	3	6	5	8	11	18	23	33	37	145	6/30/95
10	Sri Lanka	0	0	0	1	1	3	3	3	10	13	8	10	52	11/22/95
10	Thailand	1	1	0	7	5	29	54	194	728	2,402	11,340	7,374	22,135	11/22/95
	Totals for GAA10	2	3	13	26	49	66	113	306	986	2,935	12,168	8,947	25,614	
	World Totals	13,143	15,202	28,791	54,741	75,975	97,243	102,289	125,779	149,799	308,353	152,911	164,665	1,288,891	

Appendix B. Estimating the Status and Trends of the HIV/AIDS Pandemic, 1996

In 1992, *AIDS in the World* presented a method for estimating HIV infections, AIDS, and AIDS-related deaths. Based on comments and suggestions received since the publication of that book, this approach has been refined further for the present volume. As in the 1992 edition, the resulting estimates presented in this volume must be considered conservative.

Data used to estimate the prevalence of HIV and AIDS and the number of AIDS-related deaths for each of the GAAs and the world have been drawn from a large number of sources, including published literature, documents and reports issued by epidemiological units of national AIDS programs, and unpublished information collected during visits to countries and presented at meetings and conferences. An invaluable source of information was the *HIV/AIDS Surveillance Database* of the U.S. Bureau of the Census. Data obtained from this source provided many of the variables needed for *AIDS in the World II* to model the HIV/AIDS pandemic in the developing world.

HIV seroprevalence rates obtained from surveys of pregnant women were considered to be representative of the sexually active female population in urban areas. For many countries, data on pregnant women also provide the most representative picture of HIV infection in the general population. Pregnant women can be considered to be at somewhat higher risk than the general adult population, since they are likely to be more sexually active than people in older age-groups. On the other hand, they also are drawn from a limited age-range, may be biased towards those in marital (formal or informal) unions, and tend to be younger than adult women in general.

An estimated frequency distribution of HIV infections in adult women helped draw the profile of HIV infections in adults. The introduction of age-specific fertility rates then allowed for the estimation of the number of newborn infants with HIV infection. Seroprevalence rates in rural, sexually active populations were available for only a few countries. In other countries, an estimation was made of the urban:rural ratio of HIV-infected women.

The number of HIV-infected adults as of January 1, 1995, was then estimated for each country for which data were available. Estimated numbers are presented as best estimates that should be regarded as conservative. The HIV seroprevalence rates retained in calculations were obtained from studies conducted anytime during 1991–1994. In most countries, in particular in sub-Saharan Africa, more studies were available for the earlier than the later part of this period, thus providing rates which were closer to the lowest limit of the range of rates that would be expected during the 3-year time span. Indeed, in no country have studies shown any decline in the rate of HIV infection in pregnant women since the beginning of the pandemic, even in countries where the overall incidence of HIV (new infections within a calendar year) seems to have reached a plateau. In a number of countries, estimates of HIV prevalence had been made by national AIDS programs through the application of epidemiological models. In such instances, national figures obtained through a worldwide survey of governmental national AIDS programs were preferred.

Several parameters entered into the model have been modified in this update to take into account the improved—albeit still incomplete—knowledge about certain characteristics of HIV transmission. This was made in several steps, including: (a) a review of literature that provided parameters applicable to specific geographic regions or populations; (b) selection of values and creation of curves to represent current knowledge about these parameters; (c) consultation of ten panelists chosen for their expertise in HIV epidemiology; and (d) adjustment of variables based on the advice received. Opinions sometimes varied about the value of each parameter for each GAA. In these cases, a value was chosen from the best source of information or as the average of all values obtained from panelists. Tables B-1 to B-4 and Figures B-1 to B-4 present the parameters fed into the "epimodel" to derive the estimates.

Table B-1 HIV seropositivity among women of various ages, by geographic area of affinity (GAA), 1994

Ratio male:female	North America	Western Europe	Oceania	Latin America	Sub-Saharan Africa	Caribbean	Eastern Europe	SE Mediterranean	Northeast Asia	Southeast Asia
	6:1	5:1	8:1	4:1	1:1.1	1.5:1	10:1	5:1	5:1	2:1
Age in years										
15	2.0	2.0	2.0	3.0	6.0	4.7	2.0	2.0	2.0	6.6
20	5.0	4.0	3.5	4.0	9.0	6.9	3.0	3.0	3.0	10.2
25	4.0	4.0	2.5	5.0	11.5	7.8	2.0	5.0	5.0	7.7
30	2.0	3.0	1.5	4.0	9.2	7.6	1.0	4.0	4.0	4.5
35	0.5	2.0	1.0	2.0	7.0	5.5	1.0	3.0	2.0	2.5
40	0.5	1.0	0.5	1.0	4.7	3.5	0.0	0.0	1.0	1.2
45	0.0	1.0	0.0	0.5	3.0	2.5	0.0	0.0	0.0	0.6
50	0.0	0.0	0.0	0.5	2.0	1.5	0.0	0.0	0.0	0.0

Table B-2 Age-specific fertility rates*, by geographic area of affinity (GAA), 1994

Years	North America	Western Europe	Oceania	Latin America	Sub-Saharan Africa	Caribbean	Eastern Europe	SE Mediterranean	Northeast Asia	Southeast Asia
15	3.8	1.6	4.0	10.5	15.1	10.7	4.9	6.1	6.2	6.2
20	9.2	8.5	10.5	22.4	28.5	21.6	17.4	20.9	16.8	16.8
25	11.4	12.2	14.5	21.8	28.9	20.9	11.3	25.7	16.7	16.7
30	7.2	6.3	7.8	16.8	26.2	14.4	5.1	21.9	12.2	12.2
35	2.0	1.9	2.5	12.0	20.5	9.8	2.1	14.9	7.5	7.5
40	1.0	0.8	0.5	6.4	12.6	5.1	0.9	7.2	3.2	3.2
45	0.0	0.0	0.0	0.0	0.0	0.0	0.0	0.0	0.0	0.0

*x/y.

Source: *United Nations Population Report*, 1994.

Table B-3 Mother-to-child transmission rates, circa 1994*

Developing countries	Industrialized countries
30%	20%

*The likelihood that a given child born to an infected woman will be infected.

Table B-4 Urban:rural ratios of HIV-infected adults (ages 15–49), by GAA, 1994

GAA	Ratio of urban:rural
North America	3.2:1
Western Europe	5.0:1
Oceania	3.3:1
Latin America	2.3:1
Sub-Saharan Africa	2.0:1
Caribbean	3.6:1
Eastern Europe	3.2:1
SE Mediterranean	12.0:1
Northeast Asia	5.0:1
Southeast Asia	3.0:1

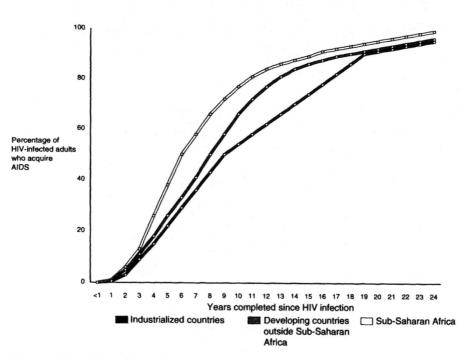

Figure B-1   Adult HIV-to-AIDS time interval.

Figure B-2   Adult AIDS-to-death time interval.

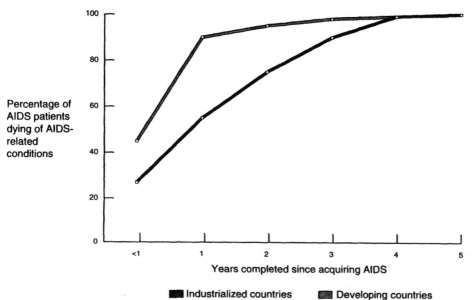

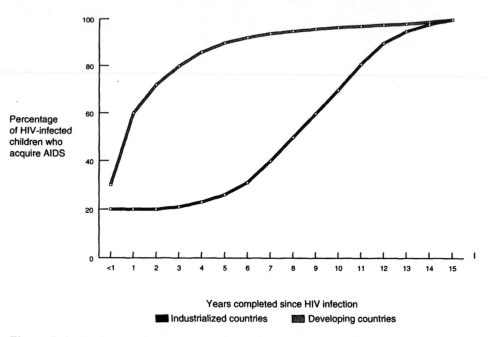

Figure B-3   Pediatric AIDS-to-death time interval.

Figure B-4   Perinatally acquired HIV-to-AIDS time interval.

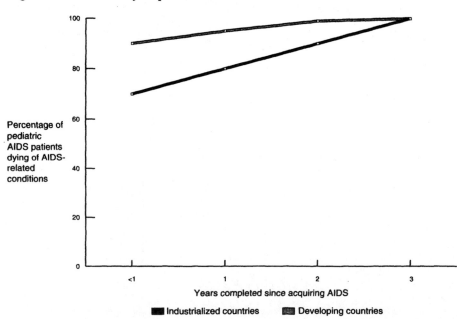

Appendix C. Estimated 1994 Adult HIV Prevalence by Country

GAA	Country	1994 population aged 15–49 yr	Estimated number of adult HIV infections: 1994	Estimated 1994 adult HIV prevalence rate (per 100 population aged 15–49 yr)
1	Canada	15,697,000	30,000	0.191
1	USA	136,303,000	700,000	0.514
	Totals for GAA1	152,000,000	730,000	0.480
2	Austria	4,059,000	8,000	0.197
2	Belgium	5,066,000	10,000	0.197
2	Cyprus	369,000	1,000	0.271
2	Denmark	2,650,000	4,000	0.151
2	Finland	2,598,000	500	0.019
2	France	29,293,000	90,000	0.307
2	Germany	40,442,000	43,000	0.106
2	Greece	5,100,000	5,000	0.098
2	Iceland	140,000	200	0.143
2	Ireland	1,803,000	1,700	0.094
2	Italy	29,190,000	90,000	0.308
2	Luxembourg	211,000	300	0.142
2	Malta	189,000	200	0.106
2	Netherlands	8,251,000	3,000	0.036
2	Norway	2,193,000	1,250	0.057
2	Portugal	5,018,000	8,000	0.159
2	Spain	20,707,000	120,000	0.580
2	Sweden	4,175,000	3,000	0.072
2	Switzerland	3,706,000	12,000	0.324
2	UK	28,758,000	25,000	0.087
	Totals for GAA2	193,918,000	426,150	0.220
3	Australia	9,533,000	11,000	0.115
3	Fiji	400,000	150	0.038
3	New Zealand	1,846,000	1,200	0.065
3	Papua New Guinea	2,104,000	4,000	0.190
	Totals for GAA3	13,883,000	16,350	0.118
4	Argentina	16,727,000	60,000	0.359
4	Belize	99,000	2,000	2.020
4	Bolivia	3,448,000	2,000	0.058
4	Brazil	84,407,000	550,000	0.652
4	Chile	7,482,000	10,000	0.134
4	Colombia	18,776,000	40,000	0.213
4	Costa Rica	1,738,000	9,000	0.518

(continued)

GAA	Country	1994 population aged 15–49 yr	Estimated number of adult HIV infections: 1994	Estimated 1994 adult HIV prevalence rate (per 100 population aged 15–49 yr)
4	Ecuador	5,720,000	16,000	0.280
4	El Salvador	2,658,000	15,000	0.564
4	Guatemala	4,673,000	20,000	0.428
4	Guyana	464,000	6,000	1.293
4	Honduras	2,551,000	40,000	1.568
4	Mexico	47,803,000	200,000	0.418
4	Nicaragua	1,906,000	1,500	0.079
4	Panama	1,353,000	8,000	0.591
4	Paraguay	2,370,000	2,600	0.110
4	Peru	12,098,000	30,000	0.248
4	Suriname	215,000	2,500	1.163
4	Uruguay	1,540,000	5,000	0.325
4	Venezuela	11,022,000	35,000	0.318
	Totals for GAA4	227,050,000	1,054,600	0.464
5	Angola	4,616,000	48,000	1.040
5	Benin	2,269,000	27,000	1.190
5	Botswana	694,000	125,000	18.012
5	Burkina Faso	4,490,000	300,000	6.682
5	Burundi	2,804,000	75,000	2.675
5	Cameroon	5,777,000	175,000	3.029
5	Central African Republic	1,467,000	85,000	5.794
5	Chad	2,793,000	75,000	2.685
5	Comoros	270,000	250	0.093
5	Congo	1,113,000	80,000	7.188
5	Côte d'Ivoire	5,763,000	390,000	6.767
5	Djibouti	266,000	8,000	3.008
5	Equatorial Guinea	175,000	2,000	1.143
5	Eritrea	1,575,000	50,000	3.175
5	Ethiopia	23,575,000	588,000	2.494
5	Gabon	572,000	13,000	2.273
5	Gambia	518,000	11,000	2.124
5	Ghana	7,642,000	172,000	2.251
5	Guinea	2,864,000	17,000	0.594
5	Guinea-Bissau	477,000	15,000	3.145
5	Kenya	12,028,000	1,000,000	8.314
5	Lesotho	909,000	28,000	3.080
5	Liberia	1,283,000	17,000	1.325
5	Madagascar	6,363,000	2,500	0.063
5	Malawi	4,771,000	650,000	13.624
5	Mali	4,601,000	58,000	1.261
5	Mauritania	1,032,000	7,000	0.678

Appendix C Estimated 1994 adult HIV prevalence by country—continued

GAA	Country	1994 population aged 15–49 yr	Estimated number of adult HIV infections: 1994	Estimated 1994 adult HIV prevalence rate (per 100 population aged 15–49 yr)
5	Mauritius	626,000	500	0.080
5	Mozambique	6,951,000	400,000	5.755
5	Namibia	697,000	45,000	6.456
5	Niger	3,823,000	40,000	1.046
5	Nigeria	48,643,000	1,050,000	2.159
5	Reunion	346,000	150	0.043
5	Rwanda	3,495,000	250,000	7.153
5	Senegal	3,689,000	50,000	1.355
5	Sierra Leone	2,004,000	60,000	2.994
5	Somalia	3,964,000	10,000	0.252
5	South Africa	20,124,000	650,000	3.230
5	Sudan	12,604,000	125,000	0.992
5	Swaziland	397,000	15,000	3.778
5	Togo	1,773,000	150,000	8.460
5	Uganda	8,940,000	1,300,000	14.541
5	United Rep. Tanzania	13,035,000	840,000	6.444
5	Zaire	18,162,000	680,000	3.744
5	Zambia	4,093,000	700,000	17.102
5	Zimbabwe	5,186,000	900,000	17.354
	Totals for GAA5	259,259,000	11,284,400	4.353
6	Bahamas	153,000	6,000	3.922
6	Barbados	144,000	4,000	2.778
6	Cuba	6,110,000	1,300	0.021
6	Dominican Republic	4,051,000	40,000	0.987
6	Haiti	3,375,000	150,000	4.444
6	Jamaica	1,312,000	12,000	0.915
6	Trinidad & Tobago	678,000	6,000	0.885
	Totals for GAA6	15,823,000	219,300	1.386
7	Albania	1,793,000	100	0.006
7	Armenia	1,803,000	20	0.001
7	Azerbaijan	3,854,000	50	0.001
7	Belarus	5,043,000	200	0.004
7	Bosnia & Hrzgvna.	1,946,000	750	0.039
7	Bulgaria	4,346,000	300	0.007
7	Croatia	2,247,000	300	0.013
7	Czech Rep.	5,390,000	2,000	0.037
7	Estonia	761,000	40	0.005
7	Georgia	2,686,000	500	0.019
7	Hungary	5,148,000	3,000	0.058
7	Kazakhstan	8,805,000	50	0.001

(continued)

GAA	Country	1994 population aged 15–49 yr	Estimated number of adult HIV infections: 1994	Estimated 1994 adult HIV prevalence rate (per 100 population aged 15–49 yr)
7	Kyrgyzstan	2,256,000	25	0.001
7	Latvia	1,247,000	100	0.008
7	Lithuania	1,838,000	200	0.011
7	Poland	19,841,000	10,000	0.050
7	Republic of Moldova	2,237,000	40	0.002
7	Romania	11,695,000	500	0.004
7	Russian Federation	75,020,000	3,000	0.004
7	Slovakia	2,798,000	250	0.009
7	Slovenia	1,002,000	150	0.015
7	Tajikistan	2,703,000	25	0.001
7	TFRY Macedonia	1,141,000	500	0.044
7	Turkmenistan	1,965,000	25	0.001
7	Ukraine	24,875,000	1,500	0.006
7	Uzbekistan	10,745,000	100	0.001
7	Yugoslavia	5,369,000	5,000	0.093
	Totals for GAA7	208,554,000	28,725	0.014
8	Afghanistan	9,065,000	50	0.001
8	Algeria	13,735,000	10,000	0.073
8	Bahrain	322,000	500	0.155
8	Egypt	30,470,000	7,500	0.025
8	Iran (Islamic Rep.)	30,002,000	1,000	0.003
8	Iraq	9,317,000	250	0.003
8	Israel	2,760,000	2,000	0.073
8	Jordan	2,466,000	600	0.024
8	Kuwait	871,000	1,000	0.115
8	Lebanon	1,505,000	1,350	0.090
8	Libyan Arab J.	2,347,000	1,300	0.055
8	Morocco	13,733,000	5,000	0.036
8	Oman	905,000	1,000	0.111
8	Pakistan	63,195,000	40,000	0.063
8	Qatar	338,000	290	0.086
8	Saudi Arabia	8,505,000	1,000	0.012
8	Syrian Arab Rep.	6,261,000	700	0.011
8	Tunisia	4,528,000	2,000	0.044
8	Turkey	31,300,000	500	0.002
8	United Arab Emirates	1,090,000	2,000	0.184
8	Yemen	6,258,000	750	0.012
	Totals for GAA8	238,973,000	78,790	0.033
9	Bhutan	760,000	75	0.010
9	Cambodia	4,645,000	90,000	1.938

Appendix C Estimated 1994 adult HIV prevalence by country—continued

GAA	Country	1994 population aged 15–49 yr	Estimated number of adult HIV infections: 1994	Estimated 1994 adult HIV prevalence rate (per 100 population aged 15–49 yr)
9	China	684,807,000	10,000	0.002
9	DPR Korea	13,540,000	100	0.001
9	Hong Kong	3,381,000	3,000	0.089
9	Japan	63,239,000	6,200	0.010
9	Lao People's Dem. Rep.	2,139,000	550	0.026
9	Mongolia	1,188,000	150	0.013
9	Republic of Korea	26,044,000	2,000	0.008
9	Vietnam	36,324,000	25,000	0.069
	Totals for GAA9	836,067,000	137,075	0.016
10	Bangladesh	58,822,000	15,000	0.026
10	Brunei Darussalam	153,000	300	0.196
10	India	464,482,000	1,750,000	0.377
10	Indonesia	102,992,000	50,000	0.049
10	Malaysia	9,841,000	30,000	0.305
10	Maldives	106,000	60	0.057
10	Myanmar	22,714,000	350,000	1.541
10	Nepal	9,863,000	5,000	0.051
10	Philippines	33,438,000	18,000	0.054
10	Singapore	1,669,000	1,200	0.072
10	Sri Lanka	9,640,000	5,000	0.052
10	Thailand	33,095,000	700,000	2.115
	Totals for GAA10	746,815,000	2,924,560	0.392
	World Totals	2,892,342,000	16,899,950	0.584

Source: World Health Organization, Global Programme on AIDS and UN Population Division; Geneva, Switzerland.
Data published in the World Health Organization's Weekly Epidemiological Record 1995, 70, 353–360, no. 50, December 15, 1995; updated February 2, 1996.

Appendix D. Government National AIDS Programs Survey

The column headings for the complex tables presented in Appendix D are defined at the end of each table.

Table D-1 AIDS policies and programs: responses of government national AIDS programs (GNAP)*

GAA	Country	3	4A	4B	4C	4D	4E	4F	5A	5B	5CD	5E	5F	5G	5H	5I	7A	#.7A	7B	#.7B	7C	#.7C	7D	#.7D	7E	#.7E	7F	#.7F	7G	#.7G	7GEXP	8	9
1	United States	+	+	+	+	–	+	–	+	+	+	+	+	+	–	–	–	–	–	–	–	–	–	–	–	–	–	–	–	–		+	+
2	Austria	–	–	–	+	–	–	–	–	–	–	–	–	–	–	–	–	–	–	–	–	–	–	–	–	–	–	–	–	–		–	–
2	Belgium	+	+	+	+	+	–	–	+	+	+	–	+	–	+	+	–	–	–	–	–	–	–	–	–	–	–	–	–	–		–	+
2	Cyprus	+	+	+	+	+	+	+	+	+	+	–	+	–	+	–	–	–	–	–	–	–	–	–	–	–	–	–	–	–		–	+
2	Denmark	+	+	+	+	–	+	–	+	+	+	–	+	+	–	–	–	–	+	–	+	–	–	–	–	–	–	–	–	–		–	+
2	Finland	–	–	–	–	–	–	–	–	–	–	–	–	–	–	–	–	–	+	3	+	1	+	1	–	–	–	–	–	–		–	–
2	France	–	–	–	–	–	–	–	–	–	–	–	–	–	–	–	–	–	–	–	–	–	–	–	–	–	–	–	–	–		–	–
2	Germany	+	+	–	–	+	–	–	+	+	+	–	+	+	+	+	–	–	+	–	–	–	–	–	–	–	–	–	–	–		–	+
2	Iceland	+	–	–	–	+	–	–	+	+	–	+	+	–	–	+	–	–	–	–	+	1	–	–	–	–	+	1	–	–		–	+
2	Liechtenstein	+	+	+	–	–	–	–	+	–	+	–	+	–	+	–	–	–	–	–	+	–	–	–	–	–	+	–	–	–		–	+
2	Luxembourg	+	+	–	–	–	+	–	+	+	–	–	+	–	–	+	+	–	+	–	+	–	–	–	–	–	+	2	+	+	some MDs test pre-op. w/out patient permission	–	+
2	Malta	–	–	–	–	–	–	–	–	–	–	–	–	–	–	–	+	–	+	–	–	–	–	–	–	–	–	–	–	–		–	+
2	The Netherlands	+	+	+	+	+	+	–	+	+	+	+	+	+	+	+	+	–	–	–	+	–	–	–	–	–	+	–	+	–	exclusion of a snookerclub	+	+
2	Norway	+	+	+	+	–	–	–	+	+	+	+	+	+	+	+	+	10	+	5	+	5	+	–	–	–	+	10	–	–		+	+
2	Spain	+	+	+	+	+	–	–	+	+	+	+	+	+	+	+	+	–	–	–	–	–	–	–	–	–	–	–	–	–		–	+
2	Sweden	+	+	–	–	+	+	+	+	+	+	+	+	+	+	+	+	–	–	–	–	–	–	–	–	–	–	–	–	–		+	+
2	Switzerland	+	+	–	–	–	+	–	+	+	+	+	+	–	–	+	–	–	+	1	–	–	+	–	+	–	–	–	–	–		–	+
2	United Kingdom	+	+	+	+	+	–	+	+	+	+	+	+	+	–	+	+	–	+	–	–	–	+	–	+	–	–	–	–	–		+	+
3	Australia	+	+	+	+	+	+	+	+	+	+	+	+	+	–	+	+	–	+	–	–	–	+	–	+	–	+	–	–	–		+	+
3	Fiji	+	+	+	+	–	+	+	+	+	+	+	+	–	–	–	–	–	–	–	–	–	–	–	–	–	–	–	+	–	insurance	+	–
3	Kiribati	+	–	–	–	–	–	–	–	–	–	+	+	–	–	–	–	–	–	–	–	–	–	–	–	–	–	–	–	–		–	–
3	Micronesia, Fed. Sts.	+	+	+	+	–	+	+	+	+	+	+	+	+	+	–	–	–	–	–	–	–	–	–	–	–	–	–	–	–		+	–
3	New Zealand	+	+	+	+	+	+	+	+	+	+	+	+	+	+	–	–	–	–	–	+	–	+	–	–	–	–	–	–	–		+	+
3	Papua New Guinea	+	+	–	–	–	+	+	+	–	+	+	+	+	–	–	–	–	–	–	–	–	–	–	–	–	–	–	–	–		–	–
3	Solomon Islands	+	+	+	–	–	–	+	+	–	–	+	+	–	+	–	–	–	–	–	–	–	–	–	–	–	–	–	–	–	no diagnosed AIDS/HIV in country	–	–
3	Vanuatu	+	+	–	–	–	+	+	+	+	+	+	+	+	+	–	–	–	–	–	–	–	–	–	–	–	–	–	–	–		+	–
3	Western Samoa	+	+	+	+	+	+	–	+	+	+	+	+	+	+	–	–	–	–	–	–	–	–	–	–	–	–	–	–	–		–	+

496

Group	Country																							Notes
4	Argentina																							
4	Belize																							
4	Brazil			20																				restriction of religious service to HIV + persons
4	Chile						2	1																
4	Colombia				2		4	1	1	2	5		2	4										
4	Costa Rica				4			1	1	4	10		15											
4	Ecuador				15																			
4	El Salvador																							
4	Guatemala										6		3											
4	Mexico	20			303			5	83	73	23		52											refuse burial 10/prisoners human right 10
4	Panama									2	1		2											
4	Peru									5														
4	Suriname									4	1													
4	Uruguay						50																	
4	Venezuela				50				2	3	2		4											
5	Angola																							
5	Benin																							
5	Botswana																							(7a: life insurance-related testing)
5	Burkino Faso												2											
5	Cameroon																							yes, but no official complaints to imply
5	Cape Verde																							
5	Chad																							
5	Comoros										4													foreigners deported/detained pre-1991
5	Congo																							
5	Côte d'Ivoire																							
5	Djibouti							1																
5	Ethiopia								2															
5	Gabon									5														
5	Ghana			+																				anecdotal: ejection of HIV + persons by landlord
5	Guinea										2													
5	Guinee-Bissau				5		+																	
5	Lesotho																							

(continued)

Table D-1 AIDS policies and programs: responses of government national AIDS programs (GNAP)*—continued

GAA	Country	3	4A	4B	4C	4D	4E	4F	5A	5B	5CD	5E	5F	5G	5H	5I	7A	#.7A	7B	#.7B	7C	#.7C	7D	#.7D	7E	#.7E	7F	#.7F	7G	#.7G	7GEXP	8	9
5	Madagascar	+	+	+	-	+	+	+	+	-	-	+	+	+	+	-	-	-	-	-	-	-	-	-	-	-	-	-	-	-		-	+
5	Mali	+	+	+	+	+	+	+	+	+	+	+	+	+	-	-	-	-	-	-	-	-	-	-	-	-	-	-	-	-		-	+
5	Mauritania	+	+	+	+	+	+	+	+	-	+	+	+	-	+	+	-	-	-	-	-	-	-	-	-	-	-	-	-	-		-	+
5	Mauritius	+	-	+	-	+	+	-	+	+	+	+	+	+	+	+	+	1	-		+	1	+	1	-		-		+	-	sailors denied employment on foreign boats	-	+
5	Rwanda	+	+	-	-	-	+	+	+	+	+	+	+	-	-	+	-		-		-		-		-		-		-			-	+
5	Senegal	+	-	+	-	-	+	-	-	-	-	+	+	+	-	+	-		-		+	4	-		-		-		-			+	-
5	Seychelles	+	-	+	+	+	+	+	+	+	+	+	+	+	-	+	+		-		-		-		-		-		-			-	-
5	South Africa	+	+	+	-	+	+	+	+	+	+	+	+	+	+	+	+		+		+		-		+		+		-			+	+
5	Tanzania	+	-	-	-	-	-	-	+	+	+	-	-	-	-	-	-		+		-		-		-		-		-			-	-
5	Togo	+	-	-	-	-	-	-	+	-	+	-	-	-	+	-	-		-		-		-		-		-		-			+	+
5	Uganda	+	+	+	+	+	+	+	+	+	+	+	+	-	+	+	+		+	-	-		-		-		-		-			-	-
5	Zaire	+	+	+	-	+	+	+	+	-	+	+	+	-	+	-	-		-		-		-		-		-		+	-	discipline problems in workplace; cases unknown to government	-	+
5	Zambia	+	+	+	+	+	+	+	+	+	+	+	+	-	+	-	-		-		-		-		-		-		-			-	-
5	Zimbabwe	+	+	+	+	+	+	+	+	+	+	+	+	-	-	+	-		-		-		-		-		-		-			-	-
6	Antigua and Barbuda	+	-	-	-	+	+	-	+	-	-	+	+	-	-	+	+	2	+	6	+	2	-		-		+		-			+	+
6	Barbados	+	+	+	+	+	+	+	+	+	-	+	+	-	-	-	-		+		+		-		+		+		-			-	-
6	Dominican Republic	+	-	-	-	-	-	-	+	+	+	+	+	-	+	+	-		-		+		+		-		+		-			+	-
6	Grenada	+	+	+	+	+	+	+	+	+	+	+	+	+	+	+	+	6	+	13	+	5	+		+	1	+		-			+	+
6	Jamaica	+	+	-	-	+	-	-	+	-	-	+	+	-	+	-	+		+		+		+		-		+		-			+	+
6	St. Lucia	+	+	+	+	-	-	+	-	-	-	+	+	-	-	-	-		+	2	+		-		-		-		+	-	workplace—leaving job because of discrimination by colleagues	+	-
6	Trinidad and Tobago	+	+	+	+	+	+	+	+	+	+	+	+	-	-	-	-		-		-		-		-		+		+	-	rumors of school discrimination/ no clear reports	-	+
7	Azerbaijan	-	-	-	-	-	-	-	-	-	-	-	-	-	-	-	-		-		-		-		-		-		-			+	-
7	Belarus	+	-	-	+	-	+	+	+	+	+	+	+	-	+	+	-		+	2	-		-		+	1	-		-			+	-
7	Bulgaria	+	+	+	+	+	+	+	+	+	+	+	+	+	+	-	-		+	11	+	5	-		+	1	+	3	-			-	-
7	Croatia	+	+	+	+	+	+	+	+	-	+	-	-	+	+	-	-		-		-		-		-		-		-			-	-
7	Czech Republic	+	+	+	+	-	-	-	+	+	+	+	+	+	-	-	-		+	1	-		-		-		-		-			+	+
7	Estonia	+	+	+	+	+	-	-	+	+	+	+	+	-	+	+	-		-		-		-		+		-		-			+	-
7	Hungary	+	+	+	+	+	-	+	+	+	-	+	+	-	+	+	+	4	-		-		-		-	2	-		-			+	+

498

Region	Country	Notes
7	Kyrgyz Republic	
7	Latvia	
7	Lithuania	
7	Moldova	
7	Russian Federation	
7	Slovenia	
7	Turkmenistan	
7	Ukraine	
7	Yugoslavia, Fed. Rep.	
8	Algeria	
8	Israel	
8	Jordan	
8	Kuwait	
8	Lebanon	
8	Morocco	some countries turned Moroccans back
8	Oman	
8	Syrian Arab Rep.	"rights never violated; protected by law"
8	Tunisia	rejected by families; shelter provided by gov't.
9	Bhutan	
9	China	
9	Hong Kong	
9	Japan	
9	Taiwan	
9	Vietnam	
10	Brunei	
10	India	
10	Malaysia	
10	Nepal	
10	Singapore	
10	Sri Lanka	police mandate test and condoms of suspected sexworkers
10	Thailand	
3	American Samoa	
3	Cook Islands	

(continued)

Table D-1 AIDS policies and programs: responses of government national AIDS programs (GNAP)*—continued

GAA	Country	Policy 3	4A	4B	4C	4D	4E	4F	5A	5B	5CD	5E	5F	5G	5H	5I	7A	#,7A	7B	#,7B	7C	#,7C	7D	#,7D	7E	#,7E	7F	7G	#,7G	7GEXP	8	9
3	Guam	—	—	—	—	—	—	—	—	—	—	—	—	—	—	—	—	—	—	—	—	—	—	—	—	—	+	—	—	1	—	—
3	New Caledonia	—	—	—	—	—	—	—	—	—	—	—	—	—	—	—	—	—	—	—	—	—	—	—	—	—	—	—	—	—	—	+
3	Niue	—	—	—	—	—	—	—	—	—	—	—	—	—	—	—	—	—	—	—	—	—	—	—	—	—	—	—	—	—	—	—
3	Tokelau	—	—	—	—	—	—	—	—	—	—	—	—	—	—	—	—	—	+	4	+	3	+	3	+	3	+	—	—	3	—	+
3	Tuvalu	+	—	—	—	—	—	—	—	—	—	—	—	—	—	—	—	—	—	—	—	—	—	—	—	—	—	—	—	—	—	—
6	Bermuda	+	—	+	—	—	—	+	+	—	—	+	+	—	—	—	—	—	+	—	+	—	—	—	+	—	—	—	—	—	—	+
6	Cayman Islands	+	+	+	+	+	+	+	+	+	—	—	+	—	+	+	—	—	+	1	+	2	+	2	+	1	—	—	—	—	+	—
6	Montserrat	+	—	+	—	+	+	+	+	—	—	+	+	+	+	—	—	—	—	—	—	—	—	—	—	—	—	—	—	—	—	—
6	Netherlands Antilles	+	+	—	+	—	+	—	+	—	+	+	+	+	—	—	—	—	—	—	—	—	—	—	—	—	—	—	—	—	—	—

*Policy abbreviations: 3, a document exists outlining the government's current policy and program on HIV/AIDS. The policy and program document includes the following: 4A, statement of national policies on HIV/AIDS; 4B, description of strategic approaches for the health sector; 4C, description of strategic approaches for health and other sectors such as the ministries of development, education, and justice; 4D, description of specific activities for health and other sectors; 4E, proposed budget for central/federal expenditures on HIV/AIDS; 4F, evaluation plan for governmental activities.

Consultations or discussions take place with the following groups in the development of the document: 5A, professionals in the health sector; 5B, person with HIV/AIDS; 5CD, state or regional (provincial or district) authorities; 5E, other government departments/ministries; 5F, other agencies (i.e., private foundations, research institutions); 5G, the Parliament.

Surveys conducted in the development of the document include: 5H, needs assessment surveys for prevention; 5I, needs assessment surveys for care.

Issues for which the GNAP received reports of allegations of human rights violations include: 7A, mandatory or compulsory HIV testing—#,7A, number of reports; 7B, violation of confidentiality of HIV status—#,7B, number of reports; 7C, discrimination in the workplace against HIV-infected persons—#,7C, number of reports; 7D, restriction of housing rights to HIV-infected persons—#,7D, number of reports; 7E, discrimination against children/youth with HIV infection in the educational system—#,7E, number of reports; 7F, restrictions of health services entitlements to people with HIV infection—#,7F, number of reports; 7G, others—#,7G, number of reports; 7G EXP, other specified.

8, GNAP has an established mechanism for dealing with human rights allegations.

9, There is at least one group or organization outside of the government which monitors human rights in the context of HIV/AIDS and reports instances where violations might have occurred.

Table D-2 Countries that responded to AIW II questionnaire on government national AIDS programs, level of economy, country population, and date of first AIDS case report*

List	GAA	Country	Code	Economy	Pop. 92	Pop. 93	Adult 92	Adult 93	Case 1
1	1	United States	USA	High	255,414	257,713	134,523	135,733	1984
1	2	Austria	AUT	High	7,906	7,953	3,991	4,015	1984
1	2	Belgium	BEL	High	10,039	10,069	4,962	4,976	1984
1	2	Cyprus	CYP	U-mid	715	722	366	369	1986
1	2	Denmark	DNK	High	5,166	5,171	2,700	2,702	1984
1	2	Finland	FIN	High	5,062	5,082	2,619	2,630	1984
1	2	France	FRA	High	57,338	57,682	28,617	28,789	1984
1	2	Germany	DEU	High	80,553	81,036	40,645	40,889	1984
1	2	Iceland	ISL	U-mid	261	264	136	138	1985
1	2	Liechtenstein	LIE	High	28	28	14	14	b
1	2	Luxembourg	LUX	High	389	392	201	203	1985
1	2	Malta	MLT	L-mid	360	363	188	190	1984
1	2	The Netherlands	NLD	High	15,167	15,273	8,252	8,310	1984
1	2	Norway	NOR	High	4,281	4,298	2,163	2,171	1984
1	2	Spain	ESP	High	39,077	39,155	19,951	19,991	1984
1	2	Sweden	SWE	High	8,707	8,759	4,216	4,241	1984
1	2	Switzerland	CHE	High	6,864	6,926	3,517	3,549	1984
1	2	United Kingdom	BGR	High	57,701	57,874	28,786	28,872	1984
1	3	Australia	AUS	High	17,540	17,821	9,265	9,413	1984
1	3	Fiji	FJI	L-mid	750	757	409	413	1989
1	3	Kiribati	KIR	L-mid	75	77	39	40	1993
1	3	Micronesia, Fed. Sts.	FSM	L-mid	108	111	57	58	1991
1	3	New Zealand	NZL	High	3,415	3,439	1,819	1,832	1984
1	3	Papua New Guinea	PNG	L-mid	4,055	4,148	1,990	2,036	1987
1	3	Solomon Islands	SLB	L-mid	335	345	175	181	a
1	3	Vanuatu	VUT	L-mid	155	159	81	83	a
1	3	Western Samoa	WSM	L-mid	162	163	85	85	1992
1	4	Argentina	ARG	U-mid	33,099	33,529	15,856	16,062	1984
1	4	Belize	BLZ	L-mid	200	205	103	106	1987
1	4	Brazil	BRA	U-mid	153,850	156,619	79,731	81,166	1984

(continued)

501

Table D-2 Countries that responded to AIW II questionnaire on government national AIDS programs, level of economy, country population, and date of first AIDS case report—*continued

List	GAA	Country	Code	Economy	Pop. 92	Pop. 93	Adult 92	Adult 93	Case 1
1	4	Chile	CHL	U-mid	13,599	13,830	7,256	7,380	1984
1	4	Colombia	COL	L-mid	33,405	34,006	17,916	18,238	1986
1	4	Costa Rica	CRI	L-mid	3,135	3,213	1,608	1,648	1984
1	4	Ecuador	ECU	L-mid	11,028	11,304	5,473	5,610	1986
1	4	El Salvador	SLV	L-mid	5,387	5,484	2,432	2,476	1985
1	4	Guatemala	GTM	L-mid	9,746	10,029	4,331	4,457	1986
1	4	Mexico	MEX	U-mid	84,967	86,496	45,963	46,790	1984
1	4	Panama	PAN	L-mid	2,514	2,567	1,311	1,339	1986
1	4	Peru	PER	L-mid	22,370	22,840	11,265	11,502	1984
1	4	Suriname	SUR	U-mid	467	478	251	257	1984
1	4	Uruguay	URY	U-mid	3,131	3,150	1,620	1,630	1986
1	4	Venezuela	VEN	U-mid	20,310	20,818	10,486	10,748	1984
1	5	Angola	AGO	L-mid	9,732	10,014	4,746	4,884	1985
1	5	Benin	BEN	Low	5,042	5,203	2,217	2,287	1985
1	5	Botswana	BWA	U-mid	1,360	1,406	595	616	1985
1	5	Burkina Faso	HVO	Low	9,537	9,804	4,345	4,466	1986
1	5	Cameroon	CMR	L-mid	12,245	12,612	5,374	5,536	1986
1	5	Cape Verde	CPV	L-mid	389	400	173	177	1985
1	5	Chad	TCD	Low	5,977	6,126	2,789	2,858	1986
1	5	Comoros	COM	Low	510	529	227	236	1988
1	5	Congo	COG	L-mid	2,428	2,508	1,076	1,112	1986
1	5	Côte d'Ivoire	CIV	Low	12,841	13,355	5,467	5,685	1985
1	5	Djibouti	DJI	L-mid	465	478	193	199	1988
1	5	Ethiopia	ETH	Low	54,790	56,653	24,159	24,980	1986
1	5	Gabon	GAB	U-mid	1,201	1,233	612	629	1986
1	5	Ghana	GHA	Low	15,824	16,346	7,150	7,386	1986
1	5	Guinea	GIN	Low	6,048	6,217	2,671	2,746	1987
1	5	Guinea-Bissau	GNB	Low	1,022	1,043	470	479	1989
1	5	Lesotho	LSO	Low	1,860	1,910	854	877	1986
1	5	Madagascar	MDG	Low	12,384	12,768	5,554	5,726	1991

1	5	Mali	MLI	Low	8,962	9,213	3,961	4,072	
1	5	Mauritania	MRT	Low	2,082	2,138	937	962	1988
1	5	Mauritius	MUS	U-mid	1,099	1,111	620	626	1987
1	5	Rwanda	RWA	Low	7,310	7,529	3,213	3,310	1984
1	5	Senegal	SEN	L-mid	7,845	8,080	3,514	3,619	1986
1	5	Seychelles	SYC	U-mid	69	70	31	31	1992
1	5	South Africa	ZAF	L-mid	39,763	40,717	18,580	19,026	1984
1	5	Tanzania	TZA	Low	25,965	26,744	11,633	11,982	1984
1	5	Togo	TGO	Low	3,899	4,043	1,735	1,799	1987
1	5	Uganda	UGA	Low	17,475	18,017	7,908	8,153	1985
1	5	Zaire	ZAR	Low	39,794	41,107	17,001	17,562	1986
1	5	Zambia	ZMB	Low	8,589	8,890	3,833	3,968	1985
1	5	Zimbabwe	ZWE	Low	10,352	10,663	4,686	4,827	1987
1	6	Antigua and Barbuda	ATG	U-mid	81	82	43	43	1988
1	6	Barbados	BRB	U-mid	259	260	136	137	1984
1	6	Dominican Republic	DOM	L-mid	7,321	7,460	3,746	3,817	1984
1	6	Grenada	GRD	L-mid	91	91	48	48	1986
1	6	Jamaica	JAM	L-mid	2,394	2,413	1,265	1,275	1984
1	6	St. Lucia	LCA	U-mid	156	159	82	83	1987
1	6	Trinidad and Tobago	TTO	U-mid	1,268	1,284	683	692	1984
1	7	Azerbaijan	AZE	L-mid	7,145	7,216	3,566	3,601	a
1	7	Belarus	BLR	U-mid	10,346	10,398	5,163	5,189	c
1	7	Bulgaria	BGR	L-mid	8,952	8,952	4,320	4,320	1987
1	7	Croatia	HRV	L-mid	4,773	4,792	2,413	2,422	c
1	7	Czech Republic	CZE	L-mid	10,383	10,393	5,215	5,220	c
1	7	Estonia	EST	U-mid	1,554	1,557	776	777	c
1	7	Hungary	HUN	U-mid	10,202	10,141	5,091	5,061	1986
1	7	Kyrgyz Republic	KGZ	L-mid	4,472	4,548	2,232	2,270	c
1	7	Latvia	LVA	L-mid	2,617	2,617	1,306	1,306	c
1	7	Lithuania	LTU	L-mid	3,754	3,780	1,873	1,886	c
1	7	Moldova	MDA	L-mid	4,359	4,385	2,175	2,188	c
1	7	Russian Federation	RUS	L-mid	148,920	149,665	74,320	74,692	c
1	7	Slovenia	SVN	U-mid	2,017	2,031	1,020	1,027	c

(continued)

503

Table D-2 Countries that responded to AIW II questionnaire on government national AIDS programs, level of economy, country population, and date of first AIDS case report—*continued

List	GAA	Country	Code	Economy	Pop. 92	Pop. 93	Adult 92	Adult 93	Case 1
1	7	Turkmenistan	TKM	L-mid	3,852	3,948	1,922	1,970	c
1	7	Ukraine	UKR	L-mid	52,118	52,274	26,010	26,088	c
1	7	Yugoslavia, Fed. Rep.	YUG	L-mid	10,597	10,682	5,357	5,400	c
1	8	Algeria	DZA	L-mid	26,375	27,087	12,141	12,469	1986
1	8	Israel	ISR	High	5,113	5,251	2,495	2,562	1984
1	8	Jordan	JOR	L-mid	3,949	4,178	1,830	1,936	1986
1	8	Kuwait	KWT	High	1,400	1,368	754	737	1986
1	8	Lebanon	LBN	L-mid	3,781	3,868	1,848	1,890	1986
1	8	Morocco	MAR	L-mid	26,262	26,919	12,636	12,952	1986
1	8	Oman	OMN	U-mid	1,647	1,710	714	742	1986
1	8	Syrian Arab Rep.	SYR	L-mid	12,951	13,378	5,697	5,885	1987
1	8	Tunisia	TUN	L-mid	8,405	8,573	4,205	4,289	1985
1	9	Bhutan	BTN	Low	1,497	1,530	716	732	a
1	9	China	CHN	Low	1,166,144	1,183,636	654,550	664,368	1985
1	9	Hong Kong	HKG	High	5,805	5,857	3,408	3,439	1985
1	9	Japan	JPN	High	124,318	124,815	64,035	64,291	1985
1	9	Taiwan	TWN	High	20,476	20,476	11,342	11,342	1991
1	9	Viet Nam	VNM	Low	69,225	70,817	33,502	34,272	1993
1	10	Brunei	BRN	High	273	282	137	141	1989
1	10	India	IND	Low	883,473	902,026	440,870	450,129	1986
1	10	Malaysia	MYS	U-mid	18,610	19,075	9,351	9,585	1986
1	10	Nepal	NPL	Low	19,892	20,409	9,089	9,325	1988
1	10	Singapore	SGP	High	2,814	2,865	1,692	1,722	1986
1	10	Sri Lanka	LKA	Low	17,396	17,622	9,132	9,251	1987
1	10	Thailand	THA	L-mid	57,992	58,978	32,270	32,818	1984
2	3	American Samoa	ASM	U-mid	39	40	20	21	a
2	3	Cook Islands	COK	L-mid	17	17	9	9	a
2	3	Guam	GUM	U-mid	150	155	79	81	1991
2	3	New Caledonia	NCL	U-mid	175	179	92	94	1988

504

2	3	Niue	NIU	L-mid	2	2	1	1	a
2	3	Tokelau	TKL	L-mid	2	2	1	1	a
2	3	Tuvalu	TUV	L-mid	10	10	5	5	a
2	6	Bermuda	BMU	High	52	52	27	27	1986
2	6	Cayman Islands	CYM	High	28	28	15	15	1987
2	6	Montserrat	MSR	L-mid	12	12	6	6	1991
2	6	Netherlands Antilles	ANT	U-mid	194	196	102	103	1991

*List, core country response (1) or subsidiary response (2); GAA, geographical area of affinity; country, territory, or region responding; code, United Nations three-letter code for the country; economy, economic division based on GNP per capita as defined by the International Bank for Reconstruction and Development in *The World Bank Atlas, 1994:* Low = $675 or less, l-mid = $676–$2695, u-mid = $2696–$8355, high = $8356 or more; pop. 92, estimated total 1992 population (thousands); pop. 93, estimated total 1993 population (thousands); adult 92, estimated 1992 adult (15–49) population (thousands); adult 93, estimated 1993 adult (15–49) population (thousands); case 1, year of first reported AIDS case (a = no. cases as of January 1, 1994; b = do not report AIDS cases; c = newly formed country).

Table D-3 Government national AIDS programs: program structure and partnership*

List	GAA	Country	PU1	PU1A	PU2	PU3	PU4A	PU4B	PU4C	PU4D	PU4E	PU4F	PU4G	PU4H	PU4I
1	1	United States	+	21	11	16	NA	+	NA	−	NA	NA	NA	+	−
1	2	Austria	+	20	5	3	−	−	−	+	−	−	−	−	−
1	2	Belgium	+	18	4	15	−	−	NA	−	NA	NA	NA	+	−
1	2	Cyprus	+	25	6	5	—	—	+	+	NA	NA	NA	+	+
1	2	Denmark	+	15	3	1	NA	NA	NA	+	NA	NA	NA	+	−
1	2	Finland	+	12	5	2	−	−	NA	−	NA	NA	NA	−	−
1	2	France	−	—	—	—	−	−	−	−	—	—	—	—	+
1	2	Germany	+	42	10	42	NA	−	NA	+	−	−	−	+	+
1	2	Iceland	+	10	6	3	NA	NA	NA	+	NA	NA	NA	NA	−
1	2	Liechtenstein	+	7	2	5	−	−	−	−	−	−	−	−	−
1	2	Luxembourg	+	10	4	3	−	−	−	−	−	−	−	−	−
1	2	Malta	+	10	2	2	−	−	−	+	−	NA	NA	−	—
1	2	The Netherlands	+	25	4	5	−	−	NA	−	—	+	—	−	+
1	2	Norway	+	10	5	5	−	NA	NA	+	NA	+	NA	−	+
1	2	Spain	+	—	—	—	—	—	—	+	—	—	—	—	+
1	2	Sweden	+	15	9	4	−	−	NA	+	NA	NA	NA	+	−
1	2	Switzerland	+	33	9	—	−	−	−	−	−	−	−	−	−
1	2	United Kingdom	+	21	7	0	+	+	−	+	−	—	—	+	+
1	3	Australia	+	11	4	—	—	—	—	+	—	—	—	+	+
1	3	Fiji	+	16	4	3	−	−	−	+	−	−	−	−	−
1	3	Kiribati	+	16	3	7	—	—	—	+	—	+	—	—	—
1	3	Micronesia, Fed. Sts.	+	12	4	3	−	NA	−	+	+	+	+	NA	−
1	3	New Zealand	+	—	—	—	NA	−	NA	+	−	NA	−	−	−
1	3	Papua New Guinea	+	17	3	3	NA	+	NA	+	—	NA	+	+	+
1	3	Solomon Islands	+	10	4	4	−	−	−	−	−	NA	−	NA	−
1	3	Vanuatu	+	10	4	4	−	−	−	+	+	NA	+	NA	NA
1	3	Western Samoa	+	14	4	5	−	−	−	−	−	−	−	−	−
1	4	Argentina	−	—	—	—	—	—	—	+	+	NA	NA	−	−
1	4	Belize	+	15	10	3	−	−	−	−	−	−	−	−	−
1	4	Brazil	+	18	5	5	−	−	−	+	−	−	−	−	−
1	4	Chile	+	9	1	—	−	−	NA	+	+	NA	−	+	+
1	4	Colombia	+	10	—	2	−	−	NA	+	NA	NA	NA	−	−
1	4	Costa Rica	+	7	3	0	−	−	—	+	−	−	−	NA	+
1	4	Ecuador	−	—	—	—	−	NA	+	+	NA	+	+	+	−
1	4	El Salvador	+	7	2	0	−	—	—	+	—	—	—	+	−
1	4	Guatemala	−	—	—	—	−	—	—	+	+	—	+	+	−
1	4	Mexico	−	—	—	—	+	NA	NA	+	NA	NA	NA	NA	NA
1	4	Panama	−	—	—	—	−	−	−	−	−	−	−	−	−
1	4	Peru	−	—	—	—	NA	−	−	−	NA	NA	NA	+	−
1	4	Suriname	+	7	2	1	−	−	−	−	−	−	−	−	−
1	4	Uruguay	+	15	9	3	NA	+	−	+	+	NA	NA	+	−
1	4	Venezuela	−	—	—	—	NA	−	−	+	−	−	−	−	—
1	5	Angola	+	0	3	0	−	NA	NA	+	NA	NA	NA	+	NA
1	5	Benin	+	17	3	5	−	−	−	+	−	−	−	+	−
1	5	Botswana	−	—	—	—	—	—	—	—	—	—	—	—	—
1	5	Burkino Faso	+	51	25	10	−	−	−	−	−	−	−	−	−
1	5	Cameroon	+	15	5	3	−	+	+	+	−	−	−	+	+

506

PU4IEXP	PU691A	PU691B	PU691C	PU691D	PU691E	PU693A	PU693B	PU693C	PU693D	PU693E
	S	S	S	S	S	S	S	S	S	S
	P	P	P	P	P	P	P	P	P	P
	S	S	S	S	S	S	S	S	S	S
Press Information Office	P	P	P	P	P	P	P	P	P	P
	P	P	P	P	P	P	P	P	P	P
	P	P	P	P	P	P	P	P	P	P
Ministry of Research	—	—	—	—	—	—	—	—	—	—
research & tech/scientific collaboration	S	S	S	S	S	S	S	S	S	S
	P	P	P	P	P	P	P	P	P	P
	P	P	P	P	P	P	P	P	P	—
	P	P	P	P	P	P	P	P	P	P
	P	P	P	P	—	P	P	P	P	—
Ministry of Social Affairs and Employment, Ministry of Development & Cooperation	P	P	P	P	P	P	P	P	P	P
Justice (for prisons)	P	S	S	S	S	P	S	S	S	S
Justice/social issues	PS	PS	PS	PS	—	PS	PS	PS	PS	—
	P	P	P	P	P	P	P	P	P	P
	P	P	P	P	P	P	P	P	P	P
ODA, Environment, Employment	S	S	S	S	S	S	S	S	S	S
Corrective Services, Social Security, Immigration and Ethnic Affairs	P	P	P	P	P	P	P	P	P	P
	P	P	P	P	P	P	P	P	P	P
	P	P	—	P	P	P	P	—	PS	P
	P	P	P	P	P	P	S	S	S	S
	P	P	P	P	P	P	P	P	P	P
Corrective Services (prisons), NGO (youth)	PS	PS	P	PS	P	PS	S	PS	PS	—
	P	P	P	P	P	P	P	P	P	P
	S	P	—	P	P	S	P	—	S	P
Broadcasting	P	P	P	P	P	P	P	P	P	P
	P	P	P	P	P	P	P	P	P	P
	P	P	P	P	P	P	P	P	P	P
	P	P	P	P	P	P	P	P	P	P
Justice	P	P	P	P	P	S	S	S	S	S
Communications/Justice	P	P	P	P	P	P	P	P	S	S
Justice	P	P	P	P	P	P	S	P	S	S
	P	P	P	P	P	S	S	S	S	S
	P	P	P	P	P	P	P	P	P	P
	P	P	P	P	P	S	S	S	S	S
	P	P	P	P	P	P	P	S	P	P
	P	P	P	P	P	S	S	P	S	P
	P	P	P	P	P	P	P	P	F	P
	P	P	P	P	P	P	P	P	P	P
	P	P	P	P	P	S	S	S	S	S
	P	P	P	P	P	P	P	P	P	P
	P	P	P	P	P	P	PS	PS	PS	P
	S	P	P	S	S	S	P	P	S	S
	P	P	P	P	P	P	S	P	S	P
	P	P	P	S	P	P	P	P	S	P
Ministry of Education (after high school)	P	P	P	P	P	S	P	P	S	S

(continued)

Table D-3 Government national AIDS programs: program structure and partnership*—continued

List	GAA	Country	PU1	PU1A	PU2	PU3	PU4A	PU4B	PU4C	PU4D	PU4E	PU4F	PU4G	PU4H	PU4I
1	5	Cape Verde	−	−	−	−	−	−	−	+	−	−	−	−	−
1	5	Chad	+	15	1	5	−	−	−	−	−	−	−	−	−
1	5	Comoros	+	15	4	1	−	−	−	−	−	−	−	−	−
1	5	Congo	+	30	—	0	—	—	+	+	—	—	+	—	—
1	5	Côte d'Ivoire	+	45	7	3	−	−	−	+	+	+	+	+	+
1	5	Djibouti	+	8	2	2	−	−	−	−	−	−	−	−	−
1	5	Ethiopia	+	14	2	—	+	+	+	+	−	+	−	—	+
1	5	Gabon	+	74	—	0	NA	NA	NA	+	+	NA	NA	NA	—
1	5	Ghana	+	25	6	7	−	−	−	−	−	−	−	−	−
1	5	Guinea	+	56	22	30	−	+	NA	+	+	+	+	+	—
1	5	Guinee-Bissau	+	20	—	—	—	—	—	—	—	—	—	—	—
1	5	Lesotho	+	30	13	15	−	−	−	−	−	−	−	−	−
1	5	Madagascar	+	20	4	2	—	—	—	+	—	—	—	+	—
1	5	Mali	+	—	—	—	+	+	+	+	+	+	+	+	+
1	5	Mauritania	+	10	2	0	−	−	−	+	+	−	+	−	—
1	5	Mauritius	—	—	—	—	—	—	—	+	+	+	+	—	—
1	5	Rwanda	+	—	—	1	−	—	—	+	+	+	—	+	—
1	5	Senegal	+	25	10	5	−	+	−	+	+	+	+	+	+
1	5	Seychelles	+	19	5	0	−	—	—	+	—	—	—	—	+
1	5	South Africa	+	—	—	—	—	—	—	+	—	—	—	+	+
1	5	Tanzania	+	19	—	2	−	+	−	+	+	NA	+	+	+
1	5	Togo	+	32	7	5	−	−	−	+	−	+	NA	+	—
1	5	Uganda	+	20	4	3	−	−	−	+	+	NA	+	+	+
1	5	Zaire	+	41	5	11	NA	NA	NA	NA	NA	NA	NA	NA	NA
1	5	Zambia	+	—	—	—	−	−	−	+	+	NA	NA	+	—
1	5	Zimbabwe	+	—	—	—	—	+	—	+	+	—	+	+	—
1	6	Antigua and Barbuda	+	14	7	6	−	−	−	−	−	−	−	−	−
1	6	Barbados	+	13	5	6	−	−	−	+	−	−	+	+	—
1	6	Dominican Republic	+	32	12	1	−	−	−	−	−	−	−	−	−
1	6	Grenada	+	25	10	6	—	—	—	+	—	—	—	—	—
1	6	Jamaica	+	64	40	58	+	−	—	+	+	NA	+	+	+
1	6	St. Lucia	+	13	8	3	−	−	−	+	+	+	+	−	—
1	6	Trinidad and Tobago	+	25	13	11	−	−	−	+	—	—	—	—	—
1	7	Azerbaijan	−	—	—	—	−	−	−	−	−	−	−	−	−
1	7	Belarus	+	8	3	0	−	−	−	+	−	−	−	−	+
1	7	Bulgaria	+	11	4	2	—	—	—	+	+	—	—	+	—
1	7	Croatia	+	15	4	2	−	−	−	−	−	−	−	−	−
1	7	Czech Republic	+	25	7	6	−	−	−	−	−	−	−	−	—
1	7	Estonia	+	10	5	3	−	+	NA	+	NA	NA	NA	+	+
1	7	Hungary	+	24	4	1	−	+	NA	−	NA	NA	NA	+	+
1	7	Kyrgyz Republic	+	12	—	0	−	−	−	−	−	NA	NA	−	−
1	7	Latvia	+	11	4	1	NA	NA	NA	NA	NA	NA	NA	NA	NA
1	7	Lithuania	−	—	—	—	−	−	−	−	−	−	−	−	−
1	7	Moldova	−	—	—	—	−	−	−	−	−	−	−	−	−
1	7	Russian Federation	−	—	—	—	+	+	—	+	—	—	—	+	—
1	7	Slovenia	+	15	8	0	−	−	NA	+	NA	−	NA	−	—
1	7	Turkmenistan	+	14	3	1	—	+	—	+	—	—	—	—	—
1	7	Ukraine	−	—	—	—	−	NA	NA	+	−	NA	NA	+	NA

PU4IEXP	PU691A	PU691B	PU691C	PU691D	PU691E	PU693A	PU693B	PU693C	PU693D	PU693E
	—	—	—	—	—	S	S	S	S	S
	P	P	P	P	P	P	P	P	P	S
	P	P	P	P	P	P	P	P	P	S
	P	P	P	P	P	S	S	S	S	S
Agriculture and Livestock	P	P	P	S	P	S	P	P	S	P
	P	P	P	S	S	S	S	P	S	S
all government ministries	P	P	P	P	P	S	S	S	S	S
	S	P	S	S	S	S	P	S	S	S
	P	P	P	P	P	P	P	P	P	P
	PS	P	S	S	P	S	P	S	S	P
	P	P	—	—	S	P	P	P	P	S
	S	S	P	S	S	S	S	P	S	S
	S	P	P	S	—	S	P	S	S	S
	P	P	S	S	P	S	S	S	S	S
	S	P	P	S	S	S	P	S	P	P
	S	S	S	S	S	S	S	S	S	S
	S	P	S	S	S	S	S	S	S	S
Foreign Affairs	S	—	P	S	S	S	P	S	S	S
Ministry of Social Affairs	S	S	P	S	P	S	S	P	S	P
(many) Admin. manpower; correctional services	S	P	P	P	P	S	S	PS	S	S
Ministry of Info./Prime Minister's office/NGOs	S	S	P	S	P	S	S	P	S	P
Communication Culture	P	P	P	P	S	S	P	P	S	S
local government	P	P	P	P	P	S	P	S	S	S
	P	P	S	S	P	—	P	S	S	P
	P	P	P	P	P	S	S	P	PS	P
	P	P	P	P	P	S	S	P	S	P
	P	—	P	P	—	P	P	P	P	—
	PS	P	P	P	P	PS	P	P	P	P
	P	P	P	P	—	P	P	P	P	—
	S	P	P	S	S	S	P	P	S	S
Ministry of Labor	P	P	P	P	P	P	P	P	P	P
	P	P	P	P	P	P	P	P	P	P
	P	P	P	P	P	P	P	P	P	P
	S	P	P	S	P	S	P	P	S	P
Culture	P	P	P	P	P	S	S	S	S	S
	P	P	P	P	P	P	P	P	P	P
	P	—	P	—	—	P	—	P	—	—
	P	P	S	P	P	P	S	S	S	P
Ministry of Social Affairs (incl Min Labor)	—	—	—	—	—	PS	PS	PS	PS	P
Ministry of Justice	P	P	P	P	P	P	P	P	P	P
	S	S	S	S	S	S	S	S	S	S
	P	P	P	P	4	P	P	P	P	4
	P	P	P	P	P	P	P	P	P	P
	P	P	P	P	P	P	P	P	P	P
	S	S	S	S	S	PS	S	P	S	S
	P	P	P	P	P	P	P	P	P	P
	S	S	S	S	S	P	P	S	S	P
	—	—	—	—	—	P	P	P	P	P

(continued)

Table D-3 Government national AIDS programs: program structure and partnership*—continued

List	GAA	Country	PU1	PU1A	PU2	PU3	PU4A	PU4B	PU4C	PU4D	PU4E	PU4F	PU4G	PU4H	PU4I
1	7	Yugoslavia, Fed. Rep.	–	—	—	—	NA	NA	NA	–	–	NA	NA	NA	—
1	8	Algeria	+	25	10	1	—	—	—	+	+	—	—	+	+
1	8	Israel	+	20	12	2	NA	NA	NA	+	NA	NA	NA	+	NA
1	8	Jordan	+	8	1	1	–	–	–	–	–	–	–	–	–
1	8	Kuwait	+	14	2	0	—	—	—	—	—	—	—	—	—
1	8	Lebanon	+	27	3	15	NA	–	–	–	–	NA	NA	–	—
1	8	Morocco	+	58	10	5	–	–	–	–	–	NA	NA	+	—
1	8	Oman	+	7	0	0	–	+	–	–	–	NA	NA	+	NA
1	8	Syrian Arab Rep.	+	70	10	35	—	+	+	—	+	+	+	+	+
1	8	Tunisia	+	29	3	6	–	+	+	+	+	+	+	+	+
1	9	Bhutan	+	16	2	1	–	–	–	–	NA	NA	NA	–	—
1	9	China	+	36	9	—	—	—	—	+	—	—	+	—	+
1	9	Hong Kong	+	20	9	7	–	–	–	–	–	–	–	–	–
1	9	Japan	+	14	4	4	—	—	NA	+	NA	NA	NA	+	+
1	9	Taiwan	—	—	—	—	—	—	—	—	—	—	—	—	—
1	9	Vietnam	+	16	4	4	—	+	+	+	+	+	+	+	+
1	10	Brunei	+	7	0	0	–	+	NA	–	–	NA	NA	–	—
1	10	India	+	7	0	3	—	+	+	+	+	+	+	—	—
1	10	Malaysia	+	15	5	2	—	—	—	+	—	—	+	+	—
1	10	Nepal	+	15	2	2	–	+	+	+	NA	NA	NA	+	+
1	10	Singapore	+	18	4	7	+	+	NA	+	NA	NA	NA	+	+
1	10	Sri Lanka	+	19	—	2	+	—	—	+	—	—	+	+	—
1	10	Thailand	+	39	3	6	+	+	NA	+	+	NA	NA	+	+
2	3	American Samoa	+	25	12	10	NA	NA	NA	+	NA	NA	+	NA	—
2	3	Cook Islands	+	6	3	1	—	—	—	+	—	—	—	—	—
2	3	Guam	+	8	6	3	–	–	–	+	–	–	–	+	+
2	3	New Caledonia	+	16	5	1	–	–	–	+	–	–	–	–	–
2	3	Niue	+	7	4	4	–	–	–	+	–	–	–	–	+
2	3	Tokelau	+	9	5	12	NA	NA	NA	+	+	NA	+	NA	—
2	3	Tuvalu	+	10	3	4	–	–	–	–	–	–	–	–	–
2	6	Bermuda	+	16	9	6	–	–	–	+	–	NA	NA	–	—
2	6	Cayman Islands	+	14	5	5	NA	NA	–	–	NA	NA	NA	NA	—
2	6	Montserrat	+	19	13	7	–	–	–	–	–	–	–	–	—
2	6	Netherlands Antilles	+	9	5	3	–	–	–	–	–	–	–	–	–

*List, core country response (1) or subsidiary response (2); GAA, geographic area of affinity; country, territory, or region responding.

Abbreviations for public sector: PU1, national AIDS advisory committee or a similar body created in the country; PU1A, number of members (total) serving on the national AIDS advisory committee; PU2, number of women members serving on the national AIDS advisory committee; PU3, number of members of the national AIDS advisory committee representing NGOs.

Ministries other than the ministry of health which have developed their own AIDS programs: PU4A, planning/economic development; PU4B, internal/home affairs; PU4C, tourism; PU4D, education; PU4E, youth; PU4F, family affairs; PU4G, women's affairs; PU4H, defense; PU4I, other; PU4IEXP, other specified.

Areas in which HIV/AIDS activities were primarily the responsibility of the GNAP (P) or were shared among other ministries (S) in 1991: PU691A, planning HIV/AIDS activities; PU691B, managing HIV/AIDS activities; PU691C, financing HIV/AIDS activities; PU691D, implementing HIV/AIDS activities; PU691E, evaluating HIV/AIDS activities.

Areas in which HIV/AIDS activities were primarily the responsibility of the GNAP (P) or were shared among other ministries (S) in 1993: A–E, same areas as for 1991.

PU4IEXP	PU691A	PU691B	PU691C	PU691D	PU691E	PU693A	PU693B	PU693C	PU693D	PU693E
	—	—	—	—	—	—	—	—	—	—
Religious Affairs/Transportation	S	P	S	P	P	S	P	S	S	P
	P	P	P	P	P	P	P	P	P	P
	P	P	P	S	P	P	P	P	S	S
	P	P	P	P	—	P	P	P	P	P
	P	P	P	P	P	P	P	P	P	P
	P	P	P	P	P	P	P	P	P	P
	P	P	P	S	P	S	P	P	S	P
National union of students; youth unions; scouts	S	S	S	S	S	S	S	S	S	S
Prof. training/Religious Affairs	P	P	P	S	P	S	S	S	S	P
	P	P	P	P	P	P	P	P	P	P
Public security; justice	P	P	P	P	P	P	P	P	S	P
	P	P	P	P	P	P	P	P	P	P
Ministry of Labour/Prime Minister's office	S	S	S	S	S	S	S	S	S	S
	—	—	—	—	—	—	—	—	—	—
Ministry of Finance/Ministry of Justice	S	P	S	S	S	S	P	S	S	S
	P	P	P	P	P	P	P	P	P	P
	P	P	P	P	P	P	P	P	P	P
	P	P	P	P	P	PS	P	P	PS	P
m/o Local development, industry, info. & communication	—	—	—	—	—	S	—	—	—	—
Law, Foreign Affairs, Labor, Information & Art	P	P	P	S	P	P	P	P	S	P
	P	P	P	P	P	P	P	P	P	P
Interior	P	P	P	S	P	S	S	P	S	P
	S	S	P	S	P	S	S	P	S	S
	S	P	P	P	P	S	P	P	P	P
CBO, private clinic, hospital, public health center	P	P	P	P	P	P	P	P	P	P
	P	P	P	P	P	P	P	P	P	P
Ministry of Religion; Ministry of Women's Affairs	P	P	P	P	P	P	P	P	P	P
	P	P	P	P	P	P	P	P	P	P
	P	P	P	P	P	P	P	P	P	P
	P	S	P	P	P	S	P	P	S	S
	P	P	P	P	P	P	P	P	P	P
	S	P	P	S	P	S	P	P	S	P
	P	P	P	P	P	P	P	P	P	P

Table D-4 Government national AIDS programs—epidemiology: estimates and projections of the numbers of HIV infections in adults and children (cumulative through the year indicated)*

List	GAA	Country	EP1	EP4	EP5	EP6	EP6NUM	EP6YR	EP7NUM	EP7YR
1	1	United States	1,300,000	1.49	6.15	—	—	—	—	—
1	2	Austria	12,000	—	3.75	—	—	—	—	—
1	2	Belgium	7,155	2.20	3.30	+	9,000	1994	500	1994
1	2	Cyprus	130	7.00	—	—	—	—	—	—
1	2	Denmark	6,000	6.00	11.60	—	—	—	—	—
1	2	Finland	650	6.00	10.00	—	—	—	—	—
1	2	France	100,000	3.00	5.30	—	—	—	—	—
1	2	Germany	55,956	4.50	10.00	—	—	—	—	—
1	2	Iceland	80	6.00	6.00	—	—	—	0	1993
1	2	Liechtenstein	150	3.00	2.00	—	—	—	0	—
1	2	Luxembourg	228	4.00	10.00	—	—	—	—	—
1	2	Malta	100	20.00	28.00	—	—	—	—	—
1	2	The Netherlands	10,000	—	13.80	+	17,000	2000	—	—
1	2	Norway	1,227	3.00	6.00	+	3,800	1995	—	—
1	2	Spain	100,000	—	4.00	—	—	—	—	—
1	2	Sweden	3,318	4.10	11.30			—	—	—	—
1	2	Switzerland	24,000	3.33	3.85	—		—	—	—
1	2	United Kingdom	32,590	—	9.36	—		—	—	—
1	3	Australia	20,000	30.00	35.00	+	20,000	1994	—	—
1	3	Fiji	20	2.33	2.25	—	—	—	—	—
1	3	Kiribati	2	—	—	—	—	—	—	—
1	3	Micronesia, Fed. Sts.	2	—	—	—	—	—	—	—
1	3	New Zealand	818	13.00	24.00	—	—	—	—	—
1	3	Papua New Guinea	2,500	1.20	1.20	—	—	—	—	—
1	3	Solomon Islands	0	—	—			—	—	—	—
1	3	Vanuatu	0	—	—	—	—	—	—	—
1	3	Western Samoa	0	—	—	—	—	—	—	—
1	4	Argentina	140,000	4.00	4.00	—	—	—	—	—

1	4	Belize	—	—	—	—	—	—	—	—
1	4	Brazil	400,000	—	4.00	+	650,000	1995	—	—
1	4	Chile	1,777	8.80	94.00	+	17,000	2000	—	—
1	4	Colombia	7,231	7.00	12.00	—	—	—	—	—
1	4	Costa Rica	10,000	—	11.00	+	24,051	1997	—	—
1	4	Ecuador	664	4.00	4.00	—	—	—	—	—
1	4	El Salvador	615	3.50	3.70	+	—	—	—	—
1	4	Guatemala	1,046	3.00	3.00	+	2,739	1994	111	1994
1	4	Mexico	500,000	—	6.00	—	—	—	—	—
1	4	Panama	14,000	—	5.00	+	25,000	1997	—	—
1	4	Peru	30,000	4.00	7.00	—	—	—	—	—
1	4	Suriname	292	2.00	2.00	—	—	—	—	—
1	4	Uruguay	3,200	4.00	6.40	+	6,600	1994	100	1994
1	4	Venezuela	—	—	12.00	—	—	—	—	—
1	5	Angola	—	—	0.94	—	—	—	—	—
1	5	Benin	465	2.00	2.00	+	101,618	1998	6,486	1998
1	5	Botswana	100,400	0.76	—	+	216,000	1998	—	—
1	5	Burkino Faso	2,886	—	1.50	—	—	—	—	—
1	5	Cameroon	2,000	0.67	0.63	+	220,000	2005	—	—
1	5	Cape Verde	82	1.00	1.00	+	104	1995	8	1993
1	5	Chad	1,597	—	—	—	—	—	—	—
1	5	Comoros	25	0.92	2.00	—	—	—	—	—
1	5	Congo	—	—	—	—	—	—	—	—
1	5	Côte d'Ivoire	14,655	—	2.50	+	935,315	1998	14,207	1998
1	5	Djibouti	3,000	0.67	2.30	—	—	—	—	—
1	5	Ethiopia	500,000	1.00	1.60	—	—	—	—	—
1	5	Gabon	520	1.00	1.00	—	—	—	—	—
1	5	Ghana	10,285	—	0.53	—	—	—	—	—
1	5	Guinea	677	3.00	4.00	—	—	—	—	—
1	5	Guinea-Bissau	—	—	1.40	—	—	—	—	—
1	5	Lesotho	17,400	—	0.89	—	—	—	—	—

(continued)

513

Table D-4 Government national AIDS programs—epidemiology: estimates and projections of the numbers of HIV infections in adults and children (cumulative through the year indicated)*—continued

List	GAA	Country	EP1	EP4	EP5	EP6	EP6NUM	EP6YR	EP7NUM	EP7YR
1	5	Madagascar	34	1.00	1.00	+	5,000	2000	600	2000
1	5	Mali	14,000	0.67	3.00	+	140,000	2000	—	—
1	5	Mauritania	50	—	6.00	+	10,732	1998	—	—
1	5	Mauritius	67	2.72	5.00	—	—	—	—	—
1	5	Rwanda	297,859	1.00	1.10	+	379,257	1998	94,905	1998
1	5	Senegal	49,853	—	2.00	+	54,042	1993	1,175	1993
1	5	Seychelles	28	1.33	—	—	—	—	—	—
1	5	South Africa	560,000	—	—	+	1,000,000	1994	15,000	1994
1	5	Tanzania	800,000	0.89	1.09	+	1,600,000	1995	—	—
1	5	Togo	2,142	—	2.00	+	392,427	1998	63,084	1998
1	5	Uganda	1,900,000	1.00	1.00	+	2,700,000	1998	410,900	1998
1	5	Zaire	18,186	—	0.68	+	870,000	1996	—	—
1	5	Zambia	870,000	1.00	1.00	+	1,273,000	1998	97,300	1998
1	5	Zimbabwe	786,993	1.20	1.30	+	885,244	1997	42,507	1997
1	6	Antigua and Barbuda	72	1.00	8.00	—	—	—	—	—
1	6	Barbados	697	2.00	3.70	+	5,000	1995	—	—
1	6	Dominican Republic	10,077	—	2.60	+	300,000	2000	—	—
1	6	Grenada	62	2.70	2.36	+	900	1993	—	—
1	6	Jamaica	10,000	—	2.00	—	—	—	—	—
1	6	St. Lucia	86	1.20	2.20	—	—	—	—	—
1	6	Trinidad and Tobago	—	—	—	—	—	—	—	—
1	7	Azerbaijan	3	—	—	—	—	—	—	—
1	7	Belarus	1,670	1.90	2.00	—	—	—	—	—
1	7	Bulgaria	111	0.50	2.00	—	—	—	—	—
1	7	Croatia	56	0.10	—	—	—	—	—	—
1	7	Czech Republic	143	9.00	—	—	—	—	—	—
1	7	Estonia	33	10.00	—	—	—	—	—	—
1	7	Hungary	2,800	10.00	14.00	—	—	—	—	—
1	7	Kyrgyz Republic	15	—	—	—	—	—	—	—

List	GAA	Country	EP1	EP4	EP5	EP6	EP6NUM	EP6YR	EP7NUM	EP7YR
1	7	Latvia	16	—	—			—	—	—
1	7	Lithuania	62	11.00	—	+	686	1997	—	—
1	7	Moldova	28	4.00	1.00	—		—	—	—
1	7	Russian Federation	612	2.00	2.00	+	2,400	1992	—	—
1	7	Slovenia	—	3.70	15.00	—		—	—	—
1	7	Turkmenistan	1	—	—	—		—	—	—
1	7	Ukraine	112	1.00	5.00	—		—	—	—
1	7	Yugoslavia, Fed. Rep.	5,000	6.00	4.00	—		—	—	—
1	8	Algeria	344	2.00	3.00	—		—	—	—
1	8	Israel	2,000	3.00	5.00	—		—	—	—
1	8	Jordan	97	4.00	3.00	—		—	—	—
1	8	Kuwait	23	3.60	1.67	—		—	—	—
1	8	Lebanon	134	5.00	6.00	—		—	—	—
1	8	Morocco	302	4.00	3.60	—		—	—	—
1	8	Oman	266	1.80	—	—		—	—	—
1	8	Syrian Arab Rep.	80	10.00	—			—	—	—
1	8	Tunisia	380	3.50	4.40	—		—	—	—
1	9	Bhutan	0	—	—	+	0-100	1993	—	—
1	9	China	969	9.80	—	+	100,000	2000	—	—
1	9	Hong Kong	7,000	15.00	72.00	—		—	—	—
1	9	Japan	2,551	1.00	—	+		1993	—	—
1	9	Taiwan	416	20.86	5.67			—	—	—
1	9	Viet Nam	11	—	—	+	190,000-330,000	2000	10-20,000	2000
1	10	Brunei	7	7.00	2.00	—		—	0	1995
1	10	India	12,000	1.33	2.00	+	10,000,000	2000	4,000,000	2000
1	10	Malaysia	7,400	9.00	9.00	+	30,000	1995	—	—
1	10	Nepal	199	1.00	1.00	—		—	—	—
1	10	Singapore	158	13.40	17.00	+	400	1995	10	1995
1	10	Sri Lanka	—	3.00	3.00	+	6,100	1994	—	—
1	10	Thailand	—	—	7.00	+	4,000,000	2000	—	—
2	3	American Samoa	0	—	—	—		—	—	—

(continued)

Table D-4 Government national AIDS programs—epidemiology: estimates and projections of the numbers of HIV infections in adults and children (cumulative through the year indicated)*—continued

List	GAA	Country	EP1	EP4	EP5	EP6	EP6NUM	EP6YR	EP7NUM	EP7YR
2	3	Cook Islands	0	—	—	—	—	—	—	—
2	3	Guam	61	7.00	13.00	—	—	—	—	—
2	3	New Caledonia	77	4.10	6.00	+	—	—	—	—
2	3	Niue	0	0.00	0.00	—	—	—	—	—
2	3	Tokelau	0	—	—	—	—	—	—	—
2	3	Tuvalu	0	—	—	—	—	—	—	—
2	6	Bermuda	436	3.00	2.50	—	—	—	—	—
2	6	Cayman Islands	23	1.20	1.00	—	—	—	—	—
2	6	Montserrat	8	—	—	—	—	—	—	—
2	6	Netherlands Antilles	579	1.30	1.90	—	—	—	—	—

*List, core country response (1) or subsidiary response (2); GAA, geographic area of affinity; country, territory, or region responding.

Epidemiology abbreviations: EP1, estimated cumulative number of HIV infections in country that have occurred since the beginning of the pandemic through January 1, 1993; EP4, estimated number of men infected with HIV per every one woman infected with HIV; EP5, estimated number of men with AIDS per every one woman with AIDS; EP6, projections of the number of HIV infections for the country as a whole beyond the year 1993 have been made; EP6NUM, projected cumulative number of adults (above the age of 15) who will have been infected with HIV; EP6YR, year for which the projection (adults) was made; EP7NUM, projected cumulative number of children (under the age of 15) who will have been infected with HIV; EP7YR, year for which the projection (children) was made.

516

Table D-5 Government national AIDS programs: development, implementation, and impact on other health programs, Program 1–Program 393A*

List	GAA	Country	PR1	PR2	PR2A	PR2B	PR2C	PR2D	PR390A	PR390B	PR390C	PR390D	PR390E	PR390F	PR390G	PR390H	PR390I	PR390J	PR390K	PR393A
1	1	United States	1993	+	100%	100%	100%	—	L	—	M	O	O	L	L	O	M	O	L	L
1	2	Austria	1983	−	—	—	—	—	L	L	L	L	L	L	L	L	L	L	L	L
1	2	Belgium	1991	+	60%	0%	10%	0%	M	O	L	M	O	O	L	M	L	O	O	M
1	2	Cyprus	1989	−	—	—	—	—	M	M	L	H	H	H	H	M	O	L	O	O
1	2	Denmark	1986	+	—	—	—	—	O	—	O	O	O	O	O	O	O	O	O	O
1	2	Finland	1985	+	—	—	—	—	L	O	O	O	O	O	L	O	L	O	O	L
1	2	France	1998	−	—	—	—	—	—	—	—	—	—	—	—	—	—	—	—	—
1	2	Germany	1987	+	5%	5%	70%	20%	L	O	O	L	O	O	L	O	L	O	O	M
1	2	Iceland	1988	−	—	—	—	—	L	O	L	L	O	L	L	O	O	O	O	L
1	2	Liechtenstein	1987	−	—	—	—	—	L	O	L	L	O	O	L	L	L	L	L	L
1	2	Luxembourg	1988	−	—	—	—	—	L	O	L	M	O	O	M	O	L	O	O	M
1	2	Malta	1986	−	—	—	—	—	L	O	O	M	L	L	M	O	H	O	L	O
1	2	Netherlands	1987	−	—	—	—	—	O	O	O	O	L	O	L	L	L	O	L	O
1	2	Norway	1986	+	100%	100%	100%	—	O	L	O	O	L	L	O	O	L	L	O	O
1	2	Spain	1985	+	—	—	—	—	L	L	L	M	L	L	M	L	L	L	L	L
1	2	Sweden	1985	+	100%	100%	100%	100%	O	O	O	O	O	O	O	L	O	O	O	O
1	2	Switzerland	1987	+	—	—	—	75%	O	—	O	O	O	O	O	O	O	O	—	O
1	2	United Kingdom	1985	+	100%	100%	100%	75%	O	O	O	O	O	O	O	O	O	O	O	O
1	3	Australia	1984	+	—	—	—	—	O	—	L	L	O	O	L	O	L	L	O	O
1	3	Fiji	1988	+	100%	25%	100%	50%	L	O	O	M	O	O	L	M	M	M	O	M
1	3	Kiribati	1988	+	25%	0%	0%	0%	H	M	L	M	—	—	M	M	M	M	O	H
1	3	Micronesia, Fed. Sts.	1987	+	100%	60%	100%	45%	H	L	M	M	M	M	M	M	M	L	M	M
1	3	New Zealand	1985	−	—	—	—	—	L	O	O	M	O	M	L	M	M	L	L	L
1	3	Papua New Guinea	1989	+	98%	10%	20%	20%	M	L	M	M	L	L	O	O	M	O	M	M
1	3	Solomon Islands	1988	−	—	—	—	—	—	O	L	H	—	L	M	M	O	O	—	—
1	3	Vanuatu	1988	−	—	—	—	—	M	L	M	M	—	M	M	H	M	M	O	M
1	3	Western Samoa	1988	+	60%	15%	5%	20%	M	L	M	M	M	M	L	O	L	M	L	M
1	4	Argentina	1987	−	—	—	—	—	H	M	H	H	M	M	H	M	H	H	H	M
1	4	Belize	—			—	—	—	—	L	L	L	M	M	M	L	L	L	L	L	L
1	4	Brazil	1985	−	—	—	—	—	H	M	M	H	H	M	H	H	M	M	H	L
1	4	Chile	1990	−	—	—	—	—	M	M	L	M	M	M	M	M	M	M	M	L

(continued)

Table D-5 Government national AIDS programs: development, implementation, and impact on other health programs, Program 1–Program 393A*—continued

List	GAA	Country	PR1	PR2	PR2A	PR2B	PR2C	PR2D	PR390A	PR390B	PR390C	PR390D	PR390E	PR390F	PR390G	PR390H	PR390I	PR390J	PR390K	PR393A
1	4	Colombia	1986	–	–	–	30%	–	H	M	H	H	M	M	L	L	L	L	H	L
1	4	Costa Rica	1988	+	100%	50%	30%	50%	L	O	M	H	M	L	H	H	M	H	O	O
1	4	Ecuador	1985	+	50%	10%	30%	20%	M	L	L	H	H	O	L	L	L	L	M	M
1	4	El Salvador	1989	+	100%	–	100%	–	M	L	M	M	M	L	L	O	M	M	M	M
1	4	Guatemala	1986	+	96%	40%	75%	–	H	L	M	L	L	O	O	L	L	M	H	H
1	4	Mexico	1988	+	15%	25%	30%	10%	M	L	H	L	L	L	M	M	H	H	L	M
1	4	Panama	1989	+	–	–	–	–	H	L	H	H	M	O	M	–	H	M	O	M
1	4	Peru	1987	+	100%	5%	60%	15%	H	L	H	H	H	O	H	H	M	H	O	M
1	4	Suriname	1988	+	100%	5%	5%	100%	L	O	O	L	O	O	L	O	L	O	O	O
1	4	Uruguay	1987	+	–	–	–	–	L	O	L	L	M	O	L	L	O	O	L	L
1	4	Venezuela	1988	+	70%	5%	15%	10%	L	M	M	M	M	M	H	L	H	M	H	M
1	5	Angola	1987	+	–	–	–	–	H	M	H	M	M	M	M	L	L	L	H	H
1	5	Benin	1988	+	100%	0%	15%	6%	M	M	O	L	L	L	M	L	L	M	–	M
1	5	Botswana	1987	+	100%	–	100%	–	M	L	H	H	L	O	M	L	M	M	O	O
1	5	Burkino Faso	1986	–	–	–	–	–	M	H	O	H	M	O	M	L	L	L	H	L
1	5	Cameroon	1988	+	100%	–	100%	–	M	O	O	O	L	O	O	O	O	L	O	M
1	5	Cape Verde	1987	–	–	–	–	–	L	O	O	M	M	L	O	O	O	O	L	L
1	5	Chad	1988	–	–	–	–	–	O	O	L	M	L	O	L	M	O	H	O	M
1	5	Comoros	1990	–	–	–	–	–	H	O	O	M	L	O	M	O	O	L	M	H
1	5	Congo	1987	–	–	–	–	–	M	L	M	O	L	L	H	H	O	L	M	M
1	5	Côte d'Ivoire	1987	+	25%	80%	80%	0%	L	L	L	M	O	O	L	M	M	L	O	O
1	5	Djibouti	1988	+	100%	60%	100%	80%	L	O	H	L	M	L	M	L	M	H	L	L
1	5	Ethiopia	1985	+	100%	50%	85%	30%	L	L	O	M	O	O	M	M	M	M	H	M
1	5	Gabon	1987	+	80%	10%	50%	0%	M	L	M	M	M	O	M	H	M	M	M	M
1	5	Ghana	1986	+	100%	10%	60%	20%	M	L	M	M	M	M	H	M	M	M	L	H
1	5	Guinea	1987	+	40%	10%	30%	40%	M	L	O	O	M	O	O	O	O	O	O	O
1	5	Guinee-Bissau	1987	+	–	–	–	–	O	O	O	O	O	L	O	O	M	L	M	H
1	5	Lesotho	1987	–	–	–	–	–	M	L	M	H	L	L	L	H	L	H	H	M
1	5	Madagascar	1988	+	14%	–	–	–	H	M	M	H	M	M	H	L	H	L	O	M
1	5	Mali	1987	+	–	–	–	–	L	L	L	L	L	L	M	M	L	L	L	L
1	5	Mauritania	1990	–	–	–	–	–	M	M	O	M	M	M	M	M	M	M	M	O
1	5	Mauritius	1987	–	–	–	–	–	L	O	O	L	L	L	M	O	L	L	O	L

Table D-5 Government national AIDS programs: development, implementation, and impact on social needs programs, programs, ...

List	GAA	Country	PR1	PR2	PR2A	PR2B	PR2C	PR2D	PR390A	PR390B	PR390C	PR390D	PR390E	PR390F	PR390G	PR390H	PR390I	PR390J	PR390K	PR393A
1	5	Rwanda	1987	–	–	–	–	–	M	L	O	M	L	L	M	M	L	M	M	H
1	5	Senegal	1986	+	65%	–	–	–	L	L	M	H	M	O	L	O	L	M	M	L
1	5	Seychelles	1987	+	100%	–	–	100%	O	O	O	L	L	O	O	O	L	O	O	L
1	5	South Africa	1989	+	–	–	–	–	L	L	L	L	L	L	L	L	L	L	L	L
1	5	Tanzania	1988	+	100%	50%	100%	5%	M	M	H	M	M	M	H	H	M	M	M	M
1	5	Togo	1987	+	13%	0%	0%	0%	L	L	M	L	L	M	M	M	M	M	M	M
1	5	Uganda	1986	+	0%	0%	100%	0%	L	L	O	L	L	O	M	L	O	L	H	L
1	5	Zaire	1985	+	75%	–	10%	15%	L	L	O	O	O	M	–	M	O	O	M	H
1	5	Zambia	1987	–	–	–	–	–	M	L	O	M	L	O	O	O	O	O	M	M
1	5	Zimbabwe	1987	+	–	–	–	–	L	L	L	L	L	L	O	L	L	L	L	L
1	6	Antigua and Barbuda	1992	–	–	–	–	–	L	M	L	M	L	M	M	M	M	M	M	M
1	6	Barbados	1987	–	–	–	–	–	H	L	H	L	L	L	L	H	H	L	H	H
1	6	Dominican Republic	1987	–	–	–	–	–	H	H	H	H	H	L	H	H	H	L	M	M
1	6	Grenada	1989	+	100%	–	–	40%	M	M	M	M	H	M	M	M	M	M	M	M
1	6	Jamaica	1987	+	100%	80%	100%	75%	L	O	M	M	L	O	M	M	M	O	L	M
1	6	St. Lucia	1985	–	–	–	–	–	H	H	H	M	L	M	L	M	M	M	L	L
1	6	Trinidad and Tobago	1987	–	–	–	–	–	O	O	M	O	O	O	M	L	M	M	L	M
1	7	Azerbaijan	–	–	–	–	–	–	L	–	H	–	–	–	–	–	H	M	H	H
1	7	Belarus	1993	+	–	–	–	–	–	L	–	–	–	O	O	M	–	–	–	L
1	7	Bulgaria	1988	–	–	–	–	–	M	M	L	L	M	M	M	M	M	M	M	M
1	7	Croatia	1993	–	–	–	–	–	H	H	O	–	M	–	M	L	H	M	H	M
1	7	Czech Republic	–	–	–	–	–	–	M	M	M	L	–	L	–	–	–	–	–	H
1	7	Estonia	1992	+	50%	10%	–	20%	–	–	–	–	L	M	M	M	H	M	O	H
1	7	Hungary	1985	–	–	–	–	–	L	L	O	L	L	–	H	L	L	M	L	M
1	7	Kyrgyz Republic	–	–	–	–	–	–	O	–	L	L	H	L	M	H	–	–	–	L
1	7	Latvia	1993	–	–	–	–	–	M	O	L	L	O	O	H	H	L	L	H	H
1	7	Lithuania	1990	–	–	–	–	–	L	H	H	O	O	–	L	O	L	–	M	M
1	7	Moldova	–	–	–	–	–	–	M	–	O	–	–	H	–	M	H	M	–	H
1	7	Russian Federation	1993	–	–	–	–	–	–	L	–	L	O	–	H	–	L	–	O	O
1	7	Slovenia	1985	–	–	–	–	–	M	–	M	–	–	–	–	–	–	–	–	O
1	7	Turkmenistan	1992	–	–	–	–	–	–	–	–	–	O	–	–	–	O	O	–	M
1	7	Ukraine	1992	+	–	–	–	–	–	–	–	–	–	–	–	M	–	–	–	H
1	7	Yugoslavia, Fed. Rep.	–	–	–	–	–	–	–	–	–	–	M	L	L	–	–	–	–	H
1	8	Algeria	1988	–	–	–	–	–	M	M	L	L	M	L	L	M	M	M	M	M

(continued)

Table D-5 Government national AIDS programs: development, implementation, and impact on other health programs, Program 1–Program 393A*—continued

List	GAA	Country	PR1	PR2	PR2A	PR2B	PR2C	PR2D	PR390A	PR390B	PR390C	PR390D	PR390E	PR390F	PR390G	PR390H	PR390I	PR390J	PR390K	PR393A
1	8	Israel	1986	—	—	—	—	—	L	O	O	O	O	O	O	L	O	O	O	L
1	8	Jordan	1986	—	—	—	—	—	M	L	L	M	L	M	M	M	M	M	L	M
1	8	Kuwait	1985	—	—	—	—	—	O	O	O	L	O	L	L	O	O	O	O	O
1	8	Lebanon	1989	+	100%	0%	—	75%	H	O	H	L	O	O	O	M	O	O	M	M
1	8	Morocco	1988	+	100%	—	—	—	L	L	L	L	L	L	L	L	O	L	L	L
1	8	Oman	1988	—	—	—	—	—	M	L	M	M	O	O	L	L	L	O	L	M
1	8	Syrian Arab Rep.	1986	+	—	—	—	—	M	M	O	O	O	O	O	O	O	H	O	O
1	8	Tunisia	1987	+	—	—	—	—	O	L	O	M	L	O	O	O	L	L	O	L
1	8	Bhutan	1988	—	—	—	—	—	L	O	O	O	L	O	L		L	L		M
1	9	China	1986	+	100%	50%	60%	50%	M	M	M	M	H	L	M	M	M	M	M	M
1	9	Hong Kong	1990	—	—	—	—	—	O		L	O	O	L				L		L
1	9	Japan	1987	+	100%	10%	100%	3%	L	O										
1	9	Taiwan	—		—	—	—	—												
1	9	Vietnam	1990	+	100%	100%	100%	100%	M	L	L	O	H	L	L	L	O	L	M	O
1	10	Brunei	1986		—	—	—	—	O		O	O	O	O	L	L	O	L	O	O
1	10	India	1985	+	90%	50%	50%	20%	H	O	O	H	M	L	O	M	O	L	M	H
1	10	Malaysia	1985	+	95%	60%	95%	70%	L	L	L	M	L	M	O	O	L	L	L	O
1	10	Nepal	1987	+	60%	5%	10%	10%	L	O	M	M	M	M	M	M	M	M	M	M
1	10	Singapore	1985	+	100%	15%	—	—	O	O	O	L	O	O	O	O	O	O	O	O
1	10	Sri Lanka	1986	+	70%	0%	70%	0%	H	O	M	M	L	M	H	M	M	M	H	M
1	10	Thailand	1987	+	—	—	—	—	L	M	L	M	L	L	M	L	M	M	L	L
2	3	American Samoa	1989	—	—	—	—	—	L	O	H	L	L	—	O		L	O	M	O
2	3	Cook Islands	1988	+	50%	50%	75%	60%	H	L	M	H	H	H	L	L	L	L	H	H
2	3	Guam	1985	+	100%	10%	—	10%	M	M	H	H	H	M	O	M	M	M	H	M
2	3	New Caledonia	1990	+	80%	10%	20%	20%	L	L	L	M	L	M	M	M	M	M	M	L
2	3	Niue	1992	—	—	—	—	—												O
2	3	Tokelau	1993	+	90%	50%	50%	90%	H	H	L	L	H	L	O	O	O	O	O	M
2	3	Tuvalu	1989	+	—	—	—	—	O	O	H	M	O	O	O	O	L	L	L	O
2	6	Bermuda	1985	—	—	—	—	—	L	O	O	H	H	L	L	O	O	L	O	L
2	6	Cayman Islands	1985	+	100%	—	—	100%	L	L	H	M	H	O	O	M	O	O	O	L
2	6	Montserrat	1989	+	25%	0%	—	0%	H	O	O	O	O	O	O	O	O	O	H	H
2	6	Netherlands Antilles	1985	+	—	—	—	—	L	O	O	L	O	O	O	O	O	O	O	L

Table D-5 Government national AIDS programs: development, implementation, and impact on other health programs, Program 393B through Program 6GSPEC*

List	GAA	Country	PR393B	PR393C	PR393D	PR393E	PR393F	PR393G	PR393H	PR393I	PR393J	PR393K	pr4/5a	pr4/5b	PR6A	PR6B	PR6C	PR6D	PR6E	PR6F	PR6G	PR6GSPEC
1	1	United States	—	L	O	O	L	L	O	M	O	L	all	few	—	—	+	+	—	—	—	—
1	2	Austria	L	L	L	O	L	L	L	L	M	L	few	few	—	—	+	+	—	—	—	—
1	2	Belgium	O	L	M	O	O	L	L	L	O	O	half+	none	—	—	+	+	—	—	—	—
1	2	Cyprus	O	L	L	O	O	O	O	O	L	O	none	—	—	—	—	—	—	—	—	—
1	2	Denmark	O	O	O	O	O	O	O	O	O	O	—	all	+	—	+	+	—	—	—	—
1	2	Finland	O	O	O	O	O	L	O	O	O	O	few	—	+	—	+	+	—	—	—	—
1	2	France	—	—	—	—	—	—	—	—	—	—	—	—	+	+	+	+	+	—	—	—
1	2	Germany	O	L	L	O	O	L	L	L	O	L	all	half+	+	+	+	+	+	—	—	—
1	2	Iceland	O	O	O	O	O	L	O	O	L	O	few	—	+	+	+	+	+	—	—	—
1	2	Liechtenstein	O	L	O	M	O	L	O	M	L	O	—	—	—	+	+	—	—	—	—	—
1	2	Luxembourg	O	M	M	O	M	M	L	L	L	O	—	—	+	+	—	+	—	+	+	+ drug treatment program
1	2	Malta	O	O	M	L	M	L	M	M	M	L	—	—	—	+	+	+	+	—	+	+ health promotion +/drugs
1	2	Netherlands	L	O	L	O	L	L	L	O	O	O	few	—	+	—	+	+	—	+	+	+ national policy on chronic diseases
1	2	Norway	—	O	O	O	O	O	O	O	O	O	—	half+	—	—	—	+	—	—	—	—
1	2	Spain	L	L	L	L	L	L	L	L	O	O	—	all	—	+	—	+	—	+	—	—
1	2	Sweden	O	O	O	O	O	L	L	L	L	O	all	none	—	—	—	+	—	+	—	—
1	2	Switzerland	—	L	L	L	O	O	O	O	O	—	few	—	—	—	—	—	—	+	—	—
1	2	United Kingdom	O	O	O	O	O	O	O	L	M	O	all	all	+	+	+	+	+	+	+	—
1	3	Australia	—	L	L	L	L	L	L	L	L	O	all	half+	—	—	+	+	+	+	—	—
1	3	Fiji	M	L	M	M	M	M	L	O	O	M	none	none	—	+	—	+	—	—	—	—
1	3	Kiribati	M	L	O	M	M	L	O	L	L	O	—	—	+	+	+	+	—	+	—	—
1	3	Micronesia, Fed. Sts.	L	M	M	M	M	O	O	L	O	M	all	—	+	+	+	+	—	+	—	—
1	3	New Zealand	O	O	O	O	L	O	O	L	L	L	none	none	—	—	—	+	—	+	—	—
1	3	Papua New Guinea	L	L	L	L	L	O	O	O	O	L	few	—	—	—	—	—	—	—	—	—
1	3	Solomon Islands	L	L	M	M	M	L	L	L	O	—	none	none	—	+	+	+	+	+	—	—
1	3	Vanuatu	L	M	H	O	O	L	L	L	—	L	none	none	+	+	+	+	—	—	—	—
1	3	Western Samoa	M	M	M	L	M	M	L	M	M	L	none	none	—	—	—	+	—	—	—	—
1	4	Argentina	L	H	M	L	M	M	L	M	M	L	all	half+	+	—	+	+	—	+	—	—
1	4	Belize	L	L	M	M	L	L	L	L	M	H	—	few	+	—	+	+	—	+	—	—
1	4	Brazil	L	L	H	L	L	H	L	M	H	H	half+	few	—	—	+	+	—	—	—	—

(continued)

Table D-5 Government national AIDS programs: development, implementation, and impact on other health programs, Program 393B through Program 6GSPEC*—continued

List	GAA	Country	PR393B	PR393C	PR393D	PR393E	PR393F	PR393G	PR393H	PR393I	PR393J	PR393K	pr4/5a	pr4/5b	PR6A	PR6B	PR6C	PR6D	PR6E	PR6F	PR6G	PR6GSPEC
1	4	Chile	M	—	L	O	O	L	L	L	L	H		all	—	—	+	—	—	+	—	dental
1	4	Colombia	M	L	L	M	M	L	L	L	L	H	half+	few	—	—	+	+	—	+	+	sex education programs
1	4	Costa Rica	O	O	H	O	O	L	O	L	L	O	—	all	+	+	+	+	+	+	—	
1	4	Ecuador	L	L	H	H	O	L	O	O	O	M	all	half+	+	—	+	+	+	—	—	
1	4	El Salvador	M	M	L	M	O	L	O	M	M	M	—	all	+	—	+	+	—	‖	L	
1	4	Guatemala	M	L	L	L	L	O	O	L	L	H	all	half+	—	+	+	+	—	+	—	
1	4	Mexico	H	M	M	L	L	L	L	M	M	M	half+	half+	—	+	+	+	—	—	—	
1	4	Panama	L	M	L	L	O	L	L	L	M	O	—	all	+	+	+	+	—	—	—	
1	4	Peru	M	M	M	M	L	M	M	M	H	M	all	half+	+	+	+	+	—	+	+	oral health
1	4	Suriname	O	O	L	O	O	L	O	O	O	O	all	—	—	—	+	+	+	—	—	
1	4	Uruguay	L	L	L	O	O	O	O	O	O	O	all	all	+	+	+	+	—	—	—	
1	4	Venezuela	H	M	M	L	L	M	M	L	M	H	half+	few	+	—	+	+	—	+	—	
1	5	Angola	L	L	M	M	M	M	H	O	M	H	few	none	+	+	+	+	—	—	+	health education
1	5	Benin	L	O	L	L	L	L	L	L	O	H	all	all	—	—	—	+	—	—	—	
1	5	Botswana	O	M	M	L	O	L	O	O	O	L	—	all	+	+	—	+	—	—	—	
1	5	Burkino Faso	M	O	M	—	L	L	L	L	L	M	—	—	+	+	—	+	—	—	—	
1	5	Cameroon	O	O	O	O	O	O	O	O	O	O	all	few	—	—	—	+	—	—	—	
1	5	Cape Verde	L	O	M	L	L	O	O	O	O	O	—	half+	+	+	+	+	—	+	—	
1	5	Chad	M	O	O	O	L	O	O	O	L	H	all	half+	—	—	—	—	—	—	—	
1	5	Comoros	H	L	H	L	O	M	O	O	M	M	all	few	+	+	+	+	—	—	—	
1	5	Congo	M	—	—	—	—	—	—	—	—	—	few	few	+	+	—	+	—	—	—	
1	5	Cote d'Ivoire	L	L	L	L	L	L	L	L	O	M	half+	half+	+	+	—	+	—	+	+	
1	5	Djibouti	M	O	O	O	O	L	L	L	L	O	all	all	—	—	—	+	—	—	—	
1	5	Ethiopia	O	O	L	O	L	L	H	L	M	M	half+	—	—	—	—	+	—	+	—	
1	5	Gabon	M	M	O	O	O	M	M	M	L	M	all	all	+	+	+	+	—	+	—	
1	5	Ghana	O	L	L	L	M	M	H	O	L	L	all	half+	—	+	‖	+	—	—	—	
1	5	Guinea	M	O	L	M	O	O	M	O	O	M	all	half+	—	+	+	+	—	+	—	
1	5	Guinee-Bissau	M	O	O	O	O	O	O	M	H	M	all	all	+	+	+	—	—	+	—	
1	5	Lesotho	H	L	M	L	L	O	O	L	L	M	—	few	+	+	+	+	+	+	+	safe motherhood/Bamako initiative
1	5	Madagascar	M	L	M	M	L	M	M	M	H	O	all	half+	+	+	+	+	+	‖	—	
1	5	Mali	O	O	L	O	O	O	O	O	O	L	—	all	+	+	+	+	+	+	—	

Table D-5 Government national AIDS programs: development, implementation, and impact on other health programs, Program 339b through Program 7 *(continued)*

List	GAA	Country	PR393B	PR393C	PR393D	PR393E	PR393F	PR393G	PR393H	PR393I	PR393J	PR393K	pr4/5a	pr4/5b	PR6A	PR6B	PR6C	PR6D	PR6E	PR6F	PR6G	PR6GSPEC
1	5	Mauritania	L	O	M	L	L	L	L	L	M	O	few	few	+	+	+	+	−	−	−	
1	5	Mauritius	L	O	M	L	O	L	L	L	O	O	−	all	−	−	−	−	−	−	−	
1	5	Rwanda	M	O	H	M	L	M	M	L	M	H	half +	−	+	−	+	+	+	−	−	
1	5	Senegal	L	L	H	L	O	L	L	L	L	M	all	all	+	+	+	+	+	−	−	
1	5	Seychelles	L	O	L	O	O	O	O	O	O	O	−	−	+	+	+	+	+	−	−	
1	5	South Africa	L	L	L	O	L	L	L	L	L	L	all	half +	+	+	+	+	+	+	+	
1	5	Tanzania	H	L	M	L	L	L	L	L	L	M	all	all	−	+	+	+	+	−	−	
1	5	Togo	L	M	M	O	O	O	O	O	L	M	all	−	+	+	+	+	−	−	−	
1	5	Uganda	L	O	O	O	L	L	L	L	L	H	all	all	+	+	+	+	−	−	+	
1	5	Zaire	M	M	O	L	L	−	O	O	M	H	all	all	+	+	+	+	+	+	+	poor hygiene/sterilization of medical equipment
1	5	Zambia	O	O	M	O	O	O	O	O	O	O	all	all	+	+	+	+	−	−	−	
1	5	Zimbabwe	L	L	L	L	L	L	L	L	L	M	all	half +	−	−	−	+	−	−	−	
1	6	Antigua and Barbuda	L	L	L	L	M	M	O	H	O	L	−	−	+	+	+	−	−	−	−	
1	6	Barbados	M	M	L	M	M	M	M	M	M	M	−	−	−	−	+	+	−	−	−	
1	6	Dominican Republic	H	L	H	L	H	H	H	H	M	H	−	few	+	+	+	+	+	−	−	
1	6	Grenada	M	M	L	L	M	M	L	M	O	M	all	all	+	+	+	+	+	+	+	chronic diseases
1	6	Jamaica	O	M	M	M	L	L	L	M	O	L	all	all	+	+	+	+	−	+	+	
1	6	St. Lucia	L	L	M	L	L	M	M	L	O	H	few	−	−	−	+	+	−	−	−	
1	6	Trinidad and Tobago	L	M	L	L	L	M	M	O	O	M	−	all	+	+	+	+	+	−	−	
1	7	Azerbaijan	H	M	O	H	O	M	M	L	L	H	all	all	+	+	+	+	+	+	+	prev HIV trans through medical instruments
1	7	Belarus	M	L	O	L	L	H	O	O	O	H	none	none	−	−	−	+	−	−	−	
1	7	Bulgaria	M	L	L	O	O	O	H	L	L	H	−	half +	+	+	+	+	−	+	−	
1	7	Croatia	H	O	L	M	H	L	M	O	O	L	few	few	−	−	−	−	−	+	−	
1	7	Czech Republic	M	M	M	M	M	M	M	M	M	M	few	few	+	+	−	+	+	+	−	
1	7	Estonia	M	M	O	L	L	O	O	L	L	M	none	none	−	−	+	+	−	−	−	
1	7	Hungary	M	L	L	L	M	L	L	M	M	O	none	none	−	−	−	+	−	−	−	
1	7	Kyrgyz Republic	M	M	H	M	H	M	M	M	L	M	all	all	−	+	−	+	+	+	+	health worker training: use of medical instrument
1	7	Latvia	L	L	L	M	−	M	L	L	L	M	none	none	−	+	−	−	−	−	−	
1	7	Lithuania	M	M	M	M	L	M	M	H	L	H	none	none	−	−	−	+	−	+	+	laboratory diagnosis
1	7	Moldova	−	−	−	H	−	−	−	−	−	−	−	−	−	−	−	−	−	+	+	
1	7	Russian Federation	O	O	O	O	O	L	O	O	O	O	all	all	−	−	−	−	−	−	−	

(continued)

Table D-5 · Government national AIDS programs: development, implementation, and impact on other health programs, Program 393B through Program 6GSPEC*—continued

List	GAA	Country	PR393B	PR393C	PR393D	PR393E	PR393F	PR393G	PR393H	PR393I	PR393J	PR393K	pr4/5a	pr4/5b	PR6A	PR6B	PR6C	PR6D	PR6E	PR6F	PR6G	PR6GSPEC
1	7	Slovenia	L	M	L	O	H	H	M	O	O	O	none	none	-	-	-	-	-	-	-	
1	7	Turkmenistan	H	M	L	H	H	H	M	O	O	O	all	all	-	-	-	+	-	-	-	
1	7	Ukraine	M	L	M	H	L	M	L	M	L	H	half+	-			+	+	+	+		
1	7	Yugoslavia, Fed. Rep.	H	M	L	H	M	M	M	L	O	L	few	few	-		-	-		-		
1	8	Algeria	M	M	M	M	M	M	M	M	M	M	half+	half+	-	-	-	+	-	-	-	
1	8	Israel	L	O	O	O	O	O	L	O	O	O	none	none	-	-	-	-	-	-	-	
1	8	Jordan	L	L	L	L	L	L	L	L	L	L	none	none			-	-			-	
1	8	Kuwait	O	O	L	O	L	L	O	O	O	O	all	-	+	-	+	+	+	-	+	kidney dialysis/heart surgery
1	8	Lebanon	L	O	L	L	O	O	O	O	O	M	none	few	-	-	-	-	-	-	-	
1	8	Morocco	L	L	L	L	O	L	O	O	L	L	all	all	+	+	+	+	+	-	-	
1	8	Oman	L	M	L	O	O	O		L	H	O	half+	none	-	-	+	+	+	-	-	
1	8	Syrian Arab Rep.	M	O	O	O	O	O	O	O	L	O	few	few	-	-	+	+	-	+	-	
1	8	Tunisia	L	O	L	O	O	O	L	O	L	O	-	half+	-	+	-	+	-	-	-	
1	9	Bhutan	L	O	L	L	O	O	L	O	O	L	none	half+	-	+	+	+	-	+	-	
1	9	China	M	L	O	M	O	M		M			half+	few	-	-	+	+	-	+	-	
1	9	Hong Kong		M	L	O	L	L	L	M	L	L	-	-	+	+	+	+	-	-	+	
1	9	Japan	O	L	L	O	L	M	M	M	L	M	all	half+	+	+	+	+	-	-	+	sex educaction
1	9	Taiwan											-	-	-							
1	9	Vietnam	M	O	L	M	O	O	M	O	O	M	all	few	+	+	-	+	+	-	-	
1	10	Brunei		O	O	O	O	L	L	O	O	O	-	-	-	-	-	+	-	-	-	
1	10	India	O	O	L	L	L	L	M	M	O	M	all	-	+	+	-	+	+	+	-	
1	10	Malaysia	O	O	L	L	O	O	O	M	M	L	few	few	+	+	+	+	+	+	-	
1	10	Nepal	M	L	M	M	O	L	M	M	M	L	-	few	-	+	+	+	-	-	-	
1	10	Singapore	O	O	O	O	O	O	O	O	O	O	all	-	+	-	-	+	-	-	-	
1	10	Sri Lanka	M	L	M	L	L	L	L	L	O	L	half+	half+	-	-	+	+	+	+	-	
1	10	Thailand	L	O		O	O	L	L	L	L	H	all	all	-	-	-	+	-	+	-	
2	3	American Samoa	O	L	L	L	L	O	L	L	L	L	all	half+	+	+	-	+	+	+	-	
2	3	Cook Islands	L	L	L	L	O	O	O	O	O	H	all	all	+	+	+	+	-	-	-	
2	3	Guam	H	H	H	H	O	M	M	H	H	H	-	-	-	-	-	+	-	-	-	
2	3	New Caledonia	L	L	M	L	L	M	L	L	L	L	half+	all	-	-	-	+	-	-	-	
2	3	Niue	O	O	O	O	O	O	O	O	O		all	all	-	-	-	-	-	-	-	

Table D-5 Government national AIDS programs: development, implementation and impact on other health programs, Program 393B through Program 6GSPEC*—continued

List	GAA	Country	PR393B	PR393C	PR393D	PR393E	PR393F	PR393G	PR393H	PR393i	PR393J	PR393K	pr4/5a	pr4/5b	PR6A	PR6B	PR6C	PR6D	PR6E	PR6F	PR6G	PR6GSPEC
2	3	Tokelau	H	L	L	H	L	O	O	L	M	O	all	all	–	–	–	–	–	–	–	–
2	3	Tuvalu	O	H	M	O	O	O	O	O	O	O	all	–	–	–	–	–	–	–	–	–
2	6	Bermuda	–	O	L	O	L	O	O	O	O	L	all	all	+	+	+	+	–	–	–	–
2	6	Cayman Islands	L	O	M	O	O	O	O	L	O	O	–	–	+	+	+	+	–	–	–	–
2	6	Montserrat	M	O	L	L	L	O	O	O	O	H	–	–	+	+	–	+	–	–	–	–
2	6	Netherlands Antilles	L	L	L	O	O	O	O	O	O	O	–	–	–	+	–	+	–	–	–	–

*List, core country response (1) or subsidiary response (2); GAA, geographic area of affinity; country, territory, or region responding.

Program abbreviations: PR1, year governmental national AIDS programs (GNAP) were officially established; PR2, GNAP conducted targeted training on how to manage HIV/AIDS programs. Proportion of the following groups having received such training: PR2A, GNAP managers; PR2B, managers of other governmental programs/departments; PR2C, region/province district managers; PR2D, nongovernmental organization managers.

Problems faced by the GNAP in implementing programs and providing services in 1990 (opinion requested: O = not a problem, L = minor problem, M = major problem, H = very severe problem): PR390A, governmental financial support; PR390B, international financial support; PR390C, political support; PR390D, personnel issues (i.e., burnout, staff turnover, recruitment); PR390E, supplies (i.e., HIV testing kits, condoms, educational materials); PR390F, internal coordination within the GNAP; PR390G, coordination with other governmental programs/departments; PR390H, coordination with NGOs; PR390I, public/social support and/or opinion; PR390J, media coverage; PR390K, capacity of government to provide care for the number of persons with HIV and AIDS.

Problems faced by the GNAP in implementing programs and providing services in 1993 (opinion requested: A–K, same program abbreviations as for 1990).

Programs on HIV/AIDS have been developed by: pr4/5a, individual states, regions, or provinces; pr4/5b, individual districts, counties, prefectures within the states, regions, or provinces.

Mobilization against AIDS has impacted on other health initiatives such as with the following health programs: PR6A, maternal and child health; PR6B, family planning; PR6C, tuberculosis; PR6D, STIs; PR6E, cancer; PR6F, other communicable diseases; PR6G, other; PR6GSPEC, other specified.

Table D-6 Government national AIDS programs: financial information*

List	GAA	Country	FI1start	FI1end	National $	Internat'l $	FI4E	FI5E	FI6A	FI6B	FI6C	FI6D
1	1	United States	1-Jul-92	1-Jun-93	$5,299,000,000	.	17%	—	—	9.0%	—	51.0%
1	2	Austria	—	—		.	—	—	—	—	—	—
1	2	Belgium	1-Jan-93	1-Dec-93	$6,085,710	.	100%	—	9.4%	39.0%	—	0.0%
1	2	Cyprus	1-Jan-93	1-Nov-93	$57,000	$29,100	—	—	—	—	—	—
1	2	Denmark	1-Jan-92	1-Dec-92	$1,920,000	.	0%	—	—	—	—	—
1	2	Finland	1-Jan-93	1-Dec-93	$600,000	.	—	—	10.0%	60.0%	—	—
1	2	France	1-Jan-92	1-Dec-92	$800,000	.	18%	—	0.8%	4.0%	—	90.0%
1	2	Germany	1-Jan-92	1-Dec-92	$30,478,000	.	−46%	—	10.0%	60.0%	0.0%	0.0%
1	2	Iceland	1-Jan-93	1-Dec-93	$100,000	.	0%	—	20.0%	50.0%	3.0%	0.0%
1	2	Liechtenstein	1-Jan-93	1-Dec-93	$116,060	.	5%	—	45.0%	30.0%	10.0%	5.0%
1	2	Luxembourg	—	—	.	.	—	—	—	—	—	—
1	2	Malta	1-Jan-93	1-Dec-93	$37,500	$5,000	25%	—	15.0%	75.0%	—	—
1	2	The Netherlands	1-Jan-93	1-Dec-93	$15,789,470	.	−6%	—	15.0%	30.0%	—	20.0%
1	2	Norway	1-Jan-92	1-Dec-92	$5,000,000	.	0%	—	—	—	—	—
1	2	Spain	1-Jan-93	1-Dec-93	$14,571,430	.	—	—	69.5%	24.5%	—	—
1	2	Sweden	1-Jul-92	1-Jun-93	$24,000,000	$0	—	—	—	—	—	—
1	2	Switzerland	1-Jan-92	1-Dec-92	$9,379,310	.	8%	—	27.0%	56.0%	0.0%	0.0%
1	2	United Kingdom	—	—	.	.	—	—	—	24.8%	—	59.8%
1	3	Australia	1-Jul-92	1-Jun-93	$62,658,010	.	7%	—	6.0%	14.0%	5.0%	9.0%
1	3	Fiji	1-Jan-93	1-Dec-93	$0	$54,330	0%	18%	13.0%	57.0%	24.0%	0.0%
1	3	Kiribati	1-Jan-93	1-Dec-93		$11,920	—	—	15.0%	25.0%	25.0%	0.0%
1	3	Micronesia, Fed. Sts.	1-Jan-93	1-Dec-93	$0	$58,000	—	−18%	15.0%	50.0%	20.0%	0.0%
1	3	New Zealand	1-Jul-93	1-Jun-94	$2,491,620	$0	0%	—	—	—	—	—
1	3	Papua New Guinea	1-Jan-93	1-Dec-93	.	.	—	—	—	—	—	—
1	3	Solomon Islands	1-Jan-93	1-Dec-93	—	—	—	—	—	—	—	—
1	3	Vanuatu	1-Jan-93	1-Dec-93	$7,700	$63,610	4%	−5%	15.0%	80.0%	5.0%	0.0%
1	3	Western Samoa	1-Jan-92	1-Dec-92	$250,000	$125,000	0%	−5%	25.0%	35.0%	30.0%	0.0%
1	4	Argentina	1-Sep-93	1-Sep-94	$10,000,000	$75,000	100%	−50%	28.0%	10.0%	30.0%	30.0%
1	4	Belize	—	—	.	.	—	—	—	—	—	—
1	4	Brazil	1-Jan-93	1-Dec-93	$637,010	$3,070	316%	—	24.7%	41.2%	34.1%	0.0%
1	4	Chile	1-Jan-93	1-Dec-93	$2,400,000	$751,020	104%	122%	2.0%	58.4%	4.5%	33.0%
1	4	Colombia	1-Jan-93	1-Jan-94	$3,125,000	$180,000	60%	—	10.0%	40.0%	10.0%	10.0%
1	4	Costa Rica	1-Jan-92	1-Dec-92	$187,780	$271,810	4%	0%	10.0%	65.0%	15.0%	10.0%
1	4	Ecuador	1-Jan-93	1-Dec-93	$65,800	.	95%	—	10.0%	55.0%	20.0%	5.0%
1	4	El Salvador	1-Jan-93	1-Dec-93	$366,470	$90,000	22%	—	10.0%	60.0%	15.0%	5.0%
1	4	Guatemala	1-Jan-93	1-Dec-93	$358,000	$350,000	15%	15%	15.0%	35.0%	15.0%	15.0%
1	4	Mexico	1-Jan-92	1-Dec-92	$2,538,000	$383,980	19%	−34%	44.7%	19.5%	10.7%	0.9%
1	4	Panama	1-Jan-93	1-Dec-93	$20,000	$149,000	—	−33%	25.0%	50.0%	15.0%	0.0%
1	4	Peru	1-Jan-93	1-Dec-93	$206,420	$150,000	600%	25%	20.0%	40.0%	20.0%	10.0%
1	4	Suriname	1-Jan-93	1-Dec-93	$8,430	$89,000	10%	15%	15.0%	45.0%	15.0%	5.0%
1	4	Uruguay	1-Mar-93	1-Dec-93	$1,300,000	$137,000	0%	—	15.0%	40.0%	22.0%	20.0%
1	4	Venezuela	1-Jan-92	1-Dec-92	$800,000	.	—	—	10.0%	20.0%	60.0%	0.0%
1	5	Angola	1-Jan-93	1-Dec-93	$46,020	$531,700	100%	71%	19.0%	29.0%	—	55.1%
1	5	Benin	1-Jan-93	1-Dec-93	$27,070	$620,000	—	32%	40.0%	30.0%	—	15.0%
1	5	Botswana	1-Jan-93	1-Dec-93	$906,680	$915,530	247%	—	13.6%	77.8%	0.0%	3.5%

FI6E	FI6F	FI6G	FI6GEXP	FI7A	FI7B	FI7C	FI7D	FI7E	FI7F	FI7FEXP	FI8	FI9	FI10
—	24.0%	16.0%	income support	+	+	+	+	+	—		Q4	Q3	Q3
—	—	—		—	—	—	—	—	—		—	—	—
39.9%	11.7%	0.0%		+	—	—	+	—	—		Q4	Q1	—
—	—	—		—	—	—	—	+	—		Q4	Q4	—
—	—	—		—	—	—	—	—	—		—	—	—
10.0%	20.0%	—		—	—	+	+	+	—		Q4	—	Q1
0.2%	5.0%	0.0%		+	+	—	+	+	+	health insurance organizations	Q1	Q4	Q1
10.0%	20.0%	0.0%		+	+	+	+	+	—		Q3	Q1	Q2
15.0%	12.0%	0.0%		—	—	+	—	—	—		Q2	Q1	Q2
10.0%	0.0%	0.0%		—	—	—	—	+	—		Q4	Q1	Q1
—	—	—		—	—	—	—	—	—		—	—	—
10.0%	0.0%	0.0%		—	—	+	—	—	—		Q4	Q4	Q4
5.0%	30.0%	—		+	—	—	+	+	—		Q4	Q1	Q4
—	—	—		—	—	—	—	—	—		—	—	—
6.0%	—	—		+	+	+	+	+	+	religious institutions	Q3	—	—
—	—	—		+	+	+	+	+	—		Q3	Q1	Q1
0.0%	4.0%	13.0%	education	+	+	+	+	+	—		Q3	Q1	Q1
0.7%	9.7%	5.0%	HIV/AIDS related drug misuse activities	+	+	+	+	+	+		Q4	Q4	Q4
6.0%	12.0%	48.0%	hospital based treatment	+	+	+	+	+	—		Q1	Q2	Q1
6.0%	0.0%	0.0%		—	—	—	—	—	—		Q4	Q1	Q1
20.0%	5.0%	0.0%		—	—	—	—	—	—		Q3	Q1	Q1
15.0%	0.0%	0.0%		—	—	—	+	—	—		Q3	Q1	Q1
—	—	—		+	+	+	—	+	—		Q4	Q4	Q4
—	—	—		—	—	+	+	—	—		Q1	Q1	Q1
—	—	—		—	—	—	—	—	—		—	—	—
0.0%	0.0%	0.0%		+	—	+	—	+	—		Q4	Q1	Q1
5.0%	5.0%	—		—	+	+	—	—	—		Q3	Q1	Q1
10.0%	2.0%	0.0%		—	—	—	—	—	—		—	—	—
—	—	—		—	—	—	—	—	—		—	—	—
0.0%	0.0%	0.0%		—	—	+	+	+	—		Q2	Q2	Q1
—	2.0%	0.0%		+	—	—	+	—	—		Q3	Q2	Q1
20.0%	10.0%	—		—	—	+	+	—	—		Q3	Q1	Q1
5.0%	5.0%	0.0%		—	—	—	—	—	—		Q3	Q1	Q1
2.0%	8.0%	0.0%		—	—	—	—	—	—		Q3	Q1	Q10
5.0%	5.0%	0.0%		—	—	+	—	+	—		Q3	Q1	Q1
15.0%	5.0%	0.0%		—	—	—	—	—	—		Q2	Q1	Q1
2.0%	22.2%	—		+	—	+	+	+	—		Q4	Q2	Q1
2.0%	8.0%	0.0%		—	—	—	—	—	—		Q2	—	Q1
5.0%	5.0%	0.0%		+	+	+	+	—	+	state hospitals through own funds	Q3	Q1	Q1
10.0%	2.5%	7.5%	special projects	—	+	+	—	+	—		Q4	Q4	Q4
3.0%	0.0%	0.0%		+	—	+	—	—	—		Q2	Q1	Q1
10.0%	0.0%	0.0%		—	—	—	+	—	—		Q3	Q1	—
0.0%	3.0%	0.0%		—	—	+	—	—	+	private enterprise link to oil sector	Q1	Q3	Q1
10.0%	5.0%	0.0%		—	—	—	—	—	—		Q4	Q4	Q4
0.0%	5.2%	0.0%		+	—	+	+	—	—		Q3	Q1	Q3

(continued)

527

Table D-6 Government national AIDS programs: financial information*—continued

List	GAA	Country	FI1start	FI1end	National $	Internat'l $	FI4E	FI5E	FI6A	FI6B	FI6C	FI6D
1	5	Burkino Faso	1-Jan-92	1-Dec-93	$87,050	$1,296,730	—	—	39.2%	35.9%	—	—
1	5	Cameroon	1-Jan-92	1-Dec-92	$21,430	$3,611,000	0%	—	20.0%	55.0%	—	5.0%
1	5	Cape Verde	1-Jan-93	1-Dec-93	.	.	—	—	—	—	—	—
1	5	Chad	1-Jan-93	1-Dec-93	$20,210	$656,000	0%	0%	35.0%	55.0%	10.0%	0.0%
1	5	Comoros	1-Jan-93	1-Dec-93	$16,000	$138,000	100%	−31%	20.0%	45.0%	—	15.0%
1	5	Congo	—	—	$0	.	—	—	—	—	—	—
1	5	Côte d'Ivoire	1-Jan-93	1-Dec-93	$200,000	$2,525,630	0%	0%	20.0%	60.0%	—	6.0%
1	5	Djibouti	1-Jan-92	1-Dec-93	.	.	—	—	—	—	—	—
1	5	Ethiopia	—	—	.	.	—	—	12.0%	33.0%	20.0%	15.0%
1	5	Gabon	1-Mar-93	1-Feb-94	$3,370,580	$188,640	−3%	—	26.8%	0.2%	—	16.3%
1	5	Ghana	1-Jan-90	1-Dec-91	$0	$1,406,710	—	73%	15.0%	55.0%	25.0%	0.0%
1	5	Guinea	1-Jan-93	1-Dec-93	$45,000	$195,000	10%	−40%	30.0%	30.0%	8.0%	2.0%
1	5	Guinee-Bissau	1-Oct-92	1-Sep-93	$60,000	.	0%	—	—	—	—	—
1	5	Lesotho	1-Jun-92	1-Sep-93	$82,000	$398,800	60%	—	28.0%	40.0%	12.0%	0.0%
1	5	Madagascar	1-Jan-92	1-Dec-92	$8,570	$532,800	0%	50%	17.0%	23.0%	—	55.0%
1	5	Mali	1-Jan-93	1-Dec-93	$1,409,000	$1,000,000	30%	100%	10.0%	60.0%	—	20.0%
1	5	Mauritania	1-Jan-92	1-Dec-92	$20,000	$336,840	100%	200%	60.0%	5.0%	—	35.0%
1	5	Mauritius	1-Jan-93	1-Dec-93	$123,480	$132,300	—	—	70.0%	20.0%	—	8.8%
1	5	Rwanda	1-Jan-93	1-Dec-93	$44,340	.	—	—	—	—	—	—
1	5	Senegal	—	—	$213,330	$1,380,000	50%	25%	23.0%	48.0%	—	10.0%
1	5	Seychelles	1-Jan-93	1-Dec-93	$79,870	$4,920	48%	−65%	25.0%	50.0%	25.0%	—
1	5	South Africa	—	—	.	.	—	—	—	—	—	—
1	5	Tanzania	1-Jul-92	1-Jun-93	$16,200	$2,039,630	0%	39%	42.0%	30.0%	18.0%	3.0%
1	5	Togo	1-Jan-92	1-Dec-92	$250,370	$626,510	0%	70%	20.0%	30.0%	—	20.0%
1	5	Uganda	1-Jul-91	1-Jun-92	$186,580	$707,350	561%	300%	20.0%	45.0%	10.0%	14.0%
1	5	Zaire	1-Jan-92	1-Dec-92	$394,130	$212,550	—	—	42.0%	15.0%	—	16.0%
1	5	Zambia	1-Jan-93	1-Dec-93	$350,000	$2,000,000	—	—	20.0%	35.0%	15.0%	15.0%
1	5	Zimbabwe	1-Jan-93	1-Dec-93			—	—	—	—	—	—
1	6	Antigua and Barbuda	1-Jan-92	1-Dec-92	$63,450	$31,000	—	—	25.0%	40.0%	20.0%	4.0%
1	6	Barbados	1-Jan-92	1-Dec-92	$128,000	$78,100	−45%	−21%	15.0%	40.0%	30.0%	13.0%
1	6	Dominican Republic	—	—	.	.	—	—	—	—	—	—
1	6	Grenada	1-Jan-92	1-Dec-92	$0	$26,310	—	60%	30.0%	20.0%	15.0%	15.0%
1	6	Jamaica	1-Jul-92	1-Jun-93	$359,970	$120,540	600%	—	60.0%	20.0%	4.0%	0.0%
1	6	St. Lucia	1-Jan-92	1-Dec-92	$92,590	$170,740	100%	20%	10.0%	45.0%	15.0%	10.0%
1	6	Trinidad and Tobago	1-Jan-92	1-Dec-92	$40,050	$207,560	—	8%	34.0%	49.0%	0.0%	0.0%
1	7	Azerbaijan	1-Jan-92	1-Dec-92	$14,030	.	−205%	—	0.0%	0.0%	100.0%	0.0%
1	7	Belarus	—	—	.	.	—	—	5.0%	22.0%	50.0%	10.0%
1	7	Bulgaria	1-Jan-92	1-Dec-92	$351,230	$51,900	—	—	0.0%	13.0%	87.0%	0.0%
1	7	Croatia	—	.	.	—	—	—	—	—	—
1	7	Czech Republic	1-Jan-93	1-Dec-93	$2,166,670	$17,500	0%	—	5.0%	10.0%	40.0%	40.0%
1	7	Estonia	1-Jan-93	1-Dec-93	$139,560	$30,000	127%	—	52.7%	7.4%	8.6%	21.5%
1	7	Hungary	1-Jan-93	1-Dec-93	$1,430,000	$18,500	37%	—	0.0%	34.0%	48.0%	14.0%
1	7	Kyrgyz Republic	1-Jan-92	1-Dec-92	$0	$0	—	—	—	—	—	—
1	7	Latvia	1-Jan-93	1-Dec-93	$285,950	$19,000	39%	—	4.0%	10.0%	80.0%	5.0%
1	7	Lithuania	1-Jan-92	1-Jan-93	$59,950	$0	457%	0%	4.0%	36.0%	17.0%	9.0%

528

FI6E	FI6F	FI6G	FI6GEXP	FI7A	FI7B	FI7C	FI7D	FI7E	FI7F	FI7FEXP	FI8	FI9	FI10
0.2%	3.7%	19.0%	training	+	+	−	−	−	+	state societies	Q4	Q1	Q4
10.0%	10.0%	0.0%		+	+	—	—	+	—		Q2	Q1	Q1
—	—	—		—	—	—	—	—	—		Q3	Q1	—
0.0%	0.0%	0.0%		−	−	−	−	−	−		Q2	Q1	Q1
0.0%	0.0%	20.0%	laboratory support	−	−	+	−	−	−		Q2	Q1	Q1
—	—	—		—	+	+	−	−	−		Q4	Q3	Q4
10.0%	4.0%	0.0%		+	+	+	+	+	—		Q3	Q2	Q2
—	—	—		−	−	+	−	−	−		—	—	—
15.0%	5.0%	—		−	−	+	−	−	−		Q3	Q1	Q1
0.0%	0.0%	56.7%		+	+	−	−	−	−		Q4	Q1	Q1
3.0%	2.0%	—		—	—	+	—	—	—		Q3	—	—
30.0%	0.0%	—		−	−	+	−	−	−		Q3	Q1	Q1
—	—	—		+	+	+	+	—	—		—	—	—
20.0%	0.0%	0.0%		+	+	+	+	+	+	missionaries	Q1	Q1	Q1
0.0%	5.0%	0.0%		−	−	−	−	−	−		Q4	—	Q4
8.0%	2.0%	0.0%		−	−	+	+	+	—		Q3	Q3	Q2
0.0%	0.0%	0.0%		−	−	−	−	−	−		Q4	Q4	Q4
1.0%	0.2%	0.0%		—	+	—	—	—	—		Q1	Q1	Q1
—	—	—		−	−	+	—	−	−		Q2	Q1	Q1
15.0%	4.0%	0.0%		−	−	+	+	−	−		Q4	Q4	Q4
—	—	—		+	+	—	−	−	−		Q4	Q4	Q4
—	—	—									—	—	—
5.0%	2.0%	0.0%		−	−	+	+	−	−		Q2	Q1	Q1
20.0%	0.0%	10.0%	epidemic surveillance	−	−	−	−	−	−		Q4	Q4	Q4
2.0%	5.0%	4.0%	patient care counselling	−	−	−	−	−	−		—	—	—
25.6%	1.4%	0.0%		+	+	+	+	+	−		Q1	Q1	Q1
0.0%	0.0%	15.0%	clinical support	−	+	+	−	−	—		Q4	Q2	Q1
—	—	—		+	+	+	+	+	—		Q2	Q3	Q1
1.0%	5.0%	5.0%	infection cont/train health prov	−	−	−	−	−	−		Q2	Q1	Q1
2.0%	0.0%	0.0%		+	+	+	—	—	—		Q3	Q1	Q1
—	—	—		—	—	—	—	—	—		—	—	—
15.0%	2.0%	3.0%	special activities -eg World AIDS Day	+	—	—	—	+	—		Q1	Q3	Q1
10.0%	6.0%	0.0%		+	+	+	−	−	—		Q4	Q1	Q4
15.0%	5.0%	—		+	−	−	−	−	+	bilateral assistance from donor gov'ts	Q2	Q1	Q1
0.0%	—	17.0%	reduction of socio-econ impact	−	−	−	−	−	−		—	—	—
0.0%	0.0%	0.0%		−	−	−	+	−	−		Q1	Q1	Q3
3.0%	10.0%	0.0%		—	—	—	—	—	—		—	—	—
0.0%	0.0%	—		−	−	−	−	−	−		Q4	Q1	Q1
—	—	—		−	+	−	—	—	—		Q4	Q4	Q1
2.5%	2.5%	—		+	+	−	+	+	—		Q1	Q2	Q1
6.4%	3.4%	—		−	+	−	+	+	—		Q1	Q2	Q1
3.0%	0.0%	1.0%	epid surveillance	−	−	−	−	−	−		Q4	—	Q2
—	—	—		−	−	−	−	+	−		—	—	—
0.0%	1.0%	0.0%		−	−	−	−	−	−		Q4	Q4	Q4
4.0%	5.0%	25.0%	salaries, communic, transport, etc	−	−	−	−	−	+	state enterprises	Q4	Q4	Q4

(continued)

529

Table D-6 Government national AIDS programs: financial information*—continued

List	GAA	Country	FI1start	FI1end	National $	Internat'l $	FI4E	FI5E	FI6A	FI6B	FI6C	FI6D
1	7	Moldova	1-Jan-93	1-Dec-93	.	.	—	—	—	—	16.8%	—
1	7	Russian Federation	1-Jan-93	1-Dec-93	$3,835,290	.	100%	—	23.4%	32.5%	18.0%	21.5%
1	7	Slovenia	—	—	.	.	—	—	—	—	—	—
1	.7	Turkmenistan	—	—			—	—	—	—	—	—
1	7	Ukraine	1-Sep-92	1-Sep-93		.	—	—	10.4%	18.2%	59.2%	2.2%
1	7	Yugoslavia, Fed. Rep.	—	—	.	.	—	—	—	—	—	—
1	8	Algeria	—	—		.	—		—	—	—	—
1	8	Israel	1-Jan-93	1-Dec-93	$1,666,670	.	10%	—	0.0%	20.0%	80.0%	0.0%
1	8	Jordan	1-Jan-93	1-Dec-93	$77,000	$113,900	−15%	−20%	26.5%	47.0%	4.5%	0.0%
1	8	Kuwait	1-Jul-92	1-Jun-93	$1,733,330	$0	15%	—	10.0%	15.0%	60.0%	5.0%
1	8	Lebanon	1-Jan-93	1-Jan-94	$0	$79,000	—	0%	15.0%	65.0%	5.0%	0.0%
1	8	Morocco	1-Jan-93	1-Dec-93	$827,720	$437,190	−29%	—	16.0%	32.0%	—	52.0%
1	8	Oman	1-Jan-93	1-Dec-93	$278,580	$29,500	—	—	25.0%	35.0%	20.0%	20.0%
1	8	Syrian Arab Rep.	—	—	.	.	—	—	—	—	—	—
1	8	Tunisia	1-Jan-93	1-Dec-93	$250,000	$300,000	25%	−3%	21.7%	34.2%	—	38.6%
1	9	Bhutan	1-Jan-93	1-Dec-93	.	$246,200	—	38%	17.0%	60.0%	15.0%	7.0%
1	9	China	—	—	.	.	—	—	—	—	—	—
1	9	Hong Kong	1-Apr-92	1-Mar-93		.	—	—	—	—	—	—
1	9	Japan	1-Apr-93	1-Mar-94	$98,398,060	.	483%	—	—	33.0%	—	0.0%
1	9	Taiwan	1-Jul-92	1-Jun-93	.	.						.
1	9	Vietnam	1-Jan-93	1-Dec-93		.						
1	10	Brunei	—	—	.	.	—	—	—	—	—	—
1	10	India	1-Apr-92	1-Mar-93	$17,000,000	$3,266,300	—	—	24.0%	46.0%	30.0%	0.0%
1	10	Malaysia	1-Jan-93	1-Dec-93	$8,888,890	.	—	—	8.0%	20.0%	4.0%	60.0%
1	10	Nepal	1-Jan-93	1-Dec-93	$2,850	$351,140	—	99%	13.0%	40.0%	30.0%	0.0%
1	10	Singapore	—	—	.	.	—	—	—	—	—	—
1	10	Sri Lanka	1-Jan-93	1-Dec-93	.	.	—	−30%	25.0%	30.0%	30.0%	5.0%
1	10	Thailand	1-Oct-92	1-Sep-93	$47,000,000	$9,000,000	240%	−30%	2.0%	15.0%	2.0%	75.0%
2	3	American Samoa	1-Jan-93	1-Dec-94	.	.	—	—	—	—	—	—
2	3	Cook Islands	1-Jul-92	1-Jun-93	$14,280	$15,340	6%	0%	20.0%	40.0%	30.0%	—
2	3	Guam	1-Jan-93	1-Dec-93	$170,000 .	.	−33%	—	80.0%	5.0%	15.0%	0.0%
2	3	New Caledonia	1-Jan-93	1-Dec-93	.	.	—	—	—	—	—	—
2	3	Niue	1-Oct-93	1-Dec-93	$0	$3,000	0%	—	85.0%	10.0%	5.0%	0.0%
2	3	Tokelau	—	—	.	.	—	—	—	—	—	—
2	3	Tuvalu	1-Jan-93	1-Dec-93	$0	$1,990	—	50%	20.0%	60.0%	10.0%	0.0%
2	6	Bermuda	1-Apr-92	1-Mar-93	.	.	—	—	2.5%	25.0%	2.5%	70.0%
2	6	Cayman Islands	1-Jan-93	1-Dec-93	$14,000	$0	0%	—	15.0%	20.0%	20.0%	30.0%
2	6	Montserrat	1-Apr-92	1-Mar-93	$75,630	$104,300	—	−24%	22.8%	24.5%	40.9%	0.0%
2	6	Netherlands Antilles	1-Jan-93	1-Dec-93	.	$19,000	—	—	—	10.0%	30.0%	10.0%

*List, core country response (1) or subsidiary response (2); GAA, geographic area of affinity; country, territory, or region responding.

Finance abbreviations: FI1start, beginning of fiscal year of data; FI1end, end of fiscal year of data; National $, funds spent by the GNAP which were received from the country's *national government* (in U.S.$); Internat'l $, funds spent by the GNAP which were received from *international sources and agencies* (in U.S.$); FI4E, percentage change in *national government* funding between this fiscal year and the previous fiscal year; FI5E, percentage change in funding from *international sources/agencies* between this fiscal year and the previous fiscal year.

Estimated distribution of total funds from national and international sources (should sum to 100%): FI6A, GNAP program management, surveillance monitoring, evaluation; FI6B, prevention (i.e., condom distribution, education); FI6C, laboratory support (HIV testing, CD4 count) (note: not asked on some survey forms); FI6D, care (i.e., drugs, housing); FI6E, support of community based organizations, AIDS support organizations, other NGOs working on AIDS; FI6F, research (i.e., clinical trials, surveys); FI6G, other; FI6GEXP, other specified.

Other sources which provide additional funds for similar HIV/AIDS activities: FI7A, private sector; FI7B, commercial sector; FI7C, NGOs; FI7D, state/province/district/local governments; FI7E, foundations; FI7F, other; FI7FEXP, other specified.

Percentage of all expenditure in the country which was spent by the GNAP on (Q1 = 0–25%, Q2 = 26–50%, Q3 = 51–75%, Q4 = 76–100%): FI8, HIV prevention; FI9, HIV care; FI10, HIV research.

FI6E	FI6F	FI6G	FI6GEXP	FI7A	FI7B	FI7C	FI7D	FI7E	FI7F	FI7FEXP	FI8	FI9	FI10
—	—	—		—	—	—	—	+	—		Q4	—	—
0.0%	4.6%	0.0%		—	—	+	+	+	—		Q4	Q4	Q4
—	—	—		—	—	+	—	—	—		—	—	—
—	—	—		—	—	+	+	—	—		—	Q4	—
—	10.0%	—		—	—	—	—	—	—		Q4	Q4	Q4
—	—	—		—	—	—	—	—	—		—	—	—
—	—	—		—	—	+	—	—	—		Q1	Q1	Q1
0.0%	0.0%	0.0%		+	+	—	—	+	—		Q4	Q1	Q1
15.0%	7.0%	0.0%		—	—	—	—	—	—		Q4	Q2	Q1
0.0%	10.0%	0.0%		—	—	—	+	+	—		Q4	Q4	Q4
10.0%	5.0%	—		+	+	+	—	—	—		Q4	Q1	Q1
—	—	—		—	—	—	—	—	—		Q4	Q4	Q1
0.0%	0.0%	0.0%		—	—	—	—	—	—		Q2	Q1	Q1
—	—	—		—	—	—	—	—	—		—	—	—
4.1%	1.4%	0.0%		—	+	+	—	—	—		Q4	Q1	Q1
3.0%	—	—		—	—	—	—	—	—		Q4	Q4	Q4
—	—	—		—	—	—	—	—	—		—	—	—
—	—	—		—	—	—	—	—	—		—	—	—
0.0%	47.0%	20.0%	subs to prefectures/ replet of treat & test	+	+	+	+	+	—		—	—	—
—	—	—		—	—	—	—	—	—		—	—	—
—	—	—		—	—	+	—	—	—		—	—	—
—	—	—		—	—	—	—	—	—		—	—	—
0.0%	0.0%	0.0%		—	—	—	—	—	—		Q4	Q1	Q1
1.0%	5.0%	2.0%		+	+	+	+	+	—		Q1	Q2	Q1
15.0%	2.0%	0.0%		—	—	—	—	—	—		—	—	—
—	—	—		—	—	+	—	—	—		—	—	—
15.0%	5.0%	0.0%		—	—	+	—	—	—		Q2	Q4	Q3
4.0%	2.0%	0.0%		+	—	+	+	+	—		Q3	Q4	Q1
—	—	—		—	—	—	—	—	+	WHO	Q4	Q1	Q1
10.0%	—	—		+	+	+	+	—	—		Q4	Q2	Q1
0.0%	0.0%	0.0%		—	—	—	—	—	—		Q4	Q1	Q1
—	—	—		—	—	—	—	—	—		—	—	—
—	0.0%	—		—	—	—	—	—	—		Q4	Q1	Q1
—	—	—		—	—	—	—	—	—		—	—	—
0.0%	10.0%	0.0%		—	—	+	—	—	—		Q4	Q3	Q1
—	—	—		—	+	+	—	+	—		Q2	Q4	—
5.0%	5.0%	5.0%	miscellaneous	—	—	+	—	—	+	SNAP (support group)	Q3	Q3	Q4
10.8%	0.0%	0.0%		—	—	+	—	—	—		Q4	Q1	Q1
10.0%	20.0%	0.0%		+	+	+	+	+	—		Q1	Q4	Q1

531

Table D-7.1 Government national AIDS programs: needs and services—information, medical care, and training; prevention needs categories 1(90)-1 through 4C*

List	GAA	Country	PN1(90)-1	PN1(90)-2	PN2(93)-1	PN2(93)-2	PN4A	PN4B	PN4C
1	1	United States	HB	ID	HB	ID	NE	SA	SA
1	2	Austria	HB	ID	ID	HT	NE	SA	SA
1	2	Belgium	HB	HT	HB	HT	SA	SA	NE
1	2	Cyprus	HB	HT	HB	HT	NE	SA	SA
1	2	Denmark	HB	HT	HB	HT	SA	SA	SA
1	2	Finland	HB	HT	HB	HT	NE	NR	NE
1	2	France	HB	ID	HB	ID	SA	SA	SA
1	2	Germany	HB	ID	HB	ID	SA	NE	SA
1	2	Iceland	HB	ID	HB	HT	NE	SA	SA
1	2	Liechtenstein	ID	HT	ID	HT	NE	SA	SA
1	2	Luxembourg	HB	ID	HB	ID	—	SA	—
1	2	Malta	HB	HT	HB	HT	NE	SA	NE
1	2	Netherlands	HB	ID	HB	ID	SA	SA	SA
1	2	Norway	HB	ID	HB	HT	NE	SA	NE
1	2	Spain	HB/ID	HB/ID	HT/ID	HT/ID	NE	NR	NE
1	2	Sweden	HB	HT	HB	HT	NE	SA	SA
1	2	Switzerland	HT	ID	HT	ID	SA	SA	NE
1	2	United Kingdom	HB	HT	HB	HT	SA	SA	SA
1	3	Australia	HB	ID	HB	ID	SA	SA	SA
1	3	Fiji	HT	HB	HT	HB	NE	SA	NE
1	3	Kiribati	—	—	HT	—	NE	NR	NE
1	3	Micronesia, Fed. Sts.	—	—	—	—	NE	NE	NE
1	3	New Zealand	HB	HT	HB	HT	NE	SA	NE
1	3	Papua New Guinea	HT	MC	HT	MC	NE	NE	NE
1	3	Solomon Islands	—	—	—	—	SA	—	SA
1	3	Vanuatu	—	—	—	—	NE	NE	NE
1	3	Western Samoa	HB	—	—	—	NE	NE	NE
1	4	Argentina	—	—	—	—	—	—	—
1	4	Belize	—	—	—	—	NE	NE	NE
1	4	Brazil	HB	ID	HB	ID	NE	SA	NE
1	4	Chile	HB	HT	HB	HT	SA	NE	NE
1	4	Colombia	HB	HT	HT	HB	SA	SA	NE
1	4	Costa Rica	HB	BT	HB	HT	NE	NE	NE
1	4	Ecuador	HB	HT	HT	HB	NE	NE	SA
1	4	El Salvador	HT	HB	HT	HB	SA	NE	NE
1	4	Guatemala	HT	HB	HT	HB	NE	—	—
1	4	Mexico	HB	HT	HB	HT	NE	NE	NE
1	4	Panama	HB	HT	HT	HB	NE	SA	NE
1	4	Peru	HB	HT	HT	HB	NE	NE	NE
1	4	Suriname	HT	HB	HT	HB	NE	NE	NE
1	4	Uruguay	HB	ID	HB	HT	SA	NE	NE
1	4	Venezuela	HB	BT	HB	ID	NE	SA	NE
1	5	Angola	HT	BT	HT	BT	SA	NE	NE

List	GAA	Country	PN1(90)-1	PN1(90)-2	PN2(93)-1	PN2(93)-2	PN4A	PN4B	PN4C
1	5	Benin	HT	MC	HT	MC	SA	NE	SA
1	5	Botswana	HT	MC	HT	MC	NE	NE	NE
1	5	Burkino Faso	HT	ID	HT	ID	NE	NE	NE
1	5	Cameroon	HT	BT	HT	BT	SA	NE	NE
1	5	Cape Verde	HT	MC	HT	MC	—	—	NE
1	5	Chad	HT	O	HT	O	SA	NE	NE
1	5	Comoros	HT	MC	HT	MC	SA	NE	NE
1	5	Congo	HT	MC	HT	MC	NE	NE	—
1	5	Côte d'Ivoire	HT	—	HT	—	NE	NE	SA
1	5	Djibouti	HT	MC	HT	MC	SA	NE	SA
1	5	Ethiopia	HT	MC	HT	MC	NE	NE	NE
1	5	Gabon	HT	MC	HT	BT	SA	NE	NE
1	5	Ghana	HT/MC	HT/MC	HT/MC	HT/MC	NE	NE	NE
1	5	Guinea	BT/MC	BT/MC	BT/MC	BT/MC	SA	NE	NE
1	5	Guinee-Bissau	HT	BT	HT	—	SA	NE	NE
1	5	Lesotho	HT	MC	HT	MC	NE	NE	NE
1	5	Madagascar	HB/HT	HB/HT	HT	HB	SA	NE	SA
1	5	Mali	HT	MC	HT	MC	SA	NE	NE
1	5	Mauritania	HT	BT	HT	BT	NE	NE	SA
1	5	Mauritius	HT	HB	HT	HB	SA	SA	SA
1	5	Rwanda	HT	MC	HT	MC	SA	NE	NE
1	5	Senegal	HT	O	HT	MC	—	NE	NE
1	5	Seychelles	HT	—	HT	—	NE	SA	NE
1	5	South Africa	HT	MC	HT	MC	SA	NE	NE
1	5	Tanzania	HT	MC	HT	MC	NE	NE	NE
1	5	Togo	HT	MC	HT	MC	SA	NE	SA
1	5	Uganda	HT	MC	HT	MC	SA	NE	NE
1	5	Zaire	HT	BT	HT	MC	NE	NE	NE
1	5	Zambia	HT	MC	HT	MC	NE	—	NE
1	5	Zimbabwe	HT	MC	HT	MC	NE	NE	NE
1	6	Antigua and Barbuda	HB	HT	HT	HB	NE	NE	NE
1	6	Barbados	HB	HT	HT	HB	SA	NE	NE
1	6	Dominican Republic	HT	HB	HT	HB	NE	NE	NE
1	6	Grenada	HT	HB	HT	HB	NE	NE	NE
1	6	Jamaica	HT	HB	HT	HB	NE	NE	NE
1	6	St. Lucia	HT	HB	HT	—	SA	NE	NE
1	6	Trinidad and Tobago	HT	HB	HT	HB	NE	NE	NE
1	7	Azerbaijan	—	—	ID	HT	NE	NE	NE
1	7	Belarus	HB	—	HT/ID	HT/ID	NE	SA	SA
1	7	Bulgaria	HT	—	ID	—	NE	NE	NE
1	7	Croatia	HB	BT	HB	ID	NE	NE	NE
1	7	Czech Republic	HB	HT	HB	HT	NE	SA	NE

(continued)

Table D-7.1 Government national AIDS programs: needs and services—information, medical care, and training; prevention needs categories 1(90)-1 through 4C*—continued

List	GAA	Country	PN1(90)-1	PN1(90)-2	PN2(93)-1	PN2(93)-2	PN4A	PN4B	PN4C
1	7	Estonia	HB/HT	HB/HT	HB/HT	HB/HT	NE	NR	NE
1	7	Hungary	HB	HT	HB	HT	NE	SA	NE
1	7	Kyrgyz Republic	HT	—	—	—	SA	NR	SA
1	7	Latvia	HB	HT	HB	HT	NE	SA	NE
1	7	Lithuania	HB	HT	HB	HT	NE	NE	NE
1	7	Moldova	HB/HT	HB/HT	HT	—	SA	NR	SA
1	7	Russian Federation	O	HB	HT	HB	SA	SA	SA
1	7	Slovenia	HB	HT	HB	HT	NE	SA	NE
1	7	Turkmenistan	—	—	—	—	NE	SA	NE
1	7	Ukraine	HT	O	HT	HB	NE	NE	NE
1	7	Yugoslavia, Fed. Rep.	—	—	—	—	NE	NE	NE
1	8	Algeria	ID	BT	ID	BT	NE	NE	SA
1	8	Israel	HB	ID	HB	ID	NE	SA	NE
1	8	Jordan	BT	HB	HB	BT	NE	NE	SA
1	8	Kuwait	HT	BT	HT	BT	NE	NE	NE
1	8	Lebanon	HT	HB	HT	HB	NE	NE	SA
1	8	Morocco	HT	ID	HT	HB	NE	SA	SA
1	8	Oman	BT	HT	HT	—	NE	NE	NE
1	8	Syrian Arab Rep.	HT	—	HT	—	—	—	—
1	8	Tunisia	ID	HT	HT	ID	NE	SA	NE
1	9	Bhutan	—	—	HT	—	NE	NE	NE
1	9	China	ID	—	HT/ID	HT/ID	NE	—	NE
1	9	Hong Kong	HB	HT	HT	HB	NE	SA	NE
1	9	Japan	BT	HB	BT	HT	SA	SA	NE
1	9	Taiwan	HB	HT	HT	HB	—	—	—
1	9	Vietnam	HT	—	ID	HT	NE	NE	NE
1	10	Brunei	BT	HB	HT	HB	NE	NR	SA
1	10	India	HT	ID	HT	ID	NE	NE	NE
1	10	Malaysia	ID	HT	ID	HT	NE	NE	NE
1	10	Nepal	HT	ID	HT	ID	NE	NR	NE
1	10	Singapore	HB	HT	HT	HB	SA	NR	SA
1	10	Sri Lanka	HT	HB	HT	HB	NE	NR	NE
1	10	Thailand	HT	ID	HT	ID	NE	NE	NE
2	3	American Samoa	—	—	—	—	NE	—	NE
2	3	Cook Islands	—	—	—	—	NE	NR	NE
2	3	Guam	HB	HT	HB	HT	NE	NE	NE
2	3	New Caledonia	HB	HT	HT	HB	NE	SA	NE
2	3	Niue	—	—	—	—	—	—	—
2	3	Tokelau	—	—	—	—	—	—	—
2	3	Tuvalu	HT	HB	HT	HB	SA	NR	SA
2	6	Bermuda	ID	HT	HB/ID	HB/ID	SA	SA	NE

List	GAA	Country	PN1(90)-1	PN1(90)-2	PN2(93)-1	PN2(93)-2	PN4A	PN4B	PN4C
2	6	Cayman Islands	HT	HB	HT	—	NE	NE	NE
2	6	Montserrat	—	—	—	—	NE	NE	NE
2	6	Netherlands Antilles	HT	HB	HT	HB	NE	SA	NE

*List, core country response (1) or subsidiary response (2); GAA, geographic area of affinity; country, territory, or region responding.

Prevention needs abbreviations: The two most prevalent modes of HIV transmission in the country (in each of 1990 and 1993) were chosen from the following: HB = homo/bisexual; HT = heterosexual; ID = injection drug use; BT = transfusion/receipt of blood products; MC = prenatal (mother—child); O = other. Note: in some cases, respondent did not distinguish between first and second mode. These are shown as code/code. PN1(90)-1, first most prevalent mode of transmission in 1990; PN1(90)-2, second most prevalent mode of transmission in 1990; PN2(93)-1, first most prevalent mode of transmission in 1993; PN2(93)-2, second most prevalent mode of transmission in 1993.

Given the most prevalent modes of transmission for country specified for 1993, prevention activities sufficiently available (SA) in the country, not required (NR), or needing expansion (NE): PN4A, targeted information campaigns; PN4B, medication and medical therapies; PN4C, training of medical personnel.

Table D-7.2 Government national AIDS programs: needs and services—reported adequacy of condom distribution, and outreach and targeted activities; prevention needs categories 4D through 4Q*

List	GAA	Country	PN4D	PN4E	PN4F	PN4G	PN4H	PN4I	PN4J	PN4K	PN4L	PN4M	PN4N	PN4O	PN4P	PN4Q
1	1	United States	—	—	SA	SA	SA	SA	NE	SA	NE	—	SA	NE	NE	SA
1	2	Austria	SA	SA	SA	SA	SA	SA	NE	NE	NE	NE	SA	SA	SA	SA
1	2	Belgium	NE	NE	SA	NE	SA	NE	NE	SA	NE	NE	NE	NE	NE	SA
1	2	Cyprus	SA	NR	SA	SA	SA	SA	NE	NE	SA	NE	NE	SA	NE	SA
1	2	Denmark	SA	SA	NE	—	SA	SA	NE	NE	SA	SA	NE	NE	NE	SA
1	2	Finland	SA	NE	SA	SA	SA	SA	NE	NE	SA	NE	SA	SA	NE	SA
1	2	France	SA	NE	SA	SA	SA	SA	SA	NE	NE	NE	NE	NE	—	SA
1	2	Germany	NE	NE	NE	NE	NE	SA	NE	SA	NE	NE	NE	NE	SA	SA
1	2	Iceland	NE	NE	SA	SA	SA	NE	NE	NE	NE	NE	NE	NE	SA	—
1	2	Liechtenstein	SA	NE	SA	NE	SA	NR	NR	NE	NE	NE	NR	NR	NE	SA
1	2	Luxembourg	SA	SA	SA	—	SA	SA	—	—	—	—	—	—	—	SA
1	2	Malta	NE	NE	NE	NE	SA	NR	NE	NE	NE	NE	NE	NE	SA	SA
1	2	Netherlands	SA	SA	SA	SA	SA	SA	SA	SA	SA	SA	SA	SA	NE	NE
1	2	Norway	SA	SA	SA	SA	SA	SA	SA	SA	SA	—	SA	—	SA	SA
1	2	Spain	NE	NE	NE	NE	NR	SA	NE	SA	NE	NE	NE	NE	NE	NR
1	2	Sweden	SA	—	SA	NE	SA	SA	NE	SA	SA	NE	SA	SA	SA	SA
1	2	Switzerland	NR	NE	SA	NE	SA	SA	NE	NE	SA	SA	SA	NE	NE	SA
1	2	United Kingdom	SA	NE	SA	SA	SA	SA	NE	NE	NE	SA	SA	SA	SA	SA
1	3	Australia	SA	SA	SA	SA	SA	SA	SA	SA	SA	SA	SA	SA	SA	NE
1	3	Fiji	NE	NR	NE	NE	SA	NE	NE	NE	NE	NE	NE	NE	NR	SA
1	3	Kiribati	NE	NR	NE	NE	NE	NR	NE	NR	SA	SA	NE	NE	NR	SA
1	3	Micronesia, Fed. Sts.	NE	NR	NE	NE	SA	NR	NE	NE	NE	NE	SA	NE	NR	NE
1	3	New Zealand	NE	SA	SA	SA	SA	SA	SA	SA	NE	NE	NE	NE	NE	SA
1	3	Papua New Guinea	NE	NR	NE	NE	NE	—	NE	NE	NE	NE	NE	NE	NR	NE
1	3	Solomon Islands	SA	—	—	SA	SA	—	—	—	—	—	SA	NR	NR	—
1	3	Vanuatu	SA	NR	SA	SA	SA	NR	NE	NE	SA	SA	NE	NE	NR	NE
1	3	Western Samoa	SA	NR	NE	NE	NE	NR	NE	NE	NE	NE	SA	NE	NR	NE
1	4	Argentina	—	—	—	—	—	—	—	—	—	—	—	—	—	—

1	4	Belize	NE	NR	NE	NE	SA	NE	NE	NE	NE	SA	NE	NE	NE	SA
1	4	Brazil	NE	NR	NE	NE	NE	NE	NE	NE	NE	NE	NE	NR	NE	SA
1	4	Chile	NE	—	NE	NE	SA	NE	NE	NE	NE	SA	NE	NE	NE	SA
1	4	Colombia	NE	NR	SA	NE	NR	NE	NE	NE	NE	SA	NE	NE	NR	SA
1	4	Costa Rica	NE	NR	SA	NE	NR	SA	SA	NE	NE	SA	NE	NE	NR	SA
1	4	Ecuador	NE	NR	SA	NE	NR	SA	NE	NE	NE	—	SA	NE	NE	NE
1	4	El Salvador	SA	SA	NE	NE	NE	NE	NE	NE	SA	NE	NE	NE	NE	NE
1	4	Guatemala	SA	NR	NE	NE	—	NE	NE	—	NE	NE	—	NE	—	—
1	4	Mexico	SA	NR	NE	NE	NE	NE	NE	NE	NE	NE	NE	NE	NR	SA
1	4	Panama	NE	NR	SA	NE	NE	NE	NE	NE	NE	NR	NE	NE	NR	NE
1	4	Peru	NE	NR	NE	NE	NR	NE	NE	SA	NE	SA	SA	NE	NR	NE
1	4	Suriname	NR	NR	SA	NE	NR	NE	NE	NE	NE	NE	NE	NE	NR	NE
1	4	Uruguay	SA	NR	NE	NE	NE	NE	SA	NE	NE	NR	NE	SA	NE	SA
1	4	Venezuela	NE	NR	SA	NE	NR	SA	NE	NE	NE	—	NE	NE	NR	SA
1	5	Angola	NE	NR	NE	NE	NE	NE	NE	SA	NE	NE	NE	NE	NR	NE
1	5	Benin	SA	NR	NE	NE	NE	SA	SA	NE	NE	SA	NE	NE	NR	SA
1	5	Botswana	SA	NR	NE	NE	NE	SA	NE	NE	NE	SA	NE	NE	NR	SA
1	5	Burkino Faso	NE	NR	NE	NE	NE	NE	NE	NE	NE	NE	NE	NE	NR	NE
1	5	Cameroon	NE	NR	NE	NE	SA	NE	NE	—	NE	NE	SA	NE	NR	NE
1	5	Cape Verde	SA	NR	—	NE	NR	SA	—	NE	NE	—	NE	NE	—	NE
1	5	Chad	NE	NE	NE	NE	NR	NE	NR	NR	NR	NR	NR	NE	—	NE
1	5	Comoros	NE	NR	NE	NE	NE	SA	NE	NE	SA	NR	NE	NE	NR	NE
1	5	Congo	SA	NR	NE	NE	NE	SA	NE	NE	NE	NE	NE	SA	NR	NE
1	5	Côte d'Ivoire	SA	NR	NE	NE	NE	NE	NE	SA	NE	NR	NE	SA	NR	SA
1	5	Djibouti	SA	—	NE	NE	NE	SA	NE	NE	NE	NR	NE	NE	NR	SA
1	5	Ethiopia	NE	NR	NE	NE	NE	NE	NE	NE	NE	NE	SA	NE	NR	NE
1	5	Gabon	SA	NR	SA	NE	—	NE	NE	NE	NE	NE	NE	NE	NE	—
1	5	Ghana	NR	NR	NE	SA	NR	NE	NE	NE	NE	SA	NE	NE	NR	NE
1	5	Guinea	SA	NE	NE	NE	SA	NE	NE	NE	NE	SA	SA	NE	NR	NE

(continued)

537

Table D-7.2 Government national AIDS programs: needs and services—reported adequacy of condom distribution, and outreach and targeted activities; prevention needs categories 4D through 4Q*—continued

List	GAA	Country	PN4D	PN4E	PN4F	PN4G	PN4H	PN4I	PN4J	PN4K	PN4L	PN4M	PN4N	PN4O	PN4P	PN4Q
1	5	Guinee-Bissau	SA	NR	NE	NE	SA	—	NE	NR	NE	NE	NE	NE	NR	SA
1	5	Lesotho	NE	NR	SA	NE	SA	—	NE	—	NE	NE	NE	SA	—	NE
1	5	Madagascar	NE	—	NE	NE	SA	—	SA	SA	SA	SA	NE	SA	—	NE
1	5	Mali	SA	NR	NE	NE	SA	NE	SA	NR	NE	NE	NE	NE	NR	SA
1	5	Mauritania	NE	NR	NE	NE	NE	NR	NE	NE	NE	—	NE	—	NR	NE
1	5	Mauritius	SA	NE	SA	SA	SA	NR	NE	NE	NE	NE	NE	SA	SA	SA
1	5	Rwanda	SA	—	NE	NE	SA	NE	NE	—	NE	NE	NE	NE	—	SA
1	5	Senegal	SA	NE	NE	NE	SA	NE	SA	NE	NE	SA	SA	NE	NE	NE
1	5	Seychelles	NE	NR	NE	NE	SA	SA	NE	NE	NE	NE	NE	SA	NR	SA
1	5	South Africa	SA	NE	SA	SA	SA	NE	NE	SA	NE	NE	SA	NE	NE	SA
1	5	Tanzania	SA	NE	NE	NE	SA	NE	NE	NR	NE	NE	NE	NE	NR	NE
1	5	Togo	SA	NR	SA	NE	SA	NE	SA	NE	SA	SA	NE	NE	NE	SA
1	5	Uganda	NE	NR	NE	NE	NE	NR	NE	NR	NE	NE	NE	SA	—	NE
1	5	Zaire	NE	NR	NE	NE	NE	NR	NE	NR	NE	NE	NE	SA	NR	NE
1	5	Zambia	SA	NR	SA	SA	NE	SA	NE	NR	NE	NE	NE	SA	NR	SA
1	5	Zimbabwe	NE	—	NE	—	SA	NE	NE	—	NE	NE	NE	SA	—	SA
1	6	Antigua and Barbuda	SA	NR	NE	NE	SA	NR	NE	NE	NE	NR	NE	SA	NR	NR
1	6	Barbados	NE	NR	SA	NE	SA	SA	NE	NE	NE	NE	NE	NE	NR	SA
1	6	Dominican Republic	NE	NR	SA	NE	NE	NR	NE	NE	NE	NE	NE	NR	NE	NE
1	6	Grenada	SA	—	SA	NE	SA	—	NE	NE	NE	NE	NE	SA	SA	—
1	6	Jamaica	NE	NR	SA	SA	SA	SA	NE	SA	NE	NE	NE	SA	NR	SA
1	6	St. Lucia	NE	NR	SA	NE	SA	NR	NE	NE	NE	NE	NE	SA	NR	NE
1	6	Trinidad and Tobago	NE	—	SA	NE	SA	—	NE	NE	NE	NE	NE	SA	—	SA
1	7	Azerbaijan	NE	NE	SA	NE	SA	NR	NE	NE	NE	NE	NE	NE	NE	NE
1	7	Belarus	NE	NE	SA	SA	SA	SA	NE	NE	NE	NE	NE	SA	NE	SA
1	7	Bulgaria	NE	NR	SA	SA	SA	SA	NE	NE	NE	NE	NE	SA	NE	SA
1	7	Croatia	NE	NE	NE	NE	NE	SA	NE	NE	NE	NE	NE	NE	NE	NE
1	7	Czech Republic	NE	NE	SA	NE	NR	NR	NE	NE	NE	NE	SA	NE	NE	NR
1	7	Estonia	NR	NE	NE	NE	NR	NR	NE	SA	NE	SA	NE	NE	—	NE

1	7	Hungary	NE	NE	SA	SA	SA	SA	SA	SA	NE	NE	NE	SA	NE	SA
1	7	Kyrgyz Republic	NE	NE	NE	NE	SA	NR	SA	NE	NE	NE	NE	SA	NR	NE
1	7	Latvia	NE	NR	SA	NE	SA	SA	NE	NE	NE	NE	NE	NE	NE	SA
1	7	Lithuania	NE	NE	NE	NE	SA	SA	NE	NE	NE	NE	NE	NE	NR	SA
1	7	Moldova	SA	NR	SA	SA	SA	SA	SA	SA	SA	SA	SA	SA	NE	SA
1	7	Russian Federation	NE	NE	SA	SA	SA	SA	NE	NE	NE	NE	NE	NE	NE	SA
1	7	Slovenia	NE	SA	SA	NE	SA	SA	NE	NE	NE	NE	NE	NE	NE	SA
1	7	Turkmenistan	NE	NR	SA	SA	SA	NR	NE	NE	NE	NE	NE	NE	NE	NE
1	7	Ukraine	NE	NE	SA	NE	NR	NR	NE	NE	NE	NE	NE	NE	NE	SA
1	7	Yugoslavia, Fed. Rep.	NE	NE	SA	NE	SA	SA	NE	NE	SA	NE	NE	NE	NE	SA
1	8	Algeria	NE	NE	SA	NE	SA	NE	SA	SA	NE	SA	NE	NE	NE	NE
1	8	Israel	NR	NR	SA	NE	SA	SA	NE	NE	—	NE	NE	NE	NE	SA
1	8	Jordan	NE	NE	NE	NE	SA	NR	—	—	NE	NE	NE	NE	NE	SA
1	8	Kuwait	—	—	SA	NE	SA	—	NE	NE	NE	NE	NE	NE	—	SA
1	8	Lebanon	NR	NR	NE	NE	SA	NR	NE	NE	NE	NE	SA	NE	NR	SA
1	8	Morocco	SA	NE	NE	NE	SA	SA	NE	NE	NE	NE	NE	SA	NE	SA
1	8	Oman	NE	NR	SA	SA	SA	NR	NR	NR	NR	NR	NE	SA	NE	SA
1	8	Syrian Arab Rep.	—	—	—	—	—	—	—	—	—	—	—	—	—	—
1	8	Tunisia	SA	NR	NE	NE	SA	SA	NE	NR	NE	NE	NE	SA	NR	NE
1	9	Bhutan	NE	—	SA	NE	SA	NE	—	—	NE	NE	SA	SA	—	SA
1	9	China	NE	—	NE	NE	NE	—	NE	NE	NE	NE	NE	NE	NE	NE
1	9	Hong Kong	NE	NE	NE	SA	SA	SA	NE	NE	SA	NE	SA	NE	SA	SA
1	9	Japan	NR	NR	SA	NE	SA	SA	SA	SA	NE	SA	NE	SA	—	SA
1	9	Taiwan	—	—	—	—	—	—	—	—	—	—	—	—	—	—
1	9	Vietnam	NE	NE	SA	NE	NE	NR	NE	NR	NE	NE	NE	NE	NE	NE
1	10	Brunei	NR	NR	SA	SA	SA	NR	NR	NR	NE	NE	NE	SA	NR	SA
1	10	India	NE	NR	SA	SA	NE	SA	NE	SA	SA	NE	SA	SA	NE	SA
1	10	Malaysia	NR	NR	NE	NE	SA	NR	NE	NE	NE	NE	NE	SA	NE	SA

(continued)

539

Table D-7.2 Government national AIDS programs: needs and services—reported adequacy of condom distribution, and outreach and targeted activities; prevention needs categories 4D through 4Q*—continued

List	GAA	Country	PN4D	PN4E	PN4F	PN4G	PN4H	PN4I	PN4J	PN4K	PN4L	PN4M	PN4N	PN4O	PN4P	PN4Q
1	10	Nepal	NE	NE	NR	NE	SA	NE	NE	NR	NE	NE	NE	SA	NE	SA
1	10	Singapore	SA	NR	SA	SA	SA	SA	SA	NE	NE	NE	SA	SA	NR	SA
1	10	Sri Lanka	NE	NR	SA	NE	SA	NR	NE	NR	NE	NE	SA	SA	NR	NE
1	10	Thailand	SA	—	NE	NE	SA	NR	NE	NR	SA	SA	NE	NE	SA	NE
2	3	American Samoa	SA	NR	SA	SA	SA	NR	NE	NE	NE	NE	NE	NE	NR	SA
2	3	Cook Islands	SA	NR	SA	SA	NE	NR	NR	NR	NE	NE	NE	SA	NR	SA
2	3	Guam	NE	NE	NE	SA	SA	SA	NE	SA	NE	NE	NE	NE	SA	SA
2	3	New Caledonia	NE	NE	NE	NE	SA	SA	NE	NE	NE	NE	NE	NE	NR	SA
2	3	Niue	—	—	—	—	—	—	—	—	—	—	—	—	—	—
2	3	Tokelau	—	—	—	—	—	—	—	—	—	—	—	—	—	—
2	3	Tuvalu	SA	NR	SA	SA	SA	NR	NR	NE	NE	NE	NE	NE	NR	NE
2	6	Bermuda	NE	NE	SA	SA	SA	SA	NE	NE	NE	SA	SA	NE	SA	SA
2	6	Cayman Islands	NE	NR	SA	SA	SA	NE	NE	NE	NE	NR	NE	NE	NR	SA
2	6	Montserrat	NE	NR	NE	NE	SA	NE	NE	NE	NE	NE	NE	SA	NE	NE
2	6	Netherlands Antilles	SA	—	SA	SA	SA	SA	SA	NE	NE	—	NE	NE	NE	SA

*List, core country response (1) or subsidiary response (2); GAA, geographic area of affinity; country, territory, or region responding. *Prevention needs abbreviations*: Given the most prevalent modes of transmission for country specified for 1993, prevention activities sufficiently available (SA) in the country, not required (NR), or needing expansion (NE): PN4D, free condom distribution; PN4E, free injection equipment distribution for drug users; PN4F, voluntary HIV testing; PN4G, voluntary HIV counseling; PN4H, HIV screening of blood and blood products; PN4I, available abortions for pregnant women infected with HIV; PN4J, outreach activities to sex workers/prostitutes; PN4K, outreach activities to gay men; PN4L, sex education in high schools; PN4M, sex education in colleges/universities; PN4N, support for community based programs/AIDS service organizations, and other NGOs working on AIDS; PN4O, integration of STI and HIV prevention services; PN4P, treatment programs for injecting drug users; PN4Q, sterilization of medical/surgical/dental equipment.

Table D-7.3 Government national AIDS programs: needs and services—projected and reported numbers of condoms distributed and achievement of target; prevention needs categories 5 through 7to6*

List	GAA	Country	PN5	PN6	PN7	PN6toad	PN7toad	PN7to6
1	1	United States	–	—	—	—	—	—
1	2	Austria	–	—	—	—	—	—
1	2	Belgium	+	250,000	250,000	0.05	0.05	1.00
1	2	Cyprus	+	20,000	15,000	0.05	0.04	0.75
1	2	Denmark	–	—	—	—	—	—
1	2	Finland	+	100,000	100,000	0.04	0.04	1.00
1	2	France	+	—	—	—	—	—
1	2	Germany	–	—	—	—	—	—
1	2	Iceland	–	—	500,000	—	3.67	—
1	2	Liechtenstein	+	5,000	4,500	0.35	0.32	0.90
1	2	Luxembourg	—	—	—	—	—	—
1	2	Malta	–	—	—	—	—	—
1	2	Netherlands	+	—	—	—	—	—
1	2	Norway	+	—	600,000	—	0.28	—
1	2	Spain	+	—	—	—	—	—
1	2	Sweden	–	—	—	—	—	—
1	2	Switzerland	–	—	14,000,000	—	3.98	—
1	2	United Kingdom	–	—	—	—	—	—
1	3	Australia	–	—	—	—	—	—
1	3	Fiji	–	—	—	—	—	—
1	3	Kiribati	+	—	—	—	—	—
1	3	Micronesia, Fed. Sts.	+	40,000	11,000	0.71	0.19	0.28
1	3	New Zealand	–	—	—	—	—	—
1	3	Papua New Guinea	+	500,000	250,000	0.25	0.13	0.50
1	3	Solomon Islands	—	—	—	—	—	—
1	3	Vanuatu	+	—	—	—	—	—
1	3	Western Samoa	+	15,000	20,000	0.18	0.24	1.33
1	4	Argentina	—	—	—	—	—	—
1	4	Belize	+	—	—	—	—	—
1	4	Brazil	+	10,000,000	1,000,000	0.13	0.01	0.10
1	4	Chile	+	500,000	500,000	0.07	0.07	1.00
1	4	Colombia	+	500,000	500,000	0.03	0.03	1.00
1	4	Costa Rica	–	—	7,000,000	—	4.35	—
1	4	Ecuador	–	—	—	—	—	—
1	4	El Salvador	+	300,000	350,000	0.12	0.14	1.17
1	4	Guatemala	+	1,000,000	1,000,000	0.23	0.23	1.00
1	4	Mexico	+	6,000,000	5,297,965	0.13	0.12	0.88
1	4	Panama	+	250,000	200,000	0.19	0.15	0.80
1	4	Peru	–	—	—	—	—	—
1	4	Suriname	+	500,000	500,000	1.99	1.99	1.00
1	4	Uruguay	+	1,220,000	1,215,900	0.75	0.75	1.00
1	4	Venezuela	+	1,000,000	1,500,000	0.10	0.14	1.50

(continued)

Table D-7.3 Government national AIDS programs: needs and services—projected and reported numbers of condoms distributed and achievement of target; prevention needs categories 5 through 7to6*—continued

List	GAA	Country	PN5	PN6	PN7	PN6toad	PN7toad	PN7to6
1	5	Angola	+	4,500,000	—	0.95	—	—
1	5	Benin	+	1,000,000	785,000	0.45	0.35	0.79
1	5	Botswana	+	—	—	—	—	—
1	5	Burkino Faso	+	2,999,993	2,252,460	0.69	0.52	0.75
1	5	Cameroon	+	—	—	—	—	—
1	5	Cape Verde	+	—	500,000	—	2.90	—
1	5	Chad	+	800,000	650,000	0.29	0.23	0.81
1	5	Comoros	+	350,000	200,000	1.54	0.88	0.57
1	5	Congo	+	—	—	—	—	—
1	5	Côte d'Ivoire	+	2,000,000	1,800,000	0.37	0.33	0.90
1	5	Djibouti	+	500,000	388,880	2.59	2.01	0.78
1	5	Ethiopia	+	4,800,000	2,900,000	0.20	0.12	0.60
1	5	Gabon	+	—	65,284	—	0.11	—
1	5	Ghana	–	—	—	—	—	—
1	5	Guinea	+	3,000,000	2,000,000	1.12	0.75	0.67
1	5	Guinee-Bissau	+	—	—	—	—	—
1	5	Lesotho	+	600,000	499,812	0.70	0.59	0.83
1	5	Madagascar	+	600,000	600,000	0.11	0.11	1.00
1	5	Mali	+	2,000,000	1,600,000	0.50	0.40	0.80
1	5	Mauritania	–	—	—	—	—	—
1	5	Mauritius	+	30,000	25,000	0.05	0.04	0.83
1	5	Rwanda	+	2,000,000	1,500,000	0.62	0.47	0.75
1	5	Senegal	+	2,500,000	2,300,000	0.71	0.65	0.92
1	5	Seychelles	+	—	200,000	—	6.53	—
1	5	South Africa	+	60,000,000	60,000,000	3.23	3.23	1.00
1	5	Tanzania	+	20,000,000	12,894,000	1.72	1.11	0.64
1	5	Togo	+	118,583	—	0.07	—	—
1	5	Uganda	+	4,440,000	4,440,000	0.56	0.56	1.00
1	5	Zaire	+	28,052,500	10,000,000	1.65	0.59	0.36
1	5	Zambia	+	28,000,000	10,000,000	7.30	2.61	0.36
1	5	Zimbabwe	+	20,000,000	35,000,000	4.27	7.47	1.75
1	6	Antigua and Barbuda	–	—	66,000	—	1.55	—
1	6	Barbados	+	—	—	—	—	—
1	6	Dominican Republic	+	500,000	—	0.13	—	—
1	6	Grenada	+	350,000	376,360	7.33	7.88	1.08
1	6	Jamaica	+	—	—	—	—	—
1	6	St. Lucia	+	—	73,000	—	0.89	—
1	6	Trinidad and Tobago	+	2,160,000	820,800	3.16	1.20	0.38
1	7	Azerbaijan	–	—	—	—	—	—
1	7	Belarus	–	—	—	—	—	—
1	7	Bulgaria	+	—	—	—	—	—
1	7	Croatia	–	—	—	—	—	—

List	GAA	Country	PN5	PN6	PN7	PN6toad	PN7toad	PN7to6
1	7	Czech Republic	–	—	—	—	—	—
1	7	Estonia	+	—	—	—	—	—
1	7	Hungary	+	—	—	—	—	—
1	7	Kyrgyz Republic	–	—	2,000,000	—	0.90	—
1	7	Latvia	–	—	—	—	—	—
1	7	Lithuania	+	500,000	10,200	0.27	0.00	0.02
1	7	Moldova	+	—	—	—	—	—
1	7	Russian Federation	—	—	—	—	—	—
1	7	Slovenia	–	—	—	—	—	—
1	7	Turkmenistan	–	—	2,000,000	—	1.04	—
1	7	Ukraine	–	—	—	—	—	—
1	7	Yugoslavia, Fed. Rep.	–	—	—	—	—	—
1	8	Algeria	+	3,000,000	3,000,000	0.25	0.25	1.00
1	8	Israel	–	—	—	—	—	—
1	8	Jordan	–	—	—	—	—	—
1	8	Kuwait	–	—	—	—	—	—
1	8	Lebanon	–	—	—	—	—	—
1	8	Morocco	+	—	1,750,000	—	0.14	—
1	8	Oman	–	—	—	—	—	—
1	8	Syrian Arab Rep.	—	—	—	—	—	—
1	8	Tunisia	+	2,000,000	3,500,000	0.48	0.83	1.75
1	9	Bhutan	+	—	18,060	—	0.03	—
1	9	China	–	—	—	—	—	—
1	9	Hong Kong	+	—	—	—	—	—
1	9	Japan	—	—	—	—	—	—
1	9	Taiwan	—	—	—	—	—	—
1	9	Viet Nam	+	80,000	3,500,000	0.00	0.10	43.75
1	10	Brunei	–	—	—	—	—	—
1	10	India	–	—	—	—	—	—
1	10	Malaysia	–	—	—	—	—	—
1	10	Nepal	+	160,000	150,000	0.02	0.02	0.94
1	10	Singapore	—	—	—	—	—	—
1	10	Sri Lanka	+	—	247,680	—	0.03	—
1	10	Thailand	+	45,000,000	—	1.39	—	—
2	3	American Samoa	+	1,000	500	0.05	0.02	0.50
2	3	Cook Islands	+	5,000	21,600	0.56	2.43	4.32
2	3	Guam	+	5,000	3,000	0.06	0.04	0.60
2	3	New Caledonia	+	100,000	80,000	1.09	0.87	0.80
2	3	Niue	+	—	—	—	—	—
2	3	Tokelau	–	—	—	—	—	—
2	3	Tuvalu	+	—	—	—	—	—
2	6	Bermuda	+	10,000	9,504	0.37	0.35	0.95

(continued)

Table D-7.3 Government national AIDS programs: needs and services—projected and reported numbers of condoms distributed and achievement of target; prevention needs categories 5 through 7to6*—continued

List	GAA	Country	PN5	PN6	PN7	PN6toad	PN7toad	PN7to6
2	6	Cayman Islands	+	5,000	4,000	0.34	0.27	0.80
2	6	Montserrat	+	—	—	—	—	—
2	6	Netherlands Antilles	+	—	—	—	—	—

*List, core country response (1) or subsidiary response (2); GAA, geographic area of affinity; country, territory, or region responding.

Prevention needs abbreviations: Given the most prevalent modes of transmission for country specified for 1993, prevention activities sufficiently available (SA) in the country, not required (NR), or needing expansion (NE): PN5, GNAP distributes condoms to regional/district programs; PN6, target number of condoms to be distributed in the country by the GNAP in 1992; PN7, actual number of condoms distributed in 1992 (best estimate requested); PN6toad, number of condoms targeted for distribution per adult (15–49 years old); PN7toad, number of condoms actually distributed per adult (15–49 years old); PN7to6, ratio of the number of condoms actually distributed to the number targeted for distribution.

Table D-7.4 Government national AIDS programs: needs and services—condom distribution sites, 1990; prevention needs categories 990A through 990K*

List	GAA	Country	PN990A	PN990B	PN990C	PN990D	PN990E	PN990F	PN990G	PN990H	PN990I	PN990J	PN990K
1	1	United States	−	−	−	−	−	−	−	−	−	−	−
1	2	Austria	−	−	−	−	−	−	−	−	−	−	−
1	2	Belgium	+	+	+	+	+	−	+	−	+	−	−
1	2	Cyprus	−	−	−	−	−	−	−	−	−	−	−
1	2	Denmark	+	+	+	+	+	+	+	+	+	+	+
1	2	Finland	+	+	+	+	−	+	+	+	+	+	−
1	2	France	+	−	−	+	−	−	+	−	+	−	−
1	2	Germany	+	+	+	+	+	+	−	+	+	+	−
1	2	Iceland	−	−	+	+	−	−	+	+	+	+	−
1	2	Liechtenstein	−	−	+	+	+	+	−	+	+	−	+
1	2	Luxembourg	+	+	+	+	+	+	+	+	+	+	−
1	2	Malta	−	−	+	+	−	−	+	+	+	+	−
1	2	Netherlands	+	+	+	+	+	+	−	−	+	+	−
1	2	Norway	+	+	+	+	+	+	+	+	+	+	+
1	2	Spain	−	−	−	−	−	−	−	−	−	−	−
1	2	Sweden	+	+	+	+	+	+	+	+	+	+	+
1	2	Switzerland	−	−	−	−	+	−	−	−	−	−	−
1	2	United Kingdom	+	+	+	+	−	+	+	+	+	+	+
1	3	Australia	+	+	+	+	−	+	+	+	+	+	+
1	3	Fiji	+	+	+	−	−	−	−	+	+	−	−
1	3	Kiribati	+	+	−	+	−	−	−	−	+	+	+
1	3	Micronesia, Fed. Sts.	+	+	−	−	−	−	+	+	−	+	−
1	3	New Zealand	+	+	+	+	+	−	+	+	+	+	+
1	3	Papua New Guinea	+	+	+	+	+	+	−	+	+	−	−
1	3	Solomon Islands	−	−	+	+	−	−	−	−	−	+	−
1	3	Vanuatu	+	+	+	+	−	+	+	+	+	+	−
1	3	Western Samoa	+	+	+	+	−	−	−	−	+	−	−
1	4	Argentina	−	−	−	−	−	−	−	−	−	−	−
1	4	Belize	−	+	+	+	+	−	−	+	+	−	−

(continued)

545

Table D-7.4. Government national AIDS programs: needs and services—condom distribution sites, 1990; prevention needs categories 990A through 990K*—continued

List	GAA	Country	PN990A	PN990B	PN990C	PN990D	PN990E	PN990F	PN990G	PN990H	PN990I	PN990J	PN990K
1	4	Brazil	+	−	−	−	+	−	−	−	−	−	−
1	4	Chile	+	+	−	−	+	−	−	−	−	−	−
1	4	Colombia	+	+	−	+	+	−	−	−	+	−	−
1	4	Costa Rica	+	+	+	+	+	−	−	+	+	−	−
1	4	Ecuador	−	−	−	−	−	−	−	−	−	+	+
1	4	El Salvador	+	+	+	+	+	+	+	−	+	+	−
1	4	Guatemala	+	+	+	+	+	−	+	+	−	−	+
1	4	Mexico	+	+	−	−	+	−	+	+	+	−	−
1	4	Panama	+	+	−	−	+	−	−	+	+	−	−
1	4	Peru	−	−	−	−	−	−	−	−	−	−	−
1	4	Suriname	+	+	+	+	+	+	+	+	+	+	+
1	4	Uruguay	+	+	+	−	+	−	−	+	+	+	+
1	4	Venezuela	+	−	−	−	−	−	−	−	+	+	+
1	5	Angola	−	−	−	−	−	−	−	−	−	−	−
1	5	Benin	+	+	+	+	+	−	+	+	+	+	−
1	5	Botswana	+	+	+	+	−	−	+	+	+	+	−
1	5	Burkino Faso	+	+	+	+	+	+	+	+	+	−	−
1	5	Cameroon	+	−	+	+	+	−	+	+	+	+	−
1	5	Cape Verde	+	+	+	+	+	+	−	+	+	+	−
1	5	Chad	−	+	+	−	−	−	−	−	−	−	−
1	5	Comoros	+	+	−	+	+	−	+	−	+	+	−
1	5	Congo	−	+	−	+	+	−	+	−	+	+	−
1	5	Côte d'Ivoire	+	+	+	+	+	+	−	+	+	−	−
1	5	Djibouti	+	+	−	+	+	−	+	−	+	+	−
1	5	Ethiopia	−	+	−	+	−	−	+	−	+	−	−
1	5	Gabon	−	+	+	+	+	+	+	+	−	−	−

546

1												
1	5	Ghana	−	−	−	−	−	−	−	−	−	−
1	5	Guinea	−	−	+	−	−	−	−	−	+	−
1	5	Guinea-Bissau	+	+	+	+	+	+	+	+	+	−
1	5	Lesotho	+	+	+	+	−	+	+	+	+	+
1	5	Madagascar	+	+	+	+	+	+	+	+	+	−
1	5	Mali	+	+	+	−	+	+	−	+	+	−
1	5	Mauritania	+	+	+	+	+	+	+	+	+	−
1	5	Mauritius	+	+	+	−	+	+	−	+	+	−
1	5	Rwanda	+	+	+	+	−	+	−	+	+	−
1	5	Senegal	+	+	+	+	+	+	+	+	+	−
1	5	Seychelles	+	+	+	+	+	+	+	+	+	−
1	5	South Africa	+	+	+	−	−	+	−	+	+	+
1	5	Tanzania	+	+	+	+	+	+	+	+	+	−
1	5	Togo	−	−	−	−	−	−	−	−	−	−
1	5	Uganda	+	+	+	+	+	+	+	+	+	+
1	5	Zaire	+	+	+	+	+	+	+	+	+	+
1	5	Zambia	+	+	+	+	+	+	+	+	+	+
1	5	Zimbabwe	+	+	+	+	+	+	+	+	+	+
1	6	Antigua and Barbuda	+	+	+	+	+	+	+	+	+	+
1	6	Barbados	+	+	+	+	+	+	+	+	+	+
1	6	Dominican Republic	+	+	+	+	+	+	+	+	+	+
1	6	Grenada	+	+	+	+	+	+	+	+	+	+
1	6	Jamaica	+	+	+	+	+	+	+	+	+	+
1	6	St. Lucia	+	+	+	+	+	+	+	+	+	+
1	6	Trinidad and Tobago	−	−	−	−	−	−	−	−	−	−
1	7	Azerbaijan	−	−	−	−	−	−	−	−	−	−
1	7	Belarus	−	−	−	−	−	−	−	−	+	−
1	7	Bulgaria	+	+	+	+	+	+	+	+	+	+
1	7	Croatia	−	−	−	−	−	−	−	−	−	−
1	7	Czech Republic	−	−	−	−	−	−	−	−	−	−

(continued)

547

Table D-7.4 Government national AIDS programs: needs and services—condom distribution sites, 1990; prevention needs categories 990A through 990K*—continued

List	GAA	Country	PN990A	PN990B	PN990C	PN990D	PN990E	PN990F	PN990G	PN990H	PN990I	PN990J	PN990K
1	7	Estonia	+	+	+	+	+	−	−	+	+	+	−
1	7	Hungary	+	+	+	+	−	+	−	+	+	+	−
1	7	Kyrgyz Republic	+	+	+	+	−	+	+	+	+	+	−
1	7	Latvia	−	−	−	−	−	−	−	−	+	−	−
1	7	Lithuania	+	+	+	+	+	+	+	+	+	+	−
1	7	Moldova	−	−	−	−	−	−	−	−	+	+	−
1	7	Russian Federation	−	−	−	−	−	−	−	−	−	−	−
1	7	Slovenia	−	−	+	+	−	−	+	+	+	+	−
1	7	Turkmenistan	−	+	+	+	−	−	+	+	+	+	−
1	7	Ukraine	−	−	−	−	−	−	−	−	−	−	−
1	7	Yugoslavia, Fed. Rep.	−	−	−	−	−	−	−	−	−	−	−
1	8	Algeria	−	+	−	−	−	−	−	+	+	+	−
1	8	Israel	+	+	+	+	+	+	+	+	+	+	−
1	8	Jordan	+	+	−	−	−	+	−	+	+	−	−
1	8	Kuwait	−	−	−	−	−	−	−	−	−	−	−
1	8	Lebanon	−	+	−	+	−	−	−	−	+	+	−
1	8	Morocco	−	+	−	−	+	−	−	+	+	−	−
1	8	Oman	−	−	−	−	−	−	−	−	−	−	−
1	8	Syrian Arab Rep.	−	−	−	−	−	−	−	−	−	−	−
1	8	Tunisia	−	+	+	+	+	−	−	+	+	−	−
1	9	Bhutan	+	+	+	+	+	−	−	+	+	−	−
1	9	China	+	+	−	−	+	−	−	+	+	−	−
1	9	Hong Kong	+	+	−	+	+	−	−	−	+	+	−
1	9	Japan	+	+	−	−	−	−	+	+	+	−	−
1	9	Taiwan	−	−	−	−	−	−	−	+	+	−	−
1	9	Vietnam	+	+	+	−	−	−	−	−	+	−	−

548

List	GAA	Country	PN990A	PN990B	PN990C	PN990D	PN990E	PN990F	PN990G	PN990H	PN990I	PN990J	PN990K
1	10	Brunei	—	—	—	—	—	—	—	—	—	—	—
1	10	India	—	—	—	—	—	—	—	—	—	—	—
1	10	Malaysia	—	+	+	+	+	+	+	—	+	+	—
1	10	Nepal	+	+	+	+	—	+	+	—	+	+	—
1	10	Singapore	+	+	+	+	+	+	+	+	+	+	—
1	10	Sri Lanka	+	—	—	—	—	+	+	+	+	+	—
1	10	Thailand	+	+	+	+	+	+	+	+	+	+	—
2	3	American Samoa	+	+	+	+	+	+	+	—	—	+	—
2	3	Cook Islands	+	+	—	—	—	+	+	—	+	+	—
2	3	Guam	+	+	+	+	+	+	+	+	+	+	—
2	3	New Caledonia	+	+	+	+	+	+	+	+	+	+	—
2	3	Niue	+	—	—	—	—	—	—	+	—	—	—
2	3	Tokelau	+	+	—	—	—	+	—	—	—	—	—
2	3	Tuvalu	+	+	—	—	—	—	—	—	—	+	—
2	6	Bermuda	+	+	+	+	+	+	+	+	+	+	—
2	6	Cayman Islands	+	+	+	+	+	+	+	—	+	+	—
2	6	Montserrat	—	—	—	—	—	—	—	—	—	—	—
2	6	Netherlands Antilles	+	+	+	+	+	+	+	+	+	+	—

List, core country response (1) or subsidiary response (2); GAA, geographic area of affinity; country, territory, or region responding. *Prevention needs abbreviations:* Sites/facilities where the federal/central government allowed the distribution of condoms in 1990: PN990A, sexually transmitted infection clinics; PN990B, other health clinics; PN990C, hotels; PN990D, bars; PN990E, brothels; PN990F, high schools; PN990G, colleges; PN990H, department stores; PN990I, pharmacies/drug stores; PN990J, public places (i.e., bathrooms, bus stations); PN990K, others.

Table D-7.5 Government national AIDS programs: needs and services—condom distribution sites, 1992; prevention needs categories 992A through 992K*

List	GAA	Country	PN992A	PN992B	PN992C	PN992D	PN992E	PN992F	PN992G	PN992H	PN992I	PN992J	PN992K
1	1	United States	+	+	+	+	–	–	+	+	+	+	+
1	2	Austria	–	–	–	–	–	–	–	–	–	–	–
1	2	Belgium	+	+	+	+	+	+	+	+	+	+	–
1	2	Cyprus	+	–	+	+	–	–	+	–	+	–	+
1	2	Denmark	+	+	+	+	+	+	+	+	+	+	+
1	2	Finland	+	+	+	+	–	+	+	+	+	+	–
1	2	France	+	+	–	+	–	+	+	+	+	+	–
1	2	Germany	+	+	+	+	+	+	+	+	+	+	–
1	2	Iceland	–	–	+	+	–	–	–	+	+	+	+
1	2	Liechtenstein	–	–	+	+	+	+	+	+	+	–	–
1	2	Luxembourg	+	+	+	+	+	+	+	+	+	+	+
1	2	Malta	–	–	+	+	–	–	–	–	+	+	–
1	2	Netherlands	+	+	+	+	+	+	+	+	+	+	–
1	2	Norway	+	–	+	+	+	+	+	+	+	+	+
1	2	Spain	+	–	–	+	–	–	–	–	+	–	–
1	2	Sweden	+	+	+	+	+	+	+	+	+	+	+
1	2	Switzerland	–	–	–	–	–	–	–	–	–	–	–
1	2	United Kingdom	+	+	+	+	+	+	+	+	+	+	+
1	3	Australia	+	+	+	+	+	+	+	+	+	+	–
1	3	Fiji	+	+	–	–	–	–	–	–	+	–	+
1	3	Kiribati	+	+	+	+	–	–	+	+	+	+	–
1	3	Micronesia, Fed. Sts.	+	+	+	+	–	–	+	+	+	+	+
1	3	New Zealand	+	+	+	+	–	–	+	+	+	+	–
1	3	Papua New Guinea	+	+	+	+	+	+	+	+	+	–	+
1	3	Solomon Islands	–	–	–	–	–	–	–	–	+	–	–
1	3	Vanuatu	+	+	+	+	+	+	+	+	+	+	–
1	3	Western Samoa	+	+	+	+	–	–	+	+	+	–	+
1	4	Argentina	–	–	–	–	–	–	–	–	–	–	–
1	4	Belize	–	+	+	+	+	–	–	+	+	–	–

		Country												
1	4	Brazil	–	–	–	–	–	+	–	–	–	–	+
1	4	Chile	–	–	–	–	–	+	–	–	–	+	+
1	4	Colombia	–	+	+	+	+	+	+	+	+	+	+
1	4	Costa Rica	–	–	+	+	+	+	+	+	+	+	+
1	4	Ecuador	–	–	–	–	–	–	–	–	–	–	–
1	4	El Salvador	–	+	+	–	–	+	+	+	–	+	+
1	4	Guatemala	+	–	+	+	+	+	+	+	+	+	+
1	4	Mexico	–	+	+	+	+	+	–	+	+	+	+
1	4	Panama	–	–	+	+	+	+	–	+	+	+	+
1	4	Peru	–	–	–	–	–	–	–	–	–	–	–
1	4	Suriname	–	+	+	+	+	+	+	+	+	+	+
1	4	Uruguay	–	+	+	+	+	+	–	+	+	+	+
1	4	Venezuela	–	–	+	–	+	+	–	+	–	+	+
1	5	Angola	+	–	+	–	–	+	–	–	–	–	–
1	5	Benin	+	+	+	+	–	+	+	+	+	+	+
1	5	Botswana	+	+	+	+	+	–	+	+	+	+	+
1	5	Burkino Faso	–	+	+	+	+	+	+	+	+	+	+
1	5	Cameroon	–	+	+	+	+	+	+	+	+	+	+
1	5	Cape Verde	–	+	+	+	+	+	+	+	+	+	+
1	5	Chad	–	–	+	–	+	+	+	–	+	–	–
1	5	Comoros	–	–	+	–	+	–	+	+	+	+	+
1	5	Congo	–	+	+	+	+	+	+	+	+	+	+
1	5	Côte d'Ivoire	–	+	+	+	+	+	+	+	+	+	+
1	5	Djibouti	–	–	–	+	+	+	+	+	–	–	+
1	5	Ethiopia	–	+	–	+	+	+	+	+	+	+	+
1	5	Gabon	–	–	+	–	+	+	+	+	–	+	–
1	5	Ghana	–	–	–	+	+	–	+	+	+	–	–
1	5	Guinea	–	–	+	–	+	+	–	–	–	–	+
1	5	Guinee-Bissau	–	+	+	+	+	–	+	+	+	+	–

(continued)

Table **D-7.5** Government national AIDS programs: needs and services—condom distribution sites, 1992; prevention needs categories 992A through 992K*—continued

List	GAA	Country	PN992A	PN992B	PN992C	PN992D	PN992E	PN992F	PN992G	PN992H	PN992I	PN992J	PN992K
1	5	Lesotho	+	+	+	+	–	+	+	+	+	–	+
1	5	Madagascar	+	+	+	+	–	–	+	+	+	–	–
1	5	Mali	+	+	+	+	+	+	+	+	+	–	–
1	5	Mauritania	+	+	–	+	–	–	–	–	+	–	–
1	5	Mauritius	+	+	+	–	+	+	+	+	+	+	–
1	5	Rwanda	+	+	+	+	–	–	+	–	+	–	–
1	5	Senegal	+	+	+	+	–	–	+	–	+	–	–
1	5	Seychelles	+	+	+	–	–	–	–	–	+	–	+
1	5	South Africa	+	+	–	–	–	–	+	+	+	+	–
1	5	Tanzania	+	+	+	+	–	–	+	+	–	+	–
1	5	Togo	+	+	+	+	+	+	+	+	+	+	+
1	5	Uganda	+	+	–	–	–	+	+	+	+	+	–
1	5	Zaire	+	+	+	+	+	–	+	–	+	+	–
1	5	Zambia	+	+	+	+	–	–	+	+	+	+	–
1	5	Zimbabwe	+	+	+	+	+	–	+	+	+	+	+
1	6	Antigua and Barbuda	+	+	–	+	+	–	+	–	–	+	+
1	6	Barbados	+	+	+	+	+	–	–	+	+	+	–
1	6	Dominican Republic	+	+	+	+	+	–	–	+	+	+	+
1	6	Grenada	+	+	+	+	–	–	–	+	+	+	–
1	6	Jamaica	+	+	–	+	+	+	–	–	+	–	–
1	6	St. Lucia	+	+	+	+	+	–	–	+	+	–	–
1	6	Trinidad and Tobago	+	+	+	+	+	–	–	–	–	–	–
1	7	Azerbaijan	–	–	–	–	–	–	–	–	–	–	–
1	7	Belarus	+	+	+	–	–	–	–	–	+	–	–
1	7	Bulgaria	+	+	+	+	–	+	+	+	+	+	–
1	7	Croatia	–	–	–	–	–	–	–	–	+	–	+
1	7	Czech Republic	–	–	–	–	+	–	–	–	–	–	–
1	7	Estonia	–	–	+	–	–	–	–	+	+	–	–
1	7	Hungary	+	+	+	+	–	+	–	+	+	+	–

552

	Group	Country										
1	7	Kyrgyz Republic	+	+	+	+	+	–	–	+	+	—
1	7	Latvia	–	–	–	–	–	–	–	–	–	—
1	7	Lithuania	+	+	+	+	+	+	+	+	+	—
1	7	Moldova	–	–	–	–	–	–	–	–	+	—
1	7	Russian Federation	—	—	—	—	—	—	—	—	—	—
1	7	Slovenia	—	+	–	–	+	–	+	+	+	—
1	7	Turkmenistan	–	+	–	+	+	–	+	+	+	—
1	7	Ukraine	—	—	—	—	—	—	—	—	—	—
1	7	Yugoslavia, Fed. Rep.	—	—	—	—	—	—	—	—	—	—
1	8	Algeria	+	+	–	–	–	–	+	+	+	—
1	8	Israel	+	+	+	+	+	+	+	+	+	—
1	8	Jordan	+	+	+	+	+	+	+	+	+	—
1	8	Kuwait	—	—	—	—	—	—	—	—	—	—
1	8	Lebanon	—	+	–	+	+	—	+	+	+	—
1	8	Morocco	—	+	–	+	+	—	+	+	+	—
1	8	Oman	—	—	—	—	—	—	—	—	—	—
1	8	Syrian Arab Rep.	—	—	—	—	—	—	—	—	—	—
1	8	Tunisia	+	+	+	+	+	+	+	+	+	—
1	9	Bhutan	+	+	–	+	+	+	+	+	+	—
1	9	China	+	+	–	+	+	+	+	+	+	—
1	9	Hong Kong	+	+	+	+	+	+	+	+	+	—
1	9	Japan	+	+	–	+	+	–	+	+	+	—
1	9	Taiwan	—	—	—	—	—	—	—	—	—	—
1	9	Vietnam	+	+	+	+	–	–	+	+	+	—
1	10	Brunei	—	—	—	—	—	—	—	—	—	—
1	10	India	—	—	—	—	—	—	—	—	—	—
1	10	Malaysia	+	+	+	+	+	–	+	+	+	—
1	10	Nepal	+	+	–	+	+	+	+	+	–	—
1	10	Singapore	+	+	+	+	+	+	+	+	+	—

(continued)

Table D-7.5 Government national AIDS programs: needs and services—condom distribution sites, 1992; prevention needs categories 992A through 992K*—continued

List	GAA	Country	PN992A	PN992B	PN992C	PN992D	PN992E	PN992F	PN992G	PN992H	PN992I	PN992J	PN992K
1	10	Sri Lanka	+	−	−	−	+	−	−	+	+	+	−
1	10	Thailand	+	+	+	+	+	−	−	+	+	+	−
2	3	American Samoa	+	+	+	+	−	−	−	−	−	−	−
2	3	Cook Islands	+	+	−	−	−	−	−	−	+	−	−
2	3	Guam	+	+	−	+	−	−	+	−	+	−	−
2	3	New Caledonia	+	+	−	+	−	−	−	+	+	+	−
2	3	Niue	+	−	−	−	−	−	−	+	−	−	−
2	3	Tokelau	+	+	−	−	−	−	−	−	−	−	−
2	3	Tuvalu	+	+	+	+	−	−	−	−	+	−	−
2	6	Bermuda	+	+	−	+	−	−	+	−	+	+	−
2	6	Cayman Islands	+	+	+	+	+	−	−	−	+	−	−
2	6	Montserrat	−	−	−	−	−	−	−	−	−	−	−
2	6	Netherlands Antilles	+	+	+	+	+	+	+	+	+	+	−

*List, core country response (1) or subsidiary response (2); GAA, geographic area of affinity; country, territory, or region responding.

Prevention needs abbreviations: Sites/facilities where the federal/central government allowed the distribution of condoms in 1992: PN992A, sexually transmitted infection clinics; PN992B, other health clinics; PN992C, hotels; PN992D, bars; PN992E, brothels; PN992F, high schools; PN992G, colleges; PN992H, department stores; PN992I, pharmacies/drug stores; PN992J, public places (i.e., bathrooms, bus stations); PN992K, others.

Table D-7.6 Government national AIDS programs: needs and services—HIV testing and counseling, sites and practices; prevention needs categories 992KEXP through 17*

List	GAA	Country	PN992KEXP	PN10	PN11	PN12	PN13A	PN13B	PN13C	PN16	PN16A	PN17
1	1	United States	community organizations (some states distr)	E	S	Q4	+++	+++	+++	—	—	—
1	2	Austria		E	S	Q4	+++	+++	+++	—	—	?
1	2	Belgium		E	S	—	+++	+++	—	1,600,000	R	++
1	2	Cyprus	military camps	E	S	Q1	++	+++	+	—	E	++
1	2	Denmark		E	S	—	+	+	+	450,000	R	---
1	2	Finland		E	S	Q4	++	+++	++	400,000	R	=
1	2	France		E	S	Q3	++	+++	++	4,000,000	E	++
1	2	Germany		E	S	Q4	+++	+++	+++	—	—	—
1	2	Iceland	yearly outdoor festivals	U	S	Q4	++	+++	++	11,903	R	=
1	2	Liechtenstein		E	S	Q1	+	++	·	300	E	++
1	2	Luxembourg	everywhere	E	S	—	—	+++	—	—	—	—
1	2	Malta		E	S	Q1	++	++	++	3,000	R	=
1	2	Netherlands		E	S	Q3	++	++	++	1,100,000	E	++
1	2	Norway	outreach IDU, sexwork, mwm	E	S	Q4	+++	+++	+++	300,000	R	=
1	2	Spain		E	S	Q4	++	+++	+	—	—	?
1	2	Sweden	petrol sta/grocery st/news stands	E	S	Q3	++	+++	++	370,000	R	=
1	2	Switzerland		E	PS	Q2	++	++	+	—	RE	—
1	2	United Kingdom		E	S	Q4	+++	+++	+++	250,000	RE	=
1	3	Australia		E	S	Q4	++	+++	++	2,000,000	R	++
1	3	Fiji		E	S	Q3	+++	+++	++	16,000	R	++
1	3	Kiribati	night clubs	U	S	Q1	+++	+++	+++	950	R	++
1	3	Micronesia, Fed. Sts.		U	S	Q2	++	++	++	3,681	R	+++
1	3	New Zealand	service stations	E	S	Q4	+++	+++	+++	—	—	—

(continued)

Table D-7.6 Government national AIDS programs: needs and services—HIV testing and counseling, sites and practices; prevention needs categories 992KEXP through 17ᵃ—continued

List	GAA	Country	PN992KEXP	PN10	PN11	PN12	PN13A	PN13B	PN13C	PN16	PN16A	PN17
1	3	Papua New Guinea		U	S	Q1	+++	++	++	35,000	E	++
1	3	Solomon Islands		U	S	—	—	—	—	—	—	—
1	3	Vanuatu		U	S	Q1	+++	—	+++	3,676	R	?
1	3	Western Samoa		U	S	Q4	+++	+++	+++	2,555	R	++
1	4	Argentina		—	—	—	—	—	—	—	—	—
1	4	Belize		E	S	Q2	+	+++	+++	—	—	—
1	4	Brazil		U	S	Q1	++	++	++	—	—	?
1	4	Chile		E	S	Q2	++	+++	++	—	R	+++
1	4	Colombia		U	P	Q3	++	+++	+	—	—	—
1	4	Costa Rica		E	S	Q2	++	+++	++	—	E	++
1	4	Ecuador		U	P	Q1	+	++	++	71,000	R	+++
1	4	El Salvador		E	S	Q1	++	+++	++	56,834	R	++
1	4	Guatemala	motels	U	—	Q1	+++	+++	+	—	—	—
1	4	Mexico		U	S	Q3	+++	+++	++	1,500,000	E	—
1	4	Panama		E	PS	Q1	+	++	++	55,079	R	++
1	4	Peru		U	P	Q1	+++	+++	+++	20,000	E	+++
1	4	Suriname	prisons	E	S	Q4	+++	+++	+++	6,564	R	++
1	4	Uruguay		E	S	Q3	++	+++	++	—	—	+++
1	4	Venezuela		E	S	Q1	++	++	+	350,000	R	=
1	5	Angola	consultation family planning	U	S	Q1	++	++	++	—	R	∷
1	5	Benin	gas stations	U	P	Q4	+++	+++	+++	12,000	R	=
1	5	Botswana	workplaces; border posts	E	S	Q4	++	+++	++	—	—	—
1	5	Burkino Faso		U	S	Q4	++	++	++	—	—	—
1	5	Cameroon	no longer distr, sold cheap soc market	U	P	Q4	+++	+++	+++	20,000	E	+++
1	5	Cape Verde		U	S	Q3	+++	+++	+++	3,000	R	=

556

		Country	Notes										
1	5	Chad		U	S	Q4	+++	+++	+++	—	8,000		
1	5	Comoros		E	PS	Q1	+++	+++	+++	++	8,000	R	—
1	5	Congo		U	PS	Q4	++	++	++	++	—		—
1	5	Côte d'Ivoire		U	S	Q4	+++	+++	+++	+++	—		—
1	5	Djibouti		E	S	—	+	++	++	+	15,000	E	+++
1	5	Ethiopia		U	S	Q3	++	++	++	+	19,660	R	++
1	5	Gabon		U	P	Q1	+	+	+	+	3,338	R	-
1	5	Ghana				—	++	+++	+++	+++	60,000	E	++
1	5	Guinea				Q1	++	+++	+++	+++	—	R	++
1	5	Guinee-Bissau		U	S	Q4	+++	++	++	+++	—		—
1	5	Lesotho	govt & nongovt depts	U	P	Q2	++	++	++	++	20,086	RE	+++
1	5	Madagascar		U	S	Q4	+++	+++	+++	+++	23,677	R	++
1	5	Mali		U	S	Q3	++	++	++	++	15,000	R	++
1	5	Mauritania		U	S	Q1	+	++	++	++	3,900	R	++
1	5	Mauritius		E	S	Q4	+++	+++	+++	+++	20,173	R	=
1	5	Rwanda		U	PS	Q4	+++	-	-	-	53,500	RE	+++
1	5	Senegal		U	S	Q3	++	+++	+++	++	23,000	R	++
1	5	Seychelles		E	S	Q4	++	+++	+++	++	5,976	R	++
1	5	South Africa	NGOs/CBOs/ASOs	E	S	—	++	++	++	+++	—		+++
1	5	Tanzania		U	S	Q1	+++	+++	+++	+++	200,000	E	=
1	5	Togo	at low price (free to some)	U	P	Q4	+++	+++	+++	+++	25,000	R	+++
1	5	Uganda	workshop participants	U	S	Q4	+	+	+	+	—		—
1	5	Zaire		U	P	Q1	+++	+	+	+	12,449	R	+++
1	5	Zambia		E	S	Q3	+++	+++	+++	+++	—		—
1	5	Zimbabwe		U	S	Q1	++	+++	+++	++	6,020	R	++
1	6	Antigua and Barbuda	groceries/barber, hair salons			—	+++	+++	+++	+++	—		—
1	6	Barbados		E	S	Q3	++	+++	+++	++	12,672	R	=
1	6	Dominican Republic	small and super markets; prisons	E		Q1	+	+	+	+	110,628	R	++
1	6	Grenada		U	S	Q3	+	++	++	+	1,847	R	++

(continued)

557

Table D-7.6 Government national AIDS programs: needs and services—HIV testing and counseling, sites and practices; prevention needs categories 992KEXP through 17*—continued

List	GAA	Country	PN992KEXP	PN10	PN11	PN12	PN13A	PN13B	PN13C	PN16	PN16A	PN17
1	6	Jamaica		E	S	Q3	++	++	++	50,000	E	++
1	6	St. Lucia		U	S	Q4	+++	+++	+++	5,000	R	+++
1	6	Trinidad and Tobago		E	S	Q4	+++	+++	++	18,718	R	—
1	7	Azerbaijan		E	S	Q4	+++	+++	+++	439,417	R	++
1	7	Belarus		E	S	Q4	+++	+++	++	2,500,000	R	- - -
1	7	Bulgaria		E	S	Q4	+++	+++	++	701,000	R	- -
1	7	Croatia		E	S	Q4	+++	+++	++	—	R	++
1	7	Czech Republic		E	—	Q3	++	++	++	600,000	—	++
1	7	Estonia		E	S	Q4	+++	+++	++	193,587	RE	=
1	7	Hungary		E	S	Q4	++	+++	++	600,000	R	- -
1	7	Kyrgyz Republic		E	S	Q3	++	—	+	7,718	R	- -
1	7	Latvia		U	S	Q2	++	++	+	470,000	R	=
1	7	Lithuania		E	P	Q1	++	+++	+	330,000	R	- -
1	7	Moldova		—	—	Q1	+++	—	—	768,638	E	=
1	7	Russian Federation		U	S	Q3	+++	++	+	24,290,472	—	=
1	7	Slovenia		E	P	Q1	+	++	+	105,000	E	++
1	7	Turkmenistan		E	S	Q1	+	+++	+	676,600	R	+++
1	7	Ukraine		E	S	Q1	++	+++	++	6,700,000	E	++
1	7	Yugoslavia, Fed. Rep.		U	P	Q2	+	+++	·	242,991	R	?
1	8	Algeria		U	S	Q1	—	++	—	—	R	++
1	8	Israel		E	S	Q4	++	+++	++	300,000	R	++
1	8	Jordan		U	PS	Q1	+	+	+	134,000	R	++
1	8	Kuwait		U	P	Q1	++	+++	++	533,868	—	+++
1	8	Lebanon		U	P	Q1	—	—	—	—	R	+++
1	8	Morocco		U	S	Q4	++	++	++	140,000	E	++
1	8	Oman		E	S	Q3	++	+++	+	250,000	R	?
1	8	Syrian Arab Rep.		E	P	—	—	—	—	—	—	- -
1	8	Tunisia		E	S	—	++	+++	+++	114,538	R	++

List	GAA	Country	PN10	PN11	PN12	PN13A	PN13B	PN13C	PN16	PN16A	No. tests	RE	Dir.
1	9	Bhutan	U	S	Q2	+++	+++	+++	++	R	5,500	R	++
1	9	China	E	P	Q1	++	+++	++	++	R	831,561	R	+++
1	9	Hong Kong	E	S	Q4	+++	+++	+++	+++	R	200,000	R	=
1	9	Japan	E	S	Q4	+++	+++	+++	+++	—	—	—	—
1	9	Taiwan	E	S	—	—	—	—	—	R	1,680,857	R	—
1	9	Vietnam	E	S	Q2	+++	+++	+++	++	R	46,916	R	=
1	10	Brunei	E	S	Q4	++	+++	+++	++	R	15,222	R	++
1	10	India	E	PS	Q1	·	+	·	·	—	—	—	+++
1	10	Malaysia	E	S	Q1	+++	+++	+++	+++	R	270,000	R	++
1	10	Nepal	U	—	—	—	—	—	—	—	—	—	—
1	10	Singapore	E	P	Q4	—	—	—	—	—	—	—	—
1	10	Sri Lanka	U	P	Q1	++	+++	+++	++	—	—	—	++
1	10	Thailand	E	PS	Q2	++	+++	+++	++	E	900,000	E	+++
2	3	American Samoa	—	S	Q2	+++	·	·	·	E	100	E	---
2	3	Cook Islands	U	S	Q3	++	—	+	+	E	500	E	+++
2	3	Guam	E	S	Q4	+++	+++	+++	+++	R	1,647	R	++
2	3	New Caledonia	E	S	Q4	++	+++	+++	++	R	—	R	=
2	3	Niue	E	S	Q1	++	++	—	=	—	—	—	—
2	3	Tokelau	N	—	—	—	—	—	—	—	—	—	—
2	3	Tuvalu	U	S	Q1	++	++	++	·	R	130	R	—
2	6	Bermuda	E	P	Q4	++	++	++	++	E	2,200	E	=
2	6	Cayman Islands	E	PS	Q3	++	+++	+++	++	E	4,500	E	++
2	6	Montserrat	E	S	Q4	+++	+++	+++	+++	R	814	R	++
2	6	Netherlands Antilles	E	S	Q1	+++	+++	+++	+++	R	20,000	R	=

*List, core country response (1) or subsidiary response (2); GAA, geographic area of affinity; country, territory, or region responding.
Prevention needs abbreviations: Sites/facilities where the federal/central government allowed the distribution of condoms in 1992: PN992KEXP, other specified. PN10, voluntary HIV testing is now offered: E = everywhere in the country; U = only in the capital or other large cities; N = nowhere in the country. PN11, where voluntary HIV testing is offered, in most cases testing costs are paid for by: P = person tested; S = subsidized by the federal/central government, NGOs, and/or other institutions: PS = both. PN12, the proportion of persons receiving voluntary HIV testing who also receive counseling (an estimate was requested): Q1 = 0–25%; Q2 = 26%–50%; Q3 = 51%–75%; Q4 = 76%–100%.

For those persons receiving HIV counselling, it is provided (+ + + = always; + + = sometimes; + = rarely; – = never): PN13A, prior to HIV testing to all persons requesting voluntary HIV testing; PN13B, after the HIV test: to those persons found to be HIV positive; PN13C, after the HIV test: to those persons found to be HIV negative. PN16, country-wide, the number of HIV tests performed in 1992; PN16A, number of HIV tests performed in 1992: PN16A, number of HIV tests performed in 1992 was obtained from reports (R), estimates (E), or both (RE). PN17, direction of change in the number of HIV tests since 1990: + + + = increased considerably (greater than 2-fold), + + = increased moderately (1- to 2-fold), = = did not increase or decrease (remained stable), – – = decreased moderately (1- to 2-fold), – – – = decreased considerably (greater than 2-fold), ? = cannot estimate.

Table D-8 Government national AIDS programs: behavioral surveys/studies conducted since 1990*

List	GAA	Country	BR1	BR1A	BR1B	BR1C	BR1D	BR1NUM
1	1	United States	+	1990	1991	1992	—	—
1	2	Austria	—	—	—	—	—	—
1	2	Belgium	+	1990	1991	1992	1993	4,000
1	2	Cyprus	—	—	—	—	—	—
1	2	Denmark	—	—	—	—	—	—
1	2	Finland	+	1991	1992	1993	—	1,500
1	2	France	+	1990	1992	1994	—	20,000
1	2	Germany	+	1990	1991	1992	1993	2,000
1	2	Iceland	+	1992	—	—	—	975
1	2	Liechtenstein	+	1992	—	—	—	400
1	2	Luxembourg	—	—	—	—	—	—
1	2	Malta	—	—	—	—	—	—
1	2	Netherlands	+	1990	1991	1992	1993	11,500
1	2	Norway	+	1992	—	—	—	10,000
1	2	Spain	—	—	—	—	—	—
1	2	Sweden	+	1990	—	—	—	2,000
1	2	Switzerland	+	1990	1991	1992	1993	2,500
1	2	United Kingdom	+	1990	1991	1992	1993	—
1	3	Australia	+	1990	1991	1992	1993	2,600
1	3	Fiji	—	—	—	—	—	—
1	3	Kiribati	+	1991	1993	—	—	250
1	3	Micronesia, Fed. Sts.	—	—	—	—	—	—
1	3	New Zealand	—	—	—	—	—	—
1	3	Papua New Guinea	+	1991	1992	—	—	—
1	3	Solomon Islands	+	1991	—	—	—	—
1	3	Vanuatu	+	1992	—	—	—	600
1	3	Western Samoa	—	—	—	—	—	—
1	4	Argentina	—	—	—	—	—	—
1	4	Belize	—	—	—	—	—	—
1	4	Brazil	+	1990	1991	—	—	2,000
1	4	Chile	—	—	—	—	—	—
1	4	Colombia	+	1993	—	—	—	—
1	4	Costa Rica	+	1989	1991	1992	1993	3,000
1	4	Ecuador	+	1989	1990	1991	1992	760
1	4	El Salvador	—	—	—	—	—	—
1	4	Guatemala	+	—	—	—	—	1,000
1	4	Mexico	+	1991	1992	1993	—	9,274
1	4	Panama	—	—	—	—	—	—
1	4	Peru	+	1990	1991	1992	1993	470
1	4	Suriname	+	1990	1991	1992	1993	4,500
1	4	Uruguay	+	1990	1991	—	—	1,500
1	4	Venezuela	—	—	—	—	—	—
1	5	Angola	—	—	—	—	—	—
1	5	Benin	+	1989	1991	1992	—	7,500

List	GAA	Country	BR1	BR1A	BR1B	BR1C	BR1D	BR1NUM
1	5	Botswana	+	1992	1993	—	—	1,190
1	5	Burkino Faso	+	1990	1991	1992	1993	5,000
1	5	Cameroon	+	1990	—	—	—	1,091
1	5	Cape Verde	+	1992	—	—	—	5,000
1	5	Chad	+	1991	1992	—	—	3,000
1	5	Comoros	+	1993	—	—	—	50
1	5	Congo	+	1991	—	—	—	200
1	5	Côte d'Ivoire	+	1990	1992	1993	—	3,000
1	5	Djibouti	+	1992	—	—	—	—
1	5	Ethiopia	+	1990	1991	1992	1993	8,000
1	5	Gabon	+	1990	—	—	—	400
1	5	Ghana	+	1991	1992	1993	—	1,973
1	5	Guinea	+	1990	1993	—	—	3,000
1	5	Guinee-Bissau	—	—	—	—	—	—
1	5	Lesotho	—	—	—	—	—	—
1	5	Madagascar	+	1989	1990	1991	1992	1,000
1	5	Mali	+	1990	1992	—	—	—
1	5	Mauritania	+	1993	—	—	—	1,500
1	5	Mauritius	+	1991	1992	1993	—	498
1	5	Rwanda	—	—	—	—	—	—
1	5	Senegal	+	—	—	—	—	5,000
1	5	Seychelles	—	—	—	—	—	—
1	5	South Africa	+	1991	1992	1993	—	—
1	5	Tanzania	—	—	—	—	—	—
1	5	Togo	+	1989	1991	1992	—	2,332
1	5	Uganda	+	1991	1992	—	—	1,000
1	5	Zaire	+	1990	1991	—	—	5,118
1	5	Zambia	+	—	—	—	—	—
1	5	Zimbabwe	+	1990	1991	1992	1993	—
1	6	Antigua and Barbuda	+	—	—	—	—	1,000
1	6	Barbados	+	1990	—	—	—	509
1	6	Dominican Republic	—	—	—	—	—	—
1	6	Grenada	+	1991	—	—	—	600
1	6	Jamaica	+	1992	—	—	—	4,000
1	6	St. Lucia	+	1990	1992	1991	—	150
1	6	Trinidad and Tobago	+	1991	1992	—	—	—
1	7	Azerbaijan	—	—	—	—	—	—
1	7	Belarus	—	—	—	—	—	—
1	7	Bulgaria	+	1991	1993	—	—	800
1	7	Croatia	—	—	—	—	—	—
1	7	Czech Republic	+	1991	1992	1993	—	100
1	7	Estonia	+	1991	—	—	—	300
1	7	Hungary	+	1991	1993	—	—	2,000
1	7	Kyrgyz Republic	+	1990	1991	—	—	4,000
1	7	Latvia	—	—	—	—	—	—
1	7	Lithuania	+	1990	1992	1993	—	900

(continued)

Table D-8 Government national AIDS programs: behavioral surveys/studies conducted since 1990*—continued

List	GAA	Country	BR1	BR1A	BR1B	BR1C	BR1D	BR1NUM
1	7	Moldova	–	—	—	—	—	—
1	7	Russian Federation	–	—	—	—	—	—
1	7	Slovenia	—	—	—	—	—	—
1	7	Turkmenistan	+	1990	—	—	—	200
1	7	Ukraine	+	—	—	—	1993	5,000
1	7	Yugoslavia, Fed. Rep.	+	1989	1990	1991	1992	800
1	8	Algeria	–	—	—	—	—	—
1	8	Israel	–	—	—	—	—	—
1	8	Jordan	+	1990	—	—	—	7,500
1	8	Kuwait	–	—	—	—	—	—
1	8	Lebanon	–	—	—	—	—	—
1	8	Morocco	+	1990	1991	—	—	2,064
1	8	Oman	–	—	—	—	—	—
1	8	Syrian Arab Rep.	—	—	—	—	—	—
1	8	Tunisia	+	1990	1991	1992	1993	1,440
1	9	Bhutan	–	—	—	—	—	—
1	9	China	+	1992	—	—	—	—
1	9	Hong Kong	+	1991	1992	1993	—	500
1	9	Japan	+	—	—	—	—	—
1	9	Taiwan	—	—	—	—	—	—
1	9	Vietnam	+	1990	1993	—	—	15,000
1	10	Brunei	–	—	—	—	—	—
1	10	India	+	1991	1992	1993	—	5,000
1	10	Malaysia	+	1992	—	—	—	2,270
1	10	Nepal	—	—	—	—	—	—
1	10	Singapore	+	1990	1992	1993	—	2,000
1	10	Sri Lanka	+	1993	1992	—	—	—
1	10	Thailand	+	1990	1991	1992	1993	2,800
2	3	American Samoa	–	—	—	—	—	—
2	3	Cook Islands	–	—	—	—	—	—
2	3	Guam	+	1989	—	—	—	116
2	3	New Caledonia	–	—	—	—	—	—
2	3	Niue	–	—	—	—	—	—
2	3	Tokelau	–	—	—	—	—	—
2	3	Tuvalu	–	—	—	—	—	—
2	6	Bermuda	+	1994	—	—	—	—
2	6	Cayman Islands	–	—	—	—	—	—
2	6	Montserrat	–	—	—	—	—	—
2	6	Netherlands Antilles	+	1991	—	—	—	432

*List, core country response (1) or subsidiary response (2); GAA, geographic area of affinity; country, territory, or region responding.

Behavioral research abbreviations: BR1, one or more surveys/studies on sexual behavior (also called sex surveys) have been carried out in the country since January 1, 1990. BR1A, BR1B, BR1C, BR1D, years in which the surveys/studies were conducted; BR1NUM, approximate number of respondents in the most extensive study/survey conducted.

Table D-9.1 Government national AIDS programs: evaluation practices; evaluation categories 1A through 5HEXP*

List	GAA	Country	EV1A	EV1B	EV1C	EV2	EV4A	EV4B	EV4C	EV4D	EV5A	EV5B	EV5C	EV5D	EV5E	EV5F	EV5G	EV5H	EV5HEXP
1	1	United States	+	+	+	1989	+	+	–	–	+	+	+	+	–	+	+	–	
1	2	Austria	+	+	+	1985	–	–	–	–	+	–	–	–	–	–	+	–	
1	2	Belgium	+	–	–	1991	–	–	–	–	+	+	–	+	+	+	–	–	
1	2	Cyprus	+	+	+	1993	+	+	+	+	+	–	–	+	+	+	+	–	
1	2	Denmark	–	–	–	—	–	–	–	–	–	–	–	+	–	–			–	
1	2	Finland	+	+	–	1986	+	–	+	–	+	+	–	+	+	+	+	–	
1	2	France	+	+	+	1989	+	+	–	+	+	+	+	+	–	+	+	–	
1	2	Germany	+	–	+	1987	+	–	–	–	+	+	–	+	+	+	+	–	distribution of education materials
1	2	Iceland	+		–	1992	+	–	+	–	+	–	–	+	–	+	–	+	
1	2	Liechtenstein	+	–		1988	–		+	–	+	–	–	+	–	+	+	–	
1	2	Luxembourg	+	+	+	1989	+	–	+	–	–	–	+	+	+	+	–	–	
1	2	Malta	–	–	–	—	–	–	–	–	–	–	+	+	+	+		–	
1	2	Netherlands	+	+	+	—	+	+	+	+	+	+	+	+	+	+	+	–	
1	2	Norway	–	+	+	1986	+	+	+	–	+	+	+	+	–	+	+	+	eval descriptive & qualitative
1	2	Spain	+	+	+	1992	+	+	+	+	+	+	+	+	+	+		–	
1	2	Sweden	+	+	+	1989	+	+	+	–	+	+	+	+	+	+	+	–	
1	2	Switzerland	+	+	+	1987	+	–	+	+	–	+	+	+	–	+	+	–	
1	2	United Kingdom	+	+	+	1987	+	+	+	+	+	+	+	+	+	+	+	–	
1	3	Australia	+	+	+	1986	+	+	+	+		+	+		+		+	+	quality assessment of health care impact on legislation, discrimination
1	3	Fiji	+	+	+	1993	+	+	+	+	–	+	–	–	+	–	–	+	program mgmt/activities funded by WHO
1	3	Kiribati	+	–		1993	+	+	+	+	+	+	+	+	+	+	–	–	
1	3	Micronesia, Fed. Sts.	+	+	+	1988	+	+	+	+	+	+	+	+	+	+	+	–	
1	3	New Zealand	–	+	+	1986	+	–	+	–	+	+	+	+	+	+	+	–	
1	3	Papua New Guinea	+	–	+	1992	+	+	+	+	–	–	+	+	+	+	+	+	capacity for program implementation at provincial and district levels
1	3	Solomon Islands	+	+	+	1989	+		–	+	+	–	–	–	–	+	–	–	
1	3	Vanuatu	+	–	+	1990	+	+	+	+	–	–	–	+	–	+	+	–	
1	3	Western Samoa	+	–	–	1992	+	+	+	+	–	+	–	+	+	+	–	–	

(continued)

Table D-9.1 Government national AIDS programs: evaluation practices; evaluation categories 1A through 5HEXP*—continued

List	GAA	Country	EV1A	EV1B	EV1C	EV2	EV4A	EV4B	EV4C	EV4D	EV5A	EV5B	EV5C	EV5D	EV5E	EV5F	EV5G	EV5H	EV5HEXP
1	4	Argentina	−	−	−	−	−	−	−	−	−	−	−	−	−	−	−	−	
1	4	Belize	−	−	−	−	−	−	−	−	−	−	−	−	−	−	−	−	
1	4	Brazil	+	+	+	1989	+	−	−	+	+	+	−	+	+	+	+	+	No. of behavior interventions/injecting drug users/AIDS at work/community programs
1	4	Chile	+	+	+	1991	+	−	−	+	+	+	−	+	+	+	+	−	
1	4	Colombia	−	−	−	−	−	−	−	−	−	−	−	−	−	−	−	−	
1	4	Costa Rica	+	−	−	1993	+	−	−	+	−	−	−	+	+	+	+	−	
1	4	Ecuador	+	−	+	1989	+	+	+	+	−	−	−	−	+	+	+	−	
1	4	El Salvador	+	+	+	1989	+	+	−	+	+	+	−	+	+	+	+	−	
1	4	Guatemala	+	−	+	1987	+	−	−	+	+	+	+	+	+	+	+	+	religious groups involved in prevention & counsel
1	4	Mexico	+	+	+	1992	+	−	+	+	+	+	−	−	+	+	+	−	
1	4	Panama	+	−	−	1991	+	−	−	+	−	−	−	+	−	−	−	+	adminin/prevention/surveil/educ
1	4	Peru	+	−	−	1992	+	−	+	+	+	+	−	−	+	+	−	−	
1	4	Suriname	+	+	−	1990	+	−	+	+	+	+	−	+	+	+	+	−	
1	4	Uruguay	+	+	+	1991	+	+	+	+	−	+	−	+	−	+	+	−	
1	4	Venezuela	+	−	+	−	−	−	−	+	+	+	−	+	−	+	−	−	
1	5	Angola	+	+	+	1991	+	−	−	+	−	+	−	+	+	+	−	−	
1	5	Benin	+	+	+	1990	+	+	+	+	−	+	−	+	+	+	+	−	
1	5	Botswana	+	−	+	1990	+	+	+	+	−	+	−	+	+	+	+	−	
1	5	Burkino Faso	+	+	+	1988	+	+	+	+	−	+	−	+	+	+	+	+	result of activities done & replanning
1	5	Cameroon	+	+	−	1989	+	+	+	+	+	+	−	+	+	+	+	+	budget allowances/program mgmt
1	5	Cape Verde	+	+	+	−	+	+	+	+	+	+	−	+	+	+	+	−	
1	5	Chad	+	+	−	1990	+	+	+	+	+	+	−	+	+	+	+	−	
1	5	Comoros	+	+	+	1991	+	−	+	+	+	+	−	+	−	+	−	+	(many) no. health care workers trained; no. info activities
1	5	Congo	+	−	−	1990	+	+	+	+	−	−	−	+	−	+	−	−	
1	5	Côte d'Ivoire	+	−	−	1990	+	+	+	+	+	−	−	+	−	+	+	−	
1	5	Djibouti	+	+	+	1989	+	+	+	+	+	+	+	+	+	+	+	−	

Table (continued). Program indicators by country. Minus sign (−) = absent/negative; plus sign (+) = present/positive. Column indicator categories (left to right across the indicator columns): "no. of radio spots & no. of people listening"; "structure & mgmt of program/ appropriateness of strategies"; "level of message acquisition"; "no. trained people/no. elaborate educational materials"; "access to care"; "effectiveness of strategies, management, infrastructure".

	Reg	Country	1	2	3	4	5	6	7	8	9	10	11	12	Year	13	14	15
1	5	Ethiopia	−	−	−	−	−	−	−	−	−	−	−	−	—	—	—	−
1	5	Gabon	−	−	−	−	−	−	−	−	+	−	+	+	—	−	−	+
1	5	Ghana	−	+	+	+	−	−	+	+	+	+	+	+	1991	−	−	+
1	5	Guinea	−	−	+	−	+	−	−	+	+	+	+	+	1992	−	−	+
1	5	Guinee-Bissau	−	+	+	−	+	−	−	−	−	−	−	−	1992	−	−	+
1	5	Lesotho	+	+	+	−	+	−	−	+	+	+	+	+	1993	+	−	+
1	5	Madagascar	−	−	+	+	+	−	+	+	+	+	+	+	1992	+	−	+
1	5	Mali	−	−	+	+	+	−	+	+	+	+	−	+	1992	+	+	+
1	5	Mauritania	+	+	+	+	+	−	+	+	+	+	+	+	1990	+	+	+
1	5	Mauritius	−	−	−	−	−	−	−	−	−	−	−	−	—	−	−	−
1	5	Rwanda	+	−	+	−	+	−	+	+	+	+	+	+	1990	−	−	+
1	5	Senegal	−	+	−	+	+	−	+	−	+	+	+	+	1989	+	+	+
1	5	Seychelles	−	−	+	+	+	−	+	−	+	+	+	+	1993	−	−	+
1	5	South Africa	−	−	−	+	+	−	−	−	+	+	+	+	1990	+	+	+
1	5	Tanzania	−	+	+	+	+	+	+	+	+	+	+	+	1989	−	−	+
1	5	Togo	+	+	+	+	+	−	+	+	+	+	+	+	1988	+	−	+
1	5	Uganda	−	+	+	−	−	−	−	+	+	−	+	+	1991	−	+	+
1	5	Zaire	−	−	+	−	+	−	+	+	+	+	+	+	1990	−	−	+
1	5	Zambia	−	+	+	+	+	−	+	+	+	+	+	+	1993	+	+	+
1	5	Zimbabwe	−	−	+	+	+	−	+	+	+	+	+	+	1990	+	+	+
1	6	Antigua and Barbuda	−	−	−	−	−	−	−	−	−	−	−	−	—	−	−	−
1	6	Barbados	−	+	+	+	+	−	+	+	+	+	+	+	1990	−	−	+
1	6	Dominican Republic	−	−	−	−	−	−	−	−	+	−	+	+	—	−	−	−
1	6	Grenada	+	+	+	+	−	−	+	+	+	+	+	+	1991	−	+	+
1	6	Jamaica	+	+	+	+	+	−	+	+	+	+	+	+	1993	+	−	+
1	6	St. Lucia	−	+	+	+	−	−	+	−	+	−	−	+	1990	+	+	+
1	6	Trinidad and Tobago	−	+	+	−	+	−	+	+	+	+	+	+	1990	−	−	+

(continued)

Table D-9.1 Government national AIDS programs: evaluation practices; evaluation categories 1A through 5HEXP*—continued

List	GAA	Country	EV1A	EV1B	EV1C	EV2	EV4A	EV4B	EV4C	EV4D	EV5A	EV5B	EV5C	EV5D	EV5E	EV5F	EV5G	EV5H	EV5HEXP
1	7	Azerbaijan	–	–	–	–	+	+	–	–	–	–	–	–	–	–	–	–	
1	7	Belarus	–	–	–	–	–	–	–	–	–	–	–	–	–	–	–	–	
1	7	Bulgaria	+	+	+	1988	+	–	–	+	+	+	–	+	+	+	+	–	
1	7	Croatia	–	–	–	–	–	–	–	–	–	+	–	–	–	–	+	–	
1	7	Czech Republic	–	–	–	–	–	–	+	–	–	–	–	–	–	–	–	–	
1	7	Estonia	–	–	–	1992	+	+	+	+	+	+	–	+	+	+	–	–	
1	7	Hungary	+	+	+	1990	+	+	+	+	+	+	–	+	+	+	–	–	
1	7	Kyrgyz Republic	–	–	–	–	+	–	–	+	–	+	–	+	+	+	–	+	medical equipment sterilization/logistics/education
1	7	Latvia	–	–	–	–	–	–	–	–	–	–	–	–	–	–	–	–	
1	7	Lithuania	–	–	–	–	–	–	–	–	–	–	–	–	–	–	–	–	
1	7	Moldova	–	–	–	–	–	–	–	–	–	–	–	–	–	–	–	–	
1	7	Russian Federation	–	–	–	–	+	+	–	–	–	–	–	–	–	–	–	–	
1	7	Slovenia	–	–	–	–	–	–	–	–	–	–	–	–	–	–	–	–	
1	7	Turkmenistan	–	–	–	–	–	–	–	–	–	–	–	–	–	–	–	–	
1	7	Ukraine	+	+	–	1992	+	+	–	+	+	+	+	–	+	+	–	–	
1	7	Yugoslavia, Fed. Rep.	–	–	–	–	–	–	–	–	–	–	–	–	–	–	–	–	
1	8	Algeria	–	–	–	–	+	–	+	+	–	–	–	+	–	–	–	–	
1	8	Israel	–	–	–	–	–	–	–	–	–	–	–	–	+	–	–	–	
1	8	Jordan	–	–	–	1993	+	+	–	+	+	+	–	–	+	+	+	–	
1	8	Kuwait	+	+	+	1988	+	–	–	+	+	+	–	+	+	+	–	–	
1	8	Lebanon	–	–	–	–	–	–	–	–	–	–	–	–	–	–	–	–	
1	8	Morocco	+	–	–	1990	+	+	+	+	+	+	–	+	+	+	–	–	
1	8	Oman	+	–	–	1989	–	+	+	–	–	+	–	–	+	–	–	–	
1	8	Syrian Arab Rep.	+	+	–	–	+	+	+	–	–	+	–	–	–	–	–	–	
1	8	Tunisia	+	+	+	1990	+	+	–	+	–	+	+	+	+	+	+	+	evolution of risk factors
1	9	Bhutan	+	–	–	1993	+	+	+	+	+	+	–	+	–	+	–	–	
1	9	China	+	+	+	1993	+	+	–	+	+	+	–	–	+	+	+	–	
1	9	Hong Kong	–	–	–	–	–	–	–	–	–	–	–	–	–	–	–	–	

program management/resources/policies/implementation

List	GAA	EV1A	EV1B	EV1C	EV2	EV4A	EV4B	EV4C	EV4D	EV5A	EV5B	EV5C	EV5D	EV5E	EV5F	EV5G	EV5HEXP
1	9	Japan	–	–	–		–	–	–	–	–	–	–	–	–	–	–
1	9	Taiwan	–	–	–		–	–	–	–	–	–	–	–	–	–	–
1	9	Vietnam	+	–	+	1991	+	+	+	+	+	+	+	+	+	+	–
1	10	Brunei	–	–	–		–	–	–	–	–	–	–	–	–	–	–
1	10	India	+	+	–	1992	+	+	+	+	+	+	+	+	+	+	+
1	10	Malaysia	+	–	+	1985	+	+	+	+	+	+	+	+	+	+	+
1	10	Nepal	–	–	–		–	–	–	–	–	–	–	–	–	–	–
1	10	Singapore	+	–	+		+	+	+	+	+	+	+	+	+	+	+
1	10	Sri Lanka	+	–	–		+	+	+	+	+	+	+	–	+	–	–
1	10	Thailand	+	+	+	1987	+	+	+	+	+	+	+	+	+	+	+
2	3	American Samoa	–	–	–	1990	+	–	+	+	+	+	+	+	+	+	+
2	3	Cook Islands	–	–	–		–	–	–	–	–	–	–	–	–	–	–
2	3	Guam	+	+	+	1989	+	+	+	+	+	+	+	+	+	+	+
2	3	New Caledonia	–	–	–		–	–	–	–	–	–	–	–	–	–	–
2	3	Niue	–	–	–		–	–	–	–	–	–	–	–	–	–	–
2	3	Tokelau	–	–	–		–	–	–	–	–	–	–	–	–	–	–
2	3	Tuvalu	+	–	+	1993	+	+	+	+	+	+	+	+	+	+	+
2	6	Bermuda	+	–	–	1990	+	+	+	+	+	+	+	+	+	+	–
2	6	Cayman Islands	+	–	–	1990	+	+	+	+	+	+	+	+	+	+	–
2	6	Montserrat	+	–	–	1993	+	+	+	+	+	+	+	+	+	+	+
2	6	Netherlands Antilles	+	+	+	1993	+	+	+	+	+	+	+	+	+	+	+

*List, core country response (1) or subsidiary response (2); GAA, geographic area of affinity; country, territory, or region responding.

Evaluation abbreviations: The governmental national AIDS program (GNAP) has: EV1A, evaluated its own HIV/AIDS programs/projects; EV1B, evaluated the groups within and outside the government which it funds; EV1C, required those groups which it funds to evaluate their HIV/AIDS programs. EV2, year since which HIV/AIDS program evaluations have taken place. EV4A, ministry of health; EV4B, staff of other ministries; EV4C, representatives of NGOs; EV4D, representatives of international agencies/funding Groups that have participated in the evaluation of the GNAP: EV4A, ministry of health; EV4B, staff of other ministries; EV4C, representatives of NGOs; EV4D, representatives of international agencies/funding agencies.

Outcomes which have been evaluated or measured: EV5A, number of people reached by the program; EV5B, number of people HIV tested; EV5C, needles/syringes exchanged; EV5D, number of condoms distributed; EV5E, number of people who are HIV positive; EV5F, number of people provided with targeted specific HIV/AIDS prevention message/education; EV5G, noted behavior change; EV5H, other; EV5HEXP, other specified.

Table D-9.2 Government national AIDS programs: use of evaluation findings; evaluation categories 6A through 6GEXP*

List	GAA	Country	EV6A	EV6AEXP	EV6B	EV6BEXP	EV6C	EV6CEXP
1	1	United States	m		m		m	
1	2	Austria	O		m		O	
1	2	Belgium	O		M	plan for FCB is being reformu- lated	O	
1	2	Cyprus	O		O		—	
1	2	Denmark	—		—		—	
1	2	Finland	—		—		—	
1	2	France	—		—		—	
1	2	Germany	O		O		—	
1	2	Iceland	m		O		O	
1	2	Liechtenstein	m		m		M	
1	2	Luxembourg	O		O		m	
1	2	Malta	—		—		—	
1	2	Netherlands	—		—		—	
1	2	Norway	O		O		O	
1	2	Spain	O		—	greater institu- tional impulse	M	direction of the plan
1	2	Sweden	O		O		O	
1	2	Switzerland	m	improvements	m		M	
1	2	United Kingdom	m		—		m	
1	3	Australia	m	functioning of nat'l strategy	m	re-allocation of nat'l program funds	m	increase in inter- national focus (SE Asia/Pacific)
1	3	Fiji	O		M		m	
1	3	Kiribati	m		O		m	
1	3	Micronesia, Fed. Sts.	M	routine & manda- tory to entertain- ment workers	M	prioritization	O	
1	3	New Zealand	O		O		O	
1	3	Papua New Guinea	O		O		O	
1	3	Solomon Islands	O		O		m	involvement of NGOs
1	3	Vanuatu	—		—		—	
1	3	Western Samoa	O		O		O	
1	4	Argentina	—		—		—	
1	4	Belize	—		—		—	
1	4	Brazil	M	participate in nat'l anti-HIV vaccine test	M	creation of strong STI program	M	dept & hiring of long-term consul- tants
1	4	Chile	—		—		—	

EV6D	EV6DEXP	EV6E	EV6EEXP	EV6F	EV6FEXP	EV6G	EV6GEXP
m		m		m		m	
M		M		m		M	
O		O		O		O	
—		—		—		—	
—		—		—		—	
—		—		—		—	
—		—		—		—	
—		M		M		M	
m		m		O		O	
—		M	involving PWH/A in the project	—		M	migrants
O		O		O		m	
—		—		—		—	
—		—		—		—	
O		O		O		M	
M	endowment of more personnel	O		O		—	epidemiological vigilance made more powerful
O		M		O		O	
m		m		O		m	
—		—		—		—	
m	integration of HIV/AIDS & STI services	M	specific additional focus for indigenous people	M	ending small national direct grants program	M	redirecting funds to states/territories
m		M		M		m	
—		—		—		—	
M	from lab & surveillance support to health education	M	from general population to specific groups	O		O	
O		O		O		O	
O		m	invite churches' participation	O		m	support to other NGOs
—		m	STI management	O		O	
—		—		—		—	
—		m	focus on high-risk groups	—		m	improve STI management
—		—		—		—	
—		—		—		—	
M	testing – in STI to diffusion of innovations	m	change counseling centers training activities	—		M	research unit established
—		—		—		—	

(continued)

Table D-9.2 Government national AIDS programs: use of evaluation findings; evaluation categories 6A through 6GEXP*—continued

List	GAA	Country	EV6A	EV6AEXP	EV6B	EV6BEXP	EV6C	EV6CEXP
1	4	Colombia	M	evaluation	M	drafting of MTP	M	payroll increase
1	4	Costa Rica	M	methodology for providing info	M	target groups?	m	increase in personnel
1	4	Ecuador	M		M		O	
1	4	El Salvador	O		O		m	coordinator P.N. administrator
1	4	Guatemala	O		O		M	NAP director
1	4	Mexico	M	develop more audio/visual materials	O		M	NAP director changed 4 times
1	4	Panama	—		—		—	
1	4	Peru	M	integration betw program & service	—		M	committees, not subregional programs
1	4	Suriname	M	activities to train trainers	O		M	more professionals reshuffling
1	4	Uruguay	M		M		O	
1	4	Venezuela	—		—		—	
1	5	Angola	M	efforts on blood & sexual transmission	M	decentralization of activities in provinces	M	reinforcement of nat'l & internat'l team
1	5	Benin	—		M		—	
1	5	Botswana	M	focus on targeting interventions	—		M	recruited IE staff for direct district support
1	5	Burkino Faso	m		m		m	
1	5	Cameroon	m		M	decentralized/ multi sector-base/community mobilization	m	
1	5	Cape Verde	M		m		O	
1	5	Chad	m		M		m	
1	5	Comoros	M	change passive screening of groups for decentralization	O		m	
1	5	Congo	M		—		M	recruit adjunct of program mgr of GNAP
1	5	Côte d'Ivoire	O		M	promote multi-sector base in program fulfillment	M	reinforce coord
1	5	Djibouti	M	targeted activities	m		m	addition of personnel

570

EV6D	EV6DEXP	EV6E	EV6EEXP	EV6F	EV6FEXP	EV6G	EV6GEXP
O		M	sexual health promotion	O		—	
m	distribution of condoms	M	give information for modification of behavior	M	follow-up of sexual contacts	M	sentry/guard study
O		m		m		O	
—		O		O		O	
O		O		M	reduction in the price of reagents	M	women & AIDS
O		O		O		M	human rights advisory office
—		—		—		—	
M	centralization of activities in counseling services	M	strengthening of info & assistance	—		M	integration of activities for STI control
M	focus on decentralized counseling services	O		O		M	social services
O		M		O		M	
—		—		—		—	
M	prevention activities focus on youth & women	O		O		M	creation of STI control component
—		—		—		—	
—		—		O		M	youth peer education by National Health Services participants
M		m		O		M	
m		m		O		M	integrate AIDS fight/TB sector/counseling
O		O		O		m	
m		m		m		m	
M		M		O		O	
—		—		—		—	
M	reinforce IEC unit of coordination	M	integrate STI control in AIDS program	O		O	
—		—		—		—	

(continued)

Table D-9.2 Government national AIDS programs: use of evaluation findings; evaluation categories 6A through 6GEXP*—continued

List	GAA	Country	EV6A	EV6AEXP	EV6B	EV6BEXP	EV6C	EV6CEXP
1	5	Ethiopia	—		—		—	
1	5	Gabon	—		—		—	
1	5	Ghana	—		—		—	
1	5	Guinea	m		m		O	
1	5	Guinee-Bissau	—		—		—	
1	5	Lesotho	M		M		M	
1	5	Madagascar	M	make other ministry/departments develop programs & NGOs participate	O	updating legal text	O	
1	5	Mali	M	decentralization of program	M		M	
1	5	Mauritania	M	targeted strategies	m	multi-sector based	O	
1	5	Mauritius	—		—		—	
1	5	Rwanda	M	decentralization	M	involvement of all sectors	O	
1	5	Senegal	m		m		m	
1	5	Seychelles	—		—		—	
1	5	South Africa	M		M		m	
1	5	Tanzania	M	decentralization	M	medium-term plan no 2	M	formation of new units
1	5	Togo	M	open policy re: AIDS fight by ministries of health	M	decentralization of laboratory activities	M	reinforcement of the team
1	5	Uganda	M	from awareness campaigns to promotion of behavior change	M		O	
1	5	Zaire	—		M	review of medium-term plan	—	
1	5	Zambia	M	multisectoral approach	M	multisectoral approach	m	
1	5	Zimbabwe	M		M		m	
1	6	Antigua and Barbuda	—		—		—	
1	6	Barbados	—		—		M	employment of a program coordinator
1	6	Dominican Republic	—		—		—	
1	6	Grenada	O		O		O	
1	6	Jamaica	M	use of culture	—		—	
1	6	St. Lucia	O		m	to be revised	M	government assumed positions of staff

EV6D	EV6DEXP	EV6E	EV6EEXP	EV6F	EV6FEXP	EV6G	EV6GEXP
—		—		—		—	
—		—		—		—	
M	provide pre-test counseling	—		—		—	
O		O		O		O	
—		—		—		—	
m		m		m		M	
O	create anonymous testing/ screening center	m	reinforce fight against STIs	—		—	
—		—		O		M	under discussion
O		O		O		M	program for the young people
—		—		—		—	
O		O		O		M	sustain psychomedico social unit
O		m		O		m	
—		—		—		—	
M		M		M		M	
—		M	youth	—	not available	M	counseling
—		—		—		—	
O		—		O		M	community based counseling
—		—		—		—	
—		—		O		O	
m		m		m		m	
—		—		—		—	
—		—		—		—	
—		—		—		—	
O		O		O		O	
M	provision of local HIV testing	—		—		m	face to face program
M	Increase social services provision islandwide	O		O		O	

(continued)

List	GAA	Country	EV6A	EV6AEXP	EV6B	EV6BEXP	EV6C	EV6CEXP
1	6	Trinidad and Tobago	M	IEC from general to specific	M	add objective to reduce socio-economic impact on society	M	staff recruitment
1	7	Azerbaijan	O		O		O	
1	7	Belarus	—		—		—	
1	7	Bulgaria	M	anonymous testing/counseling	M	shift from secondary to primary prevention	M	NGOs
1	7	Croatia	—		—		—	
1	7	Czech Republic	—		—		—	
1	7	Estonia	O		O		O	
1	7	Hungary	O		O		m	
1	7	Kyrgyz Republic	M	HIV testing	O		O	
1	7	Latvia	—		—		—	
1	7	Lithuania	—		—		—	
1	7	Moldova	—		—		—	
1	7	Russian Federation	—		—		—	
1	7	Slovenia	O		O		O	
1	7	Turkmenistan	—		—		—	
1	7	Ukraine	M	from compulsory testing to voluntary	M	formulation of measures protecting people with HIV	O	
1	7	Yugoslavia, Fed. Rep.	—		—		—	
1	8	Algeria	O		O		—	
1	8	Israel	m		M		M	
1	8	Jordan	O		m	formulation of new plan	O	
1	8	Kuwait	M		M		m	
1	8	Lebanon	—		—		—	
1	8	Morocco	M	decentralization of activities; coordination with other sectors	M	action plan (information, education, communication)	O	
1	8	Oman	—		—		—	
1	8	Syrian Arab Rep.	—		—		—	
1	8	Tunisia	M	efficient promotion of condom use	O		O	
1	9	Bhutan	O		O		O	
1	9	China	m		m		—	
1	9	Hong Kong	—		—		—	
1	9	Japan	—		—		—	
1	9	Taiwan	—		—		—	
1	9	Vietnam	—		—		—	

EV6D	EV6DEXP	EV6E	EV6EEXP	EV6F	EV6FEXP	EV6G	EV6GEXP
m	surveillance & research component of MTP	—		O		M	introduction of 3 sub-committees
O		O		O		O	
—		—		—		—	
M	STI clinics/family planning offices	M	health promotion	M	mandatory screening	—	
—		—		—		—	
—		—		—		—	
O		O		O		O	
O		O		m		m	
O		—	data not available	—	data not available	—	data not available
—		—		—		—	
—		—		—		—	
—		—		—		—	
—		—		—		—	
O		O		O		O	
—		—		—		—	
M	redirection in psychological support services	m	intensification of HIV testing quality control	O		m	organization of sentinal surveillance surveys
—		—		—		—	
O		O		O		O	
O		m		O		M	
m		m		O		O	
m		m		m		M	
—		—		—		—	
O		O		O		M	AIDS sentinel surveillance posts
—		—		—		—	
—		—		—		—	
O		M	decrease psycho/social impact on HIV/AIDS	O		O	
O		O		O		O	
—		M		—		m	
—		—		—		—	
—		—		—		—	
—		—		—		—	
—		—		—		—	

(continued)

Table D-9.2 Government national AIDS programs: use of evaluation findings; evaluation categories 6A through 6GEXP*—continued

List	GAA	Country	EV6A	EV6AEXP	EV6B	EV6BEXP	EV6C	EV6CEXP
1	10	Brunei	—		—		—	
1	10	India	O		O		O	
1	10	Malaysia	—		M	sentinel surveillance	M	increase staffing from vertical organization to integrated organization
1	10	Nepal	—		—		—	
1	10	Singapore	O		m	based on epidemiological changes	m	based on epidemiological changes
1	10	Sri Lanka	—		—		—	
1	10	Thailand	M	more expression in behavior modification	M		m	
2	3	American Samoa	m		m		M	
2	3	Cook Islands	—		—		—	
2	3	Guam	O		O		M	additional social workers
2	3	New Caledonia	—		—		—	
2	3	Niue	—		—		—	
2	3	Tokelau	—		—		—	
2	3	Tuvalu	—		—		—	
2	6	Bermuda	O		m		O	
2	6	Cayman Islands	O		O		O	
2	6	Montserrat	m	now using 5 strategic approaches	M	timetable changed from 3 yrs medium-term program to annual	M	loss of AIDS program coordinator
2	6	Netherlands Antilles	—		—		—	

EV6D	EV6DEXP	EV6E	EV6EEXP	EV6F	EV6FEXP	EV6G	EV6GEXP
—		—		—		—	
O		O		O		O	
—		M	health edu: to be specifically targeted, not general	—		—	
—		—		—		—	
O		m	emphasis on condom use in high-risk groups	O		M	AIDS education targeted at jr college/polytech
—		—		—		—	
M	STI, TB, MCH development	M	risk group to youth	m		M	social welfare service
m		M		M		m	
—		—		—		—	
O		M	focus on gay population	O		O	
—		—		—		—	
—		—		—		—	
—		—		—		—	
—		—		—		—	
O		O		O		O	
m	develop leaflet & education program	—		O		O	
m	emphasis on infection control	m	emphasis on infection control	O		M	expanding school to include 4,5,6th forms
—		—		—		—	

*List, core country response (1) or subsidiary response (2); GAA, geographic area of affinity; country, territory, or region responding.

Evaluation abbreviations: Indicated significant change in policy resulting from an evaluation of the GNAP and/or one of the organizations which it funds (M = major change, m = minor change, O = no change): EV6A, change in program strategies—EV6AEXP, change explained; EV6B, reformulation of the national HIV/AIDS plan—EV6BEXP, change explained; EV6C, personnel changes—EV6CEXP, change explained. EV6D, redirection of a specific needed service—EV6DEXP, change explained; EV6E, change of a certain project focus—EV6EEXP, change explained; EV6F, ending a program component—EV6FEXP, change explained; EV6G, beginning a new program component—EV6GEXP, change explained.

Appendix E. Laws and Practices in the Context of HIV: A Survey of Government National AIDS Program Managers

Table E.1 Government national AIDS programs: laws and practices regarding HIV/AIDS, categories 1a through 2k (as reported by GNAP managers)—obligatory testing of specified groups*

Country, by GAA	I. Countries imposing restrictions based on HIV status						II. Countries practicing obligatory (compulsory and mandatory) testing of specified groups																					
	1a P	1a L	1b P	1b L	1c P	1c L	2a P	2a L	2b P	2b L	2c P	2c L	2d P	2d L	2e P	2e L	2f P	2f L	2g P	2g L	2h P	2h L	2i P	2i L	2j P	2j L	2k P	2k L
1 North America																												
1 United States	–	–	–	–	–	–	–	–	–	–	–	–	–	–	+	–	–	–	+	+	–	–	–	–	+	+	–	–
2 Western Europe																												
2 Austria	–	–	+	+	–	–	+	–	–	–	–	–	–	–	–	–	–	–	–	–	–	–	–	–	+	+	–	–
2 Belgium	–	–	–	–	–	–	–	–	–	–	–	–	+	–	–	–	–	–	–	–	–	–	–	–	+	+	–	–
2 Cyprus	–	–	+	–	–	–	+	–	+	–	+	–	+	–	–	–	+	–	–	–	–	–	–	–	+	+	–	–
2 Denmark	–	–	–	–	–	–	–	–	–	–	–	–	–	–	–	–	+	–	–	–	–	–	–	–	+	+	–	–
2 Finland	–	–	–	–	–	–	–	–	+	–	+	–	+	–	+	–	–	+	–	–	+	–	–	+	+	+	+	+
2 France	–	–	–	–	–	–	–	–	–	–	–	–	–	–	–	–	–	–	–	–	–	–	–	–	+	–	+	+
2 Germany	–	–	–	–	–	–	–	–	–	–	–	–	–	–	–	–	–	–	–	–	–	–	–	–	+	+	–	–
2 Iceland	–	–	–	–	–	–	–	–	–	–	–	–	+	–	–	–	+	–	–	–	–	–	–	–	+	+	–	–
2 Liechtenstein	–	–	–	–	–	–	–	–	–	–	–	–	–	–	–	–	–	+	–	–	–	–	–	–	–	–	–	–
2 Luxembourg	–	–	–	–	–	–	–	–	–	–	–	–	–	–	–	–	–	–	–	–	–	–	–	–	+	+	–	–
2 Malta	–	–	+	–	–	–	–	–	–	–	–	–	–	–	–	–	–	–	–	–	–	–	+	+	+	+	–	–
2 Netherlands	–	–	–	–	–	–	–	–	–	–	–	–	–	–	–	+	–	–	–	–	–	–	–	–	+	+	–	–
2 Norway	–	–	–	–	–	–	–	–	–	–	–	–	–	–	–	–	–	–	–	–	–	–	–	–	+	+	–	–
2 Spain	–	–	–	–	–	+	–	–	–	–	–	–	–	–	–	–	–	–	–	–	–	–	–	–	+	+	–	–
2 Sweden	–	–	–	–	–	–	–	–	–	–	–	–	–	–	–	–	–	–	–	–	–	–	–	–	+	+	–	–
2 Switzerland	–	–	–	–	–	–	–	–	–	–	–	–	–	–	–	–	–	–	+	–	–	–	–	–	+	+	–	–
2 United Kingdom	–	–	–	–	–	–	–	–	–	–	–	–	–	–	–	–	–	–	–	–	–	–	–	–	+	–	–	–
3 Oceania																												
3 Australia	–	–	–	–	–	–	–	–	–	–	–	–	+	–	–	–	–	–	–	–	–	–	–	–	+	+	–	–
3 Fiji	–	–	–	–	–	–	–	–	–	–	–	–	–	–	–	–	–	–	–	–	–	–	–	–	+	+	–	–

578

Country																								
3 Micronesia, Fed. Sts.	+	+	+	+	−	+	−	−	+	+	−	−	−	−	−	−	−	+	−	−	−	−	−	−
3 New Zealand	+	+	−	+	−	−	−	−	−	−	−	−	−	−	−	−	−	−	−	−	−	−	−	−
3 Papua New Guinea	−	−	−	+	+	−	−	−	−	−	−	−	−	−	−	−	−	−	−	−	−	−	−	−
3 Solomon Islands	−	−	+	+	−	−	−	−	+	−	−	−	−	−	−	−	−	−	−	−	−	−	−	−
3 Vanuatu	−	−	−	−	−	−	−	−	−	−	−	−	−	−	−	−	−	−	−	−	−	−	−	−
3 Western Samoa	−	−	+	−	−	−	−	−	−	−	−	−	−	−	−	−	−	−	−	−	−	−	−	−
4 Latin America																								
4 Argentina	−	−	+	+	−	−	−	+	−	+	−	−	−	−	−	+	+	+	−	−	+	−	−	+
4 Belize	−	−	+	+	−	+	−	+	+	+	−	−	−	−	−	+	+	+	−	−	+	−	+	−
4 Brazil	−	−	+	+	+	−	−	−	+	−	−	+	−	−	−	+	+	+	−	−	+	−	−	+
4 Chile	−	−	+	+	−	−	−	+	−	−	+	−	−	+	−	+	+	+	−	−	+	−	−	+
4 Colombia	−	−	−	−	−	−	−	−	−	−	−	−	−	−	−	+	−	−	−	−	−	−	−	+
4 Costa Rica	−	−	+	+	−	+	−	−	−	−	−	−	−	−	−	+	+	−	−	−	−	−	−	−
4 Ecuador	−	−	+	+	−	−	−	+	−	−	−	−	−	−	−	+	−	+	−	−	−	−	−	−
4 El Salvador	−	−	+	+	−	−	−	−	+	−	−	−	−	−	−	+	+	−	−	−	−	−	−	+
4 Guatemala	−	−	−	−	−	−	−	−	−	−	−	−	−	−	−	−	−	−	−	−	−	−	−	−
4 Mexico	−	+	+	+	−	+	−	−	−	+	+	+	+	+	+	+	+	+	−	+	+	−	−	+
4 Panama	+	+	+	+	−	−	−	+	−	−	−	+	−	−	−	+	+	+	−	−	+	−	−	+
4 Peru	+	+	+	+	+	+	−	−	−	−	−	−	−	−	−	−	−	−	−	−	−	−	−	−
4 Suriname	−	−	−	−	+	−	−	−	−	−	−	+	−	−	−	−	−	−	−	−	−	−	−	−
4 Uruguay	−	−	+	+	+	−	−	+	+	+	−	−	−	−	−	+	+	+	−	−	+	−	−	+
4 Venezuela	−	−	+	+	+	+	+	+	+	+	+	+	+	+	+	+	+	+	−	−	+	−	−	+
5 Sub-Saharan Africa																								
5 Angola	−	−	−	+	−	−	−	−	−	−	−	−	−	−	−	+	−	−	−	−	−	−	−	−
5 Benin	−	−	+	+	−	+	−	+	−	+	−	−	−	−	−	+	−	−	−	−	−	−	−	−
5 Botswana	+	−	−	−	−	−	−	−	−	−	−	−	−	−	−	−	−	−	−	−	−	+	−	−
5 Burkino Faso	−	−	+	+	−	−	−	−	+	−	−	−	−	−	−	+	+	+	−	−	+	−	−	+
5 Cameroon	−	−	+	+	−	−	−	+	−	−	−	−	−	−	−	+	+	+	−	−	+	−	−	+
5 Cape Verde	−	−	+	+	−	−	−	−	−	−	−	−	−	−	−	+	+	−	−	−	−	−	−	−
5 Chad	−	−	−	−	−	−	−	−	−	−	−	−	−	−	−	−	−	−	−	−	−	−	−	−
5 Comoros	−	−	+	+	−	+	−	+	−	+	−	−	−	−	−	+	+	+	−	−	+	−	−	+

(continued)

Table E.1 Government national AIDS programs: laws and practices regarding HIV/AIDS, categories 1a through 2k (as reported by GNAP managers)—obligatory testing of specified groups*—continued

Country, by GAA	I. Countries imposing restrictions based on HIV status						II. Countries practicing obligatory (compulsory and mandatory) testing of specified groups																					
	1a		1b		1c		2a		2b		2c		2d		2e		2f		2g		2h		2i		2j		2k	
	P	L	P	L	P	L	P	L	P	L	P	L	P	L	P	L	P	L	P	L	P	L	P	L	P	L	P	L
5 Congo	–	–	–	–	–	–	–	–	–	–	+	–	–	–	–	–	–	–	+	–	–	–	–	–	+	+	–	–
5 Côte d'Ivoire	–	–	–	–	–	–	–	–	–	–	–	–	–	–	–	–	–	–	–	–	–	–	–	–	+	+	–	–
5 Djibouti	–	–	–	–	–	–	+	–	–	–	–	–	–	–	–	–	+	–	+	–	–	–	–	–	+	+	–	+
5 Ethiopia	–	–	–	–	–	–	–	–	–	–	–	–	–	–	–	–	–	–	–	–	–	–	–	–	+	+	–	–
5 Gabon	–	–	–	–	–	–	–	–	–	–	–	–	–	–	–	–	–	–	+	–	–	–	–	–	+	–	–	–
5 Ghana	–	–	–	–	–	–	–	–	–	–	–	–	–	–	–	–	–	–	–	–	–	–	–	–	–	–	–	–
5 Guinea	–	–	–	–	–	–	–	–	–	–	–	–	–	–	–	–	–	–	–	–	–	–	–	–	+	+	–	–
5 Guinee-Bissau	–	–	–	–	–	–	–	–	–	–	–	–	–	–	–	–	+	–	+	–	–	–	+	–	+	–	–	–
5 Lesotho	–	–	–	–	–	–	–	–	–	–	+	–	–	–	–	–	+	–	–	–	–	–	–	–	+	–	–	–
5 Madagascar	–	–	–	–	–	–	+	–	+	–	+	–	–	–	–	–	+	–	–	–	–	–	–	–	+	–	–	–
5 Mali	–	–	–	–	+	–	–	–	–	–	–	–	–	–	–	–	–	–	+	–	–	–	–	–	+	–	–	–
5 Mauritania	–	–	–	–	–	–	–	–	–	–	–	–	–	–	–	–	–	–	–	–	–	–	–	–	+	–	–	–
5 Mauritius	–	–	–	–	–	–	–	–	–	–	–	–	–	–	–	–	+	–	–	–	–	–	–	–	+	–	–	+
5 Rwanda	–	–	–	–	–	–	–	–	–	–	–	–	–	–	–	–	–	–	–	–	–	–	–	–	+	+	–	–
5 Senegal	–	–	–	–	+	–	+	–	–	–	–	–	–	–	–	–	+	–	+	–	–	–	+	–	+	+	–	–
5 Seychelles	–	–	–	–	–	–	–	–	–	–	–	–	–	–	–	–	–	–	–	–	–	–	–	–	+	–	–	–
5 South Africa	–	–	–	–	–	–	–	–	–	–	+	–	–	–	+	–	+	–	–	–	+	–	–	–	+	+	–	–
5 Tanzania	–	–	–	–	–	–	–	–	–	–	–	–	–	–	–	–	–	–	–	–	–	–	–	–	–	–	–	–
5 Togo	–	–	–	–	–	–	–	–	–	–	–	–	–	–	–	–	–	–	+	–	–	–	–	–	+	–	–	–
5 Uganda	–	–	–	–	–	–	–	–	–	–	–	–	–	–	–	–	–	–	–	–	–	–	–	–	+	+	–	–
5 Zaire	–	–	–	–	–	–	–	–	–	–	–	–	–	–	–	–	–	–	+	–	–	–	–	–	+	–	–	–
5 Zambia	–	–	–	–	–	–	–	–	–	–	–	–	–	–	–	–	–	–	–	–	–	–	–	–	+	–	–	–
5 Zimbabwe	–	–	–	–	–	–	–	–	–	–	–	–	–	–	–	–	–	–	–	–	–	–	–	–	+	+	–	–
6 Caribbean																												
6 Antigua and Barbuda	–	–	–	–	–	–	+	–	–	–	–	–	+	–	–	–	–	–	–	–	–	–	–	–	+	–	–	–
6 Barbados	–	–	–	–	–	–	–		–		–		–		–		–		–		–		–		+		+	

580

6 Dominican Republic

6 Grenada

6 Jamaica

6 St. Lucia

6 Trinidad and Tobago

7 Eastern Europe

7 Azerbaijan

7 Belarus

7 Bulgaria

7 Croatia

7 Czech Republic

7 Estonia

7 Hungary

7 Kyrgyz Republic

7 Latvia

7 Lithuania

7 Moldova

7 Russian Federation

7 Slovenia

7 Turkmenistan

7 Ukraine

7 Yugoslavia, Fed. Rep.

8 SE Mediterranean

8 Algeria

8 Israel

8 Jordan

8 Kuwait

8 Lebanon

8 Morocco

8 Oman

8 Syrian Arab Rep.

8 Tunisia

(continued)

581

Table E.1 Government national AIDS programs: laws and practices regarding HIV/AIDS, categories 1a through 2k (as reported by GNAP managers)—obligatory testing of specified groups*—continued

Country, by GAA	I. Countries imposing restrictions based on HIV status						II. Countries practicing obligatory (compulsory and mandatory) testing of specified groups																					
	1a		1b		1c		2a		2b		2c		2d		2e		2f		2g		2h		2i		2j		2k	
	P	L	P	L	P	L	P	L	P	L	P	L	P	L	P	L	P	L	P	L	P	L	P	L	P	L	P	L
9 Northeast Asia																												
9 Bhutan	–	–	–	–	–	–	–	–	–	–	+	–	–	–	–	–	–	–	–	–	–	–	+	–	–	–	–	–
9 China	–	–	–	–	–	–	–	–	–	–	–	–	+	–	–	–	–	–	–	–	–	–	–	–	–	–	–	–
9 Hong Kong	–	–	–	–	–	–	–	–	–	–	–	–	–	–	–	–	–	–	–	–	–	–	+	–	+	–	–	–
9 Japan	–	–	–	–	–	–	–	–	–	–	–	–	–	–	–	–	–	–	–	–	–	–	–	–	–	–	–	–
9 Viet Nam	–	–	–	–	–	–	–	–	–	–	–	–	–	–	–	–	–	–	–	–	–	–	–	–	–	–	–	–
10 Southeast Asia																												
10 Brunei	–	–	–	+	–	–	–	–	+	–	–	–	+	–	–	–	+	–	+	–	–	–	+	–	+	–	–	–
10 Malaysia	–	–	+	+	+	+	+	–	+	–	+	–	+	–	–	–	+	–	+	–	–	–	+	–	+	–	–	–
10 Nepal	–	–	–	–	–	–	+	–	–	–	–	–	–	–	–	–	–	–	+	–	–	–	–	–	+	–	–	–
10 Singapore	–	–	+	+	–	–	+	–	–	–	–	–	–	–	+	–	–	–	+	–	–	–	–	–	+	–	–	–
10 Sri Lanka	–	–	–	–	–	–	–	–	–	–	–	–	–	–	–	–	–	–	+	–	–	–	+	–	+	–	–	–
10 Thailand	–	–	–	–	–	–	–	–	–	–	–	–	–	–	–	–	–	–	+	+	–	–	–	–	+	–	–	–
World totals																												
Yes (+)	3	4	15	10	9	11	31	1	12	4	19	6	27	10	8	5	32	8	33	11	9	4	13	5	99	65	7	5
No (−)	102	99	82	88	98	98	73	5	93	91	88	92	81	85	100	93	77	89	68	78	97	89	91	92	99	33	99	91
No response (—)	10	12	18	17	8	6	11	109	10	20	8	17	7	20	6	18	14	26	9	22	11	18	7	17			9	19

*Code for column headings: P, are these activities enforced in the absence or presence of laws? L, Is there a law, regulation, or decree mandating the following activities in the country? + = yes; − = no; — = no response.

I. countries imposing restrictions based on HIV status: 1a, restrictions on persons with HIV to marry; 1b, restrictions against sex workers/prostitutes; 1c, compulsory admissions of persons with HIV or AIDS into special centers.

II. countries practicing obligatory (compulsory and mandatory) testing in specified groups: 2a, sex workers/prostitutes (note: due to survey design error, the law section of this question was not answered by a majority of respondents); 2b, gay/homosexual men; 2c, pregnant women; 2d, prisoners; 2e, health care workers; 2f, patients with tuberculosis; 2g, military recruits; 2h, nationals applying for certain employment (i.e., in the tourist sector); 2i, citizen applying for student fellowship; 2j, blood donors (note: although the question was asked about HIV testing of blood donors, some respondents may have answered about HIV testing of blood donations); 2k, prior to marriage.

Table E.2 Government national AIDS programs: laws and practices regarding HIV/AIDS, categories 3a through 4d (as reported by GNAP managers)— testing of migrants and travelers*

Country, by GAA	III. Obligatory (compulsory and mandatory) testing of migrants and travelers														IV. Testing of migrants and travelers that prevents them from entering the country							
	3a		3b		3c		3d		3e		3f		3g		4a		4b		4c		4d	
	P	L	P	L	P	L	P	L	P	L	P	L	P	L	P	L	P	L	P	L	P	L
1 North America																						
1 United States	−	−	+	+	−	+	+	+	−	−	−	−	+	+	−	−	+	+	+	−	+	+
2 Western Europe																						
2 Austria	−	−	−	−	−	−	−	−	−	−	−	−	−	−	−	−	−	−	−	−	−	−
2 Belgium	−	+	+	−	−	−	−	−	−	−	+	−	+	−	+	−	−	−	−	−	−	−
2 Cyprus	−	−	−	−	−	−	−	−	+	−	−	−	−	−	+	+	+	−	−	−	−	−
2 Denmark	−	−	−	−	−	−	−	−	−	−	−	−	−	−	−	−	−	−	−	−	−	−
2 Finland	+	+	−	+	+	−	+	+	−	−	+	+	+	+	+	+	+	+	+	+	−	+
2 France	−	−	−	−	−	−	−	−	−	−	−	−	−	−	−	−	−	−	−	−	−	−
2 Germany	−	−	−	−	−	−	−	−	−	−	−	−	−	−	−	−	−	−	−	−	−	−
2 Iceland	−	−	−	−	−	−	−	−	−	−	−	−	−	−	−	−	−	−	−	−	−	−
2 Liechtenstein	−	−	−	−	−	−	−	−	−	−	−	−	−	−	−	−	−	−	−	−	−	−
2 Luxembourg	−	−	−	−	−	−	−	−	−	−	−	−	−	−	−	−	−	−	−	−	−	−
2 Malta	−	−	−	−	−	−	−	−	−	−	+	−	−	−	−	−	−	−	−	−	−	−
2 Netherlands	−	−	−	−	−	−	−	−	−	−	−	−	−	−	−	−	−	−	−	−	−	−
2 Norway	−	−	−	−	−	−	−	−	−	−	−	−	−	−	−	−	−	−	−	−	−	−
2 Spain	−	−	−	−	−	−	−	−	−	−	−	−	−	−	−	−	−	−	−	−	−	−
2 Sweden	−	−	−	−	−	−	−	−	−	−	−	−	−	−	−	−	−	−	−	−	−	−
2 Switzerland	−	−	−	−	−	−	−	−	−	−	−	−	−	−	−	−	−	−	−	−	−	−
2 United Kingdom	−	−	−	−	−	−	−	−	−	−	−	−	−	−	−	−	−	−	−	−	−	−
3 Oceania																						
3 Australia	−	−	+	+	−	−	+	+	−	−	−	−	−	−	−	−	−	−	−	−	−	−
3 Fiji	−	−	−	−	−	−	−	−	−	−	−	−	−	−	−	−	−	−	−	−	−	−
3 Micronesia, Fed. Sts.	−	−	−	−	−	−	−	−	−	−	−	−	−	−	+	+	+	+	+	−	−	−
3 New Zealand	−	−	−	−	−	−	−	−	−	−	−	−	−	−	−	−	−	−	−	−	−	−
3 Papua New Guinea	−	−	−	−	−	−	−	−	−	−	−	−	−	−	−	−	−	−	−	−	−	−

(continued)

583

Table E.2 Government national AIDS programs: laws and practices regarding HIV/AIDS, categories 3a through 4d (as reported by GNAP managers)—testing of migrants and travelers*—continued

Country, by GAA	III. Obligatory (compulsory and mandatory) testing of migrants and travelers														IV. Testing of migrants and travelers that prevents them from entering the country							
	3a		3b		3c		3d		3e		3f		3g		4a		4b		4c		4d	
	P	L	P	L	P	L	P	L	P	L	P	L	P	L	P	L	P	L	P	L	P	L
3 Solomon Islands	–	–	–	–	–	–	–	–	–	–	–	–	–	–	–	–	–	–	–	–	–	–
3 Vanuatu	–	–	–	–	–	–	–	–	–	–	–	–	–	–	–	–	–	–	–	–	–	–
3 Western Samoa	–	–	–	–	–	–	–	–	–	–	–	–	–	–	–	–	–	–	–	–	–	–
4 Latin America																						
4 Argentina	–	–	+	+	–	–	+	+	–	–	–	–	–	–	–	–	–	–	–	–	–	–
4 Belize	–	–	+	–	–	–	+	–	+	–	–	–	+	–	–	–	–	–	–	–	–	–
4 Brazil	–	–	–	–	–	–	–	–	–	–	–	–	–	–	–	–	–	–	–	–	–	–
4 Chile	–	–	–	–	–	–	–	–	–	–	–	–	–	–	–	–	–	–	–	–	–	–
4 Colombia	–	–	–	–	–	–	–	–	–	–	–	–	–	–	–	–	–	–	–	–	–	–
4 Costa Rica	–	–	–	–	–	–	–	–	–	–	–	–	–	–	–	–	–	–	–	–	–	–
4 Ecuador	–	–	–	–	–	–	–	–	–	–	–	–	–	–	–	–	–	–	–	–	–	–
4 El Salvador	–	–	+	–	–	–	+	–	–	–	–	–	–	–	–	–	–	–	–	–	–	–
4 Guatemala	–	–	–	–	–	–	–	–	–	–	–	–	–	–	–	–	–	–	+	–	–	–
4 Mexico	–	–	–	–	–	–	–	–	–	–	–	–	–	–	–	–	–	–	–	–	–	–
4 Panama	–	–	+	+	–	–	+	–	+	+	–	–	–	–	–	–	+	+	–	–	–	–
4 Peru	–	–	–	–	–	–	–	–	–	–	–	–	–	–	–	–	+	–	–	–	–	–
4 Suriname	–	–	–	–	–	–	–	–	–	–	–	–	–	–	–	–	–	–	–	–	–	–
4 Uruguay	–	–	–	–	–	–	–	–	–	–	–	–	–	–	–	–	–	–	–	–	–	–
4 Venezuela	–	–	–	–	–	–	–	–	–	–	–	–	–	–	–	–	–	–	–	–	–	–
5 Sub-Saharan Africa																						
5 Angola	–	–	–	–	–	–	–	–	–	–	–	–	–	–	–	–	–	–	–	–	–	–
5 Benin	–	–	–	–	–	–	+	+	–	–	–	–	–	–	–	–	–	–	–	–	–	–
5 Botswana	–	–	–	–	–	–	–	+	–	–	–	–	–	–	–	–	–	–	–	–	–	–
5 Burkino Faso	–	–	–	–	–	–	–	–	–	–	–	–	–	–	–	–	–	–	–	–	–	–
5 Cameroon	–	–	–	–	–	–	–	–	–	–	–	–	–	–	–	–	–	–	–	–	–	–
5 Cape Verde	–	–	–	–	–	–	–	–	–	–	–	–	–	–	–	–	–	–	–	–	–	–

(continued)

5 Chad
5 Comoros
5 Congo
5 Côte d'Ivoire
5 Djibouti
5 Ethiopia
5 Gabon
5 Ghana
5 Guinea
5 Guinea-Bissau
5 Lesotho
5 Madagascar
5 Mali
5 Mauritania
5 Mauritius
5 Rwanda
5 Senegal
5 Seychelles
5 South Africa
5 Tanzania
5 Togo
5 Uganda
5 Zaire
5 Zambia
5 Zimbabwe
6 Caribbean
6 Antigua and Barbuda
6 Barbados
6 Dominican Republic
6 Grenada
6 Jamaica

Table E.2 Government national AIDS programs: laws and practices regarding HIV/AIDS, categories 3a through 4d (as reported by GNAP managers)—testing of migrants and travelers*—continued

Country, by GAA	III. Obligatory (compulsory and mandatory) testing of migrants and travelers														IV. Testing of migrants and travelers that prevents them from entering the country							
	3a		3b		3c		3d		3e		3f		3g		4a		4b		4c		4d	
	P	L	P	L	P	L	P	L	P	L	P	L	P	L	P	L	P	L	P	L	P	L
6 St. Lucia	–	–	–	–	–	–	–	–	+	+	–	–	–	–	–	–	–	–	–	–	–	–
6 Trinidad and Tobago	–	–	–	–	–	–	–	–	–	–	–	–	–	–	–	–	–	–	–	–	–	–
7 Eastern Europe																						
7 Azerbaijan	+	–	–	–	–	–	–	–	+	+	+	–	–	–	–	–	–	–	–	–	–	–
7 Belarus	–	–	–	–	–	–	–	–	+	+	+	–	–	–	–	–	–	–	–	–	–	–
7 Bulgaria	+	+	+	–	–	–	+	+	+	+	+	+	+	+	–	–	+	+	+	+	–	–
7 Croatia	–	–	–	–	–	–	–	–	–	–	+	–	–	–	–	–	–	–	–	–	–	–
7 Czech Republic	–	–	–	–	–	–	–	–	–	–	–	–	–	–	–	–	–	–	–	–	–	–
7 Estonia	–	–	–	–	–	–	–	–	–	–	–	–	–	–	+	+	+	+	+	+	+	+
7 Hungary	–	–	–	–	–	–	–	–	–	–	–	–	–	–	–	–	–	–	–	–	–	–
7 Kyrgyz Republic	+	+	+	+	+	+	+	+	+	+	+	+	–	–	+	+	+	+	+	+	+	+
7 Latvia	–	–	–	–	–	–	–	–	–	–	–	–	–	–	–	–	–	–	–	–	–	–
7 Lithuania	–	–	–	–	–	–	+	+	–	–	–	–	–	–	–	–	–	–	–	–	–	–
7 Moldova	+	+	+	+	+	+	+	+	+	+	+	+	+	+	+	+	+	+	+	+	–	–
7 Russian Federation	+	+	+	+	–	–	+	+	+	+	+	+	+	+	+	+	+	+	–	–	–	–
7 Slovenia	–	–	–	–	–	–	–	–	–	–	–	–	–	–	–	–	–	–	–	–	–	–
7 Turkmenistan	+	+	+	+	–	–	+	+	+	+	+	+	+	+	+	+	+	+	+	+	+	+
7 Ukraine	+	+	+	–	–	–	–	–	+	+	+	+	–	–	–	–	–	–	–	–	–	–
7 Yugoslavia, Fed. Rep.	–	–	–	–	–	–	–	–	–	–	–	–	–	–	–	–	–	–	–	–	–	–
8 SE Mediterranean																						
8 Algeria	–	–	–	–	–	–	–	–	–	–	–	–	–	–	–	–	–	–	–	–	–	–
8 Israel	–	–	+	+	–	–	–	–	+	+	+	+	–	–	–	–	+	+	–	–	–	–
8 Jordan	–	–	+	+	–	–	+	+	+	+	+	+	–	–	–	–	+	+	+	+	–	–
8 Kuwait	–	–	–	–	–	–	+	+	+	+	+	+	–	–	+	+	+	+	–	–	–	–
8 Lebanon	–	–	–	–	–	–	–	–	+	+	–	–	–	–	–	–	+	+	–	–	+	–
8 Morocco	–	–	–	–	–	–	–	–	–	–	–	–	–	–	–	–	–	–	–	–	–	–
8 Oman	–														–						–	

Country	P	L	3a	3b	3c	3d	3e	3f	3g	4a	4b	4c	4d									
8 Syrian Arab Rep.	+	−	−	−	−	−	−	−	−	−	−	−	−	−	−	−	+	−	+	−	+	−
8 Tunisia	−	−	−	−	−	−	−	−	−	−	−	−	−	−	−	−	−	−	−	−	−	−

9 Northeast Asia

Country																						
9 Bhutan	−	−	−	−	−	−	−	−	−	−	−	−	−	−	−	−	−	−	−	−	−	−
9 China	−	+	+	+	+	+	−	+	+	+	+	+	−	−	−	+	+	+	−	−	−	−
9 Hong Kong	−	−	−	−	−	−	−	−	−	−	−	−	−	−	−	−	−	−	−	−	−	−
9 Japan	−	−	−	−	−	−	−	−	+	−	−	−	−	−	−	−	−	−	−	−	−	−
9 Vietnam	−	−	−	−	−	−	−	−	−	−	−	−	−	−	−	−	−	−	−	−	−	−

10 Southeast Asia

Country																						
10 Brunei	−	−	−	−	−	−	−	−	+	−	−	−	−	−	+	+	+	−	+	+	+	−
10 Malaysia	−	−	−	−	−	−	−	+	+	+	−	−	+	−	+	+	+	+	+	+	+	+
10 Nepal	−	−	−	−	−	−	−	−	−	−	−	−	−	−	−	−	−	−	−	−	−	−
10 Singapore	−	−	−	−	−	−	+	+	+	−	−	−	+	−	−	−	−	−	−	−	−	−
10 Sri Lanka	−	−	−	−	−	−	+	+	−	−	−	−	−	−	−	−	−	−	−	−	−	−
10 Thailand	−	−	−	−	−	−	−	−	−	−	−	−	−	−	−	−	−	−	−	−	−	−
World totals																						
Yes (+)	6	5	17	11	3	3	19	16	21	13	14	10	7	5	9	7	16	12	9	4	9	6
No (−)	104	93	86	82	105	94	87	78	85	82	94	88	93	85	98	88	92	81	94	86	95	85
No response (—)	5	17	12	22	7	18	9	21	9	20	7	17	15	25	8	20	7	22	12	25	11	24

*Code for column headings: P, are these activities enforced in the absence or presence of laws? L, is there a law, regulation, or decree mandating the following activities in the country? + = yes; − = no; —— = no response.

III. obligatory (compulsory and mandatory) testing of migrants and travelers: 3a, nationals returning from abroad; 3b, immigrants; 3c, tourists/travelers; 3d, applicants for residence permits; 3e, foreign laborers applying for work permits; 3f, foreign students entering the country; 3g, asylum applicants.

IV. testing of migrants and travelers that prevents them from entering the country: 4a, HIV-infected short-term travelers; 4b, HIV-infected long-term travelers; 4c, HIV-infected asylum claimants; 4d, HIV-infected refugees.

Appendix F. Universal Declaration of Human Rights

Universal Declaration of Human Rights

Preamble

Whereas recognition of the inherent dignity and of the equal and inalienable rights of all members of the human family is the foundation of freedom, justice and peace in the world,

Whereas disregard and contempt for human rights have resulted in barbarous acts which have outraged the conscience of mankind, and the advent of a world in which human beings shall enjoy freedom of speech and belief and freedom from fear and want has been proclaimed as the highest aspiration of the common people,

Whereas it is essential, if man is not to be compelled to have recourse, as a last resort, to rebellion against tyranny and oppression, that human rights should be protected by the rule of law,

Whereas it is essential to promote the development of friendly relations between nations,

Whereas the peoples of the United Nations have in the Charter reaffirmed their faith in fundamental human rights, in the dignity and worth of the human person and in the equal rights of men and women and have determined to promote social progress and better standards of life in larger freedom,

Whereas Member States have pledged themselves to achieve, in co-operation with the United Nations, the promotion of universal respect for and observance of human rights and fundamental freedoms,

Whereas a common understanding of these rights and freedoms is of the greatest importance for the full realization of this pledge,

Now, therefore,
The General Assembly
Proclaims this Universal Declaration of Human Rights as a common standard of achievement for all peoples and all nations, to the end that every individual and every organ of society, keeping this Declaration constantly in mind, shall strive by teaching and education to promote respect for these rights and freedoms and by progressive measures, national and international, to secure their universal and effective recognition and observance, both among the peoples of Member States themselves and among the peoples of territories under their jurisdiction.

Article 1

All human beings are born free and equal in dignity and rights. They are endowed with reason and conscience and should act towards one another in a spirit of brotherhood.

Article 2

Everyone is entitled to all the rights and freedoms set forth in this Declaration, without distinction of any kind, such as race, colour, sex, language, religion, political or other opinion, national or social origin, property, birth or other status.

Furthermore, no distinction shall be made on the basis of the political, jurisdictional or international status of the country or territory to which a person belongs, whether it be independent, trust, non-self-governing or under any other limitation of sovereignty.

Article 3

Everyone has the right to life, liberty and the security of person.

Article 4

No one shall be held in slavery or servitude; slavery and the slave trade shall be prohibited in all their forms.

Article 5

No one shall be subjected to torture or to cruel, inhuman or degrading treatment or punishment.

Article 6

Everyone has the right to recognition everywhere as a person before the law.

Article 7

All are equal before the law and are entitled without any discrimination to equal protection of the law. All are entitled to equal protection against any discrimination in violation of this Declaration and against any incitement to such discrimination.

Article 8

Everyone has the right to an effective remedy by the competent national tribunals for acts violating the fundamental rights granted him by the constitution or by law.

Article 9

No one shall be subjected to arbitrary arrest, detention or exile.

Article 10

Everyone is entitled in full equality to a fair and public hearing by an independent and impartial tribunal, in the determination of his rights and obligations and of any criminal charge against him.

Article 11

1. Everyone charged with a penal offence has the right to be presumed innocent until proved guilty according to law in a public trial at which he has had all the guarantees necessary for his defence.
2. No one shall be held guilty of any penal offence on account of any act or omission which did not constitute a penal offence, under national or interna-

tional law, at the time when it was committed. Nor shall a heavier penalty be Imposed than the one that was applicable at the time the penal offence was committed.

Article 12

No one shall be subjected to arbitrary interference with his privacy, family, home or correspondence, nor to attacks upon his honour and reputation. Everyone has the right to the protection of the law against such interference or attacks.

Article 13

1. Everyone has the right to freedom of movement and residence within the borders of each State.
2. Everyone has the right to leave any country, including his own, and to return to his country.

Article 14

1. Everyone has the right to seek and to enjoy in other countries asylum from persecution.
2. This right may not be invoked in the case of prosecutions genuinely arising from non-political crimes or from acts contrary to the purposes and principles of the United Nations.

Article 15

1. Everyone has the right to a nationality.
2. No one shall be arbitrarily deprived of his nationality nor denied the right to change his nationality.

Article 16

1. Men and women of full age, without any limitation due to race, nationality or religion, have the right to marry and to found a family. They are entitled to equal rights as to marriage, during marriage and at its dissolution.
2. Marriage shall be entered into only with the free and full consent of the intending spouses.
3. The family is the natural and fundamental group unit of society and is entitled to protection by society and the State.

Article 17

1. Everyone has the right to own property alone as well as in association with others.
2. No one shall be arbitrarily deprived of his property.

Article 18

Everyone has the right to freedom of thought, conscience and religion; this right includes freedom to change his religion or belief, and freedom, either alone or in community with others and in public or private, to manifest his religion or belief in teaching, practice, worship and observance.

Article 19

Everyone has the right to freedom of opinion and expression; this right includes freedom to hold opinions without interference and to seek, receive and impart information and ideas through any media and regardless of frontiers.

Article 20

1. Everyone has the right to freedom of peaceful assembly and association.
2. No one may be compelled to belong to an association.

Article 21

1. Everyone has the right to take part in the government of his country, directly or through freely chosen representatives.
2. Everyone has the right of equal access to public service in his country.
3. The will of the people shall be the basis of the authority of government; this will shall be expressed in periodic and genuine elections which shall be by universal and equal suffrage and shall be held by secret vote or by equivalent free voting procedures.

Article 22

Everyone, as a member of society, has the right to social security and is entitled to realization, through national effort and international co-operation and in accordance with the organization and resources of each State, of the economic, social and cultural rights indispensable for his dignity and the free development of his personality.

Article 23

1. Everyone has the right to work, to free choice of employment, to just and favourable conditions of work and to protection against unemployment.
2. Everyone, without any discrimination, has the right to equal pay for equal work.
3. Everyone who works has the right to just and favourable remuneration ensuring for himself and his family an existence worthy of human dignity, and supplemented, if necessary, by other means of social protection.
4. Everyone has the right to form and to join trade unions for the protection of his interests.

Article 24

Everyone has the right to rest and leisure, including reasonable limitation of working hours and periodic holidays with pay.

Article 25

1. Everyone has the right to a standard of living adequate for the health and well-being of himself and of his family, including food, clothing, housing and medical care and necessary social services, and the right to security in the event of unemployment, sickness, disability, widowhood, old age or other lack of livelihood in circumstances beyond his control.
2. Motherhood and childhood are entitled to special care and assistance. All children, whether born in or out of wedlock, shall enjoy the same social protection.

Article 26

1. Everyone has the right to education. Education shall be free, at least in the elementary and fundamental stages. Elementary education shall be compulsory. Technical and professional education shall be made generally available and higher education shall be equally accessible to all on the basis of merit.
2. Education shall be directed to the full development of the human personality and to the strengthening of respect for human rights and fundamental freedoms. It shall promote understanding, tolerance and friendship among all nations, racial or religious groups, and shall further the activities of the United Nations for the maintenance of peace.
3. Parents have a prior right to choose the kind of education that shall be given to their children.

Article 27

1. Everyone has the right freely to participate in the cultural life of the community, to enjoy the arts and to share in scientific advancement and its benefits.
2. Everyone has the right to the protection of the moral and material interests resulting from any scientific, literary or artistic production of which he is the author.

Article 28

Everyone is entitled to a social and international order in which the rights and freedoms set forth in this Declaration can be fully realized.

Article 29

1. Everyone has duties to the community in which alone the free and full development of his personality is possible.
2. In the exercise of his rights and freedoms, everyone shall be subject only to such limitations as are determined by law solely for the purpose of securing due recognition and respect for the rights and freedoms of others and of meeting the just requirements of morality, public order and the general welfare in a democratic society.
3. These rights and freedoms may in no case be exercised contrary to the purposes and principles of the United Nations.

Article 30

Nothing in this Declaration may be interpreted as implying for any State, group or person any right to engage in any activity or to perform any act aimed at the destruction of any of the rights and freedoms set forth herein.

Acknowledgments

The editors gratefully acknowledge the following people and organizations for their contributions to *AIDS in the World II*. Without their help, and that of many other friends and colleagues throughout the world who gave their time and attention, this book could not have been written. The lack of space in this second edition of *AIDS in the World* has, in a number of instances, resulted in the condensation or the omission of data or text received from contributors. Whether the prominence accorded to their contribution is commensurate or not with the effort and time they invested in it, their support is acknowledged here with the greatest gratitude.

Authors: Shawn Aldridge, Calle Almedal, Dennis Altman, Roy Anderson, Sara Back, Henry Bagarukayo, Mariella Baldo, Tony Barnett, Ronald Bayer, Seth Berkley, Stefano Bertozzi, Bea Bezmalinovic, Timothy Brewer, Jonathan Broomberg, Françoise Brun-Vézinet, Charles Cameron, Michel Caraël, Manuel Carballo, Winne Chikafumbwa, John Cleland, Robert Colebunders, Ellen Cooper, Inge Corless, Anthony Coxon, William Cutting, Kevin de Cock, Daniel Defert, Don Des Jarlais, Anke Ehrhardt, Christopher Elias, José Esparza, Eka Esu-Williams, Nancy Fee, Benoît Ferry, Donald Francis, Samuel Friedman, Donna Futterman, A. K. Ganesh, Lisa Garbus, George Gellert, Lawrence Gelmon, Pamela Gillies, Norbert Gilmore, Erica Gollub, Lawrence Gostin, Rachel Grellier, Sofia Gruskin, Geeta Gupta, Catherine Hankins, Timothy Harding, Lori Heise, Aart Hendriks, Jody Heymann, William Heyward, Neal Hoffman, Ralf Jurgens, Arata Kochi, Louise Kuhn, Marie Laga, Marc Lallemant, Normand Lapointe, Margaret Laws, Sophie Le Coeur, Sarah Lee, Carol Levine, Jay Levy, Alan Lopez, Purnima Mane, Carola Marte, Anne Martin, Francine McCutchan, David Michaels, Ken Morrison, Ruth Gunn Mota, Roland Msiska, Daan Mulder, John Mulwa, Gerald Myers, Vinh Kim Nguyen, Paul Nunn, Richard O'Brien, James Oleske, Jeffrey O'Malley, June Osborn, Saladin Osmanov, Richard Parker, Anthony Pinching, Peter Piot, Mario Raviglione, Richard Rector, Ron Rowell, Kim Ryan, Renée Sabatier, Paul Sato, Doris Schopper, Samuel Senkusu [1940–1995], Donald Shephard, Dean Shuey, Karen Stanecki, Zena Stein, S. Sundararaman, Rose Sunkutu, Ka-

594   **Acknowledgments**

tarina Tomasevski, Rinske Van Duifhuizen, Eric van Praag, Bea Vuylsteke, Simon Watney, Maria Wawer, Peter Way, Ellen Weiss, Bruce Weniger, Daniel Whelan, Alan Whiteside, Roy Widdus, Geoffrey Woolcock, Mayada Youssef.

The Editors are grateful to members of the Steering Committee of the Global AIDS Policy Coalition (GAPC) and to the Editorial Advisory Board of *AIDS in the World*, who guided this project and reviewed sections of this volume. Our warmest thanks also go to Jeffrey House, Vice President, Oxford University Press, for his excellent collaboration. Additional reviewers and contacts in international organizations are also acknowledged with thanks: Tony Adams, Martha Ainsworth, Susan Anderson, Maxine Ankrah, Sonia Bahri, Elizabeth Belsey, Gabriel Bez, Janet Bruin, Jean-Baptiste Brunet, Tony Burton, Charles Cameron, Jim Chin, Mark Connolly, Bruce Dick, Nicholas Dodd, Peter Fasan, Arthur Fell, Lieve Fransen, Alex Gromyko, Charles Halsey, Susan Holck, Jean Hughes, Susan Hunter, Paul Jansegers, Jean-Louis Lamboray, Torben Larsen, Zita Lazzarini, Gwenyth Lewis, Patrick May, Takeshi Nakano, Jai P. Narain, Thomas Netter, Mead Over, George Petersen, Elizabeth Preble, Margaret Reinfeld, Elizabeth Reid, Wendy Roseberry, Claude Rosenfeld, Donald Shepard, Henk Smid, Michael Sweat, Karen Widhelm, Mohamed Wahdan, Fernando Zacarias.

Expert panel for epidemiological parameters: Roy Anderson, Seth Berkley, Tim Brown, Kevin De Cock, François Dabis, Marc Lallemant, Daan Mulder, Thomas Quinn, George Rutherford, David Sokal.

Questionnaire respondents: Countries of which national AIDS program managers, members of national AIDS commissions, and staff of Ministries of Health, have contributed information to the governmental national AIDS program questionnaire conducted by *AIDS in the World:* Algeria, American Samoa, Angola, Antigua and Barbuda, Argentina, Australia, Austria, Azerbaijan, Bahamas, Barbados, Belarus, Belgium, Belize, Benin, Bermuda, Bhutan, Botswana, Brazil, Brunei, Bulgaria, Burkina Faso, Cameroon, Cape Verde, Cayman Islands, Chad, Chile, China, Colombia, Comores, Congo, Cook Islands, Costa Rica, Côte d'Ivoire, Croatia, Cyprus, Czech Republic, Denmark, Djibouti, Dominican Republic, Ecuador, El Salvador, Estonia, Ethiopia, Fiji, Finland, France, Gabon, Germany, Ghana, Grenada, Guam, Guatemala, Guinea, Guinea-Bissau, Hong Kong, Hungary, Iceland, India, Israel, Jamaica, Japan, Jordan, Kiribati, Korea Republic, Kuwait, Kyrgyz Republic, Latvia, Lebanon, Lesotho, Liechtenstein, Lithuania, Luxembourg, Madagascar, Malaysia, Mali, Malta, Mauritania, Mauritius, Mexico, Micronesia (Federal States of), Moldova, Montserrat, Morocco, Namibia, Nepal, Netherlands, Netherlands Antilles, New Caledonia, New Guinea, New Zealand, Niue, Norway, Oman, Panama, Papua New Guinea, Peru, Portugal, Qatar, Russian Federation, Rwanda, St. Lucia, Senegal, Seychelles, Singapore, Slovenia, Solomon Islands, South Africa, Spain, Sri Lanka, Suriname, Sweden, Switzerland, Syrian Arab Republic, Taiwan, Tanzania, Thailand, Togo, Tokelau, Trinidad and Tobago, Tunisia, Turkmenistan, Tuvalu, Uganda, Ukraine, United Kingdom, United States, Uruguay, Vanuatu, Venezuela, Vietnam, Western Samoa, Yugoslavia, Zaire, Zambia, Zimbabwe, Zanzibar.

Non-governmental organizations: The following organizations have contributed information to the survey conducted by *AIDS in the World:* Brazil: Brazilian Interdisciplinary AIDS Association; Costa Rica: Asoçiación Demográfica Costarricense; Dominican Republic: Centro de Orientacion e Investigacion Integral; France: AIDES Federation Nationale; India: Indian Health Organization; Morocco: Association Marocaine Du Lutte Contre Le SIDA; Netherlands: HIV Association Netherlands; Nigeria: Action Health, AIDS Must Go, Christian Health Association of Nigeria, Cross River State AIDS Committee, Federation of Moslem Women, Fite AIDS, National Council of Women's Societies, Nigeria Youth AIDS Programme, Salvation Army, Society for Women and AIDS in Nigeria, STOP AIDS; Russian Federation: AIDS Infoshare Russia; Santo Domingo: Patronato De Lucha Contra El SIDA, Inc.; Senegal: Enda Tiers Monde; Spain: Conite Ciudadano Anti-SIDA; Tunisia: Tunisian Association for AIDS Control; Uganda: AIDS Information Centre, The AIDS Support Organization; United Kingdom: London Lighthouse, The Terrence Higgins Trust; United States: AIDS Action Committee of Massachusetts, Inc., National Minority AIDS Council.

Countries and organizations responding to the Official Development Assistance questionnaire conducted by *AIDS in the World:* AIDS Task Force of the E.C.; Australia, Canada, Commission of the European Communities, France, Germany, Japan, Luxembourg, Netherlands, Norway, OECD, Spain, Sweden, United Kingdom, United States, UNDP, UNESCO, UNFPA, UNICEF, WHO, World Bank.

Respondents to the survey on AIDS orphans conducted by *AIDS in the World* and The Orphan Project: Antigua: Ministry of Education; Burundi: Department de la Protection Sociale of the Burundi National AIDS Program; Côte D'Ivoire: Faculté des Sciences Economiques D'Abidjan; Kenya: CAZ Boga-Zaire, Medical Service, AIDS Orphans Support Organization of Kenya, University of Nairobi; Malawi: Ministry of Women & Children Affairs & Community Services; Papua New Guinea: Office of Health Secretary, Southern Highlands Province; Romania: Children and Family's Institute in Romania, Ecumenical Association of Churches in Romania; Rwanda: Protestant Council of Rwanda; Tanzania: Community Health Nursing Service, National AIDS Control Program, Ministry of Health, Wamata-Izigo Branch, Social Welfare Department, Preventive Health Services, Ministry of Health, Zanzibar AIDS Control Programme; Uganda: Uganda Women's Effort to Save Orphans, Church of Uganda, Mobile Home Care & Orphan's Programme, All Saints Health Services, AMREF Orphan Project; United Kingdom: Barnardo's, Department of Health, HIV/STD Division, PHLS Communicable Disease Surveillance Center, Positively Irish Action On AIDS; United States: Division of HIV/AIDS, Centers for Disease Control and Prevention; Zambia: Family Health Trust, CINDI Project.

Respondents to the sexually transmitted infection questionnaire conducted by *AIDS in the World:* Susan Allen, Josef Bogaerts, Arun Chakraborty, Shao Chang-geng, John Chikwem, Debra Cohen, Mamadou Diallo, Hilde Engels, Workneh Feleke, R.P. Fule, Asha Goyal, Delfim Guerreiro, Lazare Kaptué, Sandra Larsen, Zekeng Leopold, P.M.V. Martin, Timothy Mastro, P.G. Miotti, S. Niruthisard, Watoky Nkya, Taweesak Nopkesorn, Nzilambi Nzila, Laura Olivera, Andrew Pattullo, Teera Ramasoota, Krishna Ray, J. Ross, N.D. Samb, Jorge Sánchez, Vijay Sharma, Jana Smarajit, M.F. Smikle, Surapol Suwanagool, M. Temmerman, Akgün Yildiz.

Respondents to the care model questionnaire conducted by *AIDS in the World:* France: Laboratoire d'Économie Sociale, South Marseille Health Network; Italy: Caritas Servizio di Assistenza Domiciliare, Operatori Sanitari Associati; Uganda: The AIDS Support Organization; United Kingdom: The Salvation Army International Headquarters; United States: AID Atlanta Program; Zambia: Chikankata Hospital Home Care Program.

Private corporations that have contributed information to the survey conducted by *AIDS in the World:* Anglo-American Corporation of South Africa, Ltd.; Avon Products, Inc; Banco de Brasil; Botswana Meat Commission; British-American Tobacco Co., Ltd.; Chamber of Mines of South Africa; Debswana Diamond Company; First Pacific Company Ltd.; Gold Fields of South Africa; Heineken NV; International Business Machines (I.B.M.); Kgalagabi Breweries Ltd.; Matsushita Health Care Center; Metro Pacific Corporation; Mutondo House; Nestlé; Polaroid Corporation; Saison Palette Co.; Schlumberger; Shell International Petroleum Co.; Sony Electronics Inc.; Southwestern Bell Corporation; Sun Life of Canada; Syntex; The Tata Iron and Steel Company Ltd.; 3M Thailand; Volkswagen AG; Zambia Consolidated Copper Mines. The collaboration extended to *AIDS in the World* on this project by the **AIDS Business Coalition** is also acknowledged.

Respondents to the survey on HIV/AIDS in newborns and children conducted by *AIDS in the World:* Argentina: Celia Wainstein; Brazil: Norma Rubini; Canada: Normand Lapointe; Côte D'Ivoire: Alan Greenberg; Germany: Ilse Grosch-Worner; Italy: Carlo Giaquinto; Uganda: Denis Tindyebwa; United Kingdom: Clare Davison; United States: Elaine Abrams, James Oleske.

The staff of the François-Xavier Bagnoud Center, Harvard School of Public Health, have contributed to this project with great dedication:

Publication coordinator: Susan Grady

Data analysis: Myrna Cesar, Kathy Reinig, Maria Madison

Data management and graphics: Alex Kay

Text processing: Falu Bakrania, Ann Cortissoz, Jeremy Radtke, Robert Rogers, Jeff Suzuki, Sue Vo, Sharon Walcott

Editorial assistance: Sheila Butler, Martha Doggett, Jill Hannum, Todd Macalister

Research assistants: Paul Barese, Bea Bezmalinovic, Sujata Bose, Rebecca Bunnell, Ana Cepin, David Farrar, Lisa Garbus, Gertrud Helling-Giese, Deborah Kacanek, Ayano Kato, Sonia Lal, Margaret Laws, Lydia Mann, Naomi Mann, Azmat Maskati, T. Christopher Mast, Debra Morton, Junko Otani, Deirdre Richardson, Hassan Salah, Sophia Schlette, Juliette Simon, David Studdert, Siddhartha Ventakappa, David Vu, Michele Zachs, Laura Zanini

Translation: Ana Cepin, Gabriela Fernandez DiFranco, Catherine Galley, Nick Nesbitt, Junko Otani, Sophia Schlette, Arnaud Tarantola

Project support: Vibeke Burley, Kris Kalil, Frances Lieberthal, Mary Pat McCabe, Jacoba von Gimborn

The Editors also wish to acknowledge the following organizations for their help in providing or reviewing information presented here: Agence Nationale de Recherches sur le SIDA (France), American Foundation for AIDS Research (United States), The Appropriate Health Resources and Technologies Action Group (United Kingdom), Association François-Xavier Bagnoud (Switzerland), Business Exchange on AIDS and Development (United Kingdom), Centre Nationale de la Recherche Scientifique (France), EC Commission AIDS Program (Belgium), European Centre for the Epidemiological Monitoring of AIDS (France), Family Health International (United States), Harvard AIDS Institute (United States), Indian Health Organization (India), Institut Pasteur (France), International HIV/AIDS Alliance (United Kingdom), Istituto Superiore di Sanità/Virology Department (Italy), National Institutes of Health (United States), National Leadership Coalition (United States), Pan American Health Organization (United States), PANOS Institute (United Kingdom), Rockefeller Foundation (United States), Salvation Army (United Kingdom), Save the Children Fund (United Kingdom and United States), UNAIDS, UNICEF, UNDP, UNESCO, U.S. Bureau of Census (United States), U.S. Centers for Disease Control and Prevention (United States), World Bank (United States), World Health Organization (Switzerland).

Index

Accessory genes, 178
ACTG 175, 160–161
Activism
  by homosexual groups, 119–120, 348
  by NGOs, 347–348
  as personal care strategy, 401
  research funding and, 202
ADCC (antibody-directed cellular cytotoxicity), 179
Adolescents
  AIDS cases, by transmission method, 60f
  alcohol usage, 241–242
  barriers in making choices, 242
  changing roles of, 242
  condom usage, 238–239
  HIV-infected
    in Africa, 33–34
    perinatally-acquired, 14
  HIV seroprevalence, 237
  homosexual, 241
  information/education programs, 224
  parental conflicts, 241
  partnerships with health authorities, 243–246
  personal behavior development, 240–242
  power relationships, 240
  prevention
    approaches, 237–238
    health care and, 242–243, 243t
    peer approaches, 247–248
    sex education programs, 238–239
  risk-taking behavior, 240–241
  sexual behavior, 304–306
  societal ambivalence and, 236
  STIs and, 245, 247–248
  vulnerability to HIV/AIDS, 454–457
  youth group interventions, evaluating, 149, 151t
Adults. See also Men; Women
  AIDS cases
    by GAA, 11, 11t–13t, 13f, 22t–23t
    survival rates in industrialized countries, 15
    by transmission method, 60f

deaths, AIDS-related, 17t
HIV infections
  newly acquired, 18–19, 18t, 19f
  persons living with, 21, 24, 22t–24t
  prevalence by country, 491t–495t
young. See also Adolescents
  barriers in making choices, 242
  changing roles of, 242
  condom usage, 238–239
  group interventions, evaluating, 149, 151t
  health care and HIV prevention, 242–243,
    243t
  HIV-infected, in Africa, 33–34
  personal behavior development, 240–242
  power relationships, 240
  prevention approach, 237–238
  sex education programs, 238–239
  STIs and, 245, 247–248
  vulnerability to HIV/AIDS, 454–457
Affirmation, 119
Africa. See also specific African countries; Sub-
    Saharan Africa
  AIDS orphans, 278, 283–285
  deaths, AIDS-related, of parents, children and, 281–
    282
  HIV/AIDS pandemic, 28–35
    mobility and, 33–34
    surveillance, 34–35
  HIV infection
    epidemics, 29–30
    HIV-1 subtype, 14, 15–16
    in pregnancy, socioeconomic status and, 58, 59f
    prevalence, 28, 31–32
    in women, 59–60, 59f
  HIV seroprevalence
    in pregnant women, 44f
    tuberculosis and, 87, 88t
  publicly owned industrial enterprises in, 403
  research, 35
  sexually transmitted infections, 32–33

Africa (cont'd.)
  tuberculosis, AIDS-related, 87–89, 89*t*
  women in, 216
    HIV risk, 101
    pregnant, HIV seroprevalence of, 44*f*
African-American men
  condom usage, 260
  mistrust of, 304–305
African Medical and Research Foundation (AMREF),
    284
AIDS. *See also specific aspects of the disease*
  cases
    by GAA, 11–13
    from homosexual transmission, 254–255
    in indigenous populations, 435, 435*f*
    new, 19, 20*t*–21*t*
    in young people, 237
  demographic impact, 73, 74*f*
  early observations, 207–208
  economic impact. *See* Economic factors, impact of
    HIV/AIDS on
  global prevalence, 24, 25
  history, 464
  with HIV infection. *See* HIV/AIDS
  incidence, in Europe, 36
  incubation period
    infectiousness during, 75, 77, 76*f*
    length of, 73–74, 75, 73*f*–74*f*, 165
  prevalence, 21–23
  in prison, 268–269
  progression, cofactors in, 167
  surveillance data, 37
  tuberculosis and, 87–89, 89*t*
  vaccine development. *See* Vaccine
AIDSCAP (AIDS Control and Prevention Project), 385
AIDS Case Definition, invasive cervical carcinoma
    and, 231–232
AIDS Control and Prevention Project (AIDSCAP), 385
AIDS indicator disease, invasive cervical carcinoma
    as, 231–232
AIDS service organizations (ASOs)
  functions, 341
  human rights violations and, 329
  support, 402
  sustaining, 360
AIDS Support Organization (TASO), 341–342
Alcohol
  adolescent usage, 241–242
  in HIV transmission, 234
Americans with Disabilities Act of 1990, 336, 402
Amnesty International, 329
AMREF (African Medical and Research Foundation),
    284
Anal intercourse
  cultural influences, 139
  as female risk factor, 221–222
  gay men and, 252–253
  omission from prevention programs, 259
Angola, 171–172
Antibodies, cross-reacting, 179
Antibody-dependent enhancement (ADE), 179

Antibody-directed cellular cytotoxicity (ADCC), 179
Antidiscrimination legislation, 336
Anti-envelope antibodies, 179
Anti-gp120, 180
Antiretroviral drug therapy. *See also specific anti-*
    retroviral drugs
  availability, 404–405
  development, 159
  progress, 159
  types, 400–401
  utilization, increased, 404–405
  vaccination. *See* Vaccine
Anti-V3 antibodies, 180
Apoptosis (programmed cell death), 178
Arts/artists, AIDS and, 118–119
Asia. *See also* Northeast Asia; Southeast Asia; *specific*
    Asian countries
  expenditures on AIDS, by GNAP, 420*t*
  HIV infection, with tuberculosis, 89–90, 90*t*
Asia Watch, 329
ASOs (AIDS service organizations), 329, 341–342
Association François-Xavier Bagnoud, 284
Attributable risk, 100
Australian AIDS policy, gay community and, 354–355
Australian Human Rights and Equal Opportunity Act
    of 1986, 336
Austria, 36
Azidothymidine. *See* AZT
AZT
  clinical trials, 160–162
    ACTG 175, 160
    Concorde, 160, 210
    Delta, 160
  in combination, 160–161
  development, 159–163

Bacillus Calmette-Guerin (BCG), 92–93
Bacterial vaginosis, 104
Basic reproductive rate (R_0), 71–72
BCG (Bacillus Calmette-Guerin), 92–93
Bearing witness, 118
Behavioral sciences, theories/conceptual models,
    131–132, 133*t*–135*t*
Behavioral surveys, GNAP, 560*t*–562*t*
Benzalkonium chloride, for HIV prevention, 197*t*
Biocine prototype vaccine, 187
Bisexual transmission
  age and, 57–58
  in Australia, 354
  in Caribbean, 61–62, 61*f*
  in Europe, 36–37
  incidence, 60
  in Latin America, 61–62, 61*f*
  in United States, 60–61, 61*f*
Bleach, as virucidal agent, 269–270
Blood and blood products
  contamination, HIV transmission in Europe and, 37
  donations. *See* Blood donors
  HIV transmission
    civil litigation, 288–289

compensation for, 287–288
criminal charges, 289
public inquiries, 289–290
risks, 287
safety, 290
ELISA screening and, 291
ensuring, costs for, 415, 416*f*
p24 antigen screening and, 290–291
PCR screening and, 291
strengthening, economic impact of, 295–296
treatment, reducing demand for, 295
Blood donors
commercial, 295
HIV-infected
excluding, 294–295
incidence of, 290
HIV seroprevalence
in Caribbean, 42*f*
in Latin America, 41, 42*f*
in Southeast Asia, 54, 56
patient-recruited, 294–295
recruitment, 45
screening
methods, 293–294
by p24 antigen, 290–291
self-exclusion, 294
Botswana
HIV/AIDS in, 29, 31
primary health care system, 405–407
Brazil
minority populations, HIV/AIDS and, 465
sexual culture, 139
Work and Research Group for Sex Education, 244
Breast-feeding
benefits of, 275
HIV transmission and, 273–276
recommendations, 275–276
timing, HIV transmissibility and, 274
Breast milk characteristics, HIV transmissibility and, 274
Business coalitions, 366

Cambodia, 63
Cameroon, 113
Canada
blood-borne transmission
compensation for, 288
public inquiries on, 289
HIV/AIDS
in indigenous population, 437–438
in prisons, 270–271
Candidiasis, in HIV infection, 230, 231*f*
Care. *See* Health care
Caribbean GAA
AIDS cases
cumulative, 11, 11*t*–13*t*
new, 19, 20*t*–21*t*
prevalence, 24–25
AIDS reporting in, 6
blood donors, 42*f*

deaths, AIDS-related, 17*t*
female sex workers, HIV seroprevalence, 43*f*
HIV/AIDS, 21, 23
HIV infection
cumulative data, 26–27
newly acquired cases, 18–19, 18*t*, 19*f*
persons living with, 21, 24, 22*t*–25*t*
with tuberculosis, 89–90, 90*t*, 91*t*
HIV seroprevalence, 41, 43, 42*f*–44*f*
population estimates, 9*f*
pregnant women, HIV seroprevalence, 42*f*, 98
STI clinic patients, HIV seroprevalence, 44*f*
tuberculosis, AIDS and, 87–89, 89*t*
Case management, formalized systems
African model of home-based care, 409–410
San Francisco Model, 407–409
Case reproductive rate (R_0), 71–72
Catholic religion, 451
CBOs. *See* Community-based organizations
CDC. *See* Centers for Disease Control
CD4+ lymphocytes
count
in early-to-moderate stage disease, 160
in HIV-2 infection, 173
in early AIDS observations, 207
HIV pathogenesis and, 178–179
in incubation period, 75
in non-progressors, 165
CD8+ lymphocytes, in non-progressors, 165
Centers for Disease Control (CDC)
AIDS Case Definition, 231–232
AIDS case reports, in Native Americans, 435, 437–438, 435*f*–437*f*
AIDS reporting and, 6
Central America, AIDS reporting in, 6
Cervical cancer
in HIV-infected women, 231
HIV-1 infection and, 99
for HIV prevention, 197*t*
Cervical dysplasia, in HIV-infected women, 231
Chancroid, in women, 102
Chemoprophylaxis, for HIV-TB coinfection, 92–93
Child mortality rate (CMR), 29, 275
Children. *See also* Adolescents; Infants
AIDS, persons living with, 22–23
health care requirements, 411
HIV/AIDS impact on, 279–280
HIV-infected. *See* Pediatric HIV/AIDS
orphaned by AIDS. *See* Orphans, HIV/AIDS
protection from AIDS, 236
sexual abuse of, 244–246
China, 62, 63, 65, 66
Chinese herbs, 400–401
Chlamydial infections, 103
Chlorhexidine, for HIV prevention, 198*t*
Cholangitis, HIV-2 infection and, 173
Christianity, 448–449
Cigarette smoking, AIDS progression and, 167
Civil litigation, for blood-borne transmission, 288–289
Clades
diagnostic criteria, 181–182

Clades (cont'd.)
  geographic distribution, 182*f*
  prevalence, 182–183, 182*f*
  properties, 10
  vaccine development and, 130, 183
Clinical trials
  AZT, 160–162
  protease inhibitors, 162
  research goals for, 162
  of vaccine prototype, 187
CMR (child mortality rate), 28, 275
Coalition building, 318, 366
Cocaine trade routes, in South America, 65, 66*f*
Colostrum, HIV transmission risk, 274
Community-based organizations (CBOs)
  in Australia, 354–355
  functions, 341, 344–345
  sustaining, 360
Compensation, for blood-borne transmission, 287–288
Conceptual models, social science, 131–132, 133*t*–
    135*t*
Concorde Trial, 160, 210
Condoms
  adolescents and, 238–239
  distribution
    adequacy of, 536*t*–540*t*
    costs of, 415
    number of, 541*t*–544*t*
    1990 sites, 545*t*–549*t*
    1992 sites, 550*t*–554*t*
  female. *See* Female condoms
  for prisoners, 270, 271
  quality issues, 442
  religious views on, 448, 449
  usage
    barriers to, 260–261
    fear of, 219
    perceptions of consequences of, 260
    power, by withholding sex, 218
    by young people, 238–239
Confidentiality, 363
Contraceptives. *See also specific contraceptive
    methods*
  decision-making
    male control of, 216
    powerlessness of women and, 218
  HIV infection risk and, 98
  for HIV prevention, 197*t*, 198
  hormonal, HIV risk and, 233
Corporations. *See* Private sector corporations
Costs. *See* Health care costs
Côte d'Ivoire, 88*t*, 172–173
Council of Europe
  HIV/AIDS in prisons, guidelines for, 270–271
  nondiscrimination, 331
Counseling
  GNAP, 555*t*–559*t*
  for HIV-infected women, 261–262
  peer, 398, 400
  voluntary, GNAP and, 322, 323*f*

CPT (European Committee for the Prevention of Tor-
    ture and Inhuman or Degrading Treatment or
    Punishment), 270
Criminalization, of homosexual acts, 333–334, 467
Cryptococcal meningitis, 160
CTL. *See* Cytotoxic T-cell lymphocytes (CTL)
Culture
  entitlement and, 445
  health communication and, 304
  influence on social vulnerability, 444–446
  norms, masculine ideals and, 220–221
  power and, 445
  risk and, 445
  sexual mores and, 139, 242
  traditional values, changes in, 242
Cytomegalovirus infection (CMV), 160
  AIDS progression and, 167
  HIV-2 infection and, 173
Cytotoxic T-cell lymphocytes (CTL), HIV-specific re-
    sponse, in nonprogressors, 165

DALYs (disability-adjusted life years), 111
ddC (Zalcitabine), 159, 160
ddI (Didanosine), 159–161
Deaths, AIDS-related, 306
  by GAA, 17*t*
  of parents, children and, 281–282
  time intervals for, 489*f*–490*f*
  tuberculosis, 91
  of young people, 237
Delta trial, 160–161
Demographic and health surveys (DHS), 140
Demographics
  AIDS impact on, 73, 74*f*
  population growth, 73, 74*f*
Denmark, 37
Developing countries. *See also specific countries*
  breast-feeding transmission in, 275
  gonorrhea in, 103
  health care
    cost recovery programs, 404
    needs, 163
    resources, 394–395
    user fees, 404
  HIV-1 infection in
    incubation period for, 15–16
    survival, 15–16
  homosexuality in, 255–256
  mother-to-child transmission rate, 488*t*
  prevalence, HIV/AIDS, 24, 25, 24*t*, 25*t*
  prevention
    costs, 414–416, 416*f*
    peer approaches, 247–248
  prison populations, 268
  research, 130
    agendas, 202
    funding, 202
  simulated HIV epidemic, 82–83, 83*f*, 84*f*
  tracking ODA funding to, 382, 384–385, 385*f*
  tuberculosis in, 87

urbanization, 48–49
vaccine trials
    immediate preparatory issues, 193–195
    rationale for, 193
DHS (demographic and health surveys), 140
Diaphragm, 98, 197*t*, 198
Didanosine (ddI), 159–161
Diet, in personal care strategies, 400
Disability-adjusted life years (DALYs), 111
Discrimination, 352. *See also* Human rights
    conceptual issues, 331
    employment, 363
    legal issues, 331
    legislation against, 336
    prevention, 433
    research and, 211
    tolerance and, 466–467
    vulnerability and, 465
    World Health Assembly resolution of 1988 and, 327
Disease. *See also specific diseases*
    gynecologic, in HIV-infected women, 230–232, 231*f*
DNA sequencing, 180
Donor fatigue syndrome, 387–388
Drug abusers. *See* Injection drug users (IDUs)
Drugs
    for HIV/AIDS treatment. *See* Antiretroviral drug
        therapy
    illicit
        administration routes, 65
        law enforcement efforts, 64
Dry sex, 101
Duesberg phenomenon, 308

EAPs (employee assistance programs), 363, 364
Eastern Europe GAA. *See also specific Eastern Euro-
        pean countries*
    AIDS cases
        cumulative, 11, 11*t*–13*t*
        new, 19, 20*t*–21*t*
        prevalence, 24–25
    deaths, AIDS-related, 17*t*
    HIV/AIDS, 21, 23
    HIV infection
        cumulative data, 26, 27*t*
        newly acquired cases, 18–19, 18*t*, 19*f*
        persons living with, 21, 24, 22*t*–25*t*
        with tuberculosis, 91*t*
Economic factors
    in HIV vulnerability, 471
    impact of HIV/AIDS on, 114–115
        country case study reviews, 112–114
        disability-adjusted life years and, 111
        literature review, 110–112
        sectoral, 114
    risk, 217–218
    sexual life and, 148
    in social vulnerability, 453
Education programs
    audience for, 442
    partnerships with adolescents, 243–246

peer, cost of, 416*f*
    sex education programs, 238–239
Elderly, AIDS incubation period, 73
ELISA screening, of blood donors, 291
Employee assistance programs (EAPs), 363, 364
Employment
    accommodations of HIV-infected employees,
        365
    discrimination, 363
    HIV testing, 362–363
    informal sector, 403–404
Empowerment
    and gay community in Australia, 354–355
    prevention and, 475–476
    self-efficacy and, 475
ENDA Tiers Monde, 342
Entitlement, cultural aspects of, 445
Env gene, 180
Epidemics. *See also* HIV/AIDS pandemic
    classical curve for, 71, 72*f*
    duration, 72
        variability of infectiousness and, 75, 77, 76*f*
    mixed pattern, 77, 79–85, 78*f*–84*f*
    secondary infections and, 71
    simple, 77, 78*f*
    wave pattern, 79–85, 79*f*–84*f*
Epidemiology
    of AIDS, in indigenous populations, 434
    correlation with religious practices, 450
    GNAP, 512*t*–516*t*
    HIV, gender differences in, 98–99
    of HIV, in women, 97–98
    of sexually transmitted infections, in women, 101–
        104
    studies, 430–432
    trends, 121–122
Europe. *See also* Eastern Europe; *specific European
        countries;* Western Europe
    AIDS incidence, 36
    gonorrhea in, 103
    HIV/AIDS pandemic, 36
    HIV infection, with tuberculosis, 89–90, 90*t*
    HIV transmission
        by contaminated blood, 37
        heterosexual, 37
        homosexual/bisexual, 36–37
        injection-drug use, 36
        mother-to-child, 37
    syphilis seroprevalence rate, 102
    tuberculosis, AIDS and, 87–89, 89*t*
European Centre for the Epidemiological Monitoring
        of AIDS, 35–36
European Commission and Court of Human Rights,
        333
European Committee for the Prevention of Torture
        and Inhuman or Degrading Treatment or Pun-
        ishment (CPT), 270
European Convention of Human Rights, 331
European Court of First Instance, 334
European Union (EU), 334, 377

FACT (Fraternity for AIDS Cessation in Thailand), 256

Family
  burdens, HIV/AIDS and, 282–283
  extended, child care after parental death and, 281–282
  multigenerational AIDS effect, 14–15

Federation of Red Cross and Red Crescent Societies, 337

Female condoms, 196
  distribution, 197*t*
  effectiveness, 197*t*
  evaluation, 197*t*
  priority of, 308
  use, impediments to, 233

Female genital mutilation, 220

Female sex workers. *See also* Prostitution
  contact with young males, 241–242
  HIV-2 infections, 173
  HIV prevention, spermicides and, 199
  HIV seroprevalence, 79–81, 80*f*–82*f*, 98
    injection drug use and, 98
    Southeast Asia, 52, 53*f*–54*f*, 56
    Sub-Saharan Africa, 45*f*
  interventions, evaluating, 149, 152*t*–153*t*
  serologic reactivity, dual, 174
  sexual behavior survey, 145, 146*t*
  in Southeast Asia, 63
    HIV seroprevalence, 52, 53*f*–54*f*, 56
  syphilis seroprevalence rate, 102, 102*f*
  in Thailand, 60
  trichomoniasis, 104
  vulnerability, 234

Fertility
  age-specific rates, by GAA, 488*t*
  AIDS and, 279

Finland, 37

First aid, in workplace, 363

France, 36, 37, 88*t*, 289

François-Xavier Bagnoud Center for Health and Human Rights, 337–338

Funding
  bilateral, 377, 378*t*, 379*t*
  health care, shifts in, 403–404

GAAs. *See* Geographic Areas of Affinity

Galvanization, 119

Gay men. *See also* Homosexuality
  activism, 119–120
  in AIDS causation, 207
  anal intercourse and, 252–253
  artists, AIDS-related deaths, 118–119
  behavior changes, 252–254
  of color, 254
  contact networks, 77, 78*f*
  interventions, evaluating, 149–150, 156, 155*t*
  NGOs and, 348
  prevention programs, critical issues for, 253–254
  risk, from oral sex, 259
  sex partners, number of, 253
  sexual identities/roles, construction of, 147
  survivors, long-term, 165, 166*t*

Gay rights movement, 256

GDP (gross domestic product), 112

Gender relations, 216

Genentech prototype vaccine, 187

Genetic distance, 181

Genital herpes, 103

Genital mutilation, female, 220

Genital ulcer disease (GUD)
  acquisition of HIV and, 99
  epidemiology, in women, 102–103
  syphilis, 101–102, 102*f*

Geographic Areas of Affinity (GAAs). *See also* specific GAAs
  age-specific fertility rates, 488*t*
  concept, 9–10
    advantages of, 10
    disadvantages of, 10
  HIV infections
    adult, urban:rural ratios, 488*t*
    cumulative, 11*t*
  HIV seropositivity of women, 488*t*
  population estimates, 9*f*
  reporting by, 479*t*–486*t*

Geographic distribution, HIV-2, 171–172

Germany, 36, 37, 288–290

GIPA (greater involvement of people with HIV/AIDS), 351

Global AIDS Policy Coalition (GAPC), 327
  assessment of human rights impact, 337–338
  HIV prevalence estimates, 26
  national legislation survey, 336

Global AIDS Strategy, 369, 375, 430
  funding, 378, 378*t*, 379–380, 380*t*–383*t*, 383*f*
  human rights and, 327

Global Program on AIDS. *See under* World Health Organization

GNAP. *See* Government national AIDS programs

Gonorrhea, in developing countries, 103

Government national AIDS programs (GNAPs), 7, 312
  AIDS policy and program document, 319–320, 319*t*
  assessment criteria, 315
  behavioral surveys, 560*t*–562*t*
  coalition-building, 318
  commitment to, 317, 317*t*, 318*f*
  condom distribution, 321
    adequacy of, 536*t*–540*t*
    number of, 541*t*–544*t*
    1990 sites, 545*t*–549*t*
    1992 sites, 550*t*–554*t*
  coordination, 319–320, 320*f*
  counseling, 555*t*–559*t*
    voluntary, 322, 323*f*
  epidemiology, 512*t*–516*t*
  expenditures on AIDS
    in Asia, 420*t*
    in Pacific Island countries, 421*t*
    in Sub-Saharan Africa, 418*t*–419*t*
  financial resources
    impact on NGOs, 357–358

information on, 526t–531t
securing, 322, 325
HIV/AIDS prevention, annual per capita spending,
422t–423t
HIV testing, voluntary, 322, 323t, 555t–559t
impact
evaluation of, 324t, 325
on other health programs, 517t–525t
information/medical care training, 532t–535t
laws/practices regarding HIV/AIDS, 578t–587t
managers, 316, 318
survey of, 578t–587t
needs assessment, 321, 322t
NGOs and, 318
planning, 319–320, 319t
progress, evaluation of, 324t, 325
structure/partnership, 506t–511t
survey, 315–317, 316t, 417
AIW II questionnaire responses, 501t–505t
findings, use of, 568t–577t
of managers, 336–337, 578t–587t
practices, 563t–567t
response rate for, 316t
Governments
anti-discriminatory efforts, 442
factors, in HIV vulnerability, 469–470
NGOs and, 359–360
social vulnerability and, 452–453
Gp41, 180
Gp120, 179
Greater involvement of people with HIV/AIDS
(GIPA), 351
Greece, 36, 37
Gross domestic product (GDP), 112
Gross national product (GNP), per capita, *vs.* direct
medical care costs, 391, 394, 392f
GUD. *See* Genital ulcer disease (GUD)
Gynecologic disease, in HIV-infected women, 230–
232, 231f

Haemophilus ducreyi, 102. *See also* Chancroid
Haitian nationals, political asylum for, 329
Hate crimes, 305
Health care. *See also* Health care costs
barriers, for indigenous populations, 438
case management, 405
expenditures, 424t, 425, 426t
HIV prevention and, 242–243, 243t
home-based, African model of, 409–410
programs, partnerships with adolescents, 243–
246
requirements
for children, 411
for infants, 411
for women, 411
resources, in developing countries, 394–395
San Francisco Model, 407–409
user fees, 404
Health care costs, 312
in developing countries, 394

financing shifts, 403–404
global, 396t
estimation methods, 395, 397
trends and, 397
HIV prevention
annual per capita spending by GNAP, 422t–423t
in high economy countries, 424t
in low economy countries, 424t
of HIV prevention, 414–416, 416f
for home-based care, 406–407
hospital inpatient, 390
by illness stage, 395, 395t
in industrialized countries, 394–395
long-term facility, 390–391
medical, direct
by country, 391, 394, 392t–393t
vs. per capita GNP, 391, 394, 392f
personal care strategies, 398, 400–402, 399f
recovery programs, 404
Health communication, and AIDS epidemic in United
States, 304
Hemophilia, HIV incidence, 293
Hepatitis B, transmission, 293
Hepatitis C, transmission, 293
Heroin, 265–266
Herpes, AIDS progression and, 167
Heterosexual transmission, 117
in Africa, 29, 58, 59f
in Caribbean, 61–62, 61f
contact networks, 77, 78f
Europe, 37
global, 57
HIV-2, 172
incidence, 60
in industrialized countries, 58–62
irresponsible sex and, 305
in Latin America, 61–62, 61f
in Sub-Saharan Africa, 97
women and, 229
High-risk behavior, socioeconomic status and, 58
Hiring, corporate policies on, 364–365
HIV. *See also* HIV infection; *specific aspects of*
biologic features, 177–179
genetic variability, vaccine development and, 194
history of response
current period, 430, 434, 439
period of discovery, 429, 430f, 430–432
period of early response, 429, 432–434, 433f
incidence, by GAA, 21–24
prevalence
adult, by country, 491t–495t
trends, in Africa, 31–32
progression to AIDS, time interval, 489f
screening. *See* HIV testing
seropositivity, of women, by GAA, 488t
seroprevalence
Caribbean, 41–44
in Europe, 37
in female sex workers, 79–81, 80f–82f
informing employer of, 363
Latin America, 41–44

HIV (cont'd.)
  Southeast Asia, 50–56
  Sub-Saharan Africa, 43–48
  tuberculosis and, 87, 88*t*
  women sex workers, 45
  vaccine. *See* Vaccine
HIV-1
  biologic features, 177–179
  clades, 10, 130
  envelope gene sequences, phylogenetic tree anal-
     ysis of, 180–181, 181*f*
  genotypes, global distribution, 180–183, 181*f*, 182*f*
  geographic distribution, 10, 65*f*
  infection
     incubation period, 15–16
     survival, 15–16
     transmissibility, 10
     tuberculosis and, 87–89, 88*t*
  molecular features, 180–184, 181*f*, 182*f*
  neutralization, resistance to, 180
  serologic features, 179–180
  seroprevalence
     injection-drug users, 80*f*
     prostitutes, 80*f*
  subtypes/clades
     diagnostic criteria, 181–182
     prevalence, 182–183, 182*f*
     serologic classification of, 179
     vaccine development and, 183
  subtypes/clades, geographic distribution, 182*f*
  transmission, success of, 85
HIV-2
  biologic features, 177–179
  blood screening for, 293
  disease associations, 173
  future research, 174
  geographic distribution, 65*f*, 171–172
  geographic spread, 10
  heterosexual transmission, 172
  infection
     serologic reactivity, 173–174
     transmissibility, 10
     virology of, 173–174
  molecular features, 180–184, 181*f*, 182*f*
  natural history, 173
  neutralization, resistance to, 180
  prevalence, 171
  serologic features, 179–180
  strains, 173–174
HIV/AIDS pandemic
  in Africa, 28–35
     adolescents/young adults and, 30
  beginning, 36
  complexity, 57
  "de-gaying" of, 432
  epidemic, first peak of, 37–39, 38*f*
  in Europe, 36
  features, 3
  future course, 24, 26, 28, 37–39, 38*f*
  knowledge/insight from, 306–308
  mobility and, 33–34

  orphans, 278
  prevalence, 21, 23, 24*t*, 25*t*
  prevention. *See* Prevention, HIV/AIDS
  public health challenges, 460
  response to, country assessment and strategic
     planning, 453–454
  side-by-side epidemics, 62–63, 64*f*
  status
     in 1996, 11–14
     estimating, 487–490*t*
     in mid-1990s, 3–4
  trends, 36
     estimating, 487–490*t*
HIV/AIDS services, 344
HIV encephalitis, HIV-2 infection and, 173
HIV infection. *See also specific aspects of*
  and AIDS. *See* HIV/AIDS
  female sexuality and, 261–262
  female-to-male ratio, 97
  incubation period, 73–74, 75, 73*f*–74*f*
     infectiousness during, 75, 77, 76*f*
  individual variability of, 162
  newly acquired, 18–19, 18*t*, 19*f*
  prevalence, 21–24
  progression to AIDS, 165
  saturation, 31–32
  sentinel surveillance of, 7–8, 8*f*
  stabilization, 32
  with tuberculosis, estimation methods, 90, 91*t*
  tuberculosis and, 87–89, 88*t*
  window period, 293
HIV-1 infection
  in Africa, 14, 15–16
  cervical cancer and, 99
  sexually transmitted infections and, 99
HIVNET (HIV Vaccine Efficacy Trials Network), 194
HIV seroprevalence, of street children/youth, 237
HIV testing
  of blood donations, 293–294
  GNAP, 555*t*–559*t*
  mandatory
     human rights and, 335, 336
     as UN policy, 334
  of migrants, 335
  positive results, national reporting of, 6–7
  pre-employment, 362
  in pregnancy, 6
  voluntary, GNAP and, 322, 323*f*
HIV Vaccine Efficacy Trials Network (HIVNET), 194
Home-based health care
  in Botswana, 405–407
  in Zambia, 409–410
Homeless population
  HIV/AIDS in, 437–438
  in United States, 303–304
Homophobia, 305
Homosexuality. *See also* Gay men; Lesbians
  activism and, 119–120, 348
  adolescent, 241
  attitudes toward, in United States, 119
  in Australia, 354–355

criminalization of, 333–334, 467
in developing countries, 255–256
HIV transmission, 254
  age and, 57–58
  in Australia, 354
  in Caribbean, 61–62, 61*f*
  in Europe, 36–37
  incidence, 60
  in Latin America, 61–62, 61*f*
  in United States, 60–61, 61*f*
  of priests, 452
  religious views on, 449
  ritualized male-to-male, 255
Host range, 177
HPV (human papillomavirus), in HIV-infected women, 231
HTLV-1, AIDS progression and, 167
Human papillomavirus (HPV), in HIV-infected women, 231
Human rights. *See also* Discrimination
  core principles, 468
  current issues, 334–335
  HIV/AIDS prevention and, 327
  HIV testing and, 334, 335
  HIV vulnerability and, 464–468
    analysis of, 469–471
  impact, assessing, 337–338, 338*f*
  legislation, 331–332
  national responses to AIDS and, 335–336
  promotion, 472
  public health measures and, 327–328
  violations, 466
    international responses to, 328–334
Hypothesis, scientific, 205–206

ICCPR (International Covenant on Civil and Political Rights), 333
ICJ (International Commission of Jurists), 329
ICW (International Community of Women Living with HIV/AIDS), 350
IDUs. *See* Injection drug users (IDUs)
IGLHRC (International Gay and Lesbian Human Rights Commission), 329
ILGA (International Lesbian and Gay Association), 329
Illicit drugs
  administration routes, 65
  law enforcement efforts, 64
ILO (International Labour Organization), 311
Immuno AG prototype vaccine, 187
India
  corporate response to AIDS, 367
  HIV/AIDS impact in, 124–126
  HIV seroprevalence, 52, 56, 51*f*–55*f*
    prostitutes, 80*f*
    tuberculosis and, 88*t*
  injection drug use, 265–266
  tuberculosis, AIDS and, 89*t*
Indian Ocean Island countries, 29
Indigenous populations
  health care, barriers for, 438

HIV/AIDS spread in, 434–435, 437–439, 436*f*, 437*f*
  prevention
    barriers for, 438
    success/failures, determinants of, 438
Indinovir, 162
Industrialized countries
  AIDS incubation period, 72–73, 73*f*
  heterosexual transmission, 58–62
  HIV/AIDS in, 58
    health care costs for, 394
    newly acquired, 18, 18*t*
    prevalence, 24, 25, 24, 25
    in women, 18*t*
  HIV-1 infections, 15
  mother-to-child transmission rate, 488*t*
  risk groups, 77, 78*f*
Infants. *See also* Pediatric HIV/AIDS
  health care requirements, 411
  HIV-infected, bimodal response pattern, 14
  mortality, in Africa, 29
Infections, sexually-transmitted. *See* Sexually-transmitted infections (STIs)
Information and education programs. *See* Education programs
Injection-drug users (IDUs)
  AIDS cases, 60
  in China, 65, 66
  contact networks, 77, 78*f*
  female sex workers, 98
  HIV infection in
    epidemic types, 265
    geographic distribution of, 264
    rates for, 62
    spread of, 265–266
    women, 234
  HIV seroprevalence
    HIV-1, 80*f*
    Southeast Asia, 55*f*, 56
  intervention programs
    costs of, 415
    evaluating, 149, 154*t*
    for risk reduction, 264
  needle exchange programs, 120–121
  in prison, 269–270
  transition from heroin to semisynthetic narcotics, 265–266
  transmission via, in Europe, 36
  women, 411
Institutional response, 311–313
Intergovernmental system
  actions of, 334
  responses to human rights violations, 330–331
Interleukin-2, 159–160
International AIDS Conference, 350
International Centre Against Censorship, 329–330
International Children's Centre, Paris, 112
International Commission of Jurists (ICJ), 329
International Community of Women Living with HIV/AIDS (ICW), 350
International Conference on AIDS & STD in Africa, Kampala workshop, 28–35

International Conference on Global Impact of AIDS (1988), 110
International Covenant on Civil and Political Rights (ICCPR), 333
International Federation of Red Cross and Red Crescent Societies, 337
International Gay and Lesbian Human Rights Commission (IGLHRC), 329, 342
International HIV/AIDS Alliance, 358
International Human Rights Law Group, 329
International Labour Organization (ILO), 311
International Lesbian and Gay Association (ILGA), 329
Intrauterine device (IUD), HIV infection risk and, 98
Intravenous drug users (IVDUs). *See* Injection-drug users (IDUs)
Islamic law, 449
Italy, 36
IVDUs. *See* Injection-drug users (IDUs)

Japan, 288
Judaism, 448

KABP surveys
    for sex research, 137–138
    WHO/GPA, 140, 143t–145t
Kaposi's sarcoma, 207
KASAKA, 345
Kenya, 16, 29, 30, 80f, 81
Korea, Republic of, 114

Lamivudine, with AZT, 161
Latin America, STI clinic patients, HIV seroprevalence, 44f
Latin America GAA. *See also* Central America; South America; *specific countries*
    AIDS cases
        cumulative, 11, 11t–13t
        new, 19, 20t–21t
    blood donors, seroprevalence, 41, 42f
    deaths, AIDS-related, 17t
    female sex workers, HIV seroprevalence, 43f
    genital ulcer disease, in women, 102–103
    HIV/AIDS, 21, 23
    HIV/AIDS prevalence, 24–25
    HIV infection
        cumulative data, 26, 27t
        newly acquired cases, 18–19, 18t, 19f
        persons living with, 21, 24, 22t–25t
        with tuberculosis, 89–90, 90t, 91t
    HIV seroprevalence, 41, 43, 42f–44f
        tuberculosis and, 88t
    NGOs, 348
    population estimates, 9f
    pregnant women, HIV seroprevalence, 42f
    tuberculosis, AIDS and, 87–89, 89t
    women in, 216
Legislation
    human rights and, 332, 335–336
    national, survey of, 336–337

nondiscrimination, 336
    regarding HIV/AIDS, 578t–587t
Lesbians, risk of HIV from oral sex, 259
Lesotho, 31
Library Foundation, 256
Life expectancy, after AIDS diagnosis, 11
Light sex, 220
LIP (lymphocyte interstitial pneumonia), 14
Long-term survivors, 165–167, 166t
Lymphocyte interstitial pneumonia (LIP), 14

Macroeconomic impact of HIV/AIDS, 110, 111–112
Malawi, 29
Male sex workers, 255
Marriage, first, age of, 260
MAS (medical aid societies), 403
MDR-TB (multiple drug resistant tuberculosis), 91–92, 93
Media
    AIDS hysteria and, 401
    HIV prevention programs, costs of, 415, 416f
    misinformation from, 209
    sexual messages, 240
Medical aid societies (MAS), 403
Medical care. *See* Health care
Medical care costs, direct. *See also* Health care costs
    by country, 391, 394, 392t–393t
    vs. per capita GNP, 391, 394, 392f
Medical technology, 451
Mediterranean. *See* Southeast Mediterranean GAA
Men. *See also* Gay men
    AIDS cases, 11t, 13t
    bisexual, STD risk, 58
    cultural capital and, 450–451
    deaths, AIDS-related, 17t
    HIV infections, 21, 23
        newly acquired, 18t
        persons living with, 22–24
        in young adults, 30
    HIV risk, masculine ideals and, 220–222
    homosexual, STD risk, 58
    Native Americans, HIV/AIDS in, 436f
Menfegol, for HIV prevention, 197t
Microeconomic impact of HIV/AIDS, 110, 112
Migrants
    heterosexual relationships, 139–140
    HIV screening, 335
Migration
    AIDS-related, to rural areas, 49
    HIV/AIDS and, 33–34
    sexually transmitted infection and, 234
    urban-rural, 48–49
Military service men, 52f
Minority groups
    HIV/AIDS and, 464–465
    mistrust in, 304–305
Mistrust, of authority, 304–305, 308
Monoclonal antibodies, 179, 180
Mortality. *See* Deaths, AIDS-related
Motherhood, as feminine ideal, 220

Mother-to-child transmission. *See also* Perinatal transmission
  by breast-feeding, 273–276
  in Europe, 37
  rates, by GAA, 488*t*
Mozambique, HIV-2 infection in, 171–172
Multiple drug resistant tuberculosis (MDR-TB), 91–
  92, 93
Mutations
  nonsynonymous, 180
  synonymous, 180
Mycobacterium avium complex, 160
Mycoplasma infection, AIDS progression and, 167

NAPs. *See* Government National AIDS programs
  (GNAPs)
Narcotic analgesics, semisynthetic, 265–266
Narcotics, trade, law enforcement efforts, 64
National AIDS Control Program (NACP), 353
National AIDS programs. *See* Government national
  AIDS programs (GNAPs)
National reporting
  AIDS, 5–6
    constraints on, 5–6
  of positive HIV tests, 6–7
National Research Council (NRC), 121
Native Americans, HIV/AIDS in, 435, 437–438, 435*f*–
  437*f*
Naz project, 256
Needle-exchange programs, 120–121, 416*t*
Neisseria gonorrhoeae infections, 103
Netherlands, 36, 37
NGOs. *See* Nongovernmental organizations
Nonconsensual sex, 222
Nondiscrimination
  efforts, success of, 442
  legislation, 336
Nongovernmental organizations (NGOs), 312. *See also
  specific nongovernmental organizations*
  AIDS service organizations (ASOs), 329, 341, 347
  capacities, 346–347
  funding, 346, 356–357
    proliferation of activities and, 356–357
    trends, impact of, 357–359
  governments and, 359–360
  in home-based health care development, 410
  human rights violation responses, 328–330
  identity activism, 347–348
  linking organizations, 347, 358
  needs, 346–347
  priorities, 346–347
  public policy and, 345–346
  range/diversity, 341–344
  roles, 344–345, 356–357
  social movements and, 348
  success, 358
  sustaining community action, 360
  vulnerability and, 442
Non-nucleoside reverse transcriptase inhibitors
  (NNRTIs), 162

Nonoxynol-9, for HIV prevention, 196, 197*t*, 199
Non-progressors, 165–167
Nonsyncytia-inducing virus (NSI), 177
Norris case, 333–334
North Africa, 29
North America GAA. *See also specific countries*
  AIDS cases
    cumulative, 11, 11*t*–13*t*
    new, 19, 20*t*–21*t*
    prevalence, 24–25
  chlamydial infection, 103
  deaths, AIDS-related, 17*t*
  HIV/AIDS, 21, 23
  HIV infection
    cumulative data, 26, 27*t*
    newly acquired cases, 18–19, 18*t*, 19*f*
    persons living with, 21, 24, 22*t*–25*t*
    with tuberculosis, 89–90, 90*t*, 91*t*
  population estimates, 9*f*
Northeast Asia GAA. *See also specific countries*
  AIDS cases
    cumulative, 11, 11*t*–13*t*
    new, 19, 20*t*–21*t*
    prevalence, 24–25
  deaths, AIDS-related, 17*t*
  HIV/AIDS, 21, 23
  HIV infection
    newly acquired cases, 18–19, 18*t*, 19*f*
    persons living with, 24–25
    with tuberculosis, 91*t*
  HIV information, cumulative data, 26, 27*t*
  population estimates, 9*f*
Norway, 37
Nucleoside analogs, 159
Nutrition, in personal care strategies, 400

Occupation
  mobile, HIV risk and, 33
  sexual life and, 148
Oceania GAA
  AIDS cases
    cumulative, 11, 11*t*–13*t*
    new, 19, 20*t*–21*t*
    prevalence, 24–25
  deaths, AIDS-related, 17*t*
  HIV/AIDS, 21, 23
  HIV infection
    cumulative data, 26, 27*t*
    newly acquired cases, 18–19, 18*t*, 19*f*
    persons living with, 21, 24, 22*t*–25*t*
    with tuberculosis, 89–90, 90*t*, 91*t*
  population estimates, 9*f*
Octoxynol-9, for HIV prevention, 197*t*
ODA. *See* Official development assistance (ODA)
OECD (Organization for Economic Cooperation and
  Development), 375–376, 376*f*, 387
Official development assistance (ODA)
  donor countries, 375–376, 376*f*
    trends of, 380, 384–385, 384*t*
  donor fatigue syndrome, 387–388

Official development assistance (ODA) (cont'd.)
 financing survey data sources, 376–378
 funding, 322, 325, 358
  bilateral, 377, 378*t*, 379*t*
  disbursement channels, 378–379, 379*t*
  multi-bilateral, 377, 378*t*, 379*t*
  multilateral, 377, 378*t*, 379*t*
  recipient countries, 385–386
  tracking, 382, 384–385, 385*f*
  trends of major donors, 380, 384–385, 384*t*
 Global AIDS Strategy funding and, 378, 378*t*, 379–380, 380*t*
 recipient countries, 385–386
 supply/demand, 387–388
O group, 182
Opportunistic infections, 160. *See also specific opportunistic infections*
 in infants/children, 14
Oral candidiasis, in HIV infection, 230, 231*f*
Oral contraceptives, HIV infection risk and, 98
Oral sex, risk, 259
Organization for Economic Cooperation and Development (OECD), 375–376, 376*f*
Orphanages, 283
Orphans, HIV/AIDS
 acceptance of, 282
 estimates, projected, 278–280, 279*t*
 family burdens, 282–283
 long-term perspective, 285
 needs of
  identifying, 281
  meeting, 285
 organizational support, 283
 short-term perspective, 285
 social impacts of, 280–281
 social rejection of, 281
 in Uganda, 278, 283–285

Pacific Island countries, expenditures on AIDS, by GNAP, 421*t*
p24 antibodies, in nonprogressors, 165
p24 antigen
 absence, in nonprogressors, 165
 for blood donor screening, 290–291
Paris AIDS Summit, 351
Pasteur Vaccins, prototype vaccine, 187
Pathogenesis, biologic features in, 178–179
PCP. *See Pneumocystis carinii* pneumonia (PCP)
PCR. *See* Polymerase chain reaction (PCR)
Pediatric HIV/AIDS. *See also* Children; Infants
 AIDS incubation period, 73
 bimodal response pattern, 14
 case definition, shortcomings, living with, 5–6
 cases, cumulative by GAA, 11*t*, 13*t*
 deaths
  by GAA, 17*t*
  time intervals for, 490*f*
 etiology. *See* Mother-to-child transmission; Perinatal transmission

HIV infections, newly acquired, 18*t*
 incidence, 21, 23, 273
 multisystem impact, 14
 persons living with, 22–24
Peer support groups and counseling, 398, 400
Pelvic inflammatory disease (PID), 103
Perinatal transmission. *See also* Pediatric HIV/AIDS
 HIV-2, 172–173
 HIV-to-AIDS, time interval for, 490*f*
Peripheral blood mononuclear cells (PBMC), 177
Personal behavior development, adolescents/young adults, 240–242
Personal care strategies, 398, 400–402, 399*f*
 peer support groups and counseling, 398, 400
 ranking, 398, 399*f*
Personal vulnerability, 441, 455–456
Pharmaceutical companies
 research-based, 204, 210–211
 vaccine development, 188–189
Philippines, 256
PID. *See* Pelvic inflammatory disease
Pink Triangle, 256
Plague epidemic, in London, 72*f*
Pneumocystis carinii pneumonia (PCP), 160
 in infants/children, 14
 prophylaxis, in pregnancy, 411
Politics
 HIV infection spread and, 33, 63–65, 66*f*
 HIV vulnerability and, 469–470
 research agenda and, 204
 social vulnerability and, 452–453
Polymerase chain reaction (PCR), 180
 HIV-2-specific, 173
 screening, of blood donors, 291
Polysaccharides, sulphated, 199–200
Population
 growth, AIDS impact projections, 73, 74*f*
 size, AIDS impact projections, 73, 74*f*
Population groups. *See also specific population groups*
 epidemiological studies, 431–432
 geographic spread, 62
 mobility, HIV/AIDS and, 33–34
 new, HIV pandemic extension into, 62
 urban-rural movement. *See also* Rural areas; Urban areas
  HIV dynamics, 48–49
Portugal, 36, 171
Poverty
 AIDS and, 14
 HIV/AIDS prevention and, 459
Power
 cultural aspects of, 445
 relationships, 307
 of women, 216
Pregnancy
 HIV-infected, socioeconomic status and, 58, 59*f*
 HIV screening in, 6
 HIV seroprevalence, 51*f*, 98
 trichomoniasis, 104

Prevention, HIV/AIDS. *See also* Education programs
    for adolescents/young adults, health care and, 242–243, 243*t*
    approaches, 261
    barriers, for indigenous populations, 438
    costs
        annual per capita spending by GNAP, 422*t*–423*t*
        by country, 415–415
        expenditures, 424*t*, 425, 426*t*
        in high economy countries, 424*t*
        in low economy countries, 424*t*
    empowerment and, 475–476
    future, 427–428, 463
    human rights and, 327
    human rights approach
        advantages, 474
        disadvantages, 474
        example of, 472–473
    in indigenous populations, success/failures, determinants of, 438
    limits/failures of programs, 465
    messages, for rural communities, 49
    poverty and, 459
    programs
        development, local sexual culture and, 139
        new strategy for women, 223–225
        private sector, 362, 365
        social science evaluation of, 149, 154, 156, 150*t*–155*t*
        women and, 261
    societal dimensions, 234
    strategies, underlying assumptions, 216–217
    women-controlled methods, 233
        approaches, 196, 197*t*–198*t*
        development, 199–200
    youth-centered approach, 237–238
Primary health care system, in Botswana, 405–407
Prisoners
    AIDS in, 268–269
    condoms for, 270, 271
    HIV/AIDS international guidelines, 270–271
    HIV testing, 271
    injection drug users, 269–270
    tuberculosis, HIV-associated in, 269
    women, 268
Private sector corporations, 311
    business coalitions, 366
    corporate HIV/AIDS policies, 364–365
    employee assistance programs, 363, 364
    health care and, 359
    in India, 367
    management information needs, 365–366
    prevention programs, 362, 365
        financial information, 366
        needs assessment for, 366
    workplace HIV/AIDS guidelines, 362–363
Private voluntary organizations. *See* Nongovernmental organizations (NGOs)
Program vulnerability, 441–442, 456
Promotion, corporate policies on, 364–365

Prostitution
    HIV seroprevalence and, 45, 79–81, 80*f*–82*f*
    in indigenous populations, 435
    in Southeast Asia, 63
Protease inhibitors, 159, 162
Psychological approaches, to sexual behavior studies, 132, 133*t*–135*t*
Public health measures
    challenges of HIV/AIDS pandemic, 460
    effectiveness, HIV/AIDS and, 327
    in HIV prevention programs, 433
    human rights quality and, 337–338, 338*f*
    inaction, in societal vulnerability reduction, 463–464
Public sector. *See* Governments
Public sector corporations, research funds, 202
PWAIDS/HIV (person with HIV/AIDS)
    by GAA, 21, 24, 22*t*–25*t*
    groups, external funding, 352
    life expectancy, 390
    number of, 390
    support organizations, 350–356
    terminology, 348–349

Quality of life, 402
Qur'an, 449

Race, HIV prevalence, 63
"Reach Out," 342
Reality θ, 196
Recombinant technology, 187
Red Cross. *See* International Federation of Red Cross and Red Crescent Societies
Regulatory genes, 178, 180
Religion
    AIDS as challenge to, 447–452
    beliefs of, 400
    homosexuality and, 449
    sexuality and, 447–452
Reporting
    by GAA, 479*t*–486*t*
    national, of AIDS, 5–6
Reproductive number (R), 72
Reproductive rate (R_0), basic or case, 71
Reproductive years, HIV risk during, 220
Research
    advisory committees, 203
    in Africa, 35, 129–120
    agendas, 202
        decision-making and, 204
        politics and, 204
    behavioral, 130
    budget cycle, 204
    budget proposals, 203
    on cultural influences affecting social vulnerability, 446
    in developing countries, 130
    expenditures, 425–426, 426*t*
    features of, 208–211

Research (cont'd.)
  funding
    activism and, 202
    global annual expenditures and, 203
    for sexual behavior studies, 137
  goals, for clinical trials, 162
  HIV-2 infection, 174
  for immediate solutions, 209
  infrastructure, for vaccine development, 194
  pharmaceutical company, 204
  public sector funds, 202
  scientific process in, 205–207
  sexual behavior, methodological approaches for,
    140
  social science, 130, 131
  vaccine. *See* Vaccine
Risk
  behaviors, 431–432
  codes, culture and, 445
  factors, 431–432
    behavioral, 101
    economic, 217–218
    sociocultural, 218–225
  gender differences, 215–216
  groups, 304, 431–432
    in industrialized countries, 77, 78*f*
    mixing patterns, 77, 79, 78*f*, 79*f*, 83, 84*f*
    traditional, 57–58
  hierarchy, sexual behavior patterns and, 259–262
  for HIV/AIDS, sexually transmitted disease and, 233
  reduction, for women, 216–217
  vulnerability, HIV/AIDS, 37–39
  of women, with age, 261
  women's status and, 222–223, 222*f*, 223*f*
Risk-reduction programs, for injection drug users,
    264
Ritonavir, 162
Ritual sexual cleansing, 101
Romania, 36
Rural areas
  in Africa, HIV prevalence in, 30–31
  AIDS-related migration, 49
  HIV infection, Sub-Saharan Africa, 45–48
  urban/rural differentials, 49, 52
Rwanda, 15, 29, 293

Safe sex. *See also* Sexual behavior
  gay men and, 254
San Francisco Model, 407–409
Saquinavir, 162
Saturation, 31–32
School interventions, evaluating, 149, 150*t*–151*t*
Schools
  partnerships with adolescents, 243–246
  sex education programs, 238–239
SCID-hu mouse system, 178
Scientists, mistakes/errors of, 209–210
Self-efficacy, empowerment and, 475
Self-help organizations, 350–354
Senegal, 173, 174

Sentinel populations
  in Africa, 34–35
  surveillance systems, 7–8, 8*f*
Serology
  dual reactivity, 174
  HIV, 179–180
Sex education programs, 238–239, 244
Sex partners
  acquisition patterns, 81–82, 83
  mixing patterns, 77, 79, 78*f*, 79*f*, 83, 84*f*
  multiple, for men, 220–221
  number of, 101
    for gay men, 253
    reduction recommendations for, 465
Sex tourism, 256
Sexual abuse
  of children, 244–246
  in indigenous populations, 435
Sexual behavior
  adolescent, 304–306
  conceptual models/theories, 131–132, 133*t*–135*t*
  gay men, 252–253
  patterns, 77, 78*f*, 82
    risk hierarchy and, 259–262
  research, 137–138
    methodological approaches for, 140
    qualitative surveys, 146–147, 147*t*–148*t*
    quantitative surveys, 140, 145, 141*t*–146*t*
  social context, 139, 219, 260
  surveys, 259
  systems and, 148
  WHO/GPA surveys
    of general population, 140, 141*t*–142*t*
    of target population, 145, 146*t*
Sexual contacts
  networks, 77, 78*f*, 82
  unprotected, number of, 101
Sexual intercourse
  anal. *See* Anal intercourse
  in uncoupled relationships, 260
Sexuality
  diversity of, 307
  experiencing, 146
  in HIV-infected women, 261–262
  and religion, 447–452
Sexually-transmitted diseases (STDs) *See* Sexually
    transmitted infections (STIs)
Sexually transmitted infection clinics
  costs of, 415, 416*f*
  patients, seroprevalence of, 55*f*
  youth services, 243*t*
Sexually-transmitted infections (STIs), 98
  in Africa, 32–33, 45–46, 47
  control programs, 32–33
  epidemiology, in women, 101–104
  HIV interactions, 99–100
  HIV risk and, 233
  HIV seroprevalence, Southeast Asia, 55, 56
  in indigenous populations, 434
  knowledgeability, cultural attitudes and, 219
  migration and, 234

nonulcerative. *See also* Chlamydia; Gonorrhea;
  Trichomoniasis
  HIV-1 acquisition and, 99
  prevalence, 99
  risk, of homosexual/bisexual men, 58
  services for, 224
  sexual abuse and, 245
  surveillance data, 33
  urbanization and, 234
  youth and, 245, 247–248
Sexual risk reduction. *See* Safe sex
Sexual transmission. *See* Bisexual transmission; Heterosexual transmission; Homosexuality, HIV
  transmission
Sex workers
  female. *See* Female sex workers; Prostitution
  male, 255
Shiite fundamentalism, 449
Social aspects
  of sexual life, 148
  of vaccine development, 188–190, 189*t*
Social construction theory, 139
Social movements, NGOs and, 348
Social science
  evaluation of prevention programs, 149, 154, 156,
    150*t*–155*t*
  theories/conceptual models, 131–132, 133*t*–135*t*
Social vulnerability
  country assessment and strategic planning, 453–454
  cultural influences, research on, 446
  economic factors in, 453
  governmental factors, 452–453
  political factors, 452–453
  reduction, implementation of, 453
  risk reduction strategy, 452*t*
  sociocultural factors in, 453
Societal vulnerability
  analytical framework, 456–457
  contextual factors, 463
    human rights and, 469–471
    response and, 457–458
  cultural influence on, 444–446
  focus of, 444
  parameters, 446
  reduction, 463, 464*f*
    principles in, 458–459
    public health inaction and, 463–464
Societies
  culture, networks and, 446
  impact on personal care strategy, 401–402
  response/context to HIV/AIDS, 457–458
Society for Women and AIDS in Africa (SWAA), 342–343
Sociocultural factors
  in HIV vulnerability, 470–471
  risk and, 218–225
  in social vulnerability, 453
Socioeconomic status, high-risk behavior and, 58, 59*f*
South Africa
  HIV/AIDS in, 31, 33, 62–63
    economic impact of, 113–114
    health care costs, 394–395

migrant laborers, heterosexual relationships of,
  139–140
South America. *See also* Latin America GAA; *specific
  countries*
  cocaine trade routes, 65, 66*f*
Southeast Asia GAA
  AIDS cases
    cumulative, 11, 11*t*–13*t*
    new, 19, 20*t*–21*t*
    prevalence, 24–25
  ASOs, 256
  deaths, AIDS-related, 17*t*
  HIV infection, 21, 23
    cumulative data, 26, 27*t*
    epidemic curve for, 26
    newly acquired cases, 18–19, 18*t*, 19*f*
    persons living with, 21, 24, 22*t*–25*t*
    with tuberculosis, 91*t*
  HIV prevalence, pregnant women, 98
  HIV seroprevalence, 50–56
  population estimates, 9*f*
  prostitution, 63
  tuberculosis, AIDS and, 87–89, 89*t*
Southeast Mediterranean GAA
  AIDS cases
    cumulative, 11, 11*t*–13*t*
    new, 19, 20*t*–21*t*
    prevalence, 24–25
  deaths, AIDS-related, 17*t*
  HIV infection, 21, 23
    cumulative data, 26, 27*t*
    newly acquired cases, 18–19, 18*t*, 19*f*
    persons living with, 21, 24, 22*t*–25*t*
    with tuberculosis, 91*t*
  population estimates, 9*f*
Spain, 36, 268
Spermicides
  cervical infection prevention, 199
  for HIV prevention, 196, 197*t*, 198–199
Spirituality, 400
Stavudine, 159
STDs. *See* Sexually-transmitted infections (STIs)
Stigmatization, 401
STIs. *See* Sexually-transmitted infections
Street children
  HIV risk, 244
  HIV seroprevalence, 237
  number of, 244
  sex abuse and, 244–245
Stress reduction, as personal care strategy, 401
Sub-Commission on the Prevention of Discrimination
  and Protection of Minorities, 330–331
Subculture, 446
Sub-Saharan Africa GAA. *See also* Africa; *specific
  countries*
  AIDS cases
    cumulative, 11, 11*t*–13*t*
    new, 19, 20*t*–21*t*
    prevalence, 24–25
  chlamydial infection, 103
  clanship groupings, 139

Sub-Saharan Africa GAA (cont'd.)
deaths, AIDS-related, 17t
economic impact of HIV/AIDS, 111
expenditures on AIDS, by GNAP, 418t–419t
HIV/AIDS, 21, 23
HIV infection
cumulative data, 26, 27t
incubation period, 15–16
newly acquired cases, 18–19, 18t, 19f
prevalence, 21, 24, 22t–25t, 31
rural areas, 45–48
survival, 15–16
with tuberculosis, 89–90, 90t, 91t
in women, 97
HIV seroprevalence, 43–46, 48, 44f–47f
population estimates, 9f
surveillance, 34
syphilis seroprevalence rate, 102, 102f
trichomoniasis, 104
women, sex workers, 45
Substance abuse, in indigenous populations, 434–435
"Sugar daddy" phenomenon, 217
Sulphated polysaccharides, 199–200
Sunnite fundamentalism, 449
Surveillance
AIDS, 37
HIV/AIDS, in Africa, 34–35
Survivors, long-term, 165–167, 402
SWAA (Society for Women and AIDS in Africa), 342–343
Swaziland, 31, 113
Sweden, 6, 37
Switzerland, 36
Syncytia-inducing virus (SI), 177
Syphilis, in women, 101–102, 102f
Systems theory, 139–140

Tanzania
economic impact of HIV/AIDS, 112–113
HIV infections, 29, 30–31, 33
socioeconomic status and, 58, 59
in women, 18t
HIV seroprevalence, tuberculosis and, 88t
Tasmania, 333
TASO (The AIDS Support Organization), 341–342
Tat gene, 178, 180
Terry Beirn Community Programs for Clinical Research on AIDS, 161
Thailand
economic impact of HIV/AIDS, 113
gay rights organizations, 256
heterosexual transmission, 60
HIV seroprevalence, 50, 56, 51f–55f
injection-drug users, 80f
tuberculosis and, 88t
side-by-side epidemics, 63, 64f
tuberculosis, AIDS and, 89t
Th1 cell response, in nonprogressors, 165
Th2 cell response, in nonprogressors, 165
Theories, social science, 131–132, 133t–135t

Thrush, in HIV infection, 230, 231f
Tolerance, discrimination and, 466–467
Transgression, sexual, 139
Transmission, HIV/AIDS. See also specific transmission routes
in Africa, 29
among injection drug users, 265
biologic features in, 178
by breast-feeding, 273–274
early observations, 207
efficacy, virulence and, 85
efficiency, 72
epidemiological studies, 430
in indigenous populations, 434–435, 437–439, 436f, 437f
in Native American
men, 436f
women, 437f
scientific process applications, 207–208
theories, 208
via blood and blood products, compensation for, 287–288
viral subtypes and, 183–184
Travaux preparatoires, 336
Treatment
alternative, 400–401
drug. See Antiretroviral drug therapy
immune-based, 159–160
Trichomoniasis, 104
Tuberculin skin test, seroconversion in prisoners, 269
Tuberculosis
AIDS and, 87–89, 89t
HIV-associated, in prisoners, 269
HIV-co-infected, 89–90, 90t
deaths from, 91
estimation methods, 90, 91t
HIV infection and, 87–89, 88t
HIV-2 infection and, 173
morbidity, 92–93
mortality, 92–93
multiple drug resistant, 91–92, 93
prevalence, 87
prevention strategies, 92–93
testing, mandatory, 335
treatment costs, 94–95
Tuskegee Syphilis Study, 304–305

UDHR. See Universal Declaration of Human Rights
Uganda
AIDS in, 29, 30, 122–124
blood screening, 293
deaths, AIDS-related, 16
HIV/AIDS orphans, 278, 283–285
HIV infections
in tuberculosis patients, 87, 88t
in women, 18t
HIV prevalence, 32
Kampala HIV/AIDS workshop, 28–35
UNAIDS, 369–371, 430

UNDP (United Nations Development Program), 311, 370, 372*t*–374*t*

UNESCO (United Nations Educational, Scientific and Cultural Organization), 311, 370, 372*t*–374*t*

UNFPA (United Nations Population Fund), 311, 370, 372*t*–374*t*

UNICEF (United Nations Children's Fund), 311, 370, 372*t*–374*t*

United Kingdom, 6, 36, 72*f*

United Nations
  AIDS-related human rights issues and, 330–331
  mandatory HIV testing, 334
  response to HIV/AIDS, 369–371, 372*t*–374*t*
  Working Group on Arbitrary Detention, 329

United Nations AIDS Program (UNAIDS), 312, 369–371, 372*t*–374*t*

United Nations Children's Fund (UNICEF), 311, 370, 372*t*–374*t*

United Nations Commission on Human Rights, 330, 331, 333

United Nations Commission on Status of Women, 330

United Nations Population Fund (UNPFA), 311, 370, 372*t*–374*t*

United States. *See also specific government agencies*
  AIDS cases, 59
  AIDS epidemic
    health communication and, 304
    homelessness and, 303–304
    hubris, sense of, 302–303
  AIDS-related tuberculosis, 87–89, 88*t*, 89*t*
  attitudes toward homosexuality in, 119
  HIV epidemic, 117
  HIV seroprevalence
    injection-drug users, 80*f*
    tuberculosis and, 88*t*
  homeless population, 303–304
  homosexual/bisexual transmission, 60–61, 61*f*
  Reagan-Bush administrations, 119

Universal Declaration of Human Rights (UDHR), 450, 588–592
  contextual factors in HIV prevention, 469–471
  core principles, 468

Unlinked anonymous method (UA method), 7–8

Urban areas
  in Africa, HIV prevalence in, 30–31
  HIV infection, Sub-Saharan Africa, 45–48
  migration to, HIV dynamics and, 48–49
  sexually transmitted infections and, 234
  urban/rural differentials, 49, 52
  women sex workers, HIV seroprevalence, 45

U.S. Job Corps, 237

U.S. National Commission on AIDS, final report, 307

Vaccine
  availability, 195
  clade-specific, 130
  development
    by approach, investment in, 188, 189*t*
    clade epidemiology and, 183
    guideposts for, 186
    private sector, encouragement of, 190
    profit motives, 189
    research support and, 129
    scientific concerns for, 187–188
    scientific progress in, 186–187
    social concerns for, 188–190, 189*t*
  prototype, 187
  trials, 187
    ethical issues, 195
    future challenges, 195
    immediate issues for, 193–195
    multiple, 195
    post-licensure phase IV evaluation, 195
    rationale for, 193
    repeat phase I/II, 194–195
    social-behavioral issues, 195

Vaginal candidiasis, in HIV infection, 230, 231*f*

Vaginal drying agents, 221, 233

Vaginal intercourse, unprotected, risk of, 259

Vaginal microbial products, development, 199

Variable (V3) loop, 179

Vietnam, 63

Viral infections. *See* Sexually transmitted infections (STIs); *specific viral infections*

Virasept, 162

Virginity, value of, 219–220

Virus neutralization assays, 188

V3 loop, 179

Vulnerability
  analysis, 460
  analytical framework, 454–457
  contextual factors
    constraints/barriers, 461
    interventions for, 460
    poverty as, 459
  defined, 441
  to HIV
    empowerment and, 474–475
    human rights analysis of, 469–471
    human rights and, 467–468
    human rights approach to, 472
  to HIV/AIDS
    human rights and, 464–466
    young people and, 454–457
  to infection, consequences of, 445–446
  personal, 441
  reduction, implementing, 460
  societal
    cultural influence on, 444–446
    focus of, 444
    parameters, 446

Wasting syndrome, 160

West Africa, HIV-2 incidence, 171

Western Europe GAA. *See also specific countries*
  AIDS cases
    cumulative, 11, 11*t*–13*t*
    new, 19, 20*t*–21*t*
    prevalence, 24–25
  chlamydial infection, 103

Western Europe GAA (cont'd.)
  deaths, AIDS-related, 17*t*
  HIV/AIDS, 21, 23
  HIV infection
    cumulative data, 26, 27*t*
    newly acquired cases, 18–19, 18*t*, 19*f*
    persons living with, 21, 24, 22*t*–25*t*
    with tuberculosis, 91*t*
    population estimates, 9*f*
WHO. *See* World Health Organization
WHO/GPA. *See* World Health Organization, Global
    Program on AIDS
Window period, 293, 294
Women. *See also* Heterosexual transmission; Perina-
    tal transmission; Pregnancy
  AIDS cases, 11*t*, 13*t*
  care/support, for persons with HIV/AIDS, 234–235
  condoms for. *See* Female condoms
  deaths-AIDS related, 17*t*
  health care requirements, 411
  heterosexual transmission, 229
  HIV infections, 21, 23
    adolescent, 30
    epidemiology of, 97–98
    gynecologic disease of, 230–232, 231*f*
    knowledge gap, 229
    in Native Americans, 436*f*, 437*f*
    newly acquired, 18*t*, 19*f*
    personal experience, 349–350
    persons living with, 22–24
    in young adults, 30
  HIV seroprevalence, 230*f*
  inequality of, 308
  knowledgeability about sex, 224
  NGOs, 342–343
  powerlessness of, 218, 465
  power of, 216
  prevention strategies, 233, 261. *See also* Prevention,
    HIV/AIDS
    new, 223–225
    underlying assumptions, 216–217
  rights of, religion and, 450
  risk
    behavioral factors, 98–99, 101
    biological factors, 98–99
    feminine ideals and, 218–220
  sexually-active, HIV prevalence, 73, 74*f*
  sexually transmitted infections
    in Africa, 32
    epidemiology of, 101–104

  status, HIV risk and, 222–223, 222*f*, 223*f*, 306
  trading sex for necessities, 101
  young, HIV risk and, 261
Women's Rights Project of Human Rights Watch,
    329
Work, as personal care strategy, 401
World Bank Development Report, 111
World Bank loans, 386–387
World Health Organization (WHO)
  Adolescent Health Program, 246
  Global AIDS Strategy. *See* Global AIDS Strategy
  Global Network for HIV Isolation & Characteriza-
    tion, 194
  Global Program on AIDS (WHO/GPA), 311, 430
    grant programs, 358
    HIV prevalence estimates, 26
    human rights guidelines, 330
    KABP surveys, 140, 143*t*–145*t*
    serosurveillance method, 7–8
    sex education studies, 238
    sexual behavior surveys, 140, 141*t*–142*t*
    workplace guidelines, 362–363
  guidelines, for HIV/AIDS in prisons, 270–271
  HIV-associated tuberculosis estimates, 90
  HIV policies/programs, 370, 372*t*–374*t*
  initial response to AIDS, 311
  national governments and, 311
  nondiscrimination, 327
  pediatric AIDS case definition of, sensitivity/speci-
    ficity of, 5–6
  reporting of AIDS cases and, 5, 6. *See also* Global
    AIDS Strategy
  Steering Committee on Vaccine Development,
    194
  tuberculosis prevalence estimates, 87
  UNDP Alliance, 369
  workplace HIV/AIDS guidelines, 362

Youth. *See* Adolescents; Adults, young

Zaire, 15
Zalcitabine (ddC), 159, 160
Zambia
  home-based health care, 409–410
  tuberculosis, AIDS-related, 87, 88*t*
Zidovudine. *See* AZT
Zimbabwe, 29, 31, 293

Printed in the United Kingdom
by Lightning Source UK Ltd.
115508UKS00001B/20